Bone Diseases of Children

Bone Diseases of Children

Pierre Maroteaux
Master of Research
National Center for Scientific Research
Paris

with the collaboration of

Clément Fauré
Associate Professor of Radiology
University of Paris
Paris

Claude Fessard
Associate Professor of Pediatrics
University of Rouen
Rouen

Pierre Rigault
Associate Professor of Pediatric Orthopaedic Surgery
University of Paris
Paris

translated and adapted by

Herbert J. Kaufmann
Formerly Professor of Radiology
The University of Pennsylvania School of Medicine
Philadelphia, Pennsylvania

J. B. Lippincott Company

Philadelphia · Toronto

This book was published in French under the title *Maladies Osseuses de l'Enfant* by Flammarion Editeur © 1975

ISBN 0 397 50397 0
Library of Congress Catalog Card Number 78-21567
Printed in the United States of America

1 3 5 4 2

Library of Congress Cataloging in Publication Data

Maroteaux, P
Bone diseases of children.

Translation of Les maladies osseuses de l'enfant.
Includes bibliographies and index.
1. Bones—Diseases. 2. Pediatric orthopedia.
3. Osteal manifestations of general diseases.
I. Title. [DNLM: 1. Bone diseases—In infancy and childhood. WS270 M355m]
RJ482.B65M3713 618.9'27'1 78-21567
ISBN 0-397-50397-0

Preface and Introductory Remarks

There are a great many disorders primarily involving the skeleton during infancy and childhood, and, in the course of a large number of diseases, the skeleton may also be affected.

The underlying pathology may present clinically by a number of symptoms, but a more precise evaluation and the subsequent diagnostic labeling of a given disorder is usually only possible from radiographs. The spectrum of diseases covered in this book has as common denominator its title, chosen as general as possible, "Bone Diseases of Children."

The peculiarity of its growth conveys to skeletal pathology of infancy a special character differentiating it in many ways from that of the adult. Therefore, a special chapter has been devoted to the study of growth with illustrations documenting normal radiographic appearances possibly resulting in errors in interpretation.

Considerable space has been devoted to the discussion of constitutional skeletal disorders since their importance has grown considerably over the last fifteen years. A number of diseases seen only rarely today are described in very short paragraphs just as some types of poisoning.

In the area of constitutional disorders a strong effort was undertaken to be up to date in the discussion without speculating on disorders that may be better characterized only in the future. In spite of the attempt to offer a fairly exhaustive coverage of skeletal pathology of infancy, this book has also been conceived in a way that it can be utilized by the practicing physician. For this reason a rather schematic presentation was chosen for the introductory chapters.

This English version of the French original turned out to be quite different from the format initially planned for several reasons. The underlying manuscript was concluded during the summer of 1973. Five years imply a considerable aging process in the life of a scientific book. For this reason we have combined our forces to offer the reader a version that is already two steps removed from the original book.

Based on the original text the translation adheres closely to the arrangement of content, character of style, and, especially, the train of thought, to convey as closely and as much as possible some of its individual flavor.

A major improvement should result from a thorough and critical review of the illustrations of the book. In order to provide evenly useful documentation, virtually one out of every three figures was either completely redone, differently presented, or a new case was selected.

This introduction attempts to relate recent new knowledge and ensuing considerations. Key developments in the area of skeletal diseases of the child are summarized, and some pertinent literature references are given. No attempt is made to be exhaustive, and no documentation by figures could be added.

The terminology used throughout the book is that of the 1969 Paris nomenclature. In May 1977, a second gathering of specialists took place again in Paris resulting in an updated nomenclature. Here the reader finds the complete summary of the results of these efforts, but it was not possible to incorporate all the changes into the content of this book.

PIERRE MAROTEAUX
HERBERT J. KAUFMANN

International Nomenclature of Constitutional Diseases of Bone*

Revision, May, 1977

I

OSTEOCHONDRODYSPLASIAS

ABNORMALITIES OF CARTILAGE AND/OR BONE GROWTH AND DEVELOPMENT

A. Defects of Growth of Tubular Bones and/or Spine

a. Identifiable at Birth

1. Achondrogenesis type I (Parenti-Fraccaro)
2. Achondrogenesis type II (Langer-Saldino)
3. Thanatophoric dysplasia
4. Thanatophoric dysplasia with clover-leaf skull
5. Short rib-polydactyly syndrome type I (Saldino-Noonan) (perhaps several forms)
6. Short-rib polydactyly syndrome type II (Majewski)
7. Chondrodysplasia punctata
    a. Rhizomelic form
    b. Dominant form
    c. Other forms
    Exclude: symptomatic stippling in other disorders (e.g. Zellweger syndrome, Warfarin embryopathy)
8. Campomelic dysplasia
9. Other dysplasias with congenital bowing of long bones (several forms)
10. Achondroplasia
11. Diastrophic dysplasia
12. Metatropic dysplasia (several forms)
13. Chondro-ecto-dermal dysplasia (Ellis Van Creveld)
14. Asphyxiating thoracic dysplasia (Jeune)
15. Spondylo-epiphyseal dysplasia congenita
    a. Type Spranger-Wiedemann
    b. Other forms (see b. 11-12)
16. Kniest dysplasia
17. Mesomelic dysplasia
    a. Type Nievergelt
    b. Type Langer (probably homozygous dyschondrosteosis)
    c. Type Robinow
    d. Type Reinhardt
    e. Others
18. Acromesomelic dysplasia
19. Cleido-cranial dysplasia
20. Larsen syndrome
21. Oto-palato-digital syndrome

b. Identifiable in Later Life

1. Hypochondroplasia
2. Dyschondrosteosis
3. Metaphyseal chondrodysplasia type Jansen
4. Metaphyseal chondrodysplasia type Schmid
5. Metaphyseal chondrodysplasia type McKusick
6. Metaphyseal chondrodysplasia with exocrine pancreatic insufficiency and cyclic neutropenia
7. Spondylo-metaphyseal dysplasia
    a. Type Kozlowski
    b. Other forms
8. Multiple epiphyseal dysplasia
    a. Type Fairbanks
    b. Other forms
9. Arthro-ophthalmopathy (Stickler)
10. Pseudo-achondroplasia
    a. Dominant
    b. Recessive
11. Spondylo-epiphyseal dysplasia tarda
12. Spondylo-epiphyseal dysplasia, other forms (see a. 15-16)
13. Dyggve-Melchior-Clausen dysplasia
14. Spondylo-epi-metaphyseal dysplasia (several forms)
15. Myotonic chondrodysplasia (Catel-Schwartz-Jampel)
16. Parastremmatic dysplasia
17. Tricho-rhino-phalangeal dysplasia
18. Acrodysplasia with retinitis pigmentosa and nephropathy (Saldino-Mainzer)

B. Disorganized Development of Cartilage and Fibrous Components of Skeleton

1. Dysplasia epiphysealis hemimelica
2. Multiple cartilaginous exostoses
3. Acrodysplasia with exostoses (Giedion-Langer)
4. Enchodromatosis (Ollier)

---

* List of participants:
Drs. J. Dorst, C. Fauré, A. Giedion, J. Hall, H. J. Kaufmann, K. Kozlowski, L. Langer, L. Lenzi, P. Maroteaux, A. Murphy, A. K. Poznanski, D. Rimoin, J. Sauvegrain, F. Silverman, J. Spranger, R. Stanescu, V. Stanescu.

5. Enchodromatosis with hemangioma (Maffucci)
6. Metachondromatosis
7. Fibrous dysplasia (Jaffe-Lichenstein)
8. Fibrous dysplasia with skin pigmentation and precocious puberty (McCune-Albright)
9. Cherubism (familial fibrous dysplasia of the jaws)
10. Neurofibromatosis

C. Abnormalities of Density of Cortical Diaphyseal Structure and/or Metaphyseal Modeling

1. Osteogenesis imperfecta congenita (several forms)
2. Osteogenesis imperfecta tarda (several forms)
3. Juvenile idiopathic osteoporosis
4. Osteoporosis with pseudo-glioma
5. Osteopetrosis with precocious manifestations
6. Osteopetrosis with delayed manifestations (several forms)
7. Pycnodysostosis
8. Osteopoikilosis
9. Osteopathia striata
10. Melorheostosis
11. Diaphyseal dysplasia (Camurati-Engelmann)
12. Cranio-diaphyseal dysplasia
13. Endosteal hyperostosis
    a. Autosomal dominant (Worth)
    b. Autosomal recessive (Van Buchem)
14. Tubular stenosis (Kenny-Caffey)
15. Pachydermoperiostosis
16. Osteodysplasty (Melnick-Needles)
17. Fronto-metaphyseal dysplasia
18. Cranio-metaphyseal dysplasia (several forms)
19. Metaphyseal dysplasia (Pyle)
20. Sclerosteosis
21. Dysosteosclerosis
22. Osteo-ectasia with hyperphosphatasia

II

DYSOSTOSES

MALFORMATION OF INDIVIDUAL BONES, SINGLY OR IN COMBINATION

A. Dysostoses with Cranial and Facial Involvement

1. Craniosynostosis (several forms)
2. Cranio-facial dysostosis (Crouzon)
3. Acrocephalo-syndactyly (Apert) and others
4. Acrocephalo-polysyndactyly (Carpenter) and others
5. Mandibulo-facial dysostosis
    a. Type Treacher-Collins, Franceschetti
    b. Other forms
6. Oculo-mandibulo-facial syndrome (Hallermann-Streiff-François)
7. Nevoid basal cell carcinoma syndrome

B. Dysostoses with Predominant Axial Involvement

1. Vertebral segmentation defects (including Klippel-Feil)
2. Cervico-oculo-acoustic syndrome (Wildervanck)
3. Sprengel anomaly
4. Spondylo-costal dysostosis
    a. Dominant form
    b. Recessive forms
5. Oculo-vertebral syndrome (Weyers)
6. Osteo-onychodysostosis
7. Cerebro-costo-mandibular syndrome

C. Dysostoses with Predominant Involvement of Extremities

1. Acheria
2. Apodia
3. Ectrodactyly syndrome
4. Aglossia-adactyly syndrome
5. Congenital bowing of long bones (several forms) (see also osteochondrodysplasias)
6. Familial radio-ulnar synostosis
7. Brachydactyly (several forms)
8. Symphalangism
9. Polydactyly (several forms)
10. Syndactyly (several forms)
11. Poly-syndactyly (several forms)
12. Camptodactyly
13. Poland syndrome
14. Rubinstein-Taybi syndrome
15. Pancytopenia-dysmelia syndrome (Fanconi)
16. Thrombocytopenia-radial-aplasia syndrome
17. Oro-digito-facial syndrome
    a. Type Papillon-Leage
    b. Type Mohr
18. Cardiomelic syndrome (Holt-Oram and others)
19. Femoral facial syndrome
20. Multiple synostoses (includes some forms of symphalangism)
21. Scapulo-iliac dysostosis (Kosenow-Sinios)
22. Hand foot genital syndrome
23. Focal dermal hypoplasia (Goltz)

III

IDIOPATHIC OSTEOLYSES

1. Phalangeal (several forms)
2. Tarso-carpal
    a. Including François form and others
    b. With nephropathy
3. Multicentric
    a. Hajdu-Cheney form
    b. Winchester form
    c. Other forms

IV

CHROMOSOMAL ABERRATIONS

V

PRIMARY METABOLIC ABNORMALITIES

A. Calcium and/or Phosphorus

1. Hypophosphatemic rickets
2. Pseudo-deficiency rickets (Prader, Royer)
3. Late rickets (McCance)
4. Idiopathic hypercalciuria
5. Hypophosphatasia (several forms)
6. Pseudo-hypoparathyroidism (normo and hypocalcemic forms, include acrodysostosis).

B. Complex Carbohydrates

1. Mucopolysaccharidosis, type I (alpha L-iduronidase deficiency)
    a. Hurler form
    b. Scheie form
    c. Other forms
2. Mucopolysaccharidosis, type II—Hunter (sulfoiduronate sulfatase deficiency)
3. Mucopolysaccharidosis, type III—San Filippo
    Type A (Heparin sulfamidase deficiency)
    Type B (N-acetyl alpha-glucosaminidase deficiency)
4. Mucopolysaccharidosis, type IV—Morquio (N-acetylgalactosamine-6-sulfate-sulfatase deficiency)
5. Mucopolysaccharidosis, type VI—Maroteaux-Lamy (aryl sulfatase B deficiency)
6. Mucopolysaccharidosis, type VII (beta-glucuronidase deficiency)
7. Aspartylglucosaminuria (aspartylglucosaminidase deficiency)
8. Mannosidosis (alpha-mannosidase deficiency)
9. Fucosidosis (alpha-fucosidase deficiency)
10. GM1-Gangliosidosis (beta-galactosidase deficiency)
11. Multiple sulfatases deficiency (Austin, Thieffry)
12. Neuraminidase deficiency (formerly Mucolipidosis I)
13. Mucolipidosis II
14. Mucolipidosis III

C. Lipids

1. Niemann-Pick disease
2. Gaucher disease

D. Nucleic Acids

1. Adenosine-deaminase deficiency and others

E. Amino Acids

1. Homocystinuria and others

F. Metals

1. Menkes kinky hair syndrome and others

In order of the presentation in the course of this book we shall now comment on some recent and important new developments with respect to the following disorders:

Achondrogenesis

Heterogeneity of this disorder has already been alluded to. Two major forms can be distinguished:

1. The less severe skeletal type with the mid-diaphyseal portions of the long bones radiologically recognizable and with a normal diameter. Such patients have virtually straight extremities.

2. The Parenti-Fraccaro type with extremely short shafts of all long bones showing a minimally ossified and widened mid-diaphyseal portion.

3. There may be further subtypes of achondrogenesis that might be more clearly defined in the future.[23]

Radiological findings usually help in the differentiation. All patients have in common a discrepancy between the relatively well formed bones of the skull, mandible, clavicle, and ribs, while the bodies of the vertebrae are not ossified.

Histologic differentiation should be possible since the "less severe type" has an aspect of its growth cartilage, somewhat different from that of the Parenti-Fraccaro type.[36]

Genetically both types of achondrogenesis appear to be recessive disorders.

Dysplasia Epiphysealis Punctata

This disorder is not purely genetically determined as suggested in the discussion on p. 44. Whereas the rhizomelic type is now clearly defined,[14] it must be admitted that the Conradi-Hühnermann type actually is a heterogeneous group of separate entities, which will have to be properly subdivided in the future.*

A special problem resulting from the lack of growth of the tracheal rings has recently been recognized in patients who had calcifications within these cartilaginous structures at birth.[21]

The significance as the precipitating agent of Warfarin therapy during the early phase of pregnancy in women on anticoagulant therapy in the production of a closely similar syndrome is now well established.[31, 38] The possibility of further agents resulting in similar pathology must be considered.

Mesomelic Dwarfism

This group of disorders characterized by predominant mesomelic shortening is clearly more complex than previously thought and even as reflected in the updated Paris nomenclature of 1977.[16, 27]

In a number of patients, the additional radiographic finding of an unusually long fibula may eventually result in the definition of a separate, if not several individual entities.[24]

Without being formal, it can already be stated that the Langer type of mesomelic dysplasia can be a homozygous manifestation of dyschondrosteosis.[10] This, however, is not consistently the case in every affected patient of the respective family, even after a careful radiographic investigation of both parents.

The dominant transmission of the syndrome of Robinow is presently being questioned, since a number of observations seem to indicate a possibly autosomal recessive inheritance.[13]

Micrognathic Dysplasia

There may be several types of this disorder combining the Pierre Robin syndrome—micrognathia—with varying degrees of micromelia.

1. The Weissenbacher-Zweymüller type seems to have an unexpectedly good growth potential and an altogether fair prognosis.[5, 17]

2. Several patients described recently had severe shortening of the extremities. Some patients were born dead, others did not survive long, but there has been an occasional survivor.[8]

As an additional finding vertebrae had an abnormal ossification with two centers present. The term "dyssegmental dwarfism" has been introduced for this type.[15]

Adenosin-Deaminase Deficiency

Within the group of metaphyseal chondrodysplasias a special disorder can be defined combining with this skeletal disorder, a disturbed immunity. As an additional finding, a peculiar shape of the iliac bones and a wavy contour of the supra-acetabular region may be diagnostically helpful.[4]

Asphyxiating Thoracic Dysplasia

The individual nature of this disorder must be more clearly recognized since it has been confused especially in its milder expression with other diseases affecting ribs and long bones. An unusually narrow thorax with short ribs but with a normal pelvis was present in patients eventually diagnosed as suffering from the combination of metaphyseal chondrodysplasia, exocrine pancreatic insufficiency, and cyclic neutropenia.[7] Careful differentiation must always be made also from thanatophoric and metatropic dwarfism as well as the short rib-polydactyly syndrome, if there is severe neonatal involvement. The term "asphyxiating thoracic dysplasia" should be limited strictly to this clearly defined autosomal recessive disorder.

Pseudo-achondroplasia

Histologically this seems so far to be a uniform disorder.[16, 18] The postulated genetic homogeneity has been questioned. On the whole, however, there is dominant transmission in spite of the fact that some brother-sister observations are on record.

Thiemann's Disease

Since no such cases have been seen by the experts in the field of acrodysplasias over the last 20 years, the existence of such an entity must be questioned.

---

* One such type seems to be the combination of peripheral extremity involvement by stippling with a peculiar facial appearance.[33]

Spondylo-metaphyseal Dysplasias

This is a rather nonhomogeneous group of disorders. Clinical, radiologic, and genetic reasons will unquestionably result in the definition of a variety of types. Still, at the present there is only one entity clearly individualized, the type described by Kozlowski.[22]

Osteopetrosis

The first therapeutic trials with bone marrow transplants have resulted in encouraging initial results. Besides a marked hematologic correction and significant clinical improvement, there was, after some months, a markedly diminished radiographic density of the skeleton.[1]

This is of special interest since the reported clinical trials were undertaken based on experience gained experimentally from parabiosis and bone marrow transplants in rats and mice.

Osteoectasia With Hyperphosphatasia

The initial attempts at treating this disorder with calcitonin by Whalen and coworkers were successful.[39] On this basis it is important to recognize this disorder at the earliest possible moment before the crippling bowing deformities of the extremities have occurred.

A number of disorders with varying degrees of skeletal involvement have recently been described. We would like to select one of these especially, since it has a most typical diagnostic aspect on the AP chest film.

The Cerebro-mandibulo-costal Syndrome

This recessively inherited disorder is now clearly defined. The diagnosis can be confidently made in the presence of the characteristic, symmetrical serial posterior rib gap defects.[11, 40]

Metabolism

Since 1973 further significant progress has been made in the area of vitamin D metabolism. Even though the mechanisms resulting in hypophosphatemic familial vitamin D-resistant rickets are still in question, two types of vitamin D-dependent rickets have been defined.[2, 3, 12] The first Type-I results from a defective hydroxylation to 1,25-dihydroxyvitamin D within the kidney and Type II with severe skeletal involvement is considered to result from a local non-response within bone.[3]

Pseudo-hypo-hyper-para-thyroidism

It has now been well documented in a number of patients that some persons with pseudohypoparathyroidism will at some time develop hypocalcemia and hyperphosphatemia with radiographic evidence of hyperparathyroidism secondary to a defective mechanism of hydroxylation in the kidneys.[28, 29]

Mucopolysaccharidoses[6]

Type I-H and Type I-S both result from the same metabolic defect.

The formation of compounds I-H/S and further combinations are possible and will be identified.[20]

The enzymatic deficit in Morquio's disease has been well proven.[34] The very same deficit has also been found in some minor forms identified earlier as pseudo-Morquio's disease Type I (p. 244).

Mucolipidoses

Metabolically these disorders are quite heterogeneous.[9] Type-II and Type-III mucolipidoses seem to result from a deficit in $\alpha = 2, 6$ neuraminidase and $\alpha = 2, 3$ neuraminidase. Mucolipidosis I has as its underlying mechanism a deficit in $\alpha = 2, 5$ neuraminidase.[26, 35] The very same deficit has been noted in nephrosialidosis presenting clinically as severe mental deterioration, renal failure, and skeletal signs of abnormal storage substances within bones, usually with a fatal outcome before the fifth year[25] and in myoclonic epilepsy with a cherry red spot[30, 32], but with a normal skeletal appearance.

REFERENCES

1. Ballet, J. J., Griscelli, C., Coutris, C., Milhaud, G., and Maroteaux, P.: Bone marrow transplantation in human osteopetrosis. Lancet, *2:*1137, 1977.
2. Balsan S., Garabedian, M., Sorgniard, R., Holick, M. F., and Deluca, H. R.: 1,25-dihydroxyvitamin D_3 and 1, α-hydroxyvitamin D_3 in children: biologic and therapeutic effects in nutritional rickets and different types of vitamin D resistance. Pediatr. Res., *9:*586, 1975.
3. Brooks, M. H., *et al.:* Vitamin-D dependent rickets type II. Resistance of target organs to 1,25-Dihydroxyvitamin D. N. Engl. J. Med., *298:*996, 1978.
4. Cederbaum, S. D., Kaitila, I., Rimoin, D. L., and Stiehm, E. R.: The chondro-osseous dysplasia of adenosine deaminase deficiency with severe combined immunodeficiency. J. Pediatr., *89:*737, 1976.
5. Cortina, H., Aparici, R., Beltran, J., and Alberto, C.: The Weissenbacher-Zweymüller syndrome. A case report with review of the world literature. Pediat. Radiol., *6:*109, 1977.

6. Danes, B. S.: Variant of iduronidase deficient mucopolysaccharidoses. Further evidence for genetic heterogeneity. J. Med. Genet., *14:*346, 1977.
7. Danks, D. M., Haslam, R., Mayne, Y., Kaufmann, H. J., and Holtzapple, P. G.: Metaphyseal chondrodysplasia, neutropenia, and pancreatic insufficiency presenting with respiratory distress in the neonatal period. Arch. Dis. Child., *51:*697, 1976.
8. Dinno, N. D., Shearer, L., and Weisskopf, B.: Chondrodysplastic dwarfism, cleft palate and micrognathia in a neonatal, a new syndrome? Eur. J. Pediatr., *123:*39, 1976.
9. Durand, P., *et al.:* Sialidosis (mucolipidosis I). Helv. Paediatr. Acta, *32:*391, 1977.
10. Espiritu, C., Chen, H., and Woolley, P. V., Jr.: Mesomelic dwarfism as the homozygous expression of dyschondrosteosis. Am. J. Dis. Child., *129:*375, 1975.
11. Fauré, C., Valleur, D., and Vital, J. L.: Le syndrome cérébro-costo-mandibulaire. Nouv. Presse Med., *7:*445, 1978.
12. Fraser, D., *et al.:* Pathogenesis of hereditary vitamin-D-dependent rickets. An inborn error of vitamin D metabolism involving defective conversion of 25-hydroxyvitamin D to 1α, 25-dihydroxyvitamin D. N. Engl. J. Med., *289:*817, 1973.
13. Giedion, A., Battaglia, G. F., Bellini, F., and Fanconi, G.: The radiological diagnosis of the fetal-face (= Robinow) syndrome (mesomelic dwarfism and small genitalia). Helv. Paediatr. Acta, *30:*409, 1975.
14. Gilbert, E. F., *et al.:* Chondrodysplasia punctata—rhizomelic form. Pathologic and radiologic studies of three infants. Eur. J. Pediatr., *123:*89, 1976.
15. Gruhn, J. G., Gorlin, R. J., and Langer, L. O.: Dyssegmental dwarfism. A lethal anisospondylic camptomicromelic dwarfism. Am. J. Dis. Child., *132:*382, 1978.
16. Hall, J. G.: Pseudoachondroplasia. Disorders of connective tissue. Birth Defects: Original Article Series XI, *6:*187, 1975.
17. Haller, J. O., *et al.:* The Weissenbacher-Zweymüller syndrome of micrognathia and rhizomelic chondrodysplasia at birth with subsequent normal growth. Am. J. Roentgenol. Radium Ther. Nucl. Med., *125:*936, 1975.
18. Heselson, N. G., Cremin, B. J., and Beighton, P.: Pseudoachondroplasia, a report of 13 cases. Br. J. Radiol., *50:*473, 1977.
19. Kaitila, I. I., Leisti, J. T., and Rimoin, D. L.: Mesomelic skeletal dysplasias. Clin. Orthop., *114:*94, 1975.
20. Kajii, T., *et al.:* Hurler/Scheie genetic compound (mucopolysaccharidosis IH/IS in Japanese brothers. Clin. Genet., *6:*394, 1974.
21. Kaufmann, H. J., Mahboubi, S., Spackman, T. J., Capitanio, M. A., and Kirkpatrick, J.: Tracheal stenosis as a complication of chondrodysplasia punctata. Ann. Radiol., *19:*203, 1976.
22. Kozlowski, K., *et al.:* Spondylo-metaphyseal dysplasias. (report of a case of common type and three pairs of siblings of new varieties.) Australas. Radiol., *20:*154, 1976.
23. ———: Neonatal death dwarfism. (Report of 17 cases). Australas. Radiol., *21:*164, 1977.
24. Langer, L. O., *et al.:* A severe infantile micromelic chondrodysplasia which resembles Kniest disease. Eur. J. Pediatr., *123:*29, 1976.
25. Maroteaux, P., Humbel, R., Strecker, G., Michalski, J. C., and Mande, R.: Un nouveau type de sialidose avec atteinte rénale: la néphrosialidose. Arch. Fr. Pediatr., accepted for publication.
26. Maroteaux, P., Poissonnier, M., Tondeur, M., Strecker, G., and Lemonnier, M.: Sialidose par deficit en alpha (2-6) neuraminidase sans atteinte neurologique Mucolipidose de type I? Archives Francaises de Pediatrie, *35:*280, 1978.
27. Maroteaux, P., and Spranger, J.: Essai de classification des chondrodysplasies à predominance mesomelique. Arch. Fr. Pediatr., *34:*945, 1977.
28. Marx, S. J., and Aurbach, G. D.: Heterogeneous hormonal disorder in pseudohypoparathyroidism. N. Engl. J. Med., *20:*169, 1977.
29. Metz, S. A., Baylink, D. J., Hughes, M. R., Haussler, M. R., and Robertson, R. P.: Selective deficiency of 1,25-dihydroxycholecalciferol. A cause of isolated skeletal resistance to parathyroid hormone. N. Engl. J. Med., *297:*1084, 1977.
30. O'Brien, J. S.: Neuraminidase deficiency in the cherry red spot-myoclonus syndrome. Biochem. Biophys. Res. Commun., *79:*1136, 1977.
31. Pauli, R. M., Madden, J. D., Kranzler, K. J., Culpepper, W., and Port R.: Warfarin therapy initiated during pregnancy and phenotypic chondrodysplasia punctata. J. Pediatr., *88:*506, 1976.
32. Rapin, I., Goldfischer, S., Karzman, R., Engel, J., Jr., and O'Brien, J. S.: The cherry red spot-myoclonus syndrome. Ann. Neurol., *3:*234, 1978.
33. Sheffield, L. J., Danks, D. M., Mayne, V., and Hutchinson, L. A.: Chondrodysplasia punctate-23 cases of a mild and relatively common variety. J. Pediatr., *89:*916, 1976.
34. Singh, J., Di Ferrante, N., Niebes, P., and Tavella, D.: N-acetylgalactosamine-6-sulfate sulfatase in man. Absence of the enzyme in Morquio disease. J. Clin. Invest., *57:*1036, 1976.
35. Spranger, J., Gehler, J., and Cantz, M.: Mucolipidosis I—A sialidosis. Am. J. Med. Genet., *1:*21, 1977.
36. Stanescu, V., Stanescu, R., and Maroteaux, P.: Etude morphologique et biochemique du cartilage de croissance dans les osteochondrodysplasies. Arch. Fr. Pediatr., *34:*1, 1977.
37. Steele, R. W., Britton, H. A., Anderson, C. T., and Kniker, W. T.: Severe combined immunodeficiency with cartilage hair hypoplasia: In vitro response to thymosin and attempted reconstitution. Pediatr. Res., *10:*1003, 1976.
38. Warkany, J.: Warfarin embryopathy. Teratology, *14:*205, 1976.
39. Whalen, J. P., *et al.:* Calcitonin treatment in hereditary bone dysplasia with hyperphosphatasemia: A radiographic and histologic study of bone. Am. J. Roentgenol., Radium Ther. Nucl. Med., *129:*29, 1977.
40. Williams, H. J., and Sane, S. M.: Cerebro-costo-mandibular syndrome: long term follow up of a patient and review of the literature. Am. J. Roentgenol. Radium Ther. Nucl. Med., *126:*1223, 1976.

Acknowledgments

This book is not the result of the efforts of a single author, but rather the product of a collaboration among friends. Clément Fauré, in particular, has accepted the preparation of the chapters devoted to tumors, Claude Fessard those on the pathology of the nervous system and in the context of hematologic disorders, and Pierre Rigault wrote the chapters on osteomyelitis and pediatric orthopaedic surgery.

We would very much like to express our gratitude to all those who have helped us in the preparation of this book, particularly Professor Maurice Lamy, Professor Pierre Royer, as well as Mrs. S. Balsan. Special thanks should go to M. Broyer, J. de Grouchy, H. Mathieu, and R. Rappaport who have allowed us to benefit from their experience in the writing of several chapters particularly to those devoted to the calcium and phosphorus metabolism of bone and to chromosomal aberrations. Also, we would like to thank the Professors Jean Frézal, Jacques Lefebvre, and Jean Rey, who offered their counsel as well as V. Stanescu and all those colleagues and friends from France and abroad who have opened their archives and offered their documents such as:

J. Aicardi, M. Aussanaire, H. Boissière, J. Caffey, E. Campailla, J. Channarond, A. Cosson, J. Cukier, R. Dailly, J. C. Dayras, I. Emerit, M. Fèvre, G. Fontaine, D. Gosselin, L. Guéraud, P. Guilbaud, J. Guivarch, M. Hassan, J. F. Hirsch, J. C. Job, M. Juster, G. Kalifa (2CV), J. Kucera, J. Marie, R. Laplane, M. Laval-Jeantet, B. Le Marec, J. A. Lièvre, P. Mabille, R. Mallet, G. Malpuech, A. Mazabraud, Menget, J. Menkes, F. Moran, A. Mugnier, J. Naffah, D. Nusslé, G. Payet, B. Pépin, C. Piussan, J. Pont, J. G. Pous, M. O. Rethoré, A. Rossier, J. Sauvegrain, O. Schweisguth, P. Segond, R. Stanescu, S. Thieffry, J. Vialatte, R. Walbaum, S. Weil, H. R. Wiedemann, and J. Wittmer.

Finally, this book would not have seen publication without the assistance of Mrs. M. Henry, J. Kelley, and R. Leroy, who in a very large measure have provided the necessary effort to type the text and the bibliography.

We would also like to thank Professors R. Debré and S. De Séze, who have given permission to reproduce a number of their figures.

And last, but far from least, a very special mention must go together with our combined thanks to Mme. Novarina at Flammarion Médecine-Sciences and Suzanne Boyd, Mary Frawley, and Mr. Fred Zeller at the J. B. Lippincott Company.

PIERRE MAROTEAUX
HERBERT J. KAUFMANN

Contents

Part Five: Acquired Bone Diseases

Part Six: Bone Tumors
Clément Fauré

Part One:

Normal Bone and Its Growth

1 The Bone

DEFINITION

According to Littré the bones can be defined as the hard, solid framework of the body, the basic characteristic being the presence of calcium salts which are fixed on a protein-matrix. The study of bone, therefore, cannot be limited to anatomic, embryologic, or histologic approaches, but must also widely emcompass the analysis of its chemical interaction and the rather complex mechanisms of ossification and calcification.

Three principal types of bone are commonly distinguished. There are the long bones which constitute the skeletal part of the extremities, the short bones represented by the carpal and tarsal bones, and the flat bones.

All long bones are composed of three parts; the diaphyses, the epiphyses, and the metaphyses (Fig. 1-1). The diaphysis, the middle part of the bone, is a hollow cylinder containing the medullary cavity within its interior. The most distal parts form the epiphyses which articulate with the neighboring bones. The metaphyses separate the diaphysis from the epiphyses. During infancy, the metaphyses are limited in their distal ends by growth cartilage. Rubin has proposed to call this cartilage physis. We will return to the description of the metaphyses when we discuss its anatomic and structural study.

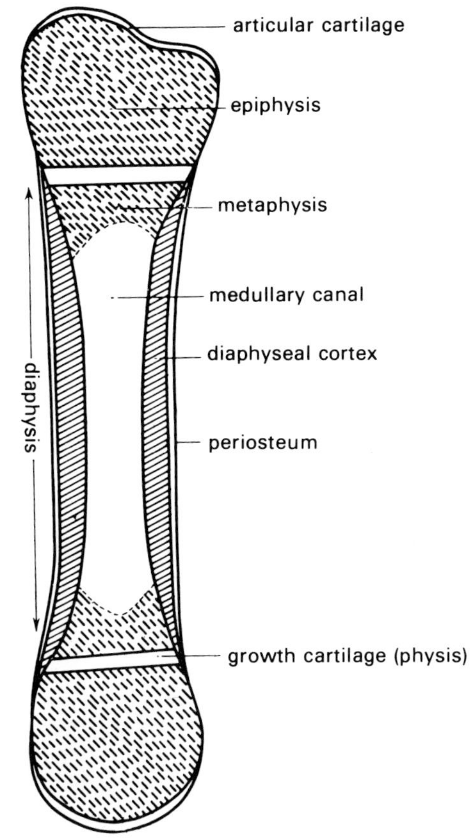

Fig. 1-1. The schematic appearance of a long bone. (Taken from: Maladies des os et des articulations. CMC, Flammarion)

EMBRYOLOGIC ORIGIN AND TYPE OF DEVELOPMENT

From the primitive mesenchyme originate the different parts of the skeletal system. The initial prelude to the appearance of bone is the condensation of mesenchymal cells. This takes place after their multiplication in conjunction with the significant synthesis of the specific macromolecules collagen and glycosaminoglycans* whose roles are still poorly understood.

If there is any understanding of the mechanism of appearance of the anlage of the extremities, which begins at the same time as does the condensation of mesenchymal cells and which is the result of interactions between mesodermal and ectodermal structures, we are still in the dark as to the induction mechanisms which precipitate this condensation. Bony induction, which will be discussed later, has been studied on ex-

* This expression refers to acid mucopolysaccharides in the old nomenclatures.

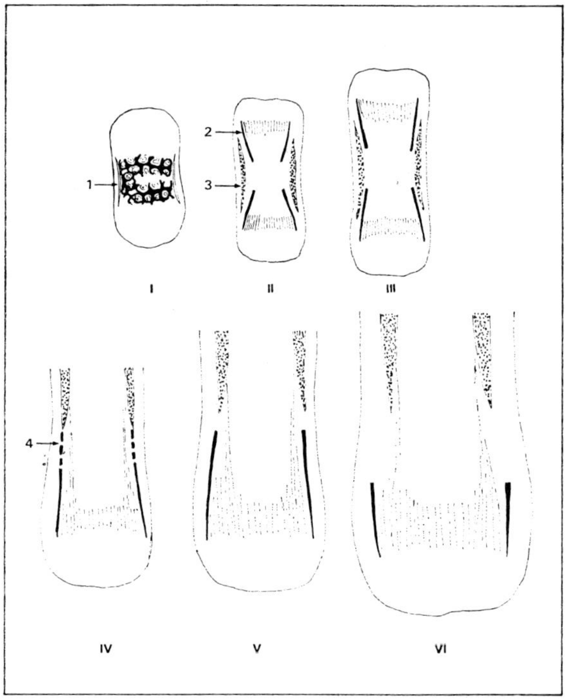

Fig. 1-2. Development of a long bone. (M. Juster and N. Balmain-Oligo: Pathologie Biologie *19*:33-42, 1971)
I: Calcified marginal membrane
II: Perichondral ring
III: Periosteal bone
IV: Osteoclastic erosion

perimental models which are far removed from the actual situation of embryogenesis.

After condensation takes place there is a transformation of the mesenchymal cells into osteoprecursors or chondroprecursors depending on the zone to be studied. The cranial vault and the facial bones originate directly from the mesenchyme. This process is referred to as membranous ossification. Long bones, the vertebrae, and the base of the skull are formed within cartilage, as a secondary ossification. This is referred to as enchondral ossification.

The factors causing cellular differentiation are still a source of mystery. While the synthesis of glycosaminoglycans will bring about chondrogenesis, and formation of tropocollagen or collagen will result in osteogenesis (Hall). High oxygen content will influence synthesis in the latter direction. Mechanical stimulation will favor chondrogenesis, possibly through intermediary piezo-electrical forces.

During the process of membranous ossification mesenchymal cells align themselves in a parallel and regular fashion. This is true, for instance, in the cranial vault in the maxillary bone, where they arrange themselves in more anarchic islands. They then produce collagenous fibers along which the osteoblasts arrange themselves.

At the center of the mesenchymal outline in long bones there occurs proliferation of larger, rounded cells. Occurring at the same time is the enlargement of intercellular spaces. This is the result of the deposition of a basophilic and homogeneous matrix, whereas the collagen fibers disappear. This cartilage will progressively invade the entire bony model and will be surrounded by a layer of fibrous tissue, known as the perichondrium. As early as the seventh week of intrauterine life this cartilaginous model has the exact formation of the bone which will later replace it. The onset of calcification occurs in the center of the cartilaginous matrix during the eighth week. This process can be recognized initially by hypertrophy, and then by the necrotic appearance of the cartilaginous cells. This will then progress out toward the periphery where a fine marginal membrane will be formed. This is the site of secondary calcification. Following this, primary resorption of the calcific zone will occur, however, formation of enchondral bone produced by osteoblasts originating from the circulating blood will replace the trabecula (Fig. 1-2 I).

Simultaneously the formation of periosteal bone will be taking place at the periphery of this marginal membrane. This is distinctly different from the above since it is produced by the osteoblasts of the deep layer of the perichondrium which becomes the periosteum. (Fig. 1-2 II).

Following this secondary resorption occurs at the center of the diaphysis which leads to the disappearance of the trabeculae of enchondral bone. Thus, the medullary cavity is formed while, according to Juster, the marginal membrane divides itself into two parts (Fig. 1-2 II, III). These latter structures will be found pushed further and further toward the ends of the bone and will eventually localize at the distal portion of the periosteal bone, which had covered them completely during their primitive phase (Fig. 1-2 IV).

The metaphyses undergo resorption in their proximal regions which neighbor the central parts of the bones, while growth occurs at the distal regions. The actual site of progression is marked by a cartilaginous band which assures the growth of the bone. See the growth zone (Fig. 1-2 IV). Laterally, according to Juster, the metaphyses are developed by the marginal membrane, which by the addition of bone to its internal and external surface will turn into the perichondrial ring (Fig. 1-2, 1-3). To others who have written on the subject (Lacroix), this structure corresponds to a portion of periosteal bone situated at the level of the zone

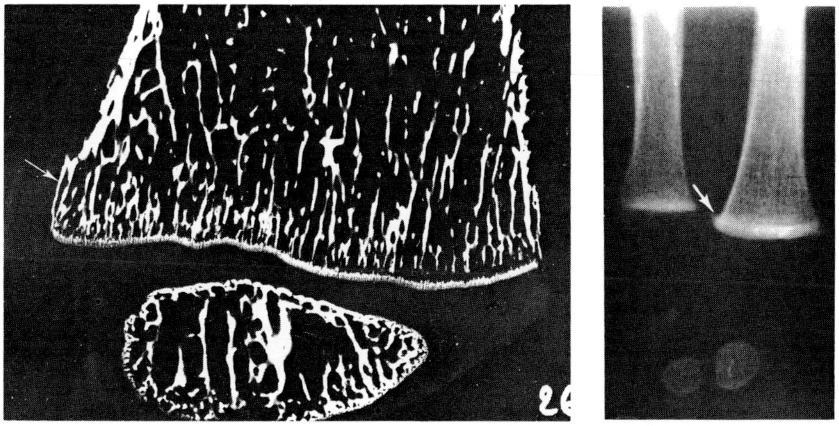

Fig. 1-3. (Left) Microradiograph of the distal end of a long bone showing the perichondrial ring. (J. Wittmer) *(Right)* This same ring can be recognized on the radiograph of a baby.

of proliferating cartilage outside the effect of modeling resorption.

Within the epiphyses there is later development of ossification centers. Their time of appearance is markedly different according to their location.

ANATOMIC AND STRUCTURAL STUDY

Schematically, one must clearly distinguish the two types of bony structure. Compact bone forms the diaphysis of long bones and the spongiosa which is composed of finely interlaced lamellae known as trabeculations. These trabeculations border on cavities which contain the bone marrow. This tissue is formed within the metaphyses of long bones, the vertebral bodies and flat bones. The periphery of the bone is covered by the periosteum which is a layer of connective tissue.

The diaphysis of a long bone is a cylinder of compact tissue. This consists of concentric layers formed by the periosteum and which are constantly being replaced by new additions of further peripheral layers, whereas the more centrally located ones are destroyed, forming the medullary cavity. Thus, both the growth in bone width as well as its modeling is assured. Primary bone is made up of immature tissue with its collagen fibers having an anarchic arrangement and the bony trabeculae without orderly lamellar architecture. This fact is well recognized on a microradiograph of the periphery of young bone.

This tissue becomes progressively more organized. Longitudinal parallel tunnels following the long axis of the bone are formed. These tunnels contain capillaries around which osseous tissue is laid down in concentric

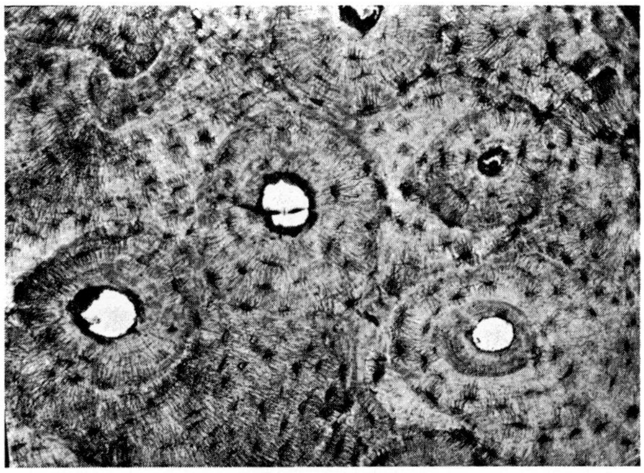

Fig. 1-4. Transverse section of a human femoral diaphysis showing the osteons with their central Haversian canal (specimen courtesy of A. Mazabraud). (Taken from: Maladies des os et des articulations, CMC Flammarion).

lamellae. Thus these lamellae are empty cylinders, one within the other. The central cavity is the Haversian canal (Fig. 1-4). The unit of the Haversian system has been given the name osteon. This system is one of the characteristic findings of mature bone. At the inner region of the Haversian system, there is communication between the individual cells or osteocytes through small canals. At a certain distance from the canal this system is recognizable only as a line called the "cement line" and beyond these structures there is no further communication.

On a microradiograph the osteons have a circular form, differing in appearance according to their degree

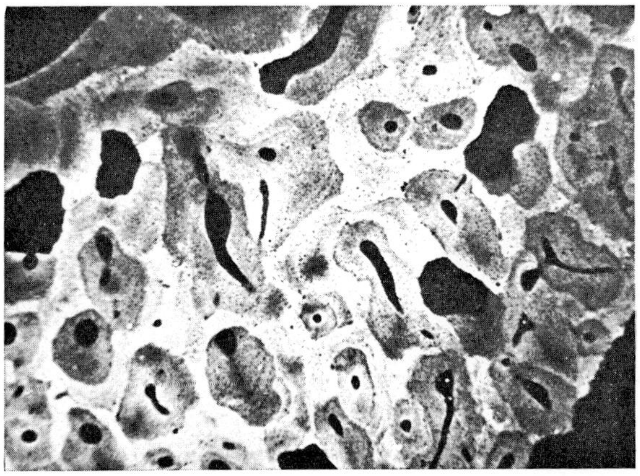

Fig. 1-5. Microradiography of a transverse section of the tibial diaphysis in a 2-year-old infant; the less mineralized secondary osteons are visible within the cortical area together with large resorptive cavities. (M. Laval-Jeantet)

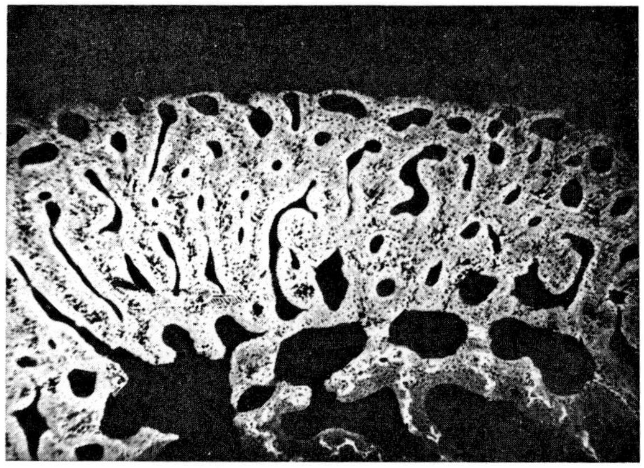

Fig. 1-6. Microradiography of the tibial diaphysis of a newborn; at the lower portion of this figure the trabeculae of spongy bone are well visualized. (J. Wittmer)

of mineralization and age. There are cavities of resorption between several of them. (Fig. 1-5). This constant process of rejuvenation has its course not only during the growth period, but it also continues in the adult as evidenced by the continuous appearance of new canals, whereas old Haversian systems undergo destruction.

There is no visible periosteum on the normal films. However, this cylinder of compact tissue can be recognized if the area has been shown tangentially leading to fine visualization of cortical bands. These bands are separated by an intermediate and less dense zone, which corresponds to the medullary canal. It should not be overlooked that anteriorly and posteriorly the x-rays have passed through dense compact bone and, therefore, bony lesions visible in the medial part of the bone are not localized within the medullary cavity.

The metaphysis is delineated toward the epiphyses by growth cartilage, which will be discussed under histology. This structure will produce a bony tissue with wide spaced lamellae separated by wide interspaces filled with bone marrow. Their structural arrangement has an anarchic appearance and the tissue formed is called spongy bone (Fig. 1-6). Radiographically, this spongiosa can be recognized as a more or less dense lace work depending on where it is located.

This meshwork is quite regular and gives to the bone a homogeneous appearance. Local thickening and an orientation which follows the lines of central forces leading to a particular structure is seen in certain areas; for example, at the level of the femoral neck. Primary and secondary spongiosa can sometimes be distinguished. Primary spongiosa is formed by bony lamellae close to the growth cartilage and results directly from the ossification of calcified cartilage while secondary spongiosa results from the turnover and growth of lamellae on the basis of the preceding layer.

The bony lamellae of enchrondral origin located at the periphery of the bone will reach toward the cortical bone without interposition of periosteal bone. The junction between this cortical zone of enchondral origin and the periosteal cortex is sometimes called the point of integration (Juster). We feel that this puts the peripheral limit of the metaphysis toward the diaphyseal side with its central border being formed by the medullary cavity. On very good radiographs one can see this point of integration, at least during early infancy. This results from the cortical bone of enchondral origin being more irregular and subject to modeling resorption, a fact which will be discussed in the following chapter (see p. 22). This point migrates toward the epiphyses during growth and continues at a somewhat faster rate when the bone approaches the adult state. This migration is paralleled by a progressive increase in length of the periosteum and of the periosteal bone.

At the periphery of the growth cartilage we must recall the existence of the perichondrial ring. This structure can be recognized in the young infant or on a microradiograph (Fig. 1-3). The actual role of this ring is still under discussion, although it does seem to play an important role in maintenance of cartilage (Oligo et al.). In between the ring, the periosteum, and the basal region of the growth cartilage, there is a grossly triangular area formed by mesenchymal tissue which has a projection of connective cells located between the ring and the periosteum. This particular region was named ossification-notch by Ranvier. Its exact function and importance have not yet been fully defined.

The epiphyses are formed by the spongiosa. They are covered by articular cartilage and protect the growth zone of the bone from secondary trauma during articular activity. This cartilage is not visible on radiographs, it can be seen indirectly as a clear space separating the distal parts of the bones. The articular line may have some variation in thickness in accordance with the joint but there is little variance from one person to another.

Vertebral bodies, along with the carpal and the tarsal bones are also formed by spongiosa and are covered by a very thin cortical layer. In contrast to this, there are two marked layers of compact tissue which are separated by the spongiosa in the area of the flat bones of the cranial vault, the scapula, and the ilium.

All bone has a rich vascular system, which is composed of nutritive arteries, as well as metaphyseal, epiphyseal, and periosteal vessels. The nutritive arteries run an oblique course entering into the diaphysis to reach the medullary cavity. There is then a division into descending and ascending branches with further subdivision and radial invasion into the bone following the Haversian canals. The venous capillaries lead into the central medullary sinus which drains through a vein accompanying the artery. On a radiograph the nutritive artery can sometimes be recognized as a small tranverse line that should never be confused with a fracture.

During the growth period there is rich vascularization of the growth zone by capillaries which originate from the nutritive artery and enter into the hypertrophic cartilage. According to Trueta the vascularization of the growth cartilage itself is assured by epiphyseal arteries. These arteries penetrate the external surface of the epiphysis, and at times its periphery. The veins take an identically parallel course, however, others feel that they have their own individual orifices.

The periosteal vascularization is still a matter of controversy. Some maintain (Brookes), that there is a blood supply from medullary arteries while others insist upon the importance of periosteal vessels. Indeed, the periosteum does have a rich network of vessels which could assure irrigation of the primary osteons and could play an important role in the repair of fractures. Furthermore it is possible, that at such a moment there is reversal of the circulation (Rhinelander), resulting in a centripetal flow. There are elements of the nervous system present within the periosteum, the marrow, and the bone itself.

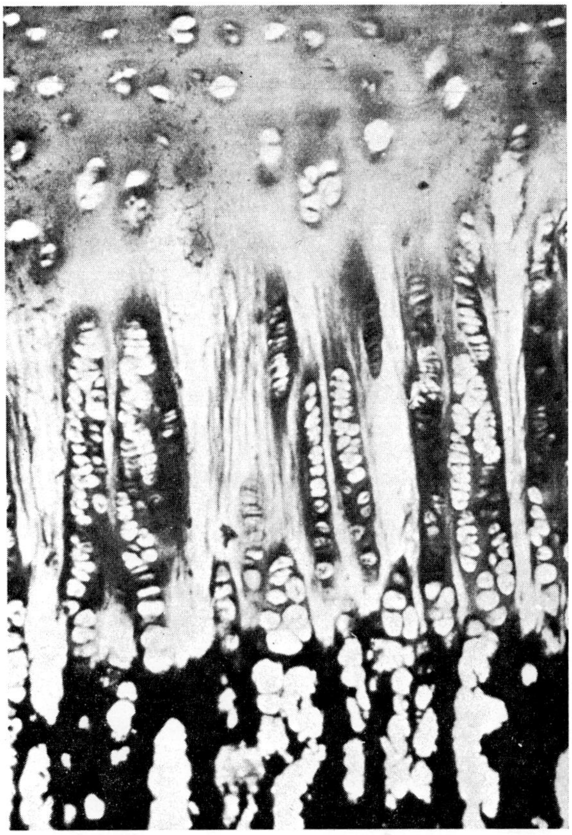

Fig. 1-7. Normal growth of human cartilage. Note especially the regular columnar arrangement of cartilage as well as that of the lines of ossification and the osseous lamellae stained in black by the von Kossa technique. (V. Stanescu)

HISTOLOGIC STUDY

In most bones the development of bony tissue arises from a cartilaginous matrix. This phenomenon of enchondral ossification we referred to earlier can be studied easily in the growth cartilage of a long bone (Fig. 1-7). The basal zone of the long bone is formed by a band of undifferentiated cartilage, sometimes referred to as the germinal layer or reserve cartilage. Below this layer there is ossification of cells and a parallel columnar arrangement which is the proliferative zone of cartilage. Subsequent to these developments there occurs hypertrophy of the cells which contain cytoplasmic vacuoles, growth in size of their nuclei and also a partial loss of the cell's chromatin. Phosphatase activity is high and they are also rich in glycogen. This defines the hypertrophic zone of cartilage.

Calcification of the ground substance begins in a narrow region, beyond which is the zone of ossifica-

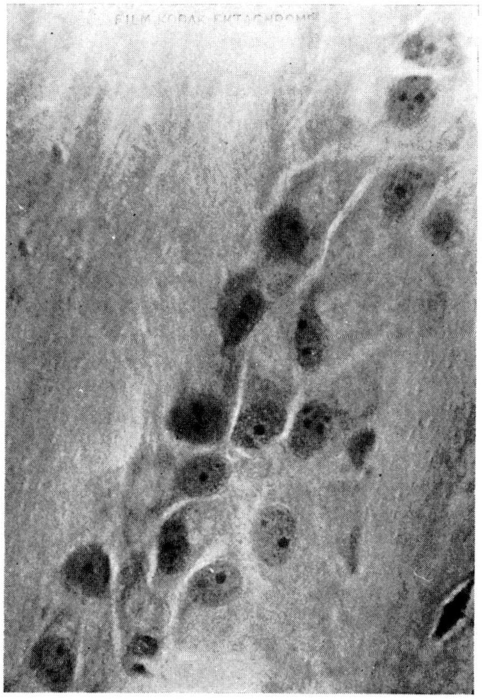

Fig. 1-8. Osteoblasts (stained with eosin hematoxyline): Note the multinucleated nucleus, cytoplasm with a clear juxtanuclear cytoplasm (specimen courtesy of A. Mazabraud). (Taken from: Maladies des os et des articulations, CMC, Flammarion)

tion, where cartilage is invaded by connective tissue-vascular structures. Much study and discussion has been devoted to the formation of these capillaries and their physiologic significance. It is presently accepted that they form from vascular buds and that their endothelial cells are distinctly different from the mesenchymal cells in their immediate vicinity. Trueta, and Little, Schenk, et al. have shown that in certain regions the continuity of the vascular wall is interrupted and that elements of blood come in a direct contact with the cartilaginous matrix. The resorption of this matrix would be under the influence of large phagocytic cells, called chondroclasts by some, because of their similarity to osteoclasts, which we will investigate later. The presence of macrophages has been documented by Anderson and Parker.

Under the influence of this vascular penetration, the transverse walls separating the individual chondrocytes will disappear. Within these tunnels which have been thus formed, bony tissue is laid down under osteoblastic influence after they have differentiated along the connective tissue-vascular axes.

The osteoblast is a quadrangular or oval cell of 20 to 30 μ in diameter whose long axis is perpendicular to the bony trabeculae (Fig. 1-8). The chromatin of its nucleus is concentrated peripherally and contains a nucleolus. Its basophilic cytoplasm has extensions forming anastomoses with the extensions of neighboring cells. It contains an abundant endoplasmic reticulum, many ribosomes, a large number of mitochondria, a Golgi apparatus, and is rich in glycogen, alkaline phosphatase, and PAS-positive material as well as nucleic acid. The origin of osteoblasts has been widely discussed; and most authors maintain that they derive from the reticular cells of the bone marrow or from the cells of the perivascular connective tissue. Trueta, however, states that they derive from the endothelial cells of capillaries.

As the osteoblast declines on its osteogenic activity, it becomes flat and its phosphatase activity and its basophilic characteristic disappear. It is then simply located in between the bony trabeculae as an osteocyte. It is also possible, that a reversal takes place, thus, the osteoblast becomes a reticular, osteoblastic, even a chondroblastic cell.

The osteocyte is the characteristic cell of bony tissue. Its form is oblong and flattened and is similar to a grain of rye. The central nucleus contains one or more nucleoli and a significant amount of chromatin. Its cytoplasm is slightly basophilic and contains some mitochondria, a small Golgi apparatus, glycogen, PAS-positive material, and fats. The osteocyte has numerous extensions which anastomose with neighboring cells. Located within the calcified substance, the osteoclast occupies a small cavity within the bony tissue called ostcoplasts and its extensions are located within fine canals (Fig. 1-9). Although the osteocytes do not undergo any further division studies by Baud have shown them to be very active cells, playing an essential role in bone metabolism. In addition to this, they do possess the capacity to put new layers of bony tissues around themselves or on the other hand, to reabsorb them.

Bone is in a constant state of renewal. A loss of calcium appears to precipitate the breakdown of old bony tissue (Bohatirchuk). Subsequently this bony resorption can lead to the intervention of specialized cells called osteoclasts (Fig. 1-10). An osteoclast is a large rounded or oval, and sometimes multilobular cell. Its diameter varies from 20 to 100 μ and the nuclei member from 10-30 or more. They are round or oval with one or two nucleoli. During at least the early part of its life the cytoplasm of the osteoclast is basophilic. Within the cytoplasm is contained PAS-positive granules and numerous vacuoles. The osteoclast is strongly attached to the bony trabeculation and is sometimes located within a lacuna. Along such trabec-

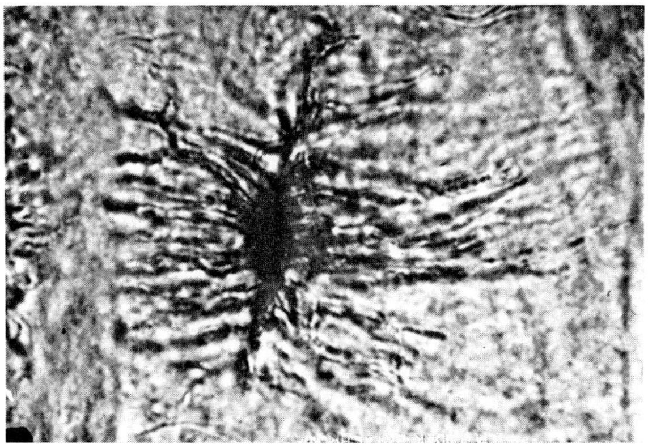

Fig. 1-9. Osteocyte with extensions (specimen courtesy of A. Mazabraud). (Taken from: Maladies des os et des articulations, CMC, Flammarion)

ulae one can observe a brush border. Osteoclasts do not contain phosphatase, but they do have the capacity to phagocytize and display a marked proteolytic activity. Because osteoclasts have a relatively short life span their origin is still under discussion. For some authors they derive from reticular cells, for others from osteoblasts.

Bony resorption is not the only type of resorption found to occur with osteoclasts. It has been noted by Duriez that another kind of resorption takes place where the osteocytes seem to play the primary role. One can observe this particular process in such adverse conditions as osteomalacia and hyperthyroidism. There are certain cases where it may be more difficult to ascertain the actual role of the osteocyte. This is referred to as halisteresis or "smooth resorption."

Within the interior of the central canal of long bones and the trabecular spongiosa, is the bone marrow which possesses an extensive network of mesenchymal tissue which contain hematopoetic cells. Hematopoetic activity is particularly strong in the newborn. There is then a subsequent reduction in activity resulting in some of the bone marrow being turned into fat. The only hematopoietic activtity in the adult involves the vertebral bodies, the ribs, and sternum, and the bones of the skull, shoulder, and pelvic girdles.

CHEMICAL STUDY

As we have stated previously bony tissue is characterized by the impregnation of calcium salts onto an organic matrix.

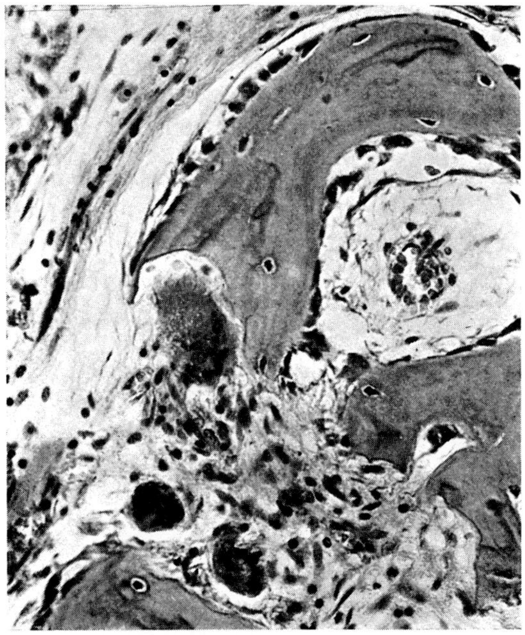

Fig. 1-10. Osteoclasts at the lower region of the bony growing lamella there is a notch containing a multinucleated osteoclast. Two others are visible at the lower left. (A. Mazabraud). (Taken from: Maladies des os et des articulations, CMC, Flammarion)

ORGANIC MATRIX

This matrix is formed by collagen fibers and a ground substance.

Collagen

There is general agreement that the basic collagen molecule is formed by three polypeptide chains. They are arranged in a triple helix and curved on itself. The collagen molecule has a length of 2800 Å and a width of 15 Å with its molecular weight being in the order of 300,000.

Several types of α-chains exist and the collagen of the bone as that of the skin contains two α_1 and one α_2 chain. In contrast to this, collagen when located within the cartilage, is composed of just three α_1 chains (Miller). This problem is not quite as simple as it may sound since there are several types of α_1 chains. We are dealing with α_1I chains within bone whereas cartilage contains α_1II chains.

Hydrogen bonds, as well as covalent bonds, define the stability of a triple helix structure (Cooper and Russell). Aggregation of these molecules form fibrils

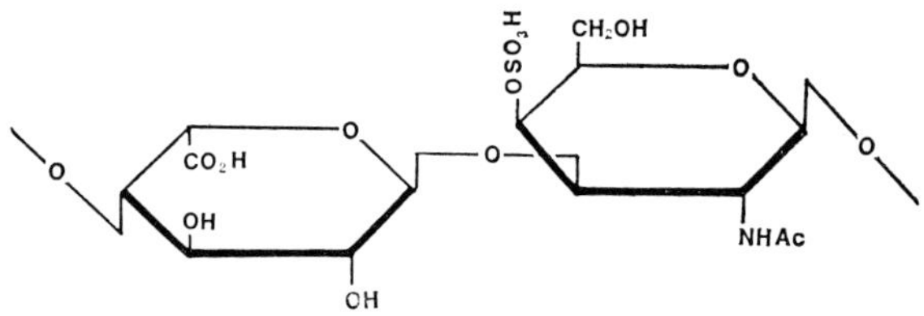

Fig. 1-11. Schematic drawing of a basic unit of a chain of dermatan-sulphate. (Courtesy of K. Meyer)

with a periodicity of 640 to 720 Å and are the basis of several rather complex theories.

The amino-acid composition of bone collagen does not significantly differ from that of other tissues. There is approximately one-third glycine, along with notable amounts of proline and hydroxypoline. Proline and hydroxyproline appear to play a fundamental role in achieving stability for the natural molecule. The presence of hydroxylysine though only present in minor amounts is constant and essential and together with hydroxyproline is considered to be indispensable for the classification of a protein under the heading of collagen.

The arrangement and morphology of collagen fibers undergo considerable variation at least in the cortical region of bone with age. During infancy their arrangement is less compact. Diameters are in the range of 150-620 Å. Contrary to this, are fibers of 1500 Å found in older individuals (Robinson and Watson).

During the period of embryonic life these fibers are smaller and further apart. It appears that there is a relationship between the dimension of the fibers and their arrangement. When they are larger, they have a greater tendency to aggregate in a close fashion.

There has been little research devoted to the collagen of abnormal bone. We shall see, however, the suggestion of a collagen anomaly in osteogenesis imperfecta. No further emphasis is placed on the value of such studies in constitutional disorders.

Osteoblasts and fibroblasts are responsible for the synthesis of collagen and will not be discussed further here. This fact has been documented by autoradiography, in vitro studies, and research involving electron microscopy. The latter technique reveals that in certain zones there is an attachment of microfibrils to cells. They seem to occasionally originate directly from the cytoplasm without any intervention by the membrane. In other areas the latter is hidden by the microfibrils.

As opposed to what one may expect collagen does not possess a particularly slow metabolism. Gerber et al., utilizing radioactively marked proline incorporation, were able to show several metabolic pathways in bone, one of which is very active, with a half life of proline being only four days.

An indirect approach to the clinical evaluation of collagen's metabolic activity is the study of the urinary excretion of hydroxyproline, which seems to be a comparable process (Lenzi). In scurvy, for example, where the synthesis of collagen is slow there is a drop in the elimination of hydroxyproline (Martin). In contrast to this parathormone will increase this elimination as the result of the increased resorption of collagen. A similar increase has been noted in osteogenesis imperfecta (Langness and Behnke).

We shall see that collagen seems to play a major role in the mineralization of bone. According to Fleisch collagen alone is capable of inducing the precipitation of hydroxyapatite in physiologic concentration. The writer suggests that there are intervening factors inhibiting calcification, and in particular pyrophosphate. Within calcified tissues a pyrophosphatase can inactivate pyrophosphate. Still, if these tissues contain a large amount of pyrophosphatase, its presence in many other tissues calls for further hypothetical explanations.

GROUND SUBSTANCE

The quantitative significance of ground substance within bone is relatively weak. According to Eastoe and Eastoe it represents only 1.2 per cent of the weight of the organic matrix, as compared to collagen fibers which make up 93 per cent. However, the ground substance does constitute 51 per cent of the organic material of cartilage. The physiologic role of ground substance, however, is of no less importance. We shall see later, that there is a group of constitutional skeletal diseases which result from a metabolic defect of mucopolysaccharides (glycosaminoglycans). Together with the glycoproteins they are an essential element.

Glycosaminoglycans are composed of long chains with a two carbohydrate base unit, one always being a hexosamine and the other a hexuronic acid (Fig. 1-11). There may be a sulfate group attached to the carbohydrates. As in the case of chondroitin-4 and -6 sulfate and keratan-sulfate, both are widespread in bone and cartilage. Keratan-sulfate, however, does not contain hexuronic acid. The glycosaminoglycans always bind themselves to proteins thus forming the complex proteoglycans. They do not occur in free form within tissues.

Proteoglycans are micromolecules which are composed of many chains of chondroitin-sulfate and keratan-sulfate. They are bound to each other by

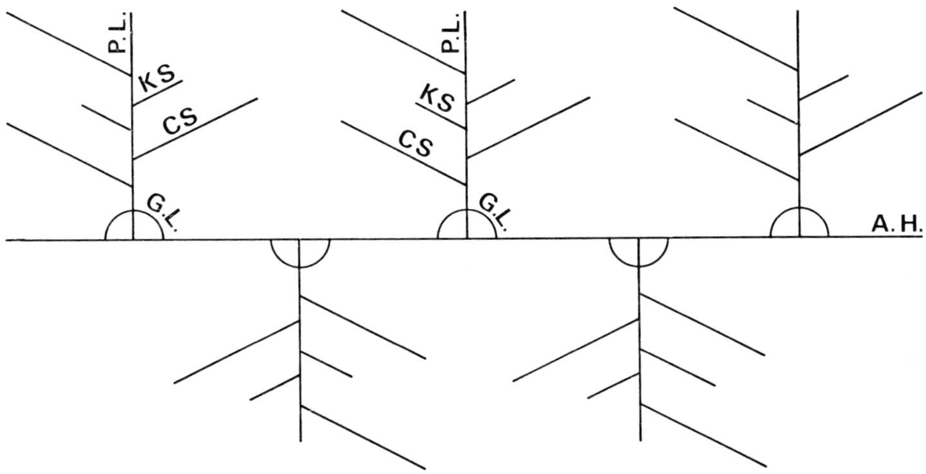

Fig. 1-12. The schematic structure of a proteoglycan. The alternating character of the chondroitin-sulphate chains and those of the keratan-sulphate which are represented here is presently under discussion.
AH: hyaluronic acid
PL: protein core
GL: protein links
CS: chondroitin-sulphate
KS: keratan-sulphate

covalent bonds and then to an intermediary unit of serine or threonine which is attached to a protein. A great deal of study has been devoted to proteoglycans found in the cartilage of the nasal septum of the bull. They are composed of subunits with an approximate molecular weight of 1.5 to 4 × 10^6. This varies in accordance with the number and the length of the mucopolysaccharide chains which are attached to the protein. The protein has a molecular weight of approximately 200,000 and a length of 3,400 Å (Rosenberg). There cannot be any dissociation of the subunits without destruction of the covalent bonds.

Within the ground substance of cartilage proteoglycans exist as aggregates of a high molecular weight. They are held together by a noncovalent association of subunits by links proteins (Fig. 1-12). While the number of subunits within the aggregates is still under discussion, there is said to be approximately 20 having a molecular weight close to 30 × 10^6.

The glycoproteins are a group of carbohydrates which are linked to proteins. They are short-chained and contain a larger variety of sugars. They can be short, straight or branched and it varies as to how many chains will bind themselves to a single protein.

Proteoglycans interefere with the formation of collagen fibrils (Mathews and Decker). Yet, on thc other hand there are numerous facts which suggest that they take an active part in the process of calcification. Their concentration increases moving from the reserve cartilage to the columnar zone (Stanescu). There is a drop within the zone of provisional calcification and most markedly within bone. However, the exact role of the proteoglycans is not well understood. It is possible, due to their strong binding capacity, that they play an important role in the transport of calcium and phosphorus in areas of ossification. In vitro experiments performed by Schubert and Pras have shown that in addition to this, they could have either an inhibitory or favorable effect on the growth of calcium phosphate crystals.

It is noteworthy that within the ground substance of bone there is a heat-resistant protein which differs in composition from that which exists in collagen (Eastoe and Eastoe), and peptides which have been studied by Leaver. The peptides could play a role in nucleation or in the blockage of the acid radicals of mucopolysaccharides. Attention has been drawn to the presence of lipids and their importance (Irving and Wuthier). Urist has maintained that they take a part in the calcification process.

Finally, the ground substance fills in the spaces between vessels and cells, allowing many metabolites to pass through it which are not a basic part of its composition. Thus, it plays an important physiologic role.

MINERALS, SALTS, AND WATER

In its normal state hydroxy-apatite $Ca_{10}(PO_4)(OH)_2$ is the only crystalline salt which can be detected in the bone utilizing crystallographic methods. A phosphate of amorphous calcium, however, having the same chemical formula is found in large quantities of bone, dentine, and cartilage (Posner). Small quantities of phosphate with a lower Ca/P ratio are said to be detectable, particularly in the zone of provisional calcification (Urist and Dowell).

Calcium carbonate is in part bound to phosphate through the substitution of CO_3 H groups by PO_4 groups. Also present is a small amount of CO_3Ca.

Hydroxyapatite crystals are of minute dimension being from 30 to 75 Å in width and thickness and 50 to 500 Å in length. According to Robinson and Watson they supposedly have the form of a polygonal plate. Other authors, however, have felt them to be more like needles (Bonucci). These crystals are located within interfibrillary spaces and form bands perpendicular to collagen fibers.

Within the crystal there are Ca, PO_4 and OH ions, with minimal changes occurring among them. There are, however, at times substitutions involving certain ions, for example, strontium. In contrast to this is its surface which contains numerous ions held in place by electrostatic surface forces, in particular, Na-, CO_3- and citrate ions. Surrounding the crystal is a shell of hydration which constitutes a zone of active exchange between the crystal's surface and its interstitial fluid. This layer of hydration has an 80-90 per cent composition of water in the adult bone.

Iso- and heteroionic changes occur in great intensity at the surface of the crystal without leading to any increase in size. Because of its considerable surface, which is in the order of 500,000 sqm in the adult (Howell), the crystal's surface constitutes a very important reserve of mobile ions. This refers not only to Ca and P, but to other ions as well. The skeleton embodies 35 per cent of the Na in the organism, 80 per cent of its carbonate, 80 per cent of its citrate, and 60 per cent of its magnesium. Water content in the bone is at its weakest concentration in the body. However, there is marked variation with the age of the tissue. The degree of hydration is greatest prior to the stage of complete mineralization when water still exists in a free state, whereas in the adults compact bone it is in bound form and does not reach 10 volume per cent (8.2 according to Robinson). The content of mineral salt and water varies inversely with the growth of bony crystals. This growth takes place in the space initially occupied by water (Cartier).

Bone contains 98 per cent of the calcium present within the body, emphasizing its importance in the role of mineral metabolism. This will be dealt with further in the chapter devoted to the metabolism of phosphorus and calcium. It is noted by Termine that the mineral activity of bone is its most active role.

OSSIFICATION

Ossification is a complex process in its induction as well as in its mechanisms.

BONY INDUCTION

It is not our purpose to present a complete overview of our understanding of the mechanisms which induce ossification. It has been shown, over a long time by several authors, that there is the possibility of inducing ossification in certain tissues whose ground substance and collagen fibers do not fundamentally differ from those of bone. Thus, since 1938 Levander has induced ectopic bone formation through the injecting of bony extracts. This has been confirmed by others. Lacroix has proposed to name the substance osteogenine. Recent work has confirmed these facts and has added to the recognition of the complexity of this process. Bony induction can be provoked by agents of markedly different types. For example, a sponge soaked with bony extract (Moss, Anderson, Dingwall et al.), millipor-chambers containing bony homografts (Goldhaber), a decalcified bony matrix, a freeze-dried bladder or placenta (Urist). However, there appears to be some specificity of the inducing agent for a given tissue. Thus, we have bone marrow inducing the formation of bone within skin (Maniatis), whereas amniontic cells are only capable of achieving this within muscle (Hancox and Wlodarski).

Urist has concluded from the accumulated information and on the basis of important research projects devoted to this problem, that there must be an induction mechanism, which he calls osseous induction. This is brought about through an interaction occurring between inducing substrates and the ground substance produced by competent mesenchymal cells. The substrate itself (bone, dentine, bladder epithelium) can react in this manner because of the presence of proteins. Their activity is not altered by the extraction of fats or of mucopolysaccharides but any substance leading to protein denaturation will destroy them. Examples of destructive substances are chelating agents, proteolytic enzymes and irradiation.

The mode of action for the induction process is still hypothetical. Action releases the repression of the genetic order of osteogenesis or semi-conduction phenomena assuring the diffusion of electrons from the inducing substrate to the competent mesenchymal cells.

It does not appear, however, that an agent of protein characteristics is the only one capable of producing induction. There are inert substances capable of bringing about the development of bony tissues. This has been shown by Winter using synthetic resins. Depolymerization suppresses their inductive action.

It remains a fact, however, that the actual physiologic problem of the bony induction by the growth cartilage has not yet been fully elucidated and it is, after all, this process that is of real interest to those studying the pathology of growth.

THE MECHANISM OF MINERALIZATION

This particular mechanism still remains a mystery and in spite of the numerous studies devoted to the problem, a schematic explanation has not been offered.

For a long time this problem has been studied almost exclusively from a physico-chemical viewpoint. Because of the orientation of the apatite crystals, whose long axis is parallel to the collagen fibers, this was thought to be the seat of initial calcification. A structural alteration of these crystals would then initiate the precipitation of calcium.

This transformation would be an act of *phosphorylation,* for which alkaline phosphotase (Robinson) and adenosine-triphosphoric acid (Cartier, Glimcher) have previously been noted. Cartier maintains that the energy liberated through glycogenolysis would bring about the synthesis of ATP; dephosphorylation to AMP would then occur and the radical pyrophosphate would become bound to the protein carrier and thus combine with calcium ions.

According to Glimcher ATP would transfer the radical phosphoryl on to collagen thus freeing the ATP. The writer believes that this would then not be an act of pyrophosphorylation but rather a fixation of an orthophosphate radical. These radicals would become fixed upon the ϵ-amines of lysine and hydroxylysine. Studies could demonstrate the decline of these groups parallel to the decrease in mineral content of the tissue.

As convincing as all those theories may sound they do not seem to sufficiently take into account the very important role played by the cells. Studies involving intramitochondrial calcium demonstrate remarkable increases which occur within the cells located in the mineralization zone. Yet the calcium deposited is clearly dependent on the collagen fibers which are within the provisional calcification zone of cartilage and bone. Though it appears that a close relationship exists it would be incorrect to assume that these fibers are the exact site of the beginnings of calcification. Electron-microscopic studies have shown that this process originates within structures of cellular origin which are situated at the exterior of cells within the matrix and between the collagen fibers (Bonucci). Subsequently, clusters of rounded or oblong crystals are formed and it would only be after this that mineralization of collagen fibers would occur.

A full explanation of the cellular mechanisms is still needed, as one is needed to define the nature and actual role of extracellular corpuscles which are said to take a part in this process. As we stated earlier the role of proteoglycans and possibly even lipids which may be involved during the course of calcification needs to be clarified.

There have been numerous theories proposed. We have made reference to Fleisch, who maintains his position on the role of collagen and the inhibiting action of pyrophosphates. Waddel, on the other hand, has suggested that macromolecules are capable of creating the microcompartments with a higher pH by fixing alkaline cations (Ca^{2+}). This raised pH would then provoke within these microcompartments and ionic concentration of PO^{3-} and OH at a sufficient high level to induce their precipitation with Ca^{2+}.

REFERENCES

Anderson (C. E.) et Parker (J.) Invasion and resorption in enchondral ossification. *J. Bone Jt Surg., 1966,* **48-A,** *899-914.*

Anderson (K. J.), Dingwall (J. A.), Schmidt (J.), LeCocq (J. F.) et Clawson (D. K.). Induced connective tissue metaplasia. I. Heterogenous bone extract implants in the rat anterior eye chamber. A preliminary report. *Transplant. Bull., 1960,* **25,** *399-405.*

Baud (C. A.). Submicroscopic structure and functional aspects of the osteocyte. *Clin. Orthop., 1968,* **56,** *227-236.*

Belanger (F.). Autoradiographic visualization of the entry and transit of ^{35}S in cartilage, bone, and dentine of young rats and the effect of hyaluronidase in vitro. *Can. J. Biochem., 1954,* **32,** *161-169.*

Bohatirchuk (F.). Calciolysis as the initial stage of bone resorption. A stain historadiographic study. *Amer. J. Med., 1966,* **41,** *836-846.*

Bonucci (E.). Fine structure of early cartilage calcification. *J. ultrastruct. Res., 1967,* **20,** *33-50.*

Bonucci (E.). The locus of initial calcification in cartilage and bone. *Clin. Orthop., 1971,* **78,** *108-139.*

BOWNESS (J. M.). Present concepts of the role of ground substance in calcification *Clin. Orthop., 1968,* **59,** *233-247.*

BROCHER (J. E. W.). Die Wirbelsäulenleiden and ihre Differentialdiagnose. *Stuttgart, 1962, Georg Thieme Verlag, éd.*

BROOKES (M.), ELKIN (A. C.), HARRISON (R. G.) et HEALD (C. B.). A new concept of capillary circulation in bone cortex. *Lancet, 1961,* **i,** *1078-1081.*

CARTIER (P.) et PICARD (J.). La minéralisation du cartilage in vitro. *Bull. Soc. Chim. biol. (Paris), 1955,* **37,** *485-490.*

CARTIER (P.). Le calcium. *In* Traité de Biochimie générale, tome III. *Paris, 1967, Masson éd., p. 489-528.*

COOPER (R. R.), MILGRAM (J. W.) et ROBINSON (R. A.). Morphology of the osteon. An electron microscopic study. *J. Bone Jt Surg., 1966,* **48-A,** *1239-1271.*

COOPER (D. R.) et RUSSELL (A. E.). Intra and intermolecular crosslinks in collagen in tendon, cartilage and bone. *Clin. Orthop., 1969,* **67,** *188-209.*

DALLEMAGNE (M. J.). Phosphate and carbonate in bone and teeth. *In H. J. J. Blackwood (Ed.), Bone and tooth. Oxford, 1964, Pergamon Press, éd.*

DURIEZ (J.) et FLAUTRE (B.). Lyse péri-ostéocytaire et phénomène de délitement. *Presse méd., 1968,* **76,** *1703-1706.*

DZIEWIATKOWSKI (D. D.). The role of sulfated proteinpolysacchiarides in calcification. *Clin. Orthop., 1964,* **35,** *189-201.*

EASTOE (J. E.) et EASTOE (B.). The organic constituents of mammalian compact bone. *Biochem. J., 1954,* **57,** *453.*

EASTOE (J. E.). Recent studies on the organic matrices of bone and teeth. *In* H. J. J. Blackwood (Ed.), Bone and tooth. *Oxford, 1964, Pergamon Press, éd., p. 269-281.*

ELLIOTT (J. C.). The problems of the composition and structure of the mineral components of the hard tissues. *Clin. Orthop., 1973,* **93,** *313-345.*

ENGFELDT (B.). Studies on the epiphysial growth zone. III. Electromicroscopic studies on the normal epiphysial growth zone. *Acta path. microbiol. scand., 1969,* **75,** *201-219.*

FITTON-JACKSON (S.) et RANDALL (J. T.). Fibrogenesis and the formation of matrix in developing bone. *In* G. E. W. Wolstenholme and C. M. O'Conner (Ed.). Bone structure and metabolism. *London, 1956. Ciba Foundation, Churchill, éd., p. 47.*

FLEISCH (H.). Role of nucleation and inhibition in calcification. *Clin. Orthop., 1964,* **32,** *170-180.*

FLEISCH (H.). Physiologie and Biocheimie der Knochenbildung. *Klin. Wschr., 1966,* **44,** *360-363.*

FLEISCH (H.), RUSSELL (R. G. G.) et STRAUMANN (F.). Effect of pyrophosphate on hydroxyapatite and its implications in calcium homeostasis. *Nature (Lond.), 1966,* **212,** *901-903.*

GERBER (G. B.), BERBER (G.) et ALTMANN (K. I.). Studies on the metabolism of tissue proteins. I. Turnover of collagen labeled with proline I-C14 in young rats. *J. biol. Chem., 1960,* **235,** *2653-2656.*

GLIMCHER (M. J.) et KRANE (S. M.). The organization and structure of bone, and the mechanism of calcification. *In* B. S. Gould (Ed.), Treatise on collagen, *2B. New York, 1968, Academic Press, éd., p. 68-251.*

GOLDHABER (P.). Osteogenic induction across millipore filters in vivo. *Science, 1961,* **133,** *2065-2067.*

HALL (B. K.). Cellular differentiation in skeletal tissues. *Biol. Rev., 1970,* **45,** *455-484.*

HANCOX (N. M.) et WLODARSKI (K.). The role of lost site in bone induction by transplanted xenogenic epithelial cells. *Calcif. Tiss. Res., 1972,* **8,** *258-261.*

HERRING (G. M.). The chemical structure of tendon, cartilage, dentin and bone matrix. *Clin Orthop., 1988,* **60,** *261-299.*

HIRSCHMAN (A.) et DZIEWIATKOWSKI (D. D.). Protein-polysaccharide loss during endochondral ossification: immunochemical evidence. *Science, 1966,* **154,** *393-395.*

HOWELL (D. S.). Current concepts of calcification. *J. Bone Jt Surg., 1963,* **6,** *250-258.*

IRVING (J. T.) et WUTHIER (R. E.). Histochemistry and biochemistry of calcification with special reference to the role of lipids. *Clin Orthop., 1968,* **56,** *372-260.*

IRVING (J. T.). Theories of mineralization of bone. *Clin. Orthop., 1973,* **99,** *225-236.*

IWATA (H.). et URIST (M. R.). Protein polysaccharide of bone morphogenetic matrix. *Clin. Orthop., 1972,* **89,** *257-274.*

JUSTER (M.) et MOSCHOFIAN (A.). Sur la formation du squelette. I. Croissance d'un os long. Apparition première d'un point de calcification. *Pathol. Biol., 1971,* **19,** *21-31.*

JUSTER (M.). et BALMAIN-OLIGO (N.). Sur la formation du squelette. II. Croissance d'un os long. Métaphyse et virole périchondrale. *Path. Biol., 1971,* **19,** *33-42.*

JUSTER (M.). BALMAIN-OLIGO (N.) et MOSCOFIAN (A.). Sur la formation du squelette. III. Croissance d'un os long. Extrémité proximale de métatarsien de rat. *Bull. Ass. Anat., 1969,* **54,** *243-256.*

JUSTER (M.). Sur la formation du squelette. IV. Croissance d'un os long. Vue d'ensemble et schéma. *Bull. Ass. Anat., 1969,* **54,** *231-242.*

KEMBER (N. F.). Cell division in enchondral ossification. A study of cell proliferation in rat bones by the method of tritiated thymidine autoradiography. *J. Bone Jt Surg., 1960,* **42-B,** *824-839.*

LACROIX (P.). L'organisation des os. *Paris, 1949, Masson, éd., et Liège, Desoer, éd.*

LACROIX (P.). Organizers and the growth of bone. *J. Bone Jt Surg., 1947,* **29,** *292-296.*

LANGNESS (U.) et BEHNKE (H.). Collagene metaholite in plasma and urine in osteogenesis imperfecta. *Metabolism, 1971,* **20,** *456-463.*

LEAVER (A. G.) et SHUTTLEWORTH (C. A.). Observations on the composition of peptides obtained from bone and dentine. *J. Bone Jt Surg., 1967,* **49B,** *381.*

LENZI (L.) et SILVIA (E.). Concetti attuali di fisiologia e nuovi orientamenti sulla patologia del tessuto connettivo. I. Il collagene. *Chir. Organi Mov., 1964,* **53,** *245-257.*

LENZI (L.) et SILVIA (E.). Concetti attuali di fisiologia e nuovi orientamenti sulla patologia del tessuto connettivo. II. La sostanza fondamentale. *Chir. Organi Mov., 1965,* **54,** *365-390.*

LEVANDER (G.). A study of bone regeneration. *Surg. Gynec. Obstet., 1938,* **67,** *705-714.*

MANIATIS (A.), TAVASSOLI (M.) et CROSBY (W. H.). Origin of osteogenic precursor cells in extramedullary marrow implants. *Blood, 1971,* **38,** *569-575.*

MARTIN (G. R.). MERGENHAGEN (S. E.) et PROCKOP (D. J.) Influence of scurvy and lathyrism (odorotism) on hydroxyproline excretion. *Nature (Lond.), 1961,* **191,** *1008 1009.*

MATHEWS (M. B.) et DECKER (L.). The effect of acid mucopolysaccharides and acid mucopolysaccharide-proteins on fibril formation from collagen solutions. *Biochem. J., 1968,* **109,** *517-526.*

MILLER (E. J.) et MARTIN (G. R.). The collagen of bone. *Clin. Orthop., 1968,* **59,** *195-232.*

MILLER (E. J.). Isolation and characterization of a collagen from chick cartilage containing three identical chains. *Biochemistry, 1971,* **10,** *1652-1659.*

Moss (M. L.). Extraction of an osteogenic inductor factor from bone. *Science, 1958,* **127,** *755-756.*

Moss (M. L.). Experimental induction of osteogenesis. *In* R. F. Sognnaes (Ed.), Calcification in biological systems. *Washington, 1960, Amer. ass. adv. Sci., éd., p. 323-328.*

Murray (D. G.). The effect of papain on epiphyseal cartilage. An electron microscopic study. *Clin. Orthop., 1987,* **55,** *191-199.*

Oligo (N.), Laval-Jeantet (M.) et Juster (M.). Le socle métaphysaire de l'os normal en croissance et ses rapports avec la virole périchondrale. *Bull. Ass. Anat., 1966,* **51,** *745-755.*

Partridge (S. M.) et Davis (H. F.). The presence in cartilage of a complex chondroitin sulphate combined with a non-collagenous protein. *In* Ciba foundation symposium on the Chemistry and Biology of Mucopolysaccharides, Boston, 1958. *1 vol., Little Brown, éd., p. 108-109.*

Posner (A. S.). Crystal chemistry of bone mineral. *Physiol. Rev., 1969,* **49,** *760-792.*

Ramachandran (G. N.). Structure of collagen at the molecular level. *In* G. N. Ramachandran (Ed.), Treatise on collagen. I. Chemistry. *London, 1967, Academic Press, éd., p. 103-183.*

Ranvier (L.). Quelques faits relatifs au développement du tissu osseux. *C. R. Acad. Sci., Paris, 1873,* **77,** *1105-1109.*

Rhinelander (F. W.). The normal microcirculation of diaphyseal cortex and its response to fracture. *J. Bone Jt Surg., 1968,* **50-A,** *784-800.*

Robinson (R. A.). Crystal-collagen-water relationships in bone matrix. *Clin. Orthop., 1960,* **17,** *69-76.*

Robinson (R. A.) et Watson (M. L.). Collagen-crystal relationships in bone as seen in the electron microscope. *Anat. Rec., 1952,* **114,** *383-410.*

Rosenberg (L.). Cartilage proteoglycan. *Fed. Proc., 1973,* **32,** *1467-1473.*

Schenk (R. K.), Wilner (J.) et Spiro (D.). Fine structural aspects of vascular invasion of the tibial epiphyseal plate of growing rats. *Acta anat. (Basel), 1968,* **69,** *1-17.*

Schubert (M.) et Pras (M.). Ground substance proteinpolysaccharides and the precipitation of calcium phosphate. *Clin. Orthop., 1968,* **60,** *235-255.*

Shaw (J. L.) et Bassett (C. A.). The effects of varying oxygen concentrations on osteogenesis and embryonic cartilage in vitro. *J. Bone Jt Surg., 1967,* **49-A,** *73-80.*

Simpson (D. R). Problems of the composition and structure of the bone minerals. *Clin. Orthop., 1972,* **86,** *260-286.*

Stanescu (V.), Stanescu (R.) et Szirmai (J. A.). Microchemical analysis of human tibial growth cartilage in various forms of dwarfism. *Acta endocr., 1972,* **69,** *659-688.*

Termine (J. D.). Mineral chemistry and skeletal biology. *Clin. Orthop., 1972,* **85,** *207-241.*

Trueta (J.) et Little (K.). The vascular contribution to osteogenesis. II. Studies with the electron microscope. *J. Bone Jt Surg., 1960,* **42B,** *367-376.*

Trueta (J.). Trauma and the living cell. *Bull. Amer. Coll. Surg., 1961,* **46,** *73-77.*

Trueta (J.). A theory of bone formation. *Acta orthop. scand., 1962,* **32,** *190-198.*

Urist (M. R.). Recent advances in physiology of calcificiation. *J. Bone Jt Surg., 1964,* **46-A,** *889-900.*

Urist (M. R.) et Dowell (T. A.). The newly deposited mineral in cartilage and bone matrix. *Clin Orthop., 1967,* **50,** *291-308.*

Urist (M. R.), Silverman (B. F.). Büring (K.), Dubuc (F. L.) et Rosenberg (J. M.). The bone induction principle. *Clin. Orthop., 1967,* **53,** *243-283.*

Urist (M. R.), Dowell (T. A.), Hay (P. H.) et Strates (B. S.). Inductive substrates for bone formation. *Clin. Orthop., 1968,* **59,** *59-96.*

Vaughan (J. M.). The physiology of bone. *Oxford, 1970, Clarendon Press éd.*

Vieillard (A.) et Borel (J.-P.). La biosynthèse du collagène et sa pathologie. *Path. Biol., 1973,* **21,** *1023-1036.*

Waddell (W. J.). A molceular mechanism for biological calcification. *Biochem. Biophys. Res. Comm., 1972,* **49,** *127-132.*

Weisman (A. M.). A review of the literature : collagen : its physical characteristic and degradation. *J. Periodont., 1969,* **40,** *53-58.*

Winter (G. D.). Heterotopic bone formation in a synthetic sponge. *Proc. roy. Soc. Med., 1970,* **63,** *1111-1118.*

Wuthier (R. E.). The role of phospholipids in biological calcification. Distribution of phospholipase activity in calcifying epiphyseal cartilage. *Clin. Orthop., 1973,* **90,** *191-200.*

2 The Growth of Bone

As the study of bone growth is indispensable for the understanding of skeletal disorders seen in children, it appears necessary to devote to it an entire chapter, in which a number of radiographs will demonstrate the typical appearance of bones at various stages of growth.

GROWTH OF LONG BONES

As we have seen, during childhood there is a clear separation of the diaphysis and the epiphyses by the growth cartilage situated in between. One can thus distinguish, successively, growth in length of the diaphysis, growth of the epiphyses, growth in the transverse diameter, and the resorptive processes of modeling and maintaining thus the typical form of the bone.

GROWTH IN LENGTH

As early as 1727 Stephen Hales postulated that the longitudinal growth of long bones occurs at the level of the growth cartilage. By drilling two holes into the diaphysis of the bone of living chicken, he noted, that those holes did not show any change in distance over time, whereas the entire bone had grown in size.

Still these facts were not fully accepted without discussion, and some authors wanted to attach a primary role to periosteal growth. Until the last decades Policard and Leveuf thought that the notch of ossification was responsible for longitudinal growth.

The role of growth cartilage in this process is a fact proven by a number of experiments. The chondrodysplasias severely affect the growth in length of the long bones and offer additional evidence, since histologic studies show that in these diseases there are dramatic abnormalities of the growth zone. Still, the physiology of the notch of ossification and of the perichondral ring is rather poorly understood. The latter grows at its distal part immediately adjacent to the epiphysis, whereas its opposite distal portion is being resorbed by the remodeling process the bone (see p. 4). The histologic appearance of the growth cartilage has been studied in the previous chapter (see p. 7).

Growth is due to the proliferation of serial cartilage cells; a number of details about the mechanism of this proliferation are still unknown. Transplantation experiments show that the cartilage maintains its potential—even under conditions where it is isolated from its natural environment—by resuming its normal development (Lacroix).

Another fact hard to understand is an unequal activity of the growth cartilage in different bones of the body; the mechanisms and forces regulating this phenomenon are still completely obscure. This fact probably allows us to explain certain growth defects seen in the human. Thus the wrist is an example, as can be seen during the course of multiple cartilagenous exostoses and in Ollier's disease. The ulna actually develops its length almost exclusively from its distal growth center. If this area is affected by local pathology, this will result in a much more severe shortening than would result from abnormality of cartilage of the corresponding radius with its growth potential present also in its proximal cartilage. In another context, we might recall that the development of the femoral neck is not exclusively under the influence of the proximal cartilage of the femur and that the trochanteric cartilage also has a very important role to play, particularly with respect to the orientation of the neck.

Toward the end of adolescence there occurs closure of the gap between metaphysis and epiphysis. The growth cartilage progressively disappears, and, likewise, the vast majority of metaphyseal spongiosa. Subsequently the base plate of the epiphysis also disappears, leading to the formation of a single medullary cavity. The actual fusion will come about at the periphery of the epiphysis. The latter develops something like hooks uniting with the cortex of the diaphysis.

The morphology of the long bones undergoes marked changes during growth, and it is necessary to be fully familiar with the radiographic aspects that present pitfalls for errors of interpretation.

At birth the aspect of the bones is quite often unusually dense (Fig. 2-1). This is due to a relative

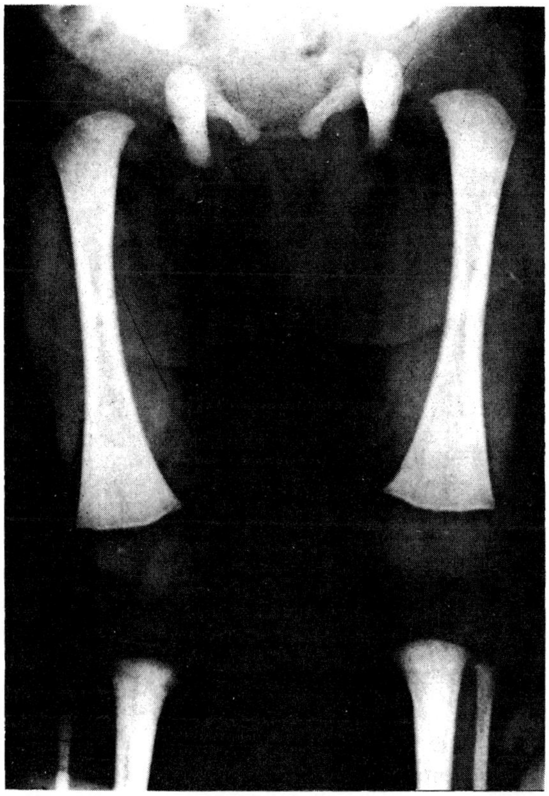

Fig. 2-1. The dense appearance of the long bones with thickening of the cortex is physiological in the newborn. Note that this infant must be premature because of the delayed skeletal maturation and because the proximal tibial ossification center normally present at birth is not visible.

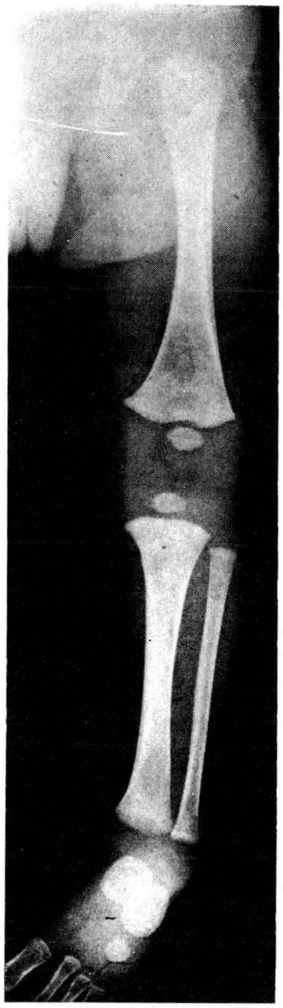

Fig. 2-2. Double contour of the cortex and hyperlucent metaphyseal zone in a 2-month-old child. (Courtesy of C. Fauré)

thickness of the cortex, the narrowness of the medullary canal, and the marked development of spongiosa. During the first weeks of life this appearance progressively changes. In the newborn one often recognizes a similar cortical thickness of the metacarpal bones.

In the normal baby there is a corticodiaphyseal ratio (sum of the widths of both cortices divided by the total width of the diaphysis) higher than 0.60 from birth to 6 months. This value will fall below 0.50 from 6 to 12 months and will then stabilize around 0.50 after about 13 months of age (Bernard and Laval-Jeantet).

It is not unusual, also, to note during the first 2 months a narrow, lucent tranversal zone immediately adjacent to the growth cartilage. This zone results, without doubt, from a discrete lack of calcium frequently seen in this age group. This interpretation seems fully confirmed, since it often occurs simultaneously with a double contour of the periosteum, together with thinning of the cortex. All these findings seem to be the result of such a deficiency, as was shown by Laval-Jeantet (Fig. 2-2).

Another abnormality of bone density, which is seen in infants older than 3 years and also in adolescents, is characterized by the presence of cortical defects localized quite typically in the distal femoral metaphysis or in the metaphyses of the tibia or fibula. These defects are located superficially, as they will show up on tangential films. They will disappear spontaneously and should not be regarded as true pathology (see Fig. 14-1).

A slightly irregular thickening of the posterior cortical aspect of the femur, which corresponds to the insertion of the adductor longus, is not so rare in adoles-

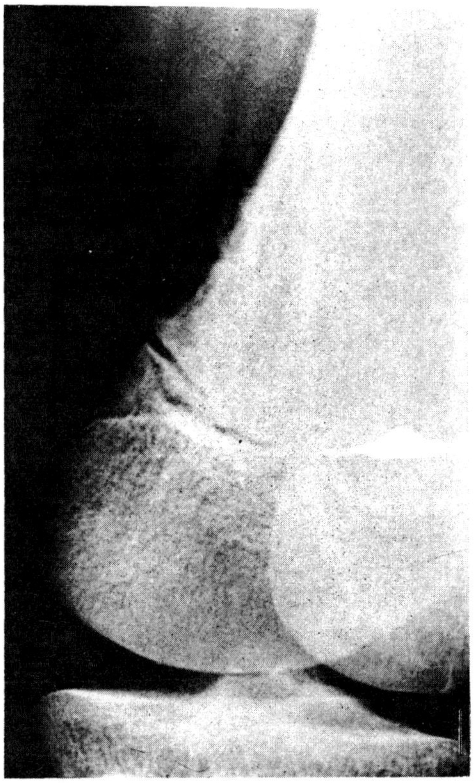

Fig. 2-3. Irregular appearance of the femoral cortex in adductur magnus tuberculum. Boy aged 14 years. (Courtesy of J. Lefebvre)

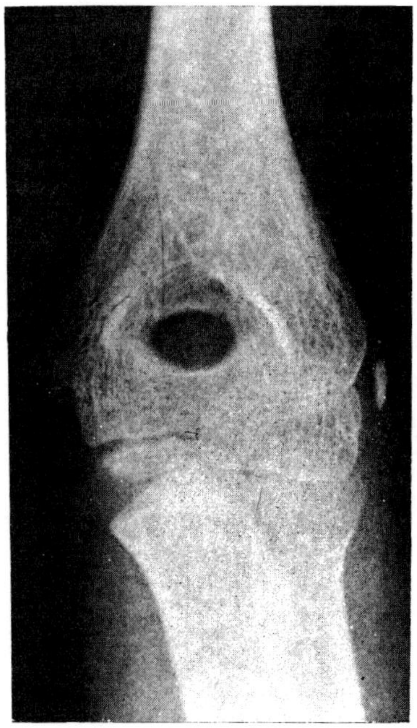

Fig. 2-4. Completely empty fossa olecrani in an 11-year-old girl. (Courtesy of J. Lefebvre)

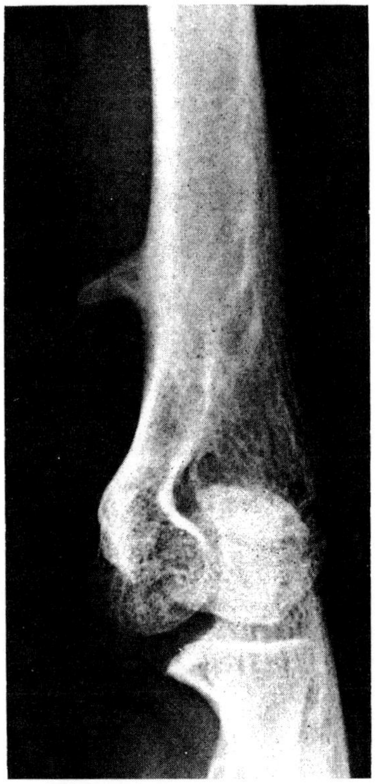

Fig. 2-5. Supracondyloid process. Girl aged 4 years. (Courtesy of J. Lefebvre)

cence and should not be confused with early changes of a local sarcoma (Fig. 2-3). Similarly one should avoid confusing a slight projectional displacement of the anterior tibial spine, due to slight rotation of the leg, with cortical thickening. At the level of the humerus on a film taken in slight external rotation one could confuse the bicipital groove with a zone of rarefaction, just as the fossa of the olecranon may occasionally appear markedly radiolucent (Fig. 2-4); a similar aspect of local rarefaction can be seen at the proximal end of the ulna. Finally it is not unusual to recognize at the lower third and on the external surface of the humerus a small bony spur referred to also as supraepitrochlear apophysis (Fig. 2-5).

At the level of the metaphyses dense striations can quite frequently be seen up to adulthood. These are arranged parallel to the growth cartilage, having a tendency to migrate during growth for a variable distance (Fig. 2-6). The actual significance of these lines, often called growth arrest lines, is still under discussion. Often multiple, they appear under many different circumstances (fracture of opposite side, infectious diseases with bed rest. . . .) and give an opportunity to appreciate the actual growth by comparing their migration on successive films.

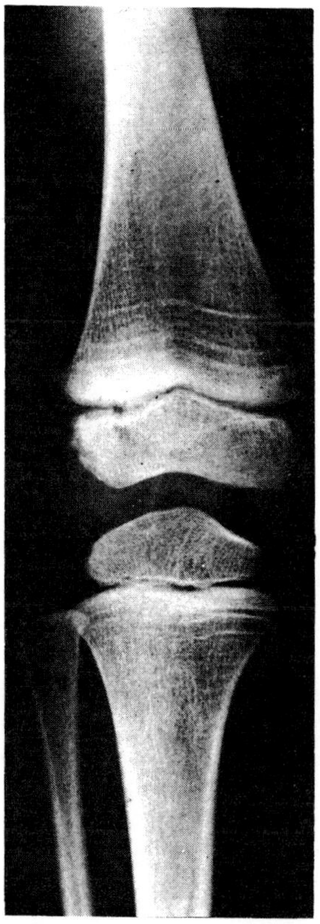

Fig. 2-6. Numerous lines of arrested growth in a 5-year-old boy. (Courtesy of C. Fauré)

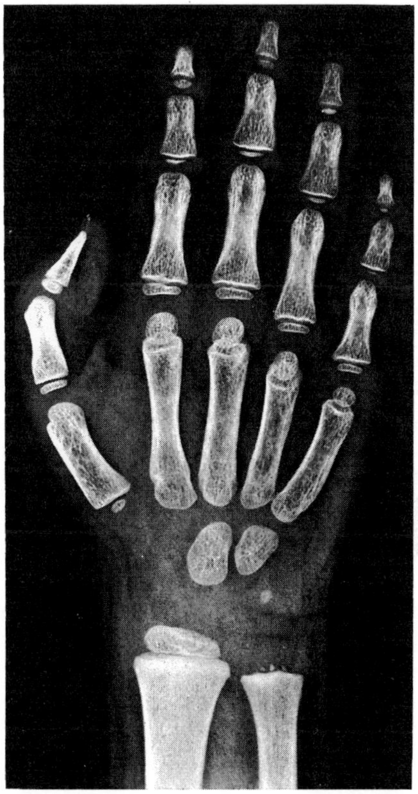

Fig. 2-7. Note the presence of fine bony spicules between the ulnar metaphysis and its epiphysis which is not yet visible. Boy 5-years-old.

The metaphyseal border close to the growth cartilage is often slightly irregular, particularly at the distal end of the tibia and fibula. In the older child there may appear a local notch, occasionally with a small extra fragment of bone present, which may simulate a fracture of this region. A notch can also be seen in the vicinity of the external border of the bone.

Irregularities of the metaphyseal border can also be seen at the femoral neck and at the distal end of the radius and ulna, where occasionally there may be minute bony bridging between metaphysis and epiphysis (Fig. 2-7). One must also be fully aware of the incidence of the radiologic view, since an oblique x-ray can be mistaken for a fracture. This particularly may be the case in the area of the uppermost part of the humerus. At the proximal region of the tibia, in the area of the anterior tuberosity, there may be a transverse radiolucent zone located 2 to 3 cm. from the growth cartilage (Fig. 2-8).

Metacarpal bones and, more rarely, phalanges may show an appearance similar to that of epiphyses at a location where none are expected; sometimes these are indeed epiphyses. The growth cartilage of the phalanges occasionally can assume the form of a V, thus

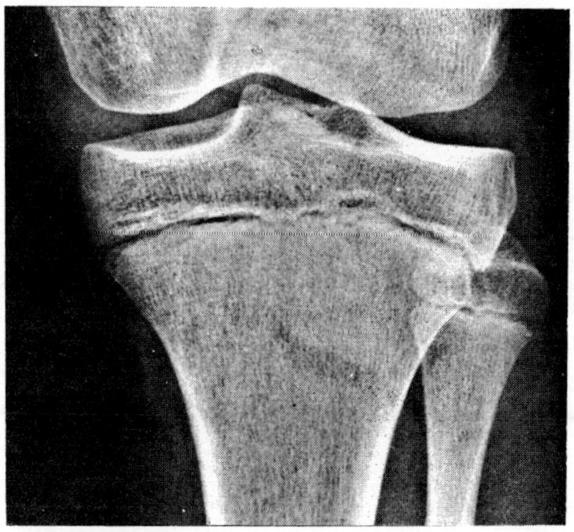

Fig. 2-8. Normal radiolucency of the anterior tibial tuberosity in a 14-year-old girl.

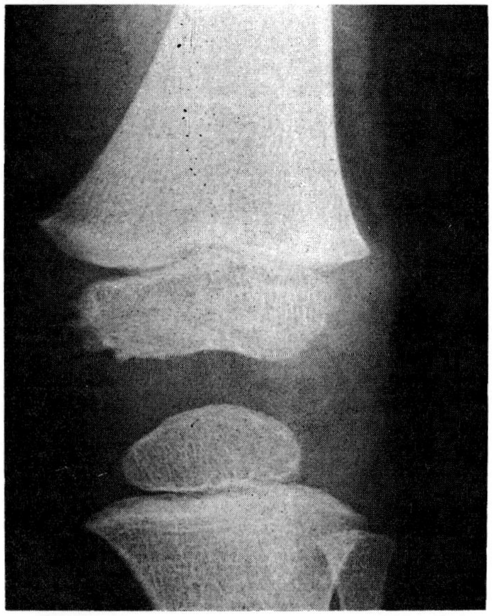

Fig. 2-9. Normal irregularity of the medial condyle of the femur. Boy aged 3 years.

giving an aspect that has been improperly interpreted as "coneshaped epiphyses" (see Fig. 3-46, p. 64).

EPIPHYSEAL GROWTH

Epiphyses initially of cartilaginous composition ossify, starting from one or several centers of ossification, with an entirely variable date of appearance according to the localization of the epiphysis under consideration. Knowledge of those dates and of the date of epiphyseal maturation is of great significance, since by careful study of the carpal and tarsal bones, it is possible to estimate the bone age (see p. 27).

Growth of the epiphysis is provided by the periphery of the center of ossification, where one finds a zone of cartilaginous cells behaving just like a growth cartilage. At its inner surface there is a similar arrangement of columnar cartilaginous cells with the described stage of maturation and their evolution towards ossification. The external layer of this cartilaginous zone guarantees the replacement of cells on the articular surface.

Epiphyseal growth could be studied on the basis of abnormal local deposits, particularly after intoxication with phosphorus (Boerema). Thus, it could be shown that growth does not occur equally in all the different directions. The center of ossification of the femoral head after 2 or 3 years will develop most at its peripheral portion and shows practically no further growth at the side of the growth plate. In the neighborhood of this cartilage the epiphysis itself is delineated by a bony plaque pierced by vascular orifices, the base plate.

Growth of the epiphyses of the bones of the hand and foot can show numerous deviations from the normal form and structure. One must be familiar with these findings. Thus, one should never consider the discrete flattening of the medial portion of the femoral head, a slight irregularity of structure of this area, as a sign of osteochondritis. The trochanters, particularly the lesser trochanter, habitually are irregular and fragmented. The condyles, especially the medial condyle, normally will show unequal contours with a somewhat spongy aspect in infants from 2 to 6 years (Fig. 2-9). In the older child there may be accessory centers of ossification near the posterior border, which one should not confuse with osteochondritis dissecans. Finally, in adolescence there may be a radiolucent oval zone located in the lateral portion of the lateral condyle corresponding to the popliteal groove.

The anterior tibial tuberosity can ossify in different ways, sometimes showing one or two different points of ossification separated somewhat from the rest of the tuberosity. Within the distal tibial epiphysis it is not rare to find an isolated center of ossification at the very tip of the medial malleolus. This finding can also be seen in the lateral malleolus, but much less frequently.

At the elbow there is usually great irregularity of the ossification center for the olecranon, sometimes with several individual centers of ossification. In the area of the wrist there is quite frequently an extra ossification center at the tip of the ulnar styloid.

We shall not at this time dwell further on anomalies or ossification in the area of either hand or foot, and particularly not on supernumerary bones (see p. 170). We would just like to remind ourselves that the pisiforme bone quite frequently has its origin from several centers of ossification, that there may be two such centers for the semilunar bone, and, finally, that the capitate bone in very young infants may offer an irregular and fragmented aspect. A similar fragmentation of the olecranon is seen with a relatively high incidence in the newborn; this finding, however, does not imply a disease process. Similarly, there may be marked irregularity in the ossification of the tarsal scaphoid, occasionally, with a dense appearance, which may be reminiscent of osteochondritis. This may be seen in an asymptomatic patient (Fig. 2-10). Extra centers of ossification can be recognized for the astragalus and the calcaneus. In the first instance there will be an extra posterior center of ossification, the os trigonum, which

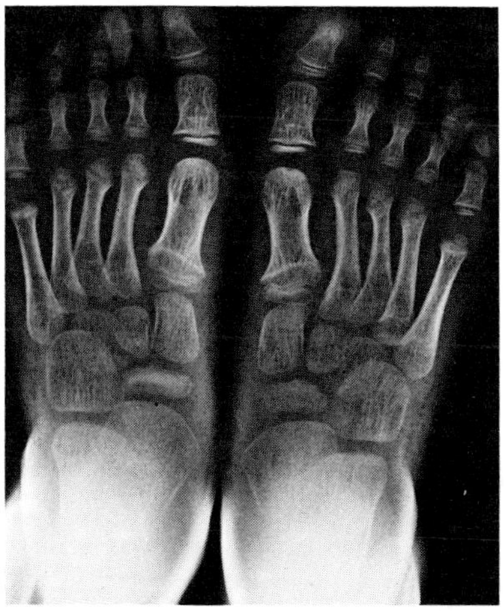

Fig. 2-10. Note that the right tarsal scaphoid is irregular and dense. This is not an abnormal finding. Boy aged 3½ years.

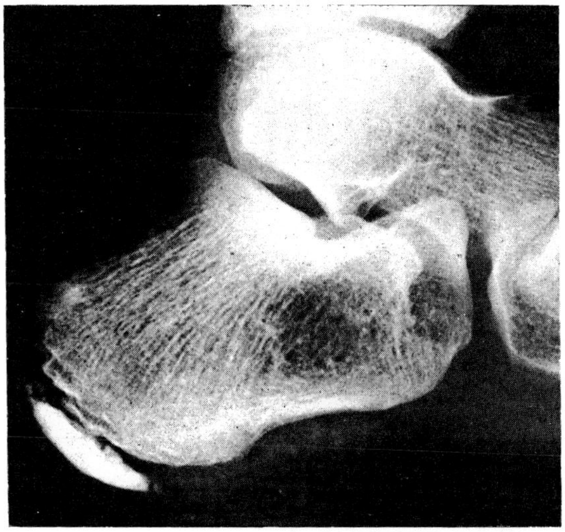

Fig. 2-11. Normal condensation of the apophysis of the calcaneus of an 8-year-old boy.

is a frequently encountered condition. The lower posterior border of the calcaneus close to the apophysis is very often irregular in its contour. The apophysis itself may be fragmented and unusually dense (Fig. 2-11).

During infancy there is usually multicentric ossification of the patella, its borders being irregular and ill defined. Toward adolescence extra centers of ossification may appear within the area anterior to the bone or of the upper or lower pole.

TRANSVERSE GROWTH

Like the matter of longitudinal growth, there are numerous controversies about transverse growth. In 1739 Duhamel, after implanting silver rings in the neighborhood of the periosteum, noted that during growth they became further imbedded within the bone. He concluded, therefore, that the periosteum had an osteoformative or "bone-forming" capacity. Von Haller and Hunter, however, completely denied such a role and placed heavy emphasis on the action of the growth cartilage.

The following is the actual composition of the periosteum; its outside is formed by the fibrous periosteum and its innermost layer of cells by osteoblasts responsible for the transverse development of the bone, a mechanism quite different from that of longitudinal growth. In effect there is no intermediary cartilaginous stage, and the bony lamellae are laid down at the peripheral surface of the cortex by direct membranous ossification. At the same time there is resorption of bone by osteoclasts at the inner surface of the cortex. We will not repeat here what has already been described about the turnover of this tissue and the formation of osteons laid down in concentric fashion (see p. 5).

The mechanism of transverse growth of the growth cartilage is still under discussion. Certain authors admit that this occurs at its periphery, through the transformation of fibroblasts into chondrocytes (Leblond and Greulich) or by the development of cartilaginous cells from periosteum (Tonna and Cronkite). This, however, is not the opinion of Langenskiöld, who bases his ideas on the observation of the growth of chondromata in Ollier's disease (see p. 97) and who admits that there is interstitial growth of cartilage. The studies of this author using ^{35}S in the rabbit seem to offer good evidence supporting this theory. Two weeks after the injection, while the bony diameter has increased considerably, there is still significant activity of the marker within the peripheral region of the cartilage. This fact would seem rather hard to accept and understand if new tissue had been laid down at this place.

MODELING

The purpose of modeling is to maintain the bone's anatomic shape at the metaphyseal region (Fig. 2-12). Longitudinal and transverse growth of the metaphysis

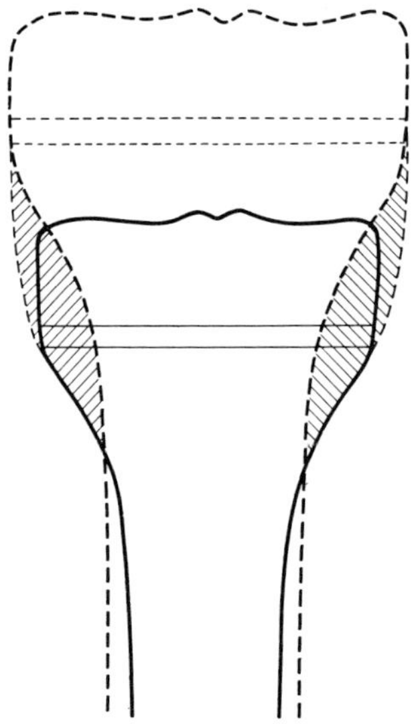

Fig. 2-12. Schematic drawing of the modeling of a long bone. (Taken from: Maladies des os et des articulations, CMC, Flammarion)

brings the perichondrial ring to the distal end of periosteal bone, over which the latter will try to advance. Thus, an erosion of the perichondrial ring is brought about together with the resorption of peripheral endochondral spongiosa.

The process of modeling resorption has been well documented with the help of coloring agents and radioactive markers. Leblond has shown in the rat, for instance, that immediately after an injection of ^{33}P there is uptake within the bony spicules throughout the entire extent of the growth zone. One week later there remain only a few marked spicules corresponding to the middle layer of the growth cartilage, from where they will subsequently migrate as a result of continuing growth, eventually becoming integrated into the diaphyseal cortex. The innermost spicules are resorbed to eventually free the space for the medullary cavity, whereas peripheral spicules disappear, in order to accomplish the normal modelling of bone.

This resorption is mainly the result of osteoclastic activity, as has been demonstrated by Arnold and Jee with radioactive plutonium (^{239}Pu) : the plutonium previously fixed to bone is found in large amounts within osteoclasts of the subperiosteal region of the metaphyses.

Some authors have suggested the possibility of a system closely relating the activity between the osteoblasts and the osteoclasts and whereby, quite possibly, then one could change into the other. This system could at the same time be effective for the construction as well as for the resorption of the bone (Rasmussen and Bordier).

GROWTH OF THE CRANIAL VAULT

This is a particularly active process during the first few years of life, since at 10 years the brain has attained 90 per cent of its adult volume. This growth is the result of proliferation of connective tissue at the sutures. This tissue is composed of several layers. The central layer, with fibers closely pressed together, is responsible for growth by the proliferation of connective tissue cells. Two peripheral layers are formed by perpendicularly oriented parallel fibers at the suture. Growth of each bone is brought about by bony apposition at its borders as well as at its surface. Here again we are dealing with membranous ossification.

The sutures are located between the frontal and parietal bones (coronal suture), between both parietal bones (sagittal suture), between the parietal and occipital bone (lambdoid suture), and between the temporal and the parietal bones. Some newborns have a interfrontal median suture which can be easily seen (metopic suture) and others exhibit accessory sutures in the lateral interoccipital (mendosal sutures), and interparietal region.

There are six fontanelles two of which are located in the midline anterior (bregma), and posterior (lambda), regions and four which are situated laterally, anteriorally (pterion), and posteriorly (asterion).

The main sutures (coronal, lambdoid and sagittal), persist throughout infancy and adolescence. They will close solidly only after the thirtieth year of life. The metopic suture normally closes prior to the third month but can remain visible in 10 per cent of all babies. Mendosal sutures do not persist longer than some weeks. The variability in closure time of the sutures does not allow us, then, to atttribute any specific significance in our attempt to estimate the developmental age of the skull.

The posterior fontanelle, if it is present at birth, closes during the first two months, and the anterior lateral fontanelles are not present beyond the third month. The posterior lateral fontanelles close during the second year, as does the bregmatic fontanelle.

In our approach to problems involving the development of the skull we must include a discussion of the muscular action which brings about growth of the external table in certain areas. This refers in particular to the external occipital protuberance and the suborbital

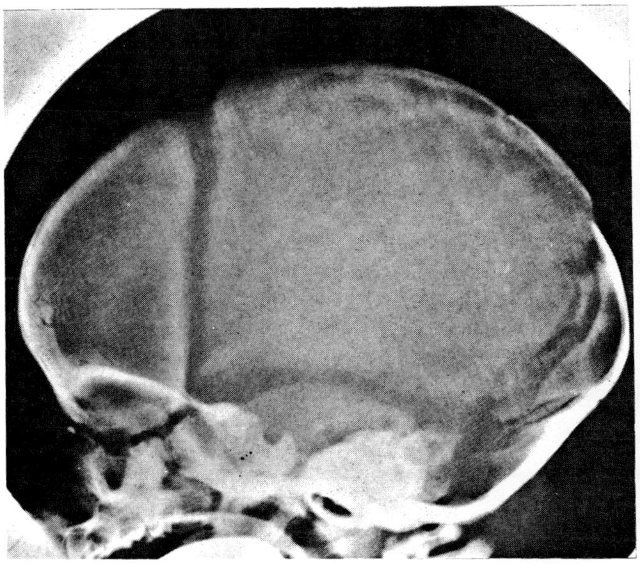

Fig. 2-13. Skull of a normal newborn baby. Note the presence of the fissure perpendicular to the sagittal suture.

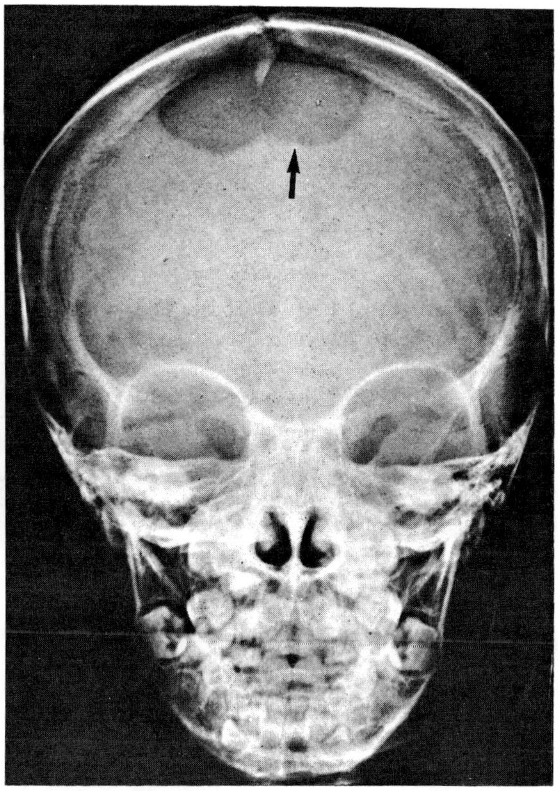

Fig. 2-14. Formina parietalia permagna. There is congenital widening of each parietal foramen.

ridge, which develop secondarily, and are not present in the newborn. Similarly, there is no mastoid apophysis present at birth and the glenoid cavity faces laterally. Its development occurs during the first 2 years of life, and the glenoid cavity will be oriented inferiorly while the external auditory canal develops.

These modalities of growth offer an explanation for the radiographic appearance of the skull in the newborn, who, in addition, may have fissures perpendicular to the sutures already described or located in close proximity (Fig. 2-13). Outside of caraniosynostoses, which we will discuss later, there are several variants of the normal growth of the skull. Bathrocephaly, which should not be considered a true malformation, characterized by a bulge of the occipital bone, is an example. The latter overlaps the parietal and looks like a step of a ladder. The parietal foramina permagna also are anatomic variants. In one out of two persons there is an emissary vein crossing through the posterior and superior angle of the parietal bone. This orifice is much larger in some people and appears radiographically as a large defect of ossification, more or less rounded in appearance (Fig. 2-14). The localization of this finding and its symmetrical presence within both parietal bones will help to avoid confusing this finding with other lacunar defects. It also appears that this morphological peculiarity is transmitted in certain families as a dominant trait.

In the larger child there are further peculiarities to which one must become familiar. Wormian bones are an example of this. They are situated within, or at the border, of sutures and fontanelles, most frequently at the lambdoid suture. In certain syndromes they may be multiple (see Fig. 3-109, p. 106), but this is generally not the case and only a few, appear as partial mosaics. In the older child it is not unusual to note a slightly dense area within the upper region of the coronal suture.

The diploe frequently is excavated by venous grooves. These occasionally can become very large and may then be confused with a depression of the internal table (see Fig. 10-7, p. 308). Vascular impressions, particularly those by the sinus of the dura mater, are variable. The most commonly seen vascular groove is caused by the middle meningeal artery which can be recognized just behind the inferior portion of the coronal suture. Imprints by Pacchioni's granulations are rarely noted before ten years of age.

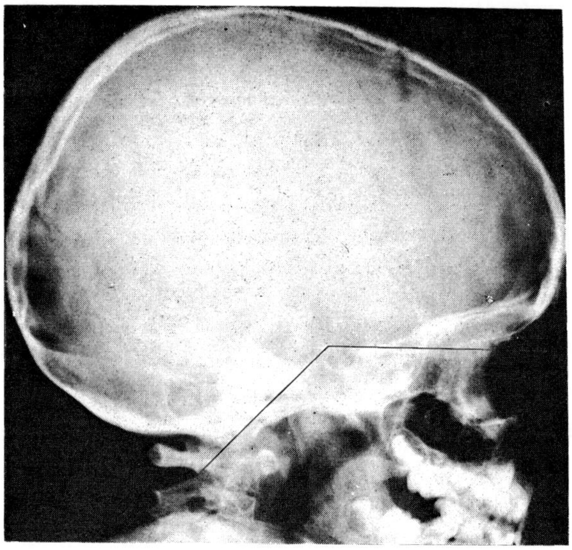

Fig. 2-15. Normal skull with an inserted schematic basal angle.

GROWTH OF THE BASE

The base of the skull develops in the manner of enchondral ossification and its growth during infancy is assured by the spheno-occipital, spheno-ethmoidal and intersphenoidal synchondroses. In relation to the cranial vault the base of the skull appears to be relatively short in the newborn. The lamina is poorly defined and the sella turcica is round with straight borders. The dorsum of the sella is short and blunt, and the clinoid processes can barely be seen (Fig. 2-13). One can easily recognize the individual parts of the internal ear in young babies within the petrous bone. The semicircular canals, cochlea and even the antrum in the newborn can be seen.

No differences are found in the basal angle when comparing the infant to the adult. This angle is formed by the clivus (the dorsal aspect of the sphenoid and of the basilar apophysis of the occipital bone), and the planum spheniodale (the upper surface of the body of the sphenoid and of the ethmoid). It measures about 120 degrees (Fig. 2-15). Closure of the spheno-occipital synchondrosis generally occurs at about puberty, and occasionally may persist into the fifteenth year.

The cartilaginous ossification of the base of the skull offers an explanation as to why the skull may show marked involvement in certain types of chondrodysplasias. This is particularly true for achondroplasia, where the insufficient development of the base of the skull is clearly the cause of the unusual cranio-facial morphology in affected patients.

GROWTH OF FACIAL BONES

The bony development of the upper maxillary region is comparable to that of the bones of the cranial vault. Growth is insured by the following three sutures: the fronto-maxillary suture found between the frontal bone and the upper apophysis of the maxillary bone, and the maxillo-malar and pterygo-palatine sutures, the latter being situated between the pterygoid apophysis of the sphenoid and the pyramidal apophysis of the palate. It is important to realize that the growth of the face occurs at a much slower rate than that of the cranial vault.

Pneumatization of the sinuses, though absent at birth develops progressively. The maxillary sinuses which can be hardly seen in newborns as a narrow notch, assumes towards the end of the first year the form of a small triangle located below the inner rim of the orbit. This structure will progressively expand, eventually reaching its lateral wall at about age 10 to 12. Similarly, we see the development of the frontal sinuses toward the end of the first decade of life with progressive enlargement superiorly and away from the anterosuperior border of the orbit.

At the end of the first year there is development of the ethmoid cells and of the sphenoid sinus both in front of and below the sella. The sphenoid sinus visible on lateral films extends posteriorly, whereas its vertical dimension grows progressively.

The development of the mandible is quite complex. In addition to the membranous ossification which is similar to the process which takes place within other facial bones, there is enchondral ossification of the mandibular angle, coronoid process and of the condyle. The latter occurs after birth and guarantees the growth of the ramus. Its role is comparable to that of a growth cartilage despite the absence of an epiphysis in this area. The two symmetric halves of the mandible will not fuse until some time in the second year. This should not be confused with a fracture of the symphysis since there may be a narrow area of persisting cartilage seen during the first few months after birth. The dental anlage for the deciduous teeth are visible at birth as are those of the first molars. The incisors and canines appear in the anlage during the first year with the premolars appearing during the second and third year.

GROWTH OF PELVIS

The pelvis is formed by three bones. They are the ilium, the pubis and the ischium. Separated at birth by cartilage, growth is achieved by enchondral ossification. Fusion occurs at variable ages. Usually the pubis and the ischium unite between the ages of 4 and 12 years. The acetabular angle, measured as the line going through the Y cartilage and the lateral edge of the acetabulum and constructed on Hilgenreiner's line measures 29 degrees in newborn girls and 26.5 degrees in boys. Its value progressively becomes lower and eventually measures only several degrees. The ossification center of the femoral head at three months should be located below the line constructed through the Y cartilage. This is known as Hilgenreiner's line. At the onset of adolescence, somewhere between the ages of 12 to 15, additional centers are formed. Epiphyses along the iliac crest and the ischium appear in the form of elongated bands along both the crest and the inferior border of the ischio-pubic rami, at the centers for the anterior superior iliac spine, the sciatic spine, the ischial tuberosity and the os acetabulare. These will insure the proper ossification of the upper and lateral region of the acetabulum. These centers will fuse between age 20 and 25.

As was true with long bones there are a number of morphologic and structural anomalies that appear during pelvic growth. Examples are irregularities of the iliac crest or the acetabulum, which quite often during early infancy give the pelvis a lacy appearance. With equal frequency one will note irregularities in the outline of the ischial tuberosity, sometimes showing areas of small lacunae. Similarly one may see a zone of temporary rarefaction just below the roof of the acetabulum. Vascular imprints also may be noted within the iliac wing. Finally, when the ischiopubic synchrondrosis closes it is common to see a local irregular hypotrophic aspect, entirely a physiologic process, which should not be thought of as osteochondritis as is occasionally done under the name of Van Neck disease (Fig. 2-16).

The development of the scapula is comparable to that of the pelvis with its growth occurring mainly along its vertebral border.

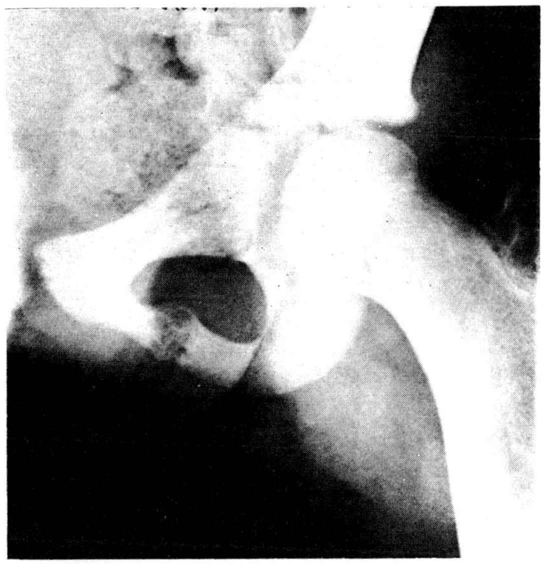

Fig. 2-16. Irregular appearance of the ischiopubic synchondrosis in a 10-year-old girl. This is a normal finding.

GROWTH OF VERTEBRAE AND RIBS

The growth of vertebral bodies occurs around the ossification center just as growth is found around an epiphyseal center. Certain authors, on the basis of studies using local irradiation, emphasize that there would be increased growth of this center near the upper plateau. Several disorders, and in particular rickets, allow us to comprehend the healing process as it takes place in vertebral bodies, showing identical growth at the upper and lower poles.

In viewing lateral films of the newborn, one can see a depression in the midportion of the anterior aspect of the vertebral bodies. There is a notch which corresponds to the vascular structures which reach to the center of ossification (Fig. 2-17). A somewhat smaller notch can be seen at the posterior border. The vertebral plateau is dense and rounded, while the intervertebral spaces are large. At about one to two months of age there may frequently be a central dense image giving the appearance of a "bone within a bone" (Brill et al.). The vertebral bodies will gradually lose their ovoid appearance as growth progresses. However, the anterior border of the vertebral body may continue to slope in its upper and lower portion giving the medial region a bullet-shaped appearance. This is seen quite frequently around the 6th year of life and should not be confused with some spondylo-epiphyseal dysplasias. Occasionally one is able to recognize in the newborn a radiolucent vertical band which appears to be a double center of ossification or the inclusion of a persistent part of the notochord or "coronal cleft vertebra" in the area where the posterior third of the vertebral body meets with the anterior two-thirds. This finding is seen more frequently in boys and disappears during the first few weeks. Though not abnormal in itself, this finding is frequently associated with other malformations (Fig. 2-17). A posterior spur can also be noticed.

Two other ossification centers are responsible for the development of the pedicles. These centers are

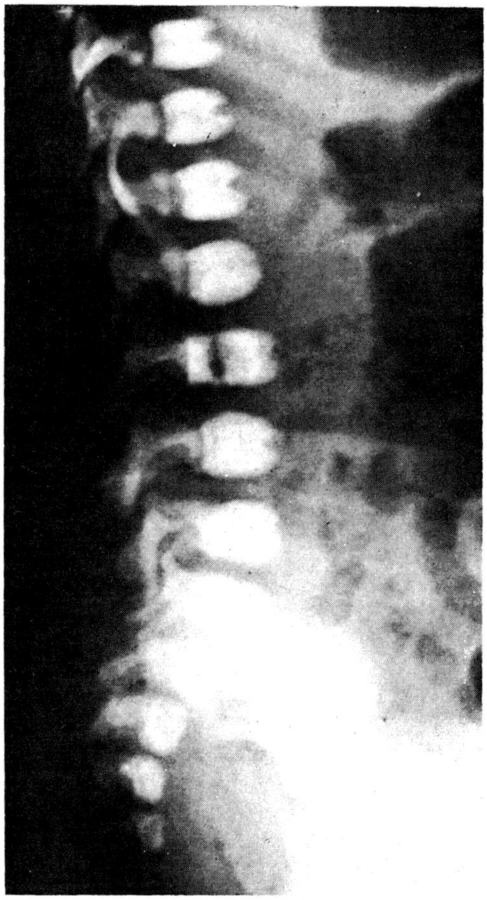

Fig. 2-17. The somewhat dense appearance of the vertebral bodies in a newborn. Note the anterior notching and the coronal cleft at L3.

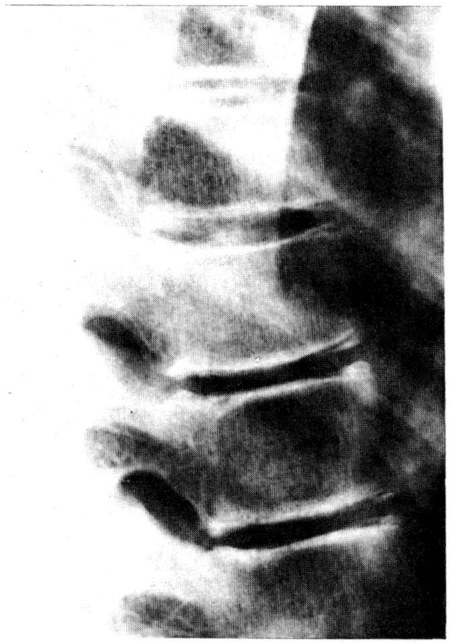

Fig. 2-18. Ossification of the marginal ring in a 14-year-old boy.

separated at birth and the two halves of the posterior arch will be united during the first two years of life. Union with the vertebral body will occur between the ages of three and six. Growth of the posterior arch will lead to proper development of the spinal canal. Its growth is extremely slow after the fifth year and stops completely at the age of ten. The posterior arch of the atlas will close later than the others. Its anterior arch is not visible at birth, which is contrary to the presence of the odontoid apophysis on the epistropheus.

Towards the ages 10 through 13 ossification of the marginal ridge will occur. We then have a cartilaginous ring comparable to a horseshoe occupying the anterior and lateral borders of the vertebral plateau. This ring does not take an active part in the growth of the vertebral body and should not be compared to an epiphysis as is occasionally suggested (Fig. 2-18).

Finally, as an individual approaches the 16th year the appearance of a number of apophyses may be noted (transverse, spinous, superior and inferior articular processes), which close approximately around the 25th year of life.

The growth of ribs occurs at the anterior cartilage and can be seen easily on a lateral film. Clavicle growth takes place at the medial end and an epiphysis appears in this location towards the 15th year. One frequently can see small notches of the inferior border corresponding towards the outside area where the conoid ligament is inserted and also towards the inside where the costo-clavicular ligament is located.

The sternum ossifies by a manubrial center and by four individual centers for the body of which the inferior two or three frequently are formed symmetrically. The center of the xiphoid process appears at around the age of six.

FACTORS AFFECTING BONE GROWTH

Before we briefly review the many factors which influence growth, it appears necessary to make some general remarks.

First of all, growth is not at all a constant phenomenon. During the first year of life statural growth is about 20 cm, subsequently slowing down rapidly to 10 cm during the second year and then stabilizing itself to about 5 cm per year. There will be a growth spurt just before puberty once again 10 cm is average. This will rapidly decrease and cease two to four years later. Growth which takes place during this period does not affect all parts of the body in a similar manner. Consequently, we see that in girls growth of the lower extremities is constant from about the fifth year on until puberty, when growth affects the upper segment of the body. Also important to note is the fact that total statural growth has increased by about 10 to 15 cm during the last century in the European and North American populations for reasons that are not yet clear. Improved hygiene and nutrition are not the only causes and the breaking up of isolates probably has also contributed to this phenomenon.

Some diseases lead to growth lags and when these conditions are corrected, the affected individuals will have the tendency to grow more rapidly in order to make up for the previous deficit. This catch-up growth spurt has been attributed to forces of homeorrhesis. We are totally in the dark when it comes to understanding this mechanism.

Factors which determine growth are many and the most important appear to be genetic. The definitive stature of a given individual is determined by a large number of genes. It should be noted that genetic factors also play a role in developing the proportions of different segments of the skeleton and of cranio-facial morphology and maturation. The mechanism behind this genetic action is not known. Some genes are susceptible to mutation thus becoming responsible for various constitutional skeletal diseases.

Metabolic maintenance of phosphorus and calcium is essential for normal harmonious skeletal development. Mechanisms regulating this metabolism are complex and depend upon the presence of vitamin D, intestinal absorption, renal regulatory mechanisms, and both thyroid and para-thyroid secretions. Endocrine organs are also responsible for secreting the hypophyseal somatotropic hormones, somatomedine and thyroxine which are indispensable for normal growth, while the adrenal glands and the gonads influence skeletal maturation.

Normal growth also requires other organs to function normally. Chronic diseases of different organ systems severely affect a child's development. Examples of this are severe congenital heart disease, chronic disturbances of the respiratory system and of the gastrointestinal canal, diseases of the nervous system and chronic hematologic disorders.

Though not yet completely defined, the role of mechanical and vascular factors is certainly noteworthy. Experiments with cultures of embryonal bone have demonstrated that muscular traction is indispensable to the normal growth as well as to the modelling of bone. We also know that a disturbed or altered blood supply can modify growth and cause circulatory stasis leading to a lengthened bone. This is found in infants who suffer from the Klippel-Trénaunay syndrome.

There are also many extrinsic factors which are capable of altering growth. Aside from nutritional deficiencies or chronic intoxication, microbial infection, tuberculosis, syphilis and trauma are capable of influencing bone growth and may cause severe and permanent damage.

Examples of this are osteomyelitis, osteitis, and certain fractures, especially those which carry a risk of injury to the growth cartilage.

METHODS OF GROWTH EVALUATION

CLINICAL FINDINGS

When evaluating a child for abnormal skeletal growth it is important to pay attention not only to the individuals total size, but also to the relative proportions of the different body segments. The latter may occasionally be difficult to measure, particularly in the baby. Radiologic study is frequently very helpful because of this difficulty.

In order to evaluate if the growth deficit is greater in the trunk or the extremities, one measures the upright height and the length of the lower segment. This is the distance between the upper limit of the symphysis pubis and the floor or the height of the individual while sitting to his or her total height while standing.

Often it is helpful to measure separately the different parts of the extremities. These measurements will allow for a better appreciation of their respective lengths and to calculate the corresponding indices. The anatomic landmarks for the upper extremity are the acromial point (lateral end of the acromion), the radial point (upper end of the radial head), styloid point (distal end of the radial styloid) and the distal end of the medius. For the lower extremity one should utilize either the trochanteric point or the anterior superior iliac spine. From here one can measure the distance to the ground while standing, the tibial point (proximal end of the medial tibial plateau), and the malleolar point (distal end of the medial malleolus).

Unfortunately, there are no reliable charts available on the different segmental relationships during infancy which are applicable to a given population. Data in the literature are derived from many different sources making their use difficult. Specific values should be es-

Table 2-1. Chronological Order of Appearance of Osseous Centers.

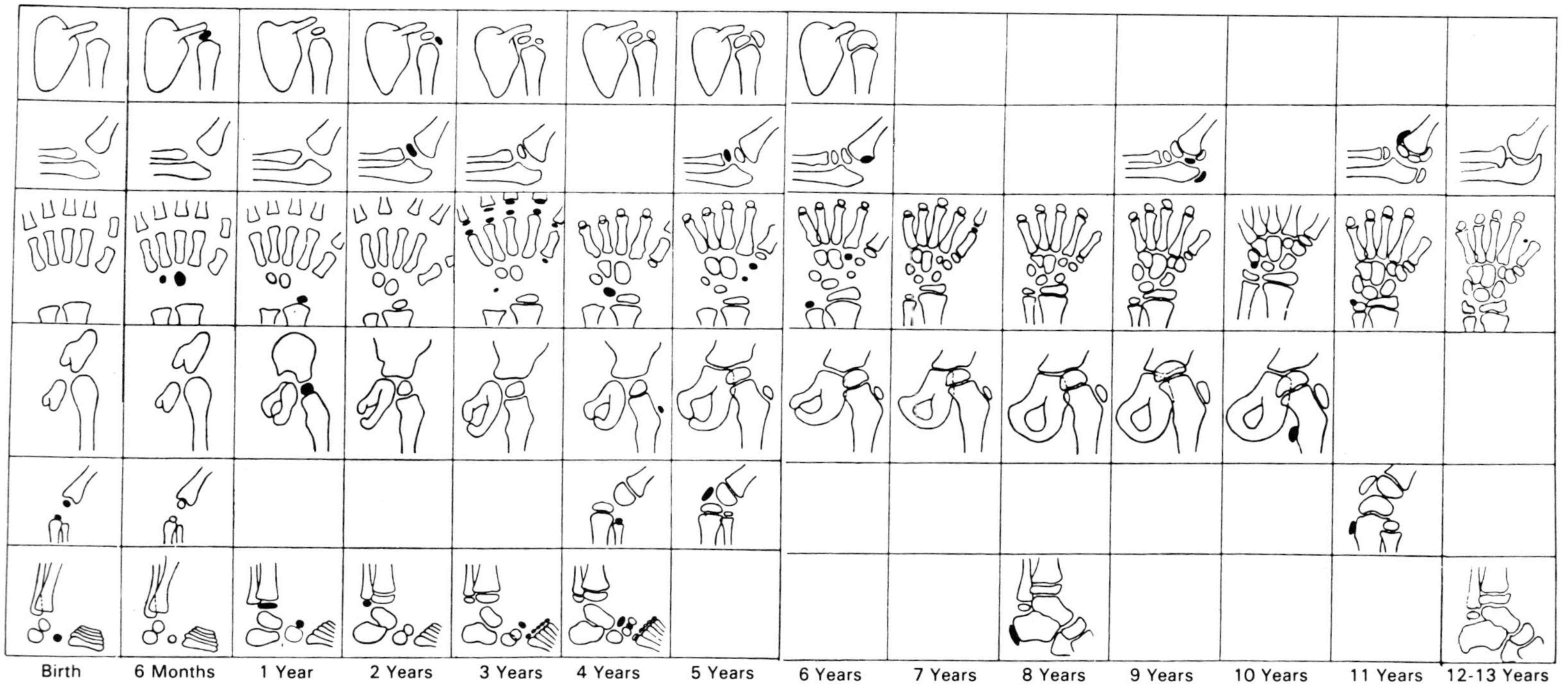

(Wikins, L. The Diagnosis and Treatment of Endocrine Disorders in Childhood and Adolescence, ed. 3. Springfield, Illinois, Charles C Thomas, 1965)

tablished for the various ethnic and racial segments of any given population.

The most frequently used charts for height are those of Scholler, and for the relationship between the lower segment and the upper segment the tables by Wilkins which were modified by Canlorbe and Scholler are used. These tables also contain information on the bi-acromial relationship (distance between both acromial points) and that of the bi-iliac crests (distance between both iliac crests) which express, in particular, the sexual orientation of the individual. It is very important to fully evaluate pubertal development in the bigger child, for it may markedly alter the conditions of growth. We will not delve into this problem, however, for it lies outside the scope of this book.

RADIOGRAPHIC FINDINGS

Radiologic study has two objects, the first is to determine exact measurements for different skeletal segments, and secondly to determine the bone age. Measuring bone length is often helpful in comprehending ratios of different segments of the body. This is particularly true in young infants as it is often quite difficult to obtain reliable clinical measurements. It is obviously necessary in this case to obtain radiographs which are reliable and reproducible and which are performed under identical conditions (teleradiography). Tables with reliable data for different age levels should be available.

Many different methods have been used in the attempt to determine bone age. Three methods are identified here: the first is based on the numbering of ossification centers, the second utilizes a numeric evaluation in order to determine the size of the different ossification centers, and the last one involves the use of an atlas (Table 2-1).

The first method simply involves counting all the centers of ossification which have been seen. This number is then compared to a value in a table, such as the one used in France by Lefebvre and Koifman. A series of radiographs must be obtained and no special attention is paid to the actual aspect of these ossification centers.

The method of numeric evaluation was proposed originally by Acheson and has been worked out in detail for the wrist by Tanner. In France Sempé has been able to modify this method and thus has corrected its shortcomings. It does have the drawback however of being a somewhat time consuming and demanding examination which requires experience to perform.

Although the atlas is less exact it is often the more practical approach. In this method one attempts to compare the radiograph of the infant under investigation with the one which appears in the atlas. Primarily used is a radiograph of the wrist. Sometimes the patient's radiograph is placed between two successive images of the atlas. There is criticism, however, directed to this technique because the reference standards need not necessarily correspond to the population which is under study.

None of the methods utilized to estimate bone age or skeletal maturation is fully perfected. Not only should the method take into account the date of appearance or the development stage of certain epiphyses, it should take into consideration these aspects of the entire skeleton. It is, however, quite difficult to assign numbers with reliability to the degree of maturation of the vertebral bodies, the skull, the pelvis and to the synchondroses.

The determination of bone age requires much training and knowledge, for the date of appearance of different ossification centers does not always carry the same significance. Silverman and his collaborators have shown that there is a much greater statistical value attached to the appearance of the metacarpal and phalangeal ossification centers, for example, than to that of the carpal bones.

It is important to critically interpret the findings of both the measurement methods and the radiographic studies. Five per cent of all individuals in the normal population have a height which is two standard deviations below the mean. One should not always consider the individuals who fall within this cagegory as abnormal, particularly if they belong to a family of small size. This small built individual may not fit into the lowest area of the normal distribution curve. There are also individual and genetic variations in skeletal maturity. For example, in the diagnosis of myxedema great vlaue can be attached to retarded bone age whereas in the majority of essential growth disturbances and in several chrondodysplasias it is only of minor importance.

REFERENCES

ACHESON (R. M.). A method of assessing skeletal maturity from radiograhpics. *J. Anat., 1954,* **88,** *498-508.*

ARNOLD (J. S.) et JEE (W. S.). Bone growth and osteoclastic activity as indicated by radioautographic distribution of plutonium. *Amer. J. Anat., 1957,* **101,** *367-417.*

BASSETT (C. A. L.). Current concepts of bone formation. *J. Bone Jt Surg., 1962,* **44-A,** *1217-1244.*

BERNARD (J.) et LAVAL-JEANTET (M.). Le rapport cortico-diaphysaire tibial pendant la croissance. *Arch. franç. Pédiat., 1962,* **19,** *805-817.*

BERNARD (J.), LAVAL-JEANTET (M.), JUSTER (M.) et DLUGATH (J.). Les structures fines de l'os diaphysaire au cours de la croissance. De la radiographie à la microradiographie. *Ann, Radiol., 1964,* **7,** *339-350.*

BOEREMA (L.). Ueber das Knockenwachstum. *Acta neerl. Morph., 1941-42,* **4,** *365-377.*

BRILL (P. W.), BAKER (D. H.) et EWING (M. L.). ≪ Bone-within-bone ≫ in the neonatal spine. Stress change or normal development. *Radiology, 1973,* **108,** *363-366.*

CAFFEY (J.). Pediatric X-ray diagnosis. *Chicago, 1967, Year Book med. publ., éd.*

CANLORBE (P.) et SCHOLLER (R.). Evaluation clinique et représentation graphique de la croissance. *Encyclopédie méd-chir. : Seconde enfance, 1957, 26001 A10.*

DUHAMEL (H. L.). Sur une racine qui a la faculté de teindre en rouge les os des amimaux vivants. *Mém. Acad. roy. Sci., Paris, 1739,* **52,** *1-13.*

DUVAL-BEAUPÈRE (G.) et COMBES (J.). Segments supérieur et inférieur au cours de la croissance physiologique des filles. Etude longitudinale de la croissance de 54 filles. *Arch. franç. Pédiat., 1971,* **28,** *1057-1071.*

EPSTEIN (J. A.) et EPSTEIN (B. S.). Deformities of the skull surfaces in infancy and childhood. *J. Pédiat., 1967,* **70,** *636-647.*

GARN (S. M.), SILVERMAN (F. N.), HERTZOG (K. P.) et ROHMANN (C. G.). Lines and bands of increased density. Their implication to growth and development. *Med. Radiogr. Photogr., 1968,* **44,** *58-89.*

GREULICH (W. W.) et PYLE (S. J.). Radiographie atlas of skeletal development of the hand and wrist. *Stanford, 1959, Stanford Univ. Press, éd.*

HALES (S.). Vegetable statics. *London, 1727, Innys and Woodward, éd.*

HALLER (von A.). Experimentora de ossium formatione. Vol. **2.** *Opera minore, Lausanne, 1763, p. 460-600.*

HERT (J.). Growth of the epiphyseal plate in circumference. *Acta anat. (Basel), 1972,* **82,** *420-436.*

HUNTER (J.). The works of John Hunter, F.R.S., with notes edited by J. F. Palmer. *London, 1835, Longman, Rees, Orme, Brown, Green and Longman, éd.*

KALAYHAN (D. B.) et COOPER (R. R.). Osteogenesis of the epiphysis. A light and electron microscopic study. *Clin. Orthop., 1972,* **85,** *242-256.*

KOHLER (A.) et ZIMMER (E. A.). Rœntgenologie. Les limites du normal et les débuts du pathologique dans la radiologie du squelette. *Berne, 1956, Delachaux et Niestlé, éd.*

LACROIX (P.). L'organisation des os. *Paris, 1949, Masson, éd., et Liège. Desoer, êd.*

LANGENSKIÖLD (A.). Normal and pathological bone growth in the light of the development of cartilagenous foci in chondrodysplasia. *Acta chir. scand., 1947,* **95,** *367-385.*

LANGENSKIÖLD (A.), RYTÖMAA (T.). An autoradiograhpic study with ^{35}S-sulphate on the growth in diameter of epiphyseal cartilage in rabbits. *Acta orthop. scand., 1967, suppl.,* **106,** *3-25.*

LAVAL-JEANTET (M.). Appositions sous-périostées avec aspect de double contour radiographique des os longs du nourrisson. *Presse méd., 1961,* **68,** *2623-2626.*

LEBLOND (C. P.), WILKINSON (G. W.), BELANGER (L. F.) et ROBICHON (J.). Radioautographic visualization of bone formation in the rat. *Amer. J. Anat., 1950,* **86,** *289-341.*

LEBLOND (C. P.) et GREULICH (R. C.). Autoradiographic studies of bone formation and growth. *In* G. H. Bourne (Ed.), The biochemistry and physiology of bone. *London, 1956, Academic Press, éd., p. 325-358.*

LEFEBVRE (J.) et KOIFMAN (A.). Etude de l'apparition des points osseux secondaries et détermination de l'âge osseux. *Arch. franç. Pédiat., 1956,* **13,** *1101-1105.*

LELONG (M.), JOSEPH (R.), CANLORBE (P.) et SCHOLLER (R.). Une nouvelle méthode de représentation graphique de la croissance. *Presse méd., 1954,* **62,** *701-704.*

LELONG (M.), JOSEPH (R.), CANLORBE (P.) et SCHOLLER (R.). Les méthodes d'évaluation du développement osseux. *Ann. Pédiat., 1955,* **31,** *63-68.*

LEVEUF (J.). Le problème de la croissance de l'os en longueur étudié à la lumière de la maladie exostosante. *Rev. Orthop., 1946,* **32,** *5-14.*

NAHUM (H.) et SAUVEGRAIN (J.). Croissance osseuse. *Encyclopédie méd.-chir., 1965, 30900 A10-30900 B50.*

POLICARD (A.). A propos des mécanismes de la croissance osseuse. *Presse méd., 1930,* **38,** *345-348.*

RASMUSSEN (H.) et BORDIER (Ph.). The cellular basis of metabolic bone disease. *New Engl. J. Med., 1973,* **289,** *25-32.*

ROCHE (A. F.), EYMAN (S. L.) et DAVILA (G. H.). Skeletal age prediction. *J. Pediat., 1971,* **78,** *998-1003.*

RUBIN (P.). Dynamic classification of bone dysplasias. *Chicago, 1964, Year Book med publ., éd.*

SCHWAGER GINDHART (P.). The frequency of appearance of transverse lines in the tibia in relation to childhood illnesses. *Amer. J. Phys. Anthrop., 1969,* **31,** *17-22.*

SEMPÉ (P.), SEMPÉ (M.) et PÉDRON (G.). Croissance et maturation osseuse. *Paris, 1971, Théraplix, éd.*

SHAPIRO (R.). Anomalous parietal sutures and the bipartite parietal bone. *Amer. J. Roentgenol., 1972,* **115,** *569-577.*

SIMON (H.). Medial distal metaphyseal femoral irregularity in children. *Radiology, 1968,* **90,** *258-260.*

SIZONENKE (P. C.). Détermination et interprétation de l'âge osseux. *Rev. Pé*diat., 1972, **8,** *587-598.*

SWISCHUK (L. E.). The normal pediatric skull varaations and artefacts. *Radiol. clin. N. Amer., 1972,* **10,** *277-290.*

SWISCHUK (L. E.). The normal newborn skull. *Seminars in Roentgenol., 1974,* **9,** *101-113.*

SWISCHUK (L. E.). The growing skull. *Seminars in Roentgenol., 1974,* **9,** *115-124.*

TANNER (J. M.). Education et croissance. Applications pédagogiques des connaissances sur la croissance de l'enfant. *Paris, 1964. Delanchaux et Nestlé, éd.*

TONNA (E. A.) et CRONKITE (E. P.). The periosteum : autoradiographic studies on cellular prolifération and transformation utilizing tritiated thymidine. *Clin. Orthop., 1963,* **30,** *218-232.*

VANDENBERG (S. G.) et FALKNER (F.). Hereditary factors in human growth. *Hum. Biol., 1965,* **37,** *357-365.*

WHALEN (J. P.), WINCHESTER (P.), KROOK (L.), DISCHE (R.) et NUNEZ (E.). Mechanisms of bone resorption in human metaphyseal remodeling. A roentgenographic and histologic study. *Amer. J. Roentgenol., 1971,* **112,** *526-531.*

WILKINS (L.). The diagnosis and treatment of endocrine disorders in childhood and adolescence, *3e édit., Springfield, 1966, C. C. Thomas éd.*

Part Two:

Constitutional Skeletal Diseases

In this opening chapter all the constitutional diseases which affect the growth, structure or the morphology of the skeleton are grouped together. Such disorders may be secondary to genetic action or that of intrauterine factors about which we know very little. In some cases these abnormalities of the bone are recognized at birth, while others will manifest themselves later. The majority of the diseases are seen during infancy, childhood and adolescence. Only rarely will one of these disorders be recognized in an adult. Numerous attempts have been made to classify these diseases. Not a single one is without drawbacks. This is an expression of the fact that we know little of the pathophysiology of these diseases.

Rubin has proposed to isolate four groups of disorders, based on whether they electively affect the epiphysis, the physis, the metaphysis or the diaphysis. Within each group, he defines hypoplasias and hyperplasias. This classification is founded upon experimentation in which lesions have been induced in rats through the irridation of their growing bones. It is not necessary here to prove the actual value of the work of Rubin in understanding disorders of bone growth. His method is not, however, sufficiently adaptable for the classification of the extremely complex findings seen in human disease. This author has been forced to discuss diseases which appear to be related to one another in widely separate chapters, such as Ollier's dyschondroplasia and multiple cartilaginous exostoses, and to group together others in an artificial manner. Thus, a new complexity has been introduced here. Rubin's classification is difficult to use in either clinical or radiologic practice.

A completely different approach, proposed and worked out at an international meeting, is devoted to the nomenclature of constitutional skeletal diseases. There is a clear distinction between those diseases where the pathogenesis is known and those where we have fragmentary understanding at best regarding their basic mechanisms. These are primary metabolic disturbances (calcium-phosphorus metabolism, mucopolysaccharide metabolism and lipid metabolism in particular), chromosomal aberrations and severe disorders of other organ systems. The latter will be discussed in the second or third part of this book.

Diseases of unknown pathogenesis can be subdivided into two large groups: the osteochondrodysplasias and the dysostoses. Acro-osteolyses which find themselves within this group will also be discussed. Osteochondrodysplasias are all those anomalies of growth which affect the structure of bone or cartilage. In the dysostoses there is malformation of a single bone or this in a regular association with some others. We are fully aware that this classification also has its drawbacks, particularly due to its somewhat schematic character. At this stage of our knowledge, however, we feel that it will be very difficult to propose a more accurate approach. Only progress in the understanding of the pathogenetic mechanisms will allow us to do this.

3 The Osteochondrodysplasias

INTRODUCTION

This group of constitutional diseases are the primary disorders of growth and development of bone and cartilage. Three lengthy chapters have been separately prepared. The first contains the anomalies of growth which have radiographic evidence of variable involvement of the spine, the pelvis, and the epiphyses or metaphyses of long bones. The second chapter concerns itself with disorders which lead to anarchic development of cartilaginous or fibrous tissue. In a third chapter there is discussion of the anomalies of modelling or bone density, two findings which occasionally appear together as seen in Albers-Schönberg's disease.

Part 1: Abnormalities of Growth

This is a complex chapter and we will successively distinguish those diseases which manifest themselves at birth as opposed to those diagnosed only later.

DYSPLASIAS RECOGNIZABLE AT BIRTH

The two groups which will be discussed are the chondrodysplasias which are always incompatible with life and the chondrydysplasias with normal chances for survival.

CHONDRODYSPLASIAS INCOMPATIBLE WITH SURVIVAL

These disorders were most often confused with achondroplasia. However, at this time there are two distinctly different and well defined disorders: thanatophoric dwarfism and achondrogenesis. Other, more rare types are possible.

Thanatophoric Dwarfism

A disorder which manifests itself at birth, it sometimes can be recognized even earlier on intrauterine radiograms which have been taken because of the small size of the fetus. In direct contrast to the extreme shortness of the extremities is the markedly voluminous skull. Though narrow, the trunk is normal in length and measures approximately 40 cm. There is an abnormal facies with marked bossing of the forehead and flattening of the nasal base coupled with protruding eyes (Fig. 3-1).

Infants with this disorder are frequently still-born. There are sometimes a few respiratory movements, however, if they do survive, it is only for a few hours or days. In such patients one notes marked muscular hypotonia and persisting cyanosis with rapid and labored respiration. There are soon obvious phases of apnea which lead to death.

Radiographic examination reveals extremely short ribs with anterior flaring. The vertebral bodies, are markedly reduced in height and have normally developed pedicles, which gives some vertebrae an aspect of an H or U on AP films. This is in contrast to the lateral view which will show considerable enlargement of the intervertebral spaces. The interpedicular distance of the lower lumbar vertebrae is reduced. (Fig. 3-2). The iliac wings have a rectangular form and are insufficiently developed, particularly in the vertical direction, and there is a very narrow sciatic notch. The roof of the acetabulum is horizontal and is elongated by a medial and sometimes lateral spur. The scapulae are small. The diaphysis of the long bones is broad, very short, almost rectangular and frequently curved. The border of the metaphysis is deformed, irregular and oblique; sometimes it is extended in the shape of a

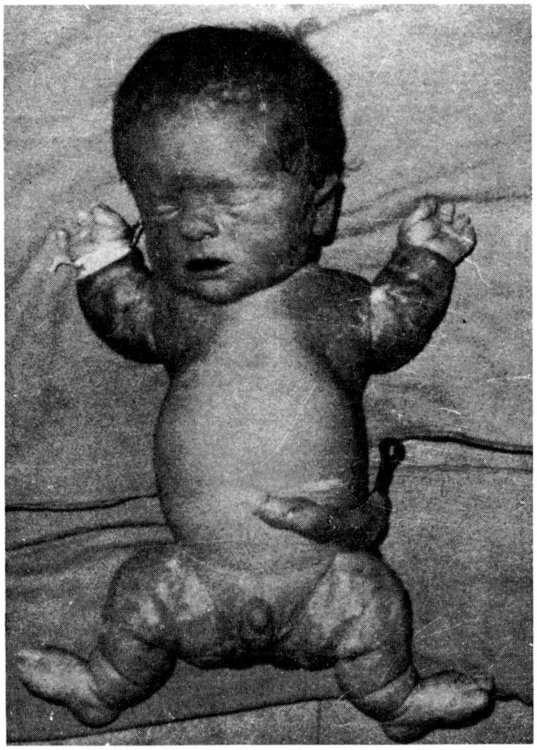

Fig. 3-1. A thanatophoric dwarf. Note the extreme shortness of all four limbs. (Courtesy of J. Robert)

cone, which can best be seen at the proximal humeral or femoral end. All the bones of the hand and foot are similarly shortened and square. Phalanges frequently are only partially ossified with irregular and wavy borders. Whereas the development of the vault of the skull is excessive, the base of the skull is markedly reduced in its length.

In several instances anatomic examination of the brain has revealed the existence of rather peculiar malformations of the temporal lobe with microgyria (Goutières et al.). Histologic studies of the growth cartilage reveal a total lack of organization which is shown by a total absence of columnar arrangement with the growth zone lacking the metachromatic staining quality to toluidine blue, in contrast to normal cartilage. The line of ossification is irregular. One must note particularly the enlarged perichondrial ring which appears to have a tendency to fold towards the central zone of the cartilage, and which sometimes obstructs it completely. Still, cartilage persists most frequently in its central portion (Fig. 3-3), with considerable variation in the degree of this process in a given patient depending on the cartilage studied. Finally, a fibrous band, which originates at the place of contact of the ring, can cross the reserve cartilage.

Almost without exception thanatophoric dwarfism has occurred in isolated instances. Although there have been several published observations referring to siblings, these are of a somewhat doubtful nature. We have had the opportunity to study one sibship, where there is no doubt. Spontaneous abortions seem to occur more frequently in these families and maternal age is significantly higher. Still, it remains difficult to ascertain whether or not a recessive gene with variable manifestation lies at the base of this disorder.

The association of thanatophoric dwarfism with a clover-leaf skull (Kleeblattschädel) has been described (see p. 152). This anomaly is well recognized on an AP view of the skull as seen by a marked protrusion of both temporal regions, resulting in an aspect of the vault reminiscent of a clover leaf. There is so far only one report on two patients in the same family with this association (Partington et al.).

Achondrogenesis

This disorder was first described under the name of anosteogenesis by Parenti in 1936, who reported on a particularly severe form of this disease. In the majority of cases, however, the skeletal involvement is less severe. The name of the disorder has been coined by Fracarro.

The clinical aspect is somewhat similar to that of thanatophoric dwarfism: excessive volume of the skull, extremely short extremities, and a somewhat shortened trunk which is broader than that seen in thanatotorphic dwarfism. These, however, lead to a more severe type of dwarfism with a total body length of from 25 to 35 cm. The evolution is always rapidly fatal (Fig. 3-4).

Radiographic examination reveals a severely inadequate ossification of the vertebral bodies and sacrum, leaving them both at times unrecognizable. The pedicles are also sometimes poorly ossified, however, the interpediculate distance of the lowest lumbar vertebrae is not diminished. The iliac wings are small with a concave internal border. The acetabular roof is horizontal and at times slightly concave inferiorly. The ischio-pubic rami are poorly ossified if they are at all. The scapulae are small (Fig. 3-5).

The membranous bones are very short, their metaphyseal ends broad and wavy with a lateral spur formation and an irregular line of ossification. The bones of the hands and feet are equally short and square. There is, at times, a more severe involvement of ossification in the bones of the extremities (Parenti).

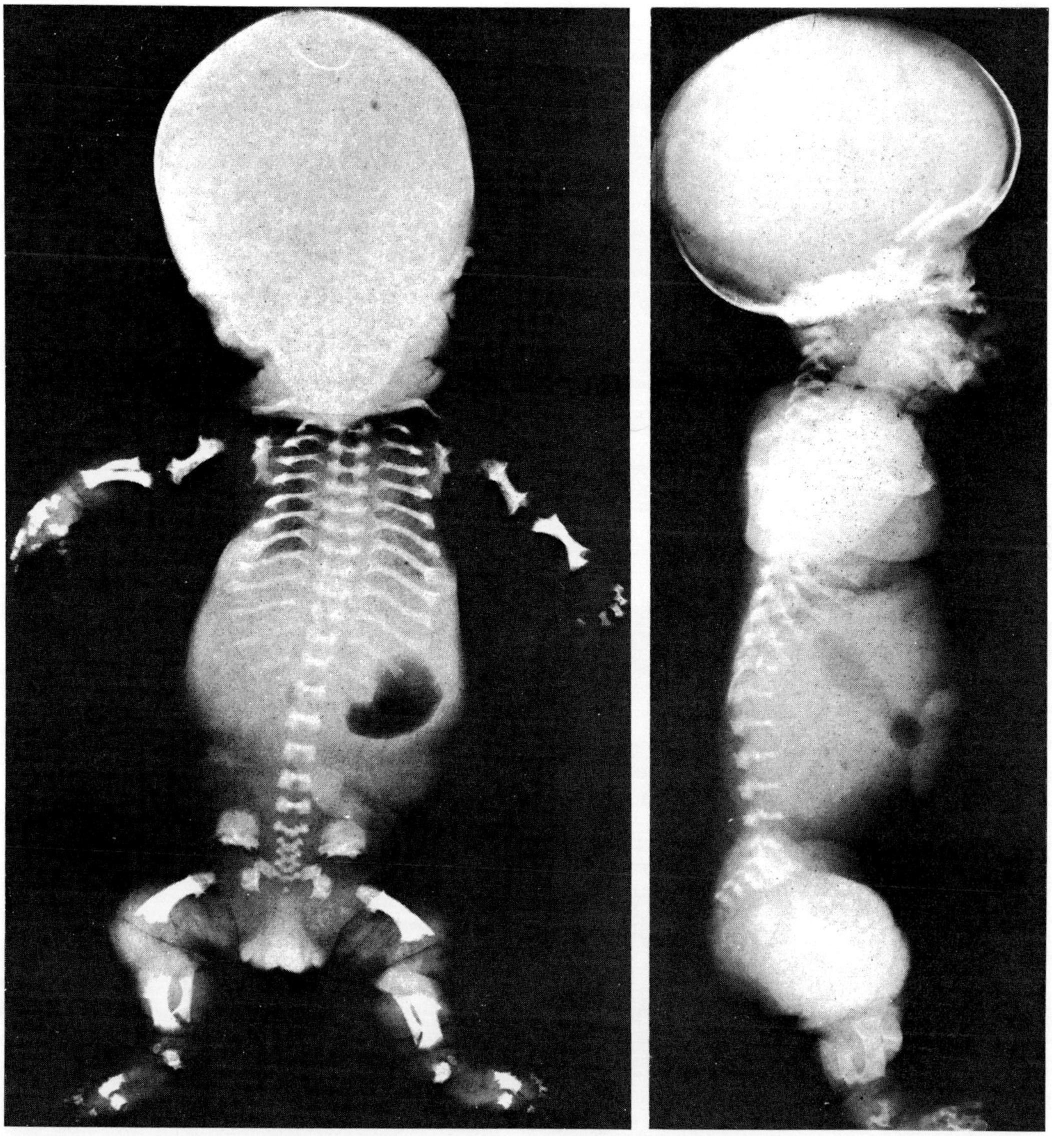

Fig. 3-2. Thanatophoric dwarfism. Note the narrow thorax, the reduced height of all the vertebral bodies, and the rectangular shape of the iliac wings. (Courtesy of J. Robert)

Histologic study of the growth cartilage reveals an increase in the volume of cartilaginous cells and a reduction in the matrix. This can be seen across the entire level of cartilage. Thus, the name achondrogenesis given to this disorder appears questionable (Fig. 3-6). Cell density is similar to that which is seen during an earlier fetal stage. There is also a degree of sclerosis of the vascular channels which is normally present in the newborn. The line of ossification is irregular. The perichondrial ring, however, appears entirely normal, which is in contrast to what we have seen in thanatophoric dwarfism. In fibroblast cultures Laxova has observed lipid granulations. The importance and meaning of such a finding remains a question.

This disorder occurs with equal incidence in both sexes and it follows an autosomal recessive transmission. Certain authors (Harris et al.) have suggested distinguishing two separate disease types based on radio-

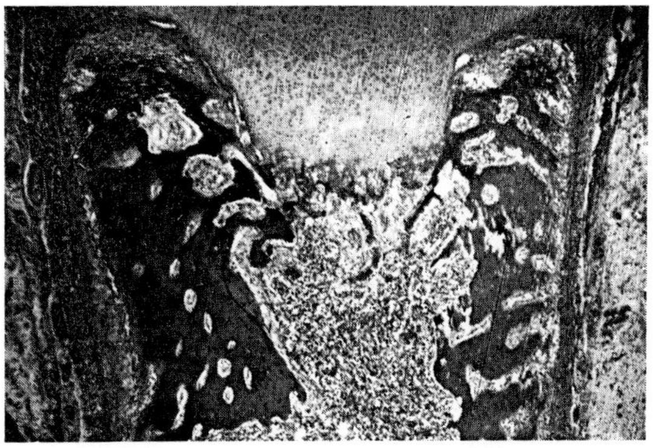

Fig. 3-3. Growth cartilage in a thanatophoric dwarf. Note the hypertrophy of the perichondral ring. (Courtesy of V. Stanescu)

logic differences, in particular if there are different areas of callus formation in the ribs indicating the occurrence of fractures in utero. Histologic appearance, however, is identical.

Similar thoughts can be voiced about the different degrees of clinical expression involving achondrogenesis. The initial publication by Parenti refers to findings more severe than those we have described here. He describes a type of achondrogenesis where there is almost total absence of ossification in the long bones. There is, however, a much less dramatic type which is somewhat close in appearance to congenital spondyloepiphyseal dysplasia. A postmortem histologic study of involved cartilage in such a case confirms its identity with achondrogenesis (Walker).

Other Types of Lethal Chondrodysplasias

There are a number of other individual lethal chondrodysplasias. These are however much rarer. We are, referring for example, to the type described by La Chapelle et al., which is characterized by electively shortened middle segments of the extremities and the bowing of long bones with an autosomal recessive transmission.

We would also like to note the two published observations by Saldino with short ribs and polydactyly. Close in its appearance to chondroectodermal dysplasia, this condition is distinguishable by severe additional malformations. These are urogenital anomalies, an imperforated anus and abnormal radiographic characteristics. The metaphyseal ends of the different long bones are characterized by resembling the narrowing distal tongue of a candle flame (Fig. 3-7). Another variant quite similar but considered as a distinct entity by Spranger et al. has been described by Majewski. In

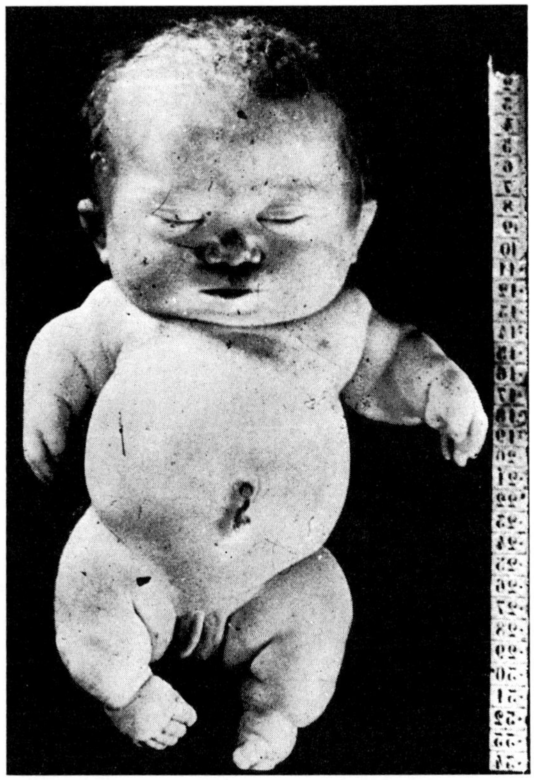

Fig. 3-4. Achondrogenesis. Note the shortness of the limbs as well as the trunk. (Courtesy of J. Legrand)

this disorder there is a particularly dramatic hypoplasia of the tibia without any major changes involving the pelvis. Further studies are needed to document these facts because there are very noticeable differences and variations from one observation to another.

There are other types of severe, and potentially fatal, chondrodysplasias. Diastrophic dwarfism, metatropic dwarfism, chondroectodermal dysplasia, and particularly, asphyxiating thoracic dysplasia which is frequently confused with thanatophoric dwarfism will be discussed later.

CHONDRODYSPLASIAS WITH SURVIVAL

The oldest and most frequently occurring disease under this heading is achondroplasia. For a long time practically all chondrodysplasias with micromelia were grouped together under this heading, however, a large number of individual disorders have now been clearly defined.

The clinical appearance and the manner in which

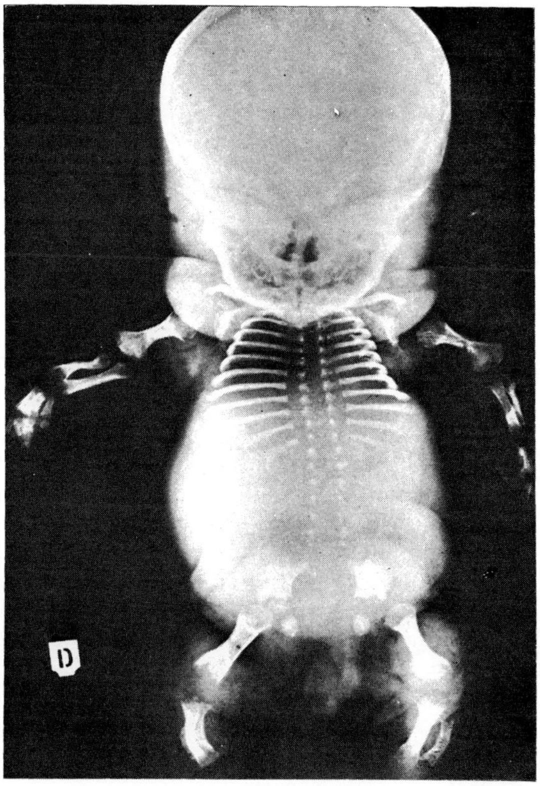

Fig. 3-5. Illustrated here is achondrogenesis, an ossification defect involving all the vertebral bodies. (Courtesy of J. Legrand)

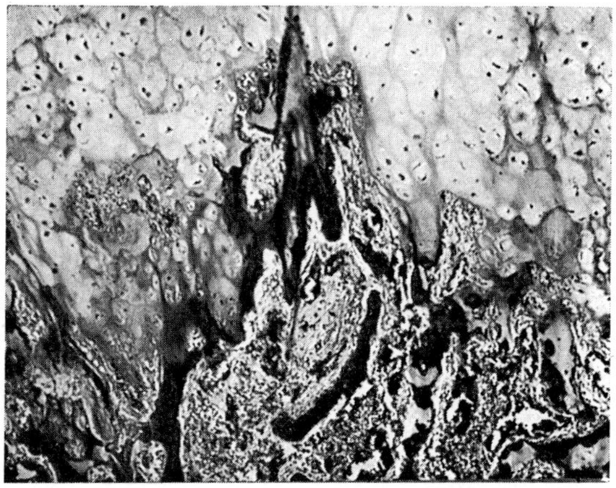

Fig. 3-6. Achondrogenesis in the growth cartilage. Notice the hypertrophy of the chondrocytes and the irregular ossification line. (Courtesy of V. Stanescu)

these disorders are recognized varies. We shall schematically divide them into three groups. In the first group are all those diseases which are responsible for strikingly shortened extremities, in the second we have those diseases which simultaneously involve the growth of the trunk and the extremities, and in the third are those skeletal dysplasias where the growth disturbance is usually not recognized.

DYSPLASIAS USUALLY RECOGNIZED BECAUSE OF MICROMELIA

This group is composed of:

achondroplasia most noted clinically by its facial features, especially the deeply set nasal bridge;

punctate chondrodysplasia frequently showing an asymmetrical shortening of an extremity;

diastrophic dwarfism which is associated with a club-foot;

metatropic dwarfism with the unusual clinical finding of palpable metaphyses in the presence of an excessively long trunk often deformed by early scoliosis;

and *mesomelic dwarfism* electively involving elements of the middle portion of the arms and legs.

ACHONDROPLASIA

The particular nature of this disease was suspected by Depaul in 1851, but it was Parrot who defined the disease and named it in 1878. In 1898 Kaufmann performed a complete histologic study of this disorder in the fetus. Pierre Marie further defined the clinical findings present during adolescence and adulthood in 1900, and it was several years later that Porak and Durante emphasized the difference between achondroplasia from the severe forms of osteogenesis imperfecta. Among the most important papers and investigations devoted to this disorder are those by Rischbieth and Barrington, Morch, Grebe and Schiemann.

Clinical Findings

Achondroplasia manifests itself in the association of micromelic dwarfism and craniofacial alterations. At birth there is a striking shortening of the extremities with a much less dramatic reduction in overall height, approximately 47 cm. The skull is large and, for this reason, may cause obstetrical problems. The bridge of the nose is flat and retracted, giving these patients a characteristic facial appearance. One must be familiar with the marked muscular hypotonicity of babies with achondroplasia. This may very well lead to the suspicion of psycho-motor retardation. Due to this

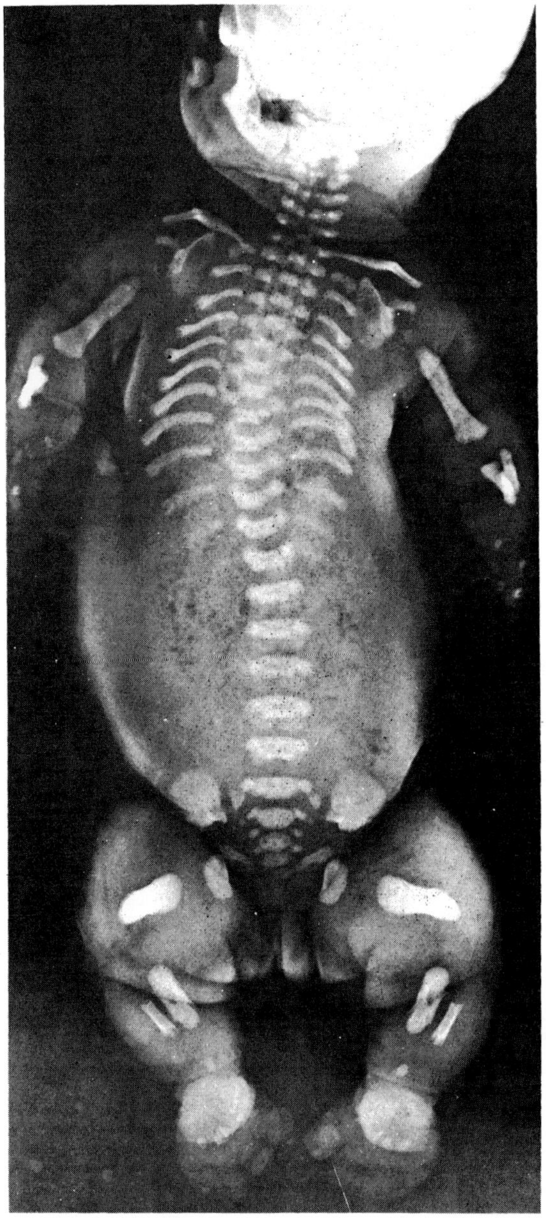

Fig. 3-7. Micromelic dwarfism together with polydactyly. Note the long bones with their tapering ends. (Courtesy of J. Kucera)

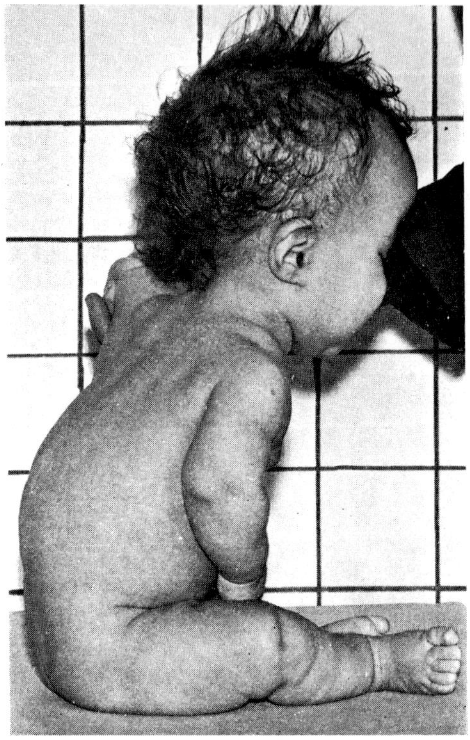

Fig. 3-8. An infant with achondroplasia. The dorsolumbar kyphosis is secondary to the hypotonia.

hypotonicity patients may show a marked dorso-lumbar kyphosis when attempting to sit. Active measures should be instituted to correct this (Fig. 3-8). Excessive sweating is often present.

During later periods of childhood and in adulthood dwarfism becomes more marked with a definitive height of 1.25 m in the male and 1.20 m in the female. The shortened extremities are most marked in the proximal segments, particuarly affecting the humerus, but other segments are also involved. The hand is squat, however, the fingers are not as plump as those seen in certain types of spondyloepiphyseal dysplasias. The third and fourth fingers are frequently somewhat separated, which has led to the term "trident hand." Occasionally there is a slight limitation of joint movements, especially during extension of the elbows.

The trunk appears to be relatively long with a slight deformity due to lumbar hyperlordosis. Frequently there is a dorsolumbar kyphosis which can coexist with an immediately adjacent lordosis.

The craniofacial morphology of achondroplasts is clearly defined. Besides brachycephaly with slight bossing of the forehead there is marked flattening of the bridge of the nose (Fig. 3-9). Sometimes these findings may be less noticeable, but rarely are these craniofacial findings absent in true achondroplasia.

Aside from the growth deficit the overall prognosis of such patients is usually quite good. Upon reaching adulthood these patients are prone to develop spinal cord and cauda equina compression due to the narrowing of the spinal canal. Secondary problems may result

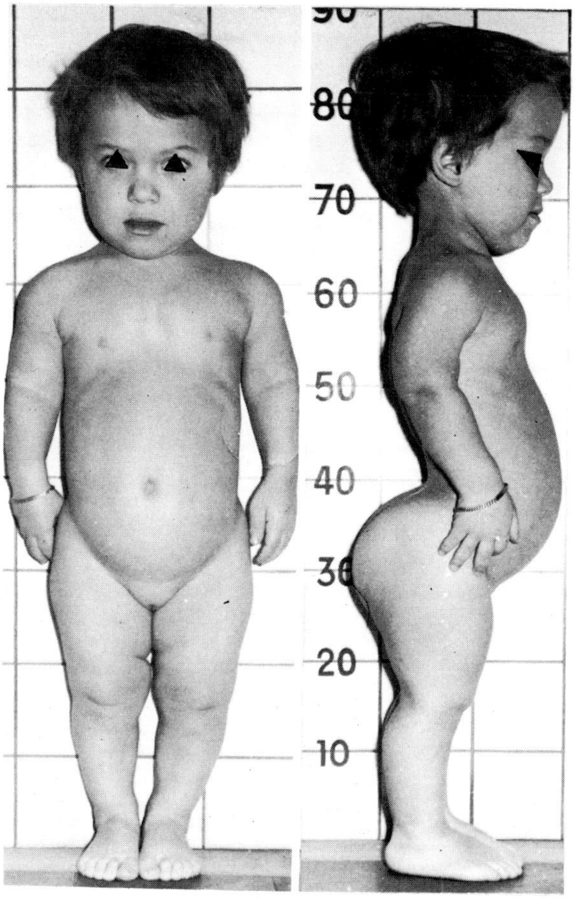

Fig. 3-9. This child has achondroplasia. Note the deep rooted nose, the short extremities, and the marked lumbar lordosis.

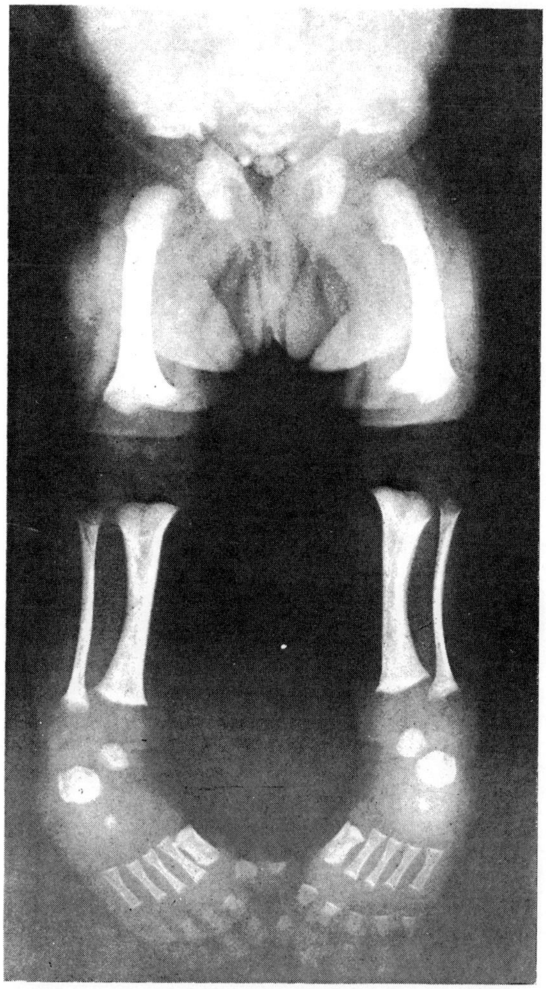

Fig. 3-10. An achondroplastic newborn. The acetabular roof is in a horizontal position. There is metaphyseal eversion with a mild degree of adjacent hyperlucency.

from a discus hernia or arthrosis. Compression, according to Bailey, can be seen in 12 per cent of all cases and will be seen most frequently in those types which exhibit marked dorso lumbar kyphosis. One should also note the marked obstetrical difficulties achondroplastic women encounter as a result of their very narrow pelvis. Hydrocephalus and respiratory problems due to shortened ribs have occasionally been seen.

Radiographic Findings

The skeletal anomalies are fully manifested in the newborn period. The bones of the extremities are short and squat and there is abrupt widening of the metaphyseal ends. This widening is less marked at the upper end of the femur and appears on AP views to be clearly abnormal, as does the humerus (Fig. 3-10). The density of the other metaphyses may also be slightly decreased. This is due to the obliquity of the growth cartilage and can be seen well on lateral films. Proximal and medial phalanges are somewhat plump. Pelvic length is reduced, the iliac wings have a square form and the acetabular roofs are horizontal with a medial spur and a middle region convexing slightly downwards. The interpediculate distances of the lower lumbar vertebrae are smaller than the value for L1, whereas normally there is an increase of the distance from L1 to L5. On lateral views these pedicles appear to be short. The development of the cranial vault is often excessive, whereas, it may be somewhat difficult at that age to fully appreciate the lack of growth at the base. At times the thorax is slightly narrow and on lat-

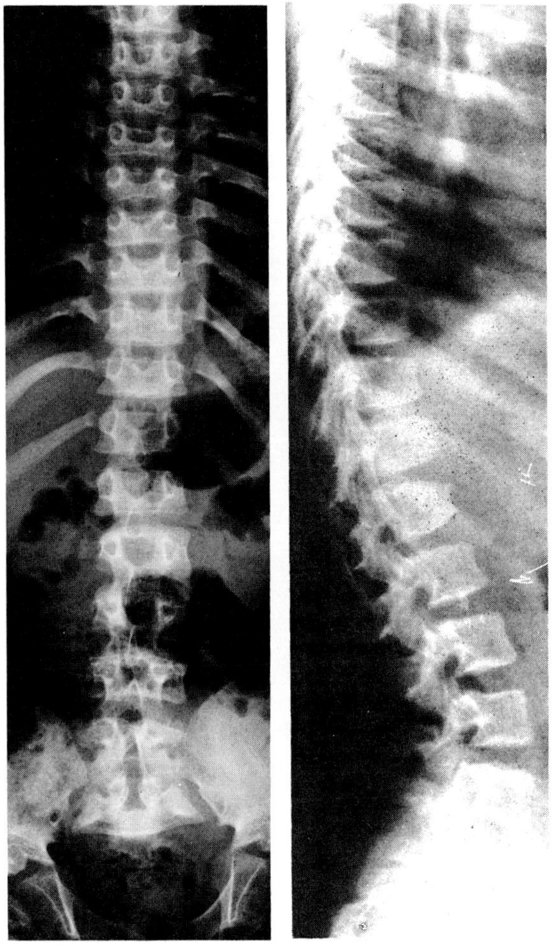

Fig. 3-11. A 6-year-old boy with achondroplasia. Note the reduction in the interpedicular distances from L1 to L5 on the AP view, and the shortness of the pedicles on the lateral view.

eral views there may be shortness of ribs with cupping of the anterior ends.

In the growing child all of these findings will continue to exist with the exception of the increased transparence of the metaphyses. Longitudinal growth of the bones is slow. The diaphyses are plump and occasionally will be slightly curved. This is particularly true of the radius. The growth cartilage at the lower end of the femur sometimes appears like an inverted V with the epiphysis drawn into the center of the cartilage. The upper tibial cartilage may also be similarly affected. The femoral neck often assumes a valgus position and may be almost vertical. The neck of the humerus can be unusually long. Epiphyseal development, often appearing with some delay, is quite satisfactory. However, the femoral condyles are small and asymmetrical

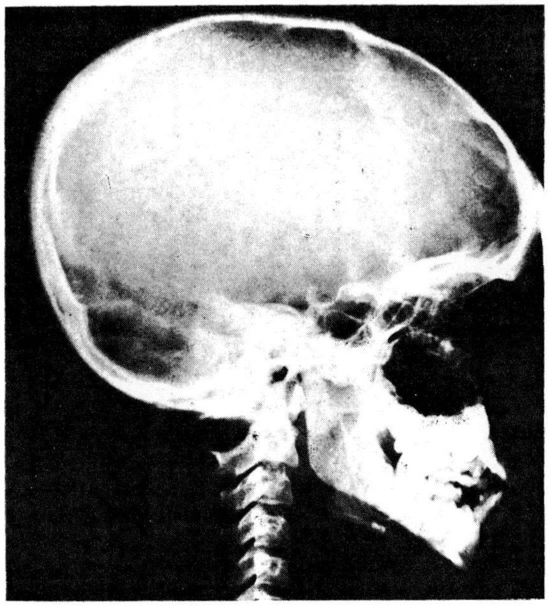

Fig. 3-12. Achondroplasia in a 9-year-old girl. Note the small size of the base of the skull, the flat basal angle, and the mild degree of basilar impression.

and are in keeping with the small dimensions of the internal condyle.

On lateral films of the spine the short pedicles are recognizable with a concave posterior border of the vertebral bodies, often exhibiting a narrow anteroposterior diameter (Fig. 3-11). It is not uncommon to find one or two wedged lumbar vertebrae. While beginning to walk during infancy, the relation of the sacrum to the spine may exhibit acute angulation sometimes approaching 90 degrees. The craniocaudal reduction of the interpediculate distances of the lower lumbar vertebral bodies is a key radiographic finding along with the pelvic changes seen on AP films. Together they form essential criteria for a positive diagnosis (Fig. 3-11).

Investigation of the skull, aside from the excessive growth of the vault, will show a shortened base resulting from the premature closure of the sphenooccipital suture along with a closing of the basal angle which is normally more than 100° (Fig. 3-12). Tomographic studies may demonstrate a basilar impression and a narrow spinal canal.

During adolescence and adulthood the skeletal changes that we have just described persist after the disappearance of the growth cartilage. During growth the aspect of the long bones becomes more massif, the areas of muscular insertions particularly the deltoid groove visible and the minor and major trochanter abnormally large (Fig. 3-13). The fibula is often unusually long in relation to the tibia. This finding, however, is not limited to achondroplasia. Occasionally epiphyseal size is reduced, and occasionally may be slightly deformed. The metacarpals, metatarsals, and phalanges are short although not unusually plump. Developmental deficiencies of pelvic bones explain their narrow characteristics. These result in considerable obstetrical difficulties which were pointed out for the first time by Porak. This narrowing is usually predominant in the AP diameter.

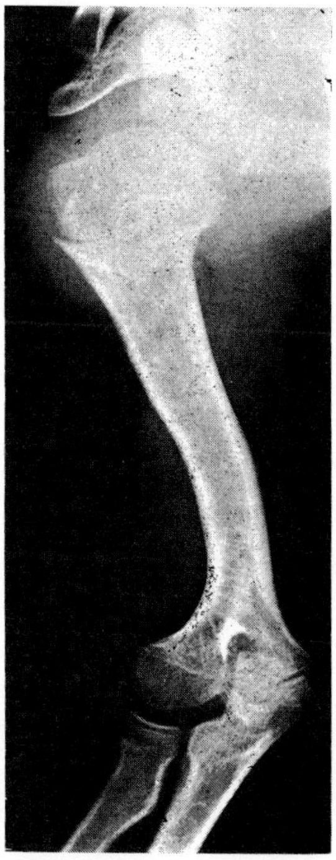

Fig. 3-13. A 17-year-old boy with achondroplasia. Note that the humerus is short and plump with an increased deltoid groove.

Genetic Data

The dominant transmission of achondroplasia cannot be doubted since there are numerous pedigrees showing this. Still, considering the relatively infrequent reproduction of such individuals there are many observations of recent mutations. The calculation of the number of mutations by Morch is given as 4×10^{-5}. This is, most likely, an excessive figure due to the heterogenicity of the material studied. Since a number of observations included are patients with thanatophoric dwarfism or pseudoachondroplastic forms of spondyloepiphyseal dysplasia, which may follow an autosomal recessive transmission. Several publications now make reference to homozygote forms of this disease (Hall and Bailey). These patients show clinical findings that fall somewhere in between those of anchondroplasia and thanatophoric dwarfism. Due to respiratory insufficiency these infants usually die within the first days or weeks of life. Radiographically the lesions are similar to those described for achondroplasia. In addition, there is a lack of height in the vertebral bodies, shortened ribs, which is somewhat reminiscent of what we see in chrondroectodermal dysplasia.

The question of whether there is a recessive form of achondroplasia has been the object of numerous discussions. At the time it appears possible to formally reject this mode of transmission. However, the observation that where the disorder appears as a recent mutation there is a significantly elevated paternal age should not be overlooked. This finding has been reported and emphasized by several authors (Bouvet et al.).

Clinical Forms

Ravenna and Léri have proposed the term *hypochondroplasia* to describe a disease similar to achondroplasia although not presenting the craniofacial features and with less dramatic radiographic findings. As a dominant, it most likely represents a distinct entity. It may sometimes be difficult to properly distinguish it from achondroplasia.

Although there are many clinical similarities the face is not involved. The medium height, which in the adult is close to 1.30 m, is slightly above the mean for achondroplasia. Radiographically, the long bones will appear similar to those in achondroplasia, somewhat squat, with mild metaphyseal flaring, and accentuated contours. The interpedicular distances of the lower vertebral bodies are narrow. Frequently, the pelvis is small with only mild reduction in the length of the iliac wings. Radiographs of the skull are usually within normal limits with an occasional, slight reduction in the size of the base.

Genetic transmission is dominant and this disease could be due to a gene allelic to that for achondroplasia: this theory however must still be proven. The hyperplastic form of achondroplasia described on the basis of histologic findings by Kaufmann seems to correspond to the recently described metatropic dwarfism (p. 48). Caffey also affirms this descriptive subdivision basing himself on radiographic findings. It is our belief that in these particular cases we are

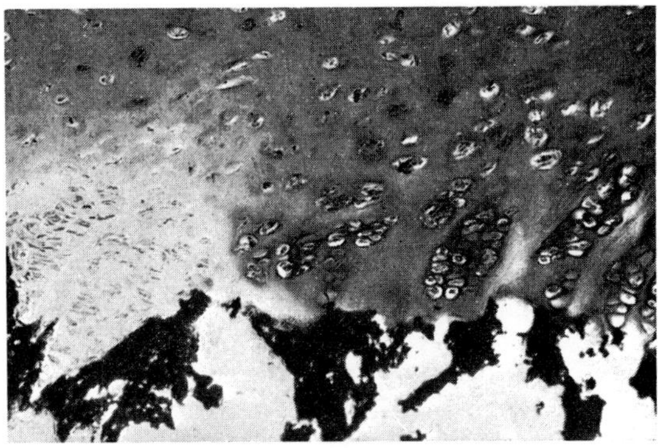

Fig. 3-14. Growth cartilage in achondroplasia. Note the reduced height of the columns with their widened septa between the columns and the zones of fibrosis. (Courtesy of V. Stanescu)

dealing with the pseudoachondroplastic type of the spondyloepiphyseal dysplasia (p. 74).

Pathogenesis

The histological abnormalities of achondroplasia are primarily found within the growth cartilage. Cell division leading to the development of the columnar cartilage is markedly disturbed. The entire layer of columnar cartilage is composed of only a very small amount of cells. The septa between the collagen-rich columns are generally enlarged and zones of fibrosis appear within cartilage (Fig. 3-14). There is sometimes a fibrous band separating the reserve zones and the proliferation of the cartilage. Rimoin has voiced a different theory which is based on the study of the chondrocostal junction of the iliac crest. In this location the anomalies appear much less marked than those involving long bones (Ponseti).

Histochemical and microchemical studies (Stanescu et al.) have confirmed that there are several anomalies of which the most striking is a considerable increase in the amount of collagen.

The interpretation of pathogenetic studies performed in achondroplasia is very difficult because reference is made to several different species which have been studied (Creeper's mutation of the chick, brachypod mutation of the mouse and the fatal achondroplasia of the rabbit). Thus, the material studied is entirely heterogeneous as has been proven by the results of the ultrastructural studies involving different mutations (Johnson and Wise, Seegmiller et al.).

The somewhat old experiments performed by Hamburger and by Rudnik utilizing chickens speak in favor of primary genetic action upon growth cartilage formation and exclude the possibility that the disease is of central origin. In the mouse these studies have been confirmed by Konyukhov and Paschin in the brachypod mutation by organ culture and for the achondroplast mutation by the use of transplants. In the latter case, the growth of the transplanted normal extremity within the achondroplastic mouse has been clearly reduced. Using embryonal extracts of the Creeper chicks, Wolff and collaborators were able to demonstrate that they do have an inhibitory action on the growth of normal tibias which have been cultivated in vitro. This has been verified in a diplopod mutation performed by Kieny and Abbott and in brachypod mutation of the mouse. The release of an inhibiting substance within the culture medium has been suggested by cultures taken from tibia of the Creeper chicks and normal chickens affected by the same culture medium (Elmer and Pierro).

Shepard and collaborators who have been working with the achondroplastic rabbit have insisted that there is an elective involvement of the cartilage's central parts. The cells of this cartilage in organ culture utilize increased amounts of glucose, and Bargman has shown that the liver of the same animal has a oxidative phosphorylation defect (lack of phosphorylation of cytochrom oxydase). However, achondroplasia in the rabbit is a lethal recessive disorder entirely different from the human disease in spite of the fact that the authors believe that they have demonstrated the same defect in the latter (Mackler et al.).

Treatment

The treatment of achondroplasia is limited to the careful attention given to a number of skeletal deformities. During infancy it is of special importance to counteract the dorsal kyphosis which is secondary to hypotonia. During this age period, as has been noted, the vertebral wedging deformity is an exceptional occurrence. We believe that a normal alignment of the vertebral column can be achieved which would avoid the appearance of such deformities. In these attempts one must apply appropriate gymnastic measures, possibly in combination with postural therapy (ventral position) and of a plaster of Paris shell. Occasionally, it will be necessary for the patient to wear a light supportive corset for a limited period of time. Surgical correction of a genu varum may later become necessary.

A number of achondroplastic patients were treated with somatotropin. The results obtained are rather questionable and do not seem to justify the therapeutic trials. Although anabolic steroids may provoke a growth spurt they carry the inherent risk of the growth cartilage's premature closure and should be avoided.

Neurosurgical interventions thought to have an effect on a latent hydrocephalus in order to improve growth should also be avoided.

Regular neurologic checkups should be offered to the adult patient. As soon as there are signs of medullary compression it will be necessary to perform a laminectomy. The fact that this procedure may run into difficulties should not be overlooked (Werner).

PUNCTATE CHONDRODYSPLASIA (CHONDRODYSPLASIA CALCIFICANS PUNCTATA, STIPPLED EPIPHYSES)

Originally described by Conradi in 1914 this disorder was first considered to be a variant of achondroplasia with premature ossification. Hünermann, who was one of the next describers in 1931, also discusses it as an abortive form of achondroplasia. The determination of the individuality of this disorder and the definition of its symptomatology result from a number of studies. In France important contributions have come from Jeune, Montlouis, and Saugier. It is to the credit of Silverman to have put special emphasis on the late effects of this disease and for the great difficulty in properly recognizing this disorder in the older child or adult.

Clinical Findings

Symptomatology, as well as the localization of this disease, is variable. Aside from the morphologic anomalies certain types are also associated with cataracts, cutaneous lesions, and cardiac defects.

In more than half of the cases there is early recognition of the disease during the first few days of life, due to a shortened extremity or a local defect. Micromelia is seen in two-thirds of the cases and is usually rhizomelic and often asymmetrical in character. In some instances there is only an isolated shortening of one or two extremities. Study of articular function may show limitation of movement, especially of extension with a fixed position in semiflexion. Unilateral and more rarely, bilateral dislocation of the hip has been described repeatedly.

Anomalies of the fingers and toes, squareness and deformity of the hand, along with clubbed feet are frequently associated with shortened extremities.

Kyphoscoliosis and shortening of the neck have occasionally been seen. In more than half of the patients there is an unusual facies. Frequently described as "mongoloid facies," this is characterized by an unusually deep nasal bridge often combined with hypoplasia of the mandible. These facial alterations may lead to confusing this disorder with achondroplasia, however, the volume of the skull is rarely excessive and there is no frontal bossing.

Cataracts are not always recognized, and in particular, when there is a lack of systematic and careful ophthalmologic investigation. Its incidence is close to 30 per cent. Commonly there is a total cataract with an occasional nuclear cataract with scalariform striae. Both eyes are usually involved from birth.

Cutaneous manifestations are seen with the same incidence as cataracts. These are thickening of the skin, ichthyosis, hyperkeratosis, erythrodermia, and scaling. The variability of these cutaneous anomalies must be emphasized. Furthermore they can occur either simultaneously or successively in the same patient.

Congenital heart disease is present in 10 per cent of these patients. There are several types on record: ASD, VSD, PDA or other, more complex defects.

Emphasis must be placed on the overall weakness of infants who suffer from chondrodysplasia punctate. The prognosis is particularly poor for patients who are suffering from cutaneous lesions or cataracts. Half of these will die during the first year of life. The presence of a congenital cardiac defect poses a particularly bad threat.

Among the surviving infants there will be many with a persisting defect of growth leading to dwarfism and deformities. Examples of this are a shortened extremity, coxa vara, a dislocated hip, genu valgum, and kyphoscoliosis.

In addition to these more or less generalized forms with involvement that is not limited exclusively to the skeletal system there are observations on record with more localized and discrete lesions. There may only be mild deformity or shortening of a single extremity as an isolated manifestation. These forms are not always recognized at birth and it is possible that quite a number of these due to their mild symptoms and the absence of all other manifestations are only recognized during the stage of late sequelae when a retrospective diagnosis is often impossible.

Radiographic Findings

A reliable diagnosis can only be established on the basis of a radiographic investigation showing the presence of calcifications, the characteristic finding of this disease (Fig. 3-15). Normally these are of small dimension, ranging from the size of a pinhead to a small grain of lead. There may be a large number of calcifications and they may appear in clusters, as bands, or punctate. Occasionally they may even appear as an irregular mass. These calcifications, distributed in an entirely chaotic manner, are in the area of enchondral bone or its vicinity. The principle site is

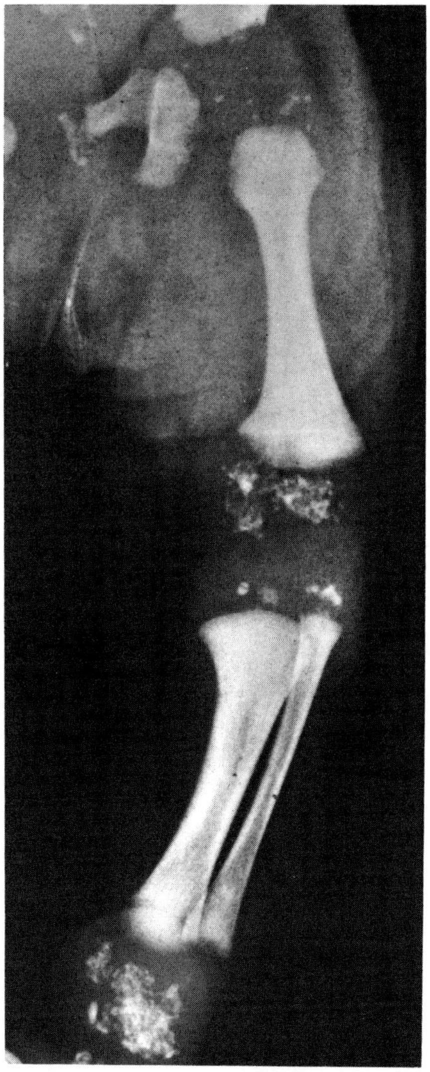

Fig. 3-15. Punctate epiphyseal dysplasia in a newborn. Note the numerous calcifications both in the pelvic region and beyond the ends of the long bones.

the epiphyseal area of the long bones and the adjacent periarticular tissues in the region of the hand, foot, vertebral column, pelvis, and patella. Other areas that may be involved are the scapula, the costal cartilages, the ribs, the intervertebral discs, the bones of the hand, and the base of the skull. The thyroid and cricoid cartilages are occasionally involved along with the tracheal rings and those of the large bronchi. These calcifications are primarily seen in multiple areas, even where the shortening of the extremities is unilateral. In certain patients, however, one side only is involved. Sometimes this involves only one extremity or just one of its segments.

Calcifications present at birth have a tendency to disappear progressively. Towards the third or fourth years, and sometimes even earlier, they vanish completely. In certain patients there may be an extension of the calcifications in the first few days of life. There will, however, be a period of regression later. Shortening of long bones, predominantly rhizomelic, is occasionally associated with these calcifications. At times asymmetric, the diaphyses appear coarse, occasionally bowed, with an acute enlargement of the metaphyseal region. Often there is an irregular, abnormally oriented growth line. Other cases may present with virtually normal bone morphology. At the time of their appearance there may be fragmentation of the epiphyseal centers or an irregular contour or structure. It is not unusual to find a dislocated hip.

In the grown child there is a noticeable radiographic similarity with the changes seen in multiple epiphyseal dysplasia as has been pointed out by Silverman. We must insist, however, on finding an asymmetrical and more anarchic distribution of the lesions which will occasionally lead to a correct retrospective diagnosis. Admittedly, this may be a difficult, and in some instances, an outright impossible task. Long bone growth varies, with an often noticeable disturbance leading to micromelia or an asymmetry of the long bones. Frequently, one has to deal with scoliosis or kyphoscoliosis, and in patients whose early examination revealed multiple spinal calcifications the follow-up will often reveal disturbed growth of the vertebral bodis. Their shape and contour may be irregular and they may have the appearance usually seen in certain types of spondyloepiphyseal dysplasias.

Genetic Data, Pathogenesis, and Treatment

Today it is accepted that chondrodysplasia punctate does not represent a single disease entity, but a heterogeneous group of disorders. Spranger and collaborators have proposed a means to distinguish between the two large groups. The Conradi-Hünermann type where the calcifications involve the epiphyses besides the spinal column together with moderate, usually asymmetrical, shortening of long bones. Genetic transmission is dominant (Bergström et al.), however, in the majority of cases there seems to be a recent mutation. In the rhizomelic, and rare type, the shortening involves predominantly the femur and humerus. The calcifications spare the spine and frequently there is an associated finding of coronal cleft vertebrae at birth as exhibited on lateral films. Most patients with this form also suffer from cataracts. Autosomal recessive inheritance seems to be the rule and these patients frequently show psycho-motor retardation.

Other authors have repeatedly emphasized the find-

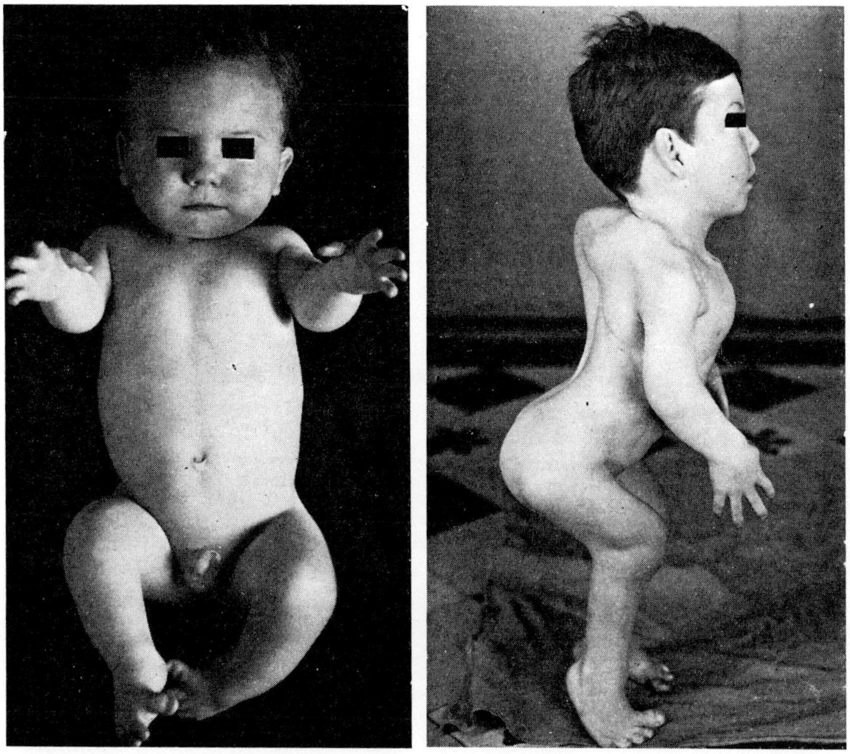

Fig. 3-16. Pictured here is a child with diastrophic dwarfism at (*left*) 10 months, and (*right*) 10 years.

ing of abnormal thyroid function in the mother and placental abnormalities. This disorder has been seen in several babies with trisomy 21.

Histologic examination confirms the presence of calcifications without any signs of ossification. The most striking feature is the presence of islands within the epiphysis of excessively large cartilaginous cells that are separated from normal cartilage by a zone which contains very few cells and is slightly metachromatic. Such islands are recognized on nondecalcified sections and do not always correspond to calcifications. This was the opinion of Sarrut who originally described them together with Cohen-Solal and his collaborators. The growth cartilage may appear at times almost normal, and at other times rather disturbed, occasionally there is even a fibrous band noted.

The pathogenesis of this disease still remains a mystery and its unique evolution attracts special attention. Its genetic origin should be accepted with caution, and, at least in some cases, it appears entirely possible that there might be an acquired etiology.

Treatment is palliative. It is limited to antiinfectious therapy and to orthopedic treatment of possible deformities of the extremities, and a direct approach to the cataracts.

DIASTROPHIC DWARFISM

Isolated in 1960 this disease had previously been confused with achondroplasia. The name is derived from the Greek word διαστροφος, meaning tortuous, It refers to the striking deformity of the trunk and extremities which characterize this disorder. A recent study makes reference to 51 observations (Walker et al.).

Clinical Findings

Diastrophic dwarfism is recognizable from birth and is based on the association of clubbed feet and micromelia (Fig. 3-16). Examination of the newborn will reveal shortening of the extremities with very marked equinovarus feet and the typical hitchhiker thumb. This is an abnormal origin of the thumb too high in location and usually held in adduction. The fingers are occasionally in a fixed extension due to blocked interphalangeal joints. In the more severe forms the joints of the extremities exhibit limited movement. The trunk is frequently normal at birth as is the head. However, one-third of all patients may exhibit a cleft palate, which is occasionally associated with hypoplasia of

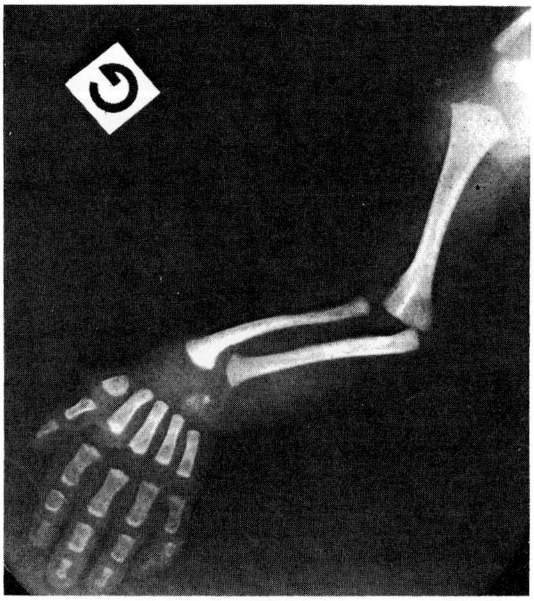

Fig. 3-17. Diastrophic dwarfism in a newborn. Note the abnormal position of the elbow and the presence of the two carpal centers.

the mandible, thus presenting the signs of the Pierre-Robin syndrome. Quite regularly towards the end of the first month of life a cyst appears on the external ear which later leads to a cauliflower deformity of the pinna.

Growth is quite slow and in the majority of patients there will be a severe and progressive scoliosis. The extremities are short and curved with marked deformity around the joints, while the hands and feet are squat (Fig. 3-16). There is usually significant limitation of joint movements, and in particular of the knee.

In the adult, who may reach a height of 1.20 m, dwarfing is due simultaneously to the shortening, the deformities of the extremities, as well as to the lack of height of the trunk secondary to scoliosis. There is often great difficulty found in walking.

The course of diastrophic dwarfism can assume a particularly serious character. It may be further aggravated by a number of complications, in particular those involving the respiratory or nervous systems, even though these do not occur with the frequency one might expect from the spinal involvement.

Radiographic Findings

At birth there is considerable similarity with changes which take place in the long bones in achondroplasia, thus explaining the confusion that has existed for a long time. The bones are short and broad with widened and flaring metaphyses, however, the distal femoral and proximal tibial epiphyses are prematurely irregular and deformed while the pelvis and spine have none of the characteristic anomalies seen in achondroplasia. The distal ends of the metacarpals have a tendency to broaden with the first metacarpal, and sometimes the first metatarsal bone having an ovoid appearance. Although these findings are not constantly seen, if they are present it is entirely characteristic of diastrophic dwarfism just as when the abnormal proximal end of the radius is in a subluxed position. Emphasis should be placed on the frequent presence of radiographically recognizable carpal points of ossification from birth (Fig. 3-17). Careful study of the vertebral column can already reveal a slight deviation from the normal and it is not at all uncommon to note abnormal development of cervical vertebral bodies which are easily recognized on the lateral film (bullet-shaped vertebral body, signs for anterior subluxation of the second or third cervical vertebral body). Hypoplasia of the mandible may complete the radiographic spectrum. In the growing child a number of abnormal findings will appear affecting both the epiphyses and metaphyses. The proximal end of the femur is broadened, its density is somewhat diminished, the neck may be absent and the femoral head has almost completely disappeared. The distal growth cartilage of the femur forms an acute angle open distally, there is an uneven structure of the adjacent metaphysis as well as an asymmetry of the condyles (Fig. 3-18). The distal end of the radius shows acute enlargement and, as we have described it for the first metacarpal bone, this element frequently appears as an ovoid or grossly triangular center. The diaphyses of the long bones are short and massive. The bones of the hand are similarly affected and occasionally the phalanges are of unequal length. Scoliosis is accompanied by marked spinal changes. Several vertebral alterations, flattening, and a cuneiform shape have all been described along with elective involvement of cervical vertebrae. Occasionally, one can see a minor reduction in the interpedicular distance of the last lumbar vertebrae. The skull is normal, although occasionally there is an increased basal angle.

During adolescence, this disorder is easily recognized because of the extremely shortened long bones and the deformity of the distal parts in association with the scoliosis (Fig. 3-18).

Genetic Data, Pathogenesis, and Treatment

Diastrophic dwarfism is transmitted as an autosomal recessive disease. This has been proven by the obser-

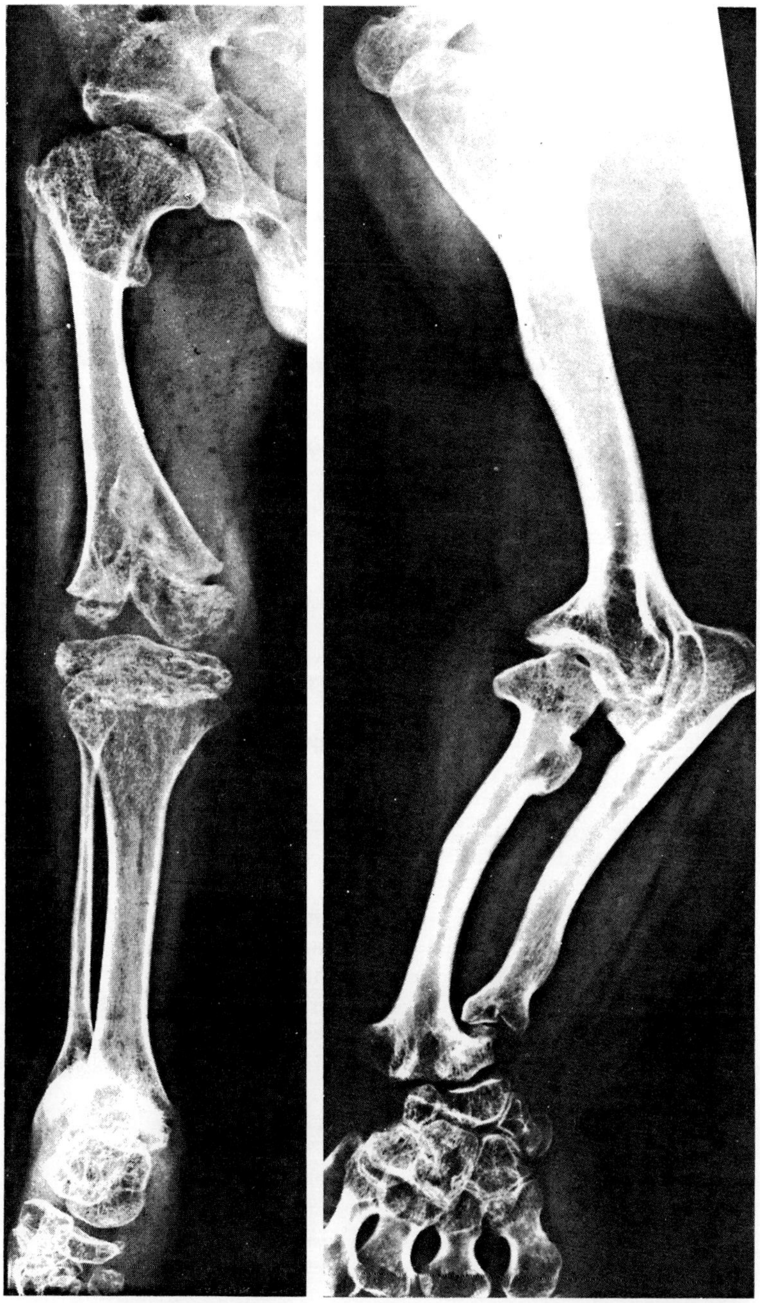

Fig. 3-18. Diastrophic dwarfism in, (*left*) a 7-year-old boy with severe epiphyseal and metaphyseal deformity, and, (*right*) a young adult with markedly shortened long bones and deformed epiphyses.

vation of several affected members of sibships. However, parental consanguinity does not appear to be markedly elevated. Seegmiller has described a recessive mutant gene in mice leading to a cleft palate and the shortening of long bones. Death seems to be the result of asphyxiation secondary to anomalies of tracheal cartilage. It appears to us that caution should be exercised in relating this disorder to diastrophic dwarfism as the author has proposed.

Histologic and histochemical studies of the growth

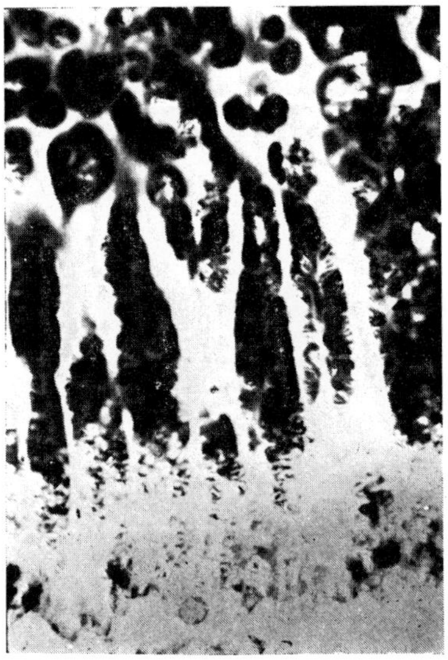

Fig. 3-19. Histochemical study of a congealed section of growth cartilage in a diastrophic dwarf after azure blue staining. In the lower portion of the columns note that metachromasia has disappeared. (Courtesy of R. Stanescu)

cartilage reveal small islands of ballooned cells at the base of the columns, the height of which is somewhat reduced, on the other hand there is marked reduction of metachromasia in the zone of proliferating cells (Fig. 3-19). This fact suggests that in this disorder there must be an anomaly of proteoglycans or of the glycoproteins of cartilage (Stanescu et al.).

Some authors have proposed to distinguish, aside from the typical form of diastrophic dwarfism, a more moderate variant sometimes referred to as pseudodiastrophic dwarfism (Bailey). We feel that this distinction should not be encouraged. There are without any discussion patients with very mild skeletal involvement, still, studies of the growth cartilage will reveal the identical findings especially the weak metachromasia of the columnar zone.

Therapy for clubbed feet must be initiated at birth. One should not overlook the great difficulty encountered here. The marked shortening of the bony elements will render the effectiveness of plaster casts questionable. It is often necessary to remove the astragalus. Difficulties of swallowing which are secondary to the anomalies of the palate and the mandible sometimes necessitate urgent measures but more often will not cause such concern. Careful attention must be paid to the position of the cervical spine so as not to miss a dislocation of cervical vertebrae. Due to its progressive characteristic it is of the utmost importance to initiate measures against the dorsolumbar scoliosis as soon as it becomes clinically manifest. The development of this complication may sometimes be late and its total absence at birth should not lead one to express an unjustifiable optimism! Treatment of these precocious types of scolioses continues to lack a uniform therapeutic approach and, furthermore, they are unusually difficult. Regular efforts to mobilize the joints will help to avoid movement limitation. Surgery should be utilized to correct the cleft palate after the patient reaches the age of 18 months. Later on it may become necessary to offer further corrective surgical interventions for the improvement of lesions in the extremities.

METATROPIC DWARFISM

First isolated in 1966 this disorder has been given this name (μεταтροπος which means variable) because of a change seen in its symptomatology during its evolution. At birth there is marked shortening of the extremities, a finding which previously led to the classification of this disorder as hyperplastic achondroplasia. In the older child there appears a progressive and impressive kyphoscoliosis subsequently resulting in a shortened trunk leading to confusion with Morquio's disease.

Clinical Findings

This disease is most frequently recognized at birth or after a few days as the morphologic anomalies are already visible. The most striking clinical finding during this phase is the marked contrast between the length of the trunk and the relative shortness of the extremities. It must be emphasized, however, that the total height is within normal limits. The thorax is long and narrow. The back, which may already be affected by a kyphoscoliosis, is usually already recognizable at this age. This can be sufficiently disturbing for the parents to seek medical advice.

It is not unusual to find at the sacral end of the spine a "tail" measuring 1-3 cm, sometimes there is just a small cutaneous fold present. The extremities are short, and abnormal protrusions of knotty character may be visible or palpable in the neighbourhood of joints, primarily near the knees (Fig. 3-20). The joint movements may be limited. Fingers and toes are long and slender with one or several interphalangeal joints frequently freezing. The craniofacial appearance is somewhat unusual with a high forehead and a flat and broad nose.

In the older child there will be a progressively more severe lack of height characterized by shortening and

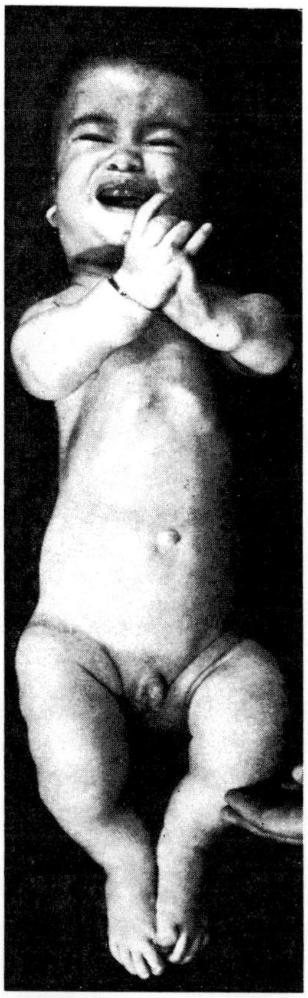

Fig. 3-20. Metatropic dwarfism in an infant. Notice the relative shortening of the extremities, the narrow thorax, and the visible prominence of the metaphyses in the region of the forearms.

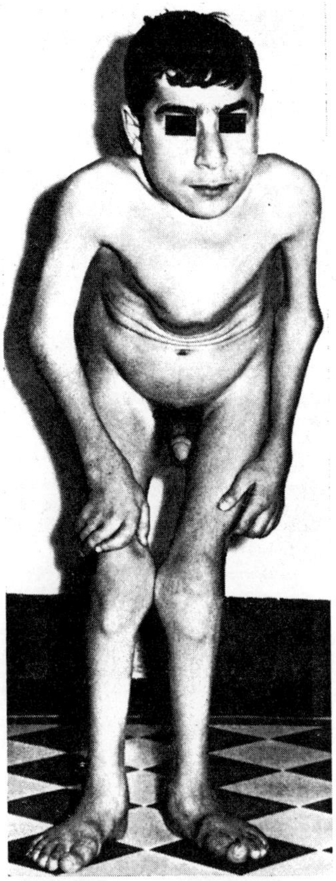

Fig. 3-21. The extreme shortness of the thorax results from marked kyphoscoliosis in this 17-year-old boy with metatrophic dwarfism.

deformity of the trunk, secondary to a rapidly progressive kyphoscoliosis accompanied by anterior bowing of the sternum. Frequently, one notes a firmly fixed flexion of the hip, the knee, and the elbow. In the severe forms this may be extreme. Hands and feet are short and square (Fig. 3-21).

The prognosis of metatropic dwarfism varies. It must always be guarded because of the very progressive character of kyphoscoliosis. The adult height of an individual will rarely be more than 1.20 m. Certain types of this disorder are rapidly fatal.

Radiographic Findings

At birth there is shortening of the long bones of the extremities along with marked widening of the metaphysis with a degree of irregularity which varies. This widening may be a rather sudden manifestation, for example, that which is seen at the distal end of the tibia or radius. It can also be accompanied by markedly swollen metaphyses, giving them the appearance of a club (Fig. 3-22*A*). The metaphyseal region, next to a widened growth zone, may be unusually dense. This is a frequent and characteristic finding, seen particularly in the bones of the hand and foot which appear short and in the form of a diabolo. This can even be seen occasionally at the nongrowing end, sometimes revealing an irregular outline (Fig. 3-22*C*). The cortex of the bones can form a protrusion, which is seen primarily in the radius and ulna. The development of the vertebral bodies is markedly reduced, often presenting only as a thin central layer. The size of the pedicles is affected mildly, and a considerable enlargement of the intervertebral spaces results (Fig. 3-22*B*). Associated with these disturbances of vertebral ossification is a kyphoscoliosis already present. The thorax is unusually long and narrow with short ribs. Its appearance is similar to that of asphyxiating

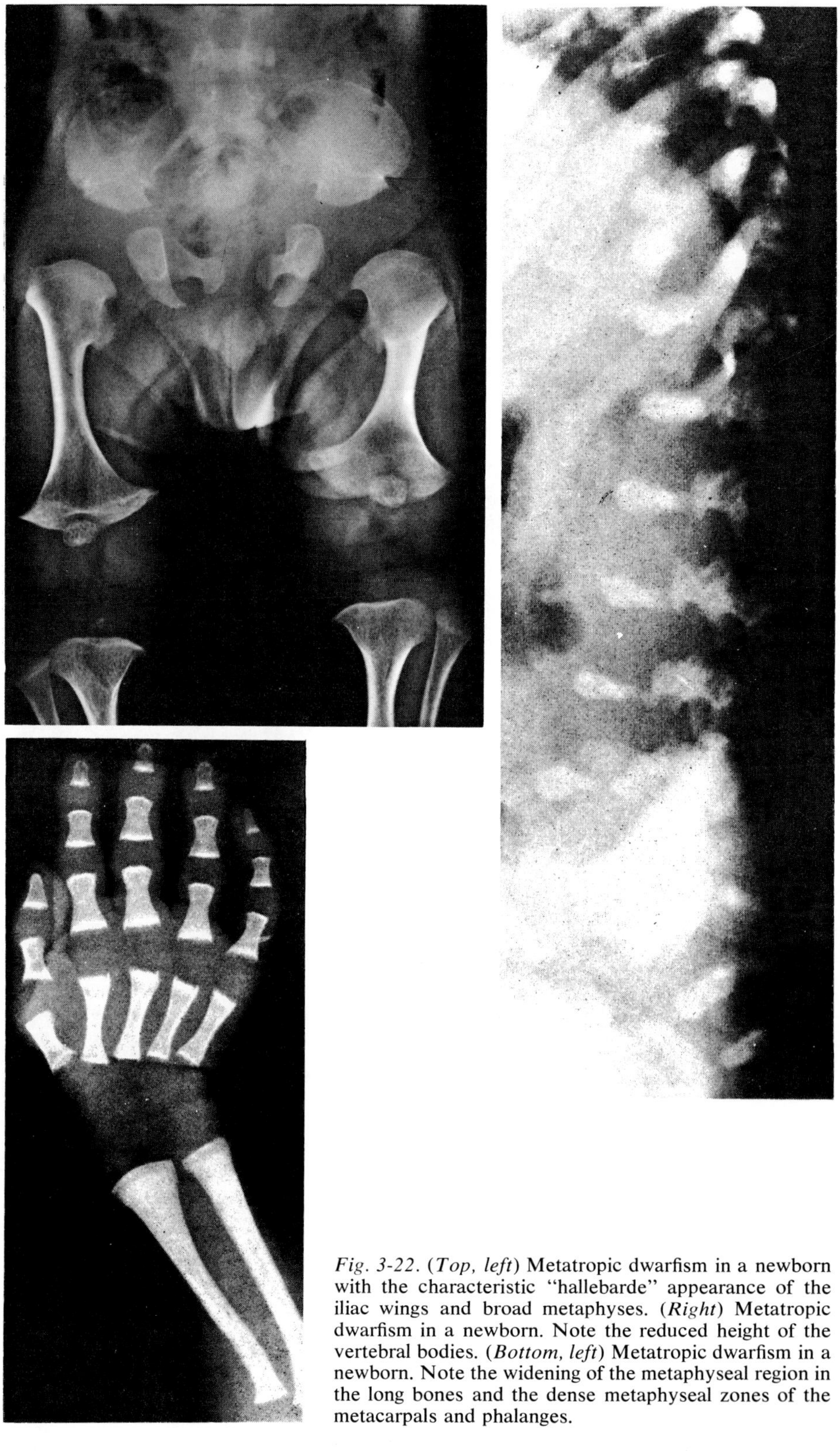

Fig. 3-22. (*Top, left*) Metatropic dwarfism in a newborn with the characteristic "hallebarde" appearance of the iliac wings and broad metaphyses. (*Right*) Metatropic dwarfism in a newborn. Note the reduced height of the vertebral bodies. (*Bottom, left*) Metatropic dwarfism in a newborn. Note the widening of the metaphyseal region in the long bones and the dense metaphyseal zones of the metacarpals and phalanges.

thoracic dysplasia. The iliac wings are plump and have the form of a hallebarde. A notch of the external border is frequently seen just above the lateral rim of the acetabulum, which may occasionally be horizontal. In addition to this, a lacunar structure of the occipital region has been noted in several severe cases.

During the first years of life the deformity in the metaphyseal region of the long bones persists. These findings, however, will become progressively milder and eventually will disappear during growth. The individual is sometimes less affected than one might have feared from the initial appearance (Fig. 3-23). The epiphyses and carpal bones appear with some delay, are diminished in size and often have an irregular structure. The metacarpals and phalanges are square, sometimes showing the presence of supernumerary epiphyses. The kyphoscoliosis will lead to significant spinal deformity. The vertebral bodies are flattened, and sometimes slightly wedged with irregular surfaces. The atlantooccipital region is just as abnormal, the cervical and vertebral bodies are of reduced length, with the characteristic pyramid appearance. In addition to this, the apophysis of the odontoid bone has an enlarged base.

In both the adolescent and adult there are, along with spinal changes and shortening of the long bones, persistence of a modeling defect, of epiphyseal abnormalities, especially of the femoral head, and excessive development of bony contours, particularly the trochanters.

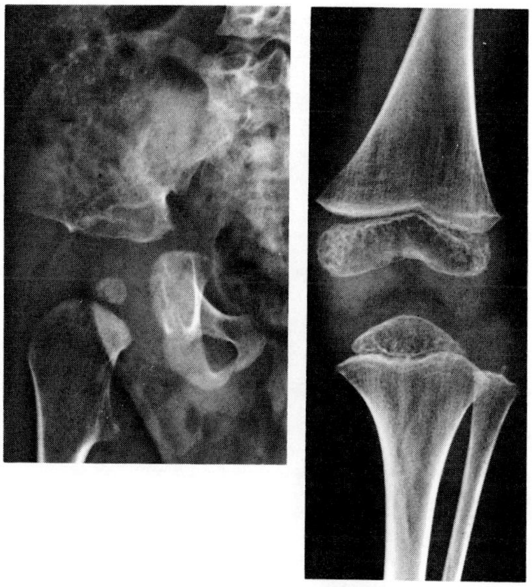

Fig. 3-23. Shown here is a three-year-old child with metatropic dwarfism. Note that the epiphyseal and metaphyseal changes are moderate and that the center for the femoral head is well developed.

Genetic Data, Pathogenesis, and Treatment

Most likely, metatropic dwarfism follows an autosomal recessive mode of transmission, however, this has not been proven because the majority of cases have been isolated observations.

The pathogenetic mechanism remains unknown. Histologic examinations reveal an irregular arrangement of the growth cartilage. The columns are poorly oriented and are formed by a few round cells with a markedly reduced zone of hypertrophic cartilage along with a small number of invading capillaries. The most striking finding is the presence of trabeculae which are formed in considerable number from cartilaginous matrix with a more generous local mineralization than occurs in the adjacent lamellar bone.

Therapy must be directed towards the prevention of the development of the kyphoscoliosis, the most limiting complication of the disease. Measures should be started very early, and as stated for diatrophic dwarfism, one should never ignore the great difficulties encountered. In cases of suboccipital instability Bailey recommends surgical fixation of the atlas and axis. Severe limb deformity may also justify corrective osteotomies.

Care should be taken so as not to confuse metatropic dwarfism with Kniest's disease during infancy. This disorder exhibits a more severe developmental defect of the proximal, femoral epiphysis, but is never responsible for such severe disorders of the spine (see p. 55. Certain types of spondyloepiphyseal dysplasias may also appear very similar to metatropic dwarfism. However, they have not yet been sufficiently defined to use the term pseudometatropic dwarfism as has been done by some.

MESOMELIC DWARFISM

Besides dyschondrosteosis, which is never recognized at birth and which will be studied later on page 86, there is a group of chondrodysplasias which electively affect the growth of the midsegment of the extremities, the forearm, and the leg. A number of these cases have not yet been clearly classified (Lamy and Bienenfeld), but a special place can already be assigned to the autosomal recessive type studied by Langer, to the syndrome described by Nievergelt, to acromesomelic dwarfism, and to the syndrome de-

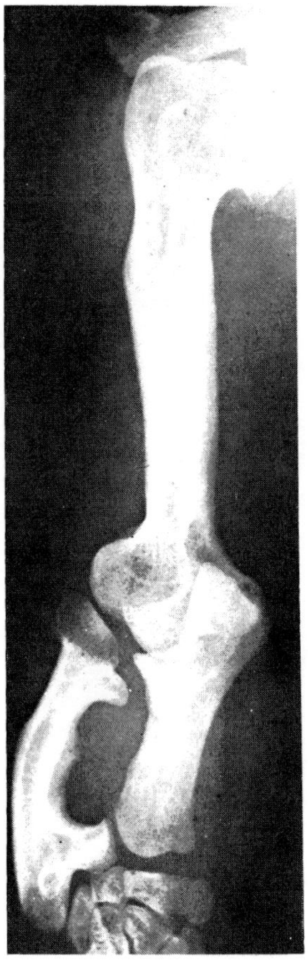

Fig. 3-24. Langer's mesomelic dwarfism. The long bones, especially the forearms, are extremely short.

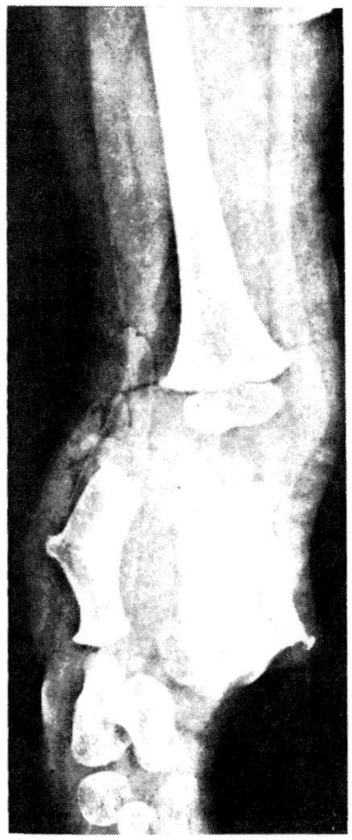

Fig. 3-25. Nievergelt's mesomelic dwarfism. Note the triangular shape of the lower leg bones. (Courtesy of J. G. Pous)

scribed by Robinow. The form of mesomelic dwarfism described by Langer as the hypoplastic ulna fibular mandible type is characterized by an extreme degree of micromelia, electively affecting the forearms and lower leg. The fibula is totally absent, and the bones of the forearms are short, abnormally shaped, and curved. The most distal parts of all four extremities are not involved (Fig. 3-24). It is our impression that hypoplasia of the mandible is not a constant finding. The transmission is autosomal recessive.

In the syndrome of Nievergelt, there is an association of an extreme degree of shortening in both bones of the lower leg with unusual, and severe changes in the shape, which is at times almost triangular, of the tibia and fibula (Fig. 3-25). The growth line of the tibia is oblique and the fibula is too long. The upper extremity may also be affected with involvement of the elbows by a subluxation of the radial head and a radioulnar synostosis. Other deformities seen are brachydactyly, and clinodactyly fusions of the carpal and tarsal bones. Genetic transmission is dominant.

It appears possible that the dominant form described by Reinhardt and Pfeiffer is really only a minor form of the Nievergelt syndrome. In this disorder there is a triangular shape of the fibula along with extreme shortness. The equally shortened ulna has a similar appearance, whereas, the radius is curved and subluxed.

Acromesomelic dwarfism may be recognized at birth or when the baby is only a few months old, because of the shortened forearm and lower leg, and the square shape of the hands and feet. In the adult, height will be at its maximum at 1.20 m. The hands are short and broad with the fingers shaped like sausages as in pseudoachondroplasia.

On a radiograph one can see the shortened diaphyses and well visualized contours. The epiphyses are normal, with the ulna shorter than the curved radius. Occasionally, there is subluxation of the radial head. All the bones of the hands and feet are unusually squat, the phalanges are square, and there is precocious fusion of the epiphyses (Fig. 3-26). The vertebral bodies show a minimal loss of height. The skull appears scaphocephalic with an increased basal angle.

This disorder follows an autosomal recessive mode of transmission and care should be taken not to confuse it with pseudoachondroplasia, where the epiphyses and metaphyses are severely affected.

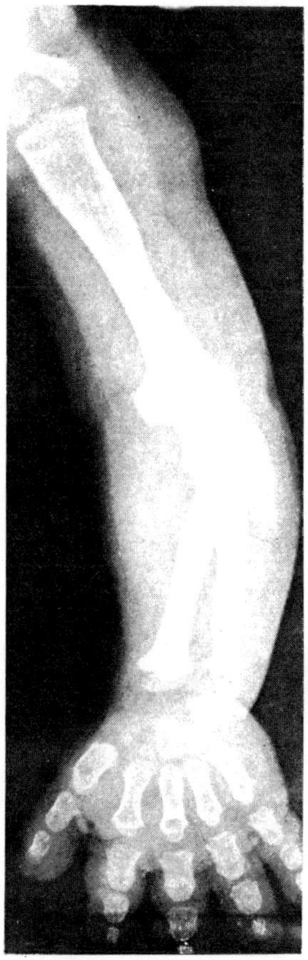

Fig. 3-26. Acromesomelic dwarfism in a 4-year-old girl. (Courtesy of E. Campailla)

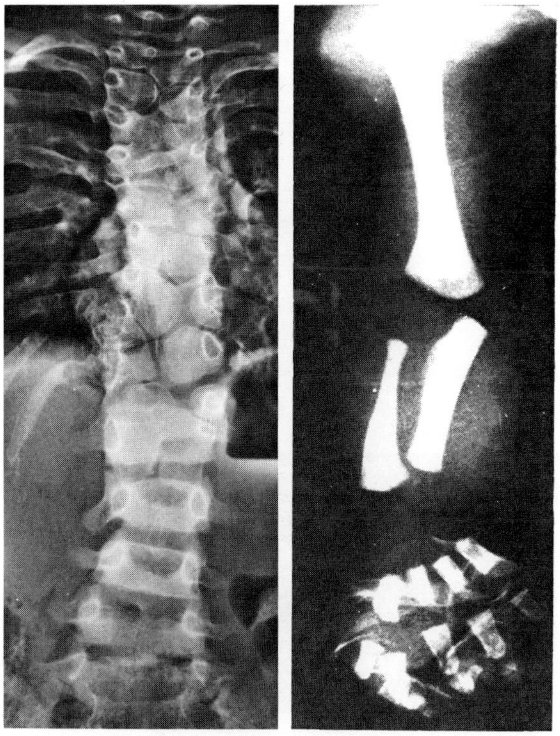

Fig. 3-27. Robinow's syndrome. Note the severely disordered spinal segmentation combined with the shortened middle segment of the limbs. (Courtesy of J. Cukier)

Another syndrome described by Robinow refers to the combination of mesomelic dwarfism with a severe disturbance of vertebral segmentation. Clinically, there are impressive changes of the facial structures. They include hypertelorism, a short nose, and a flat facial profile along with genital anomalies—micropenis. The transmission is likely to be dominant with a markedly variable genetic manifestation (Fig. 3-27).

CHONDRODYSPLASIAS LEADING TO MICROMELIC DWARFISM

In the preceding paragraph we have indicated that a number of chondrodysplasias, although fully manifested at birth are poorly defined and are under discussion as to their proper identity. Several times we have had the opportunity to study patients with severe micromelia with radiographic findings markedly different from achondroplasia. In our previous book, we have shown an example of a probable autosomal recessive transmission (Fig. 3-28). Other authors have reported similar observations, however, some are clearly different (Dürr, Rupprecht).

Among these dysplasias a special place must be reserved for micrognathic dwarfism which combines micromelia with the Pierre Robin syndrome (Fig. 3-29). Radiographically there is frequently an impressive appearance of the metaphyseal ends of the long bones and the vertebrae may occasionally be transversely enlarged. In some patients we have seen flattening and smallness of the femoral head. Mandibular hypoplasia and a cleft palate are the striking clinical findings of this disorder which is likely to be autosomal recessive.

DYSPLASIAS RECOGNIZED BECAUSE OF SHORT STATURE

Two disorders fall under this heading. They are congenital spondyloepiphyseal dysplasia and the Kniest syndrome.

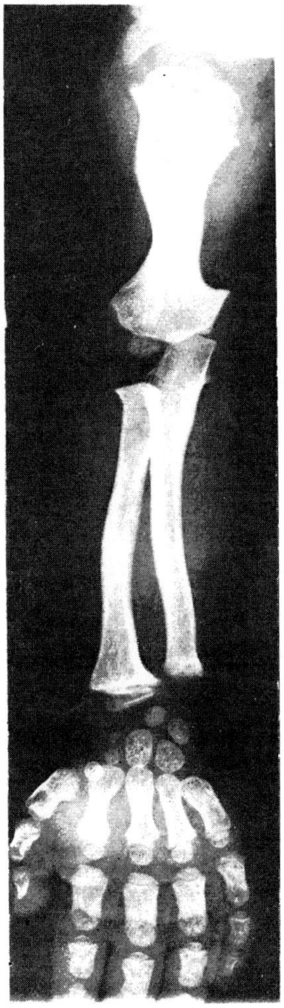

Fig. 3-28. Shown here is micromelic autosomal recessive dwarfism in a 3-year-old boy.

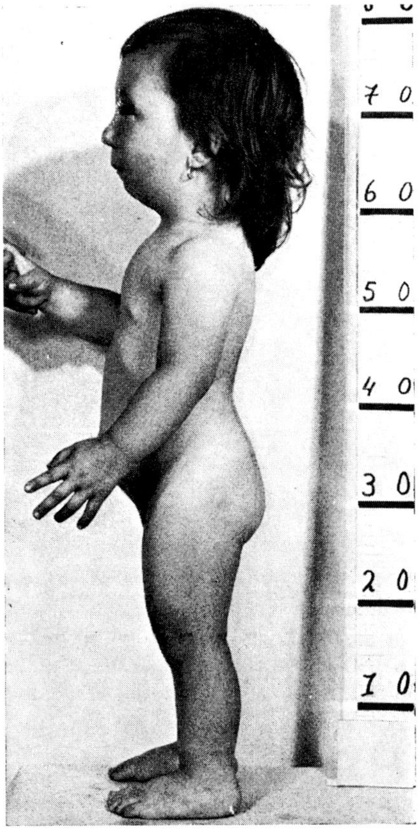

Fig. 3-29. Micrognathic dwarfism.

CONGENITAL SPONDYLOEPIPHYSEAL DYSPLASIA

This disorder, studied in particular by Spranger and Wiedemann, derives its name from the fact that it is usually recognized during the first few days, which is unusual in the group of spondyloepiphyseal dysplasias.

From birth there is an obvious deficit of stature due equally to the abnormal growth of the spine and the extremities (Fig. 3-30). During growth there is a progressive dorsal kyphosis and kyphoscoliosis may also be present. Besides the shortness of the spine, there is protrusion of the sternum, lumbar hyperlordosis, and an anterior tilt of the pelvis. The extremities are somewhat short, but the hands and feet are normal. Often, limitation of movements will be noted at the level of the hips and shoulders. The craniofacial structures are normal in the presence of a short neck. Ocular anomalies are seen with an unusually high incidence, and in particular, myopia. In the adolescent and adult, the height is variable, and most frequently reaches approximately 1.35 m. Severe involvement of the hips is a strong factor for a cautious prognosis.

Radiographic changes are limited to the spine and hips. In the newborn there is delayed bony maturation, and the slightly trapezoid appearance of vertebral bodies is due to the shortened length of the posterior border (Fig. 3-31), which is a characteristic finding. The pelvis reveals delayed ossification of the ischiopubic rami and a square iliac appearance. The ribs are somewhat short with an anterior prominence. The long bones are also somewhat shortened and the proximal end of the femora is slightly uneven and widened (Fig. 3-32). During growth vertebral irregularities of the body may be noted and result from reduced height, primarily of the thoracic and upper lumbar region, occasionally, with a slight deformity of a corner of a body. The major anomaly is found in the head and

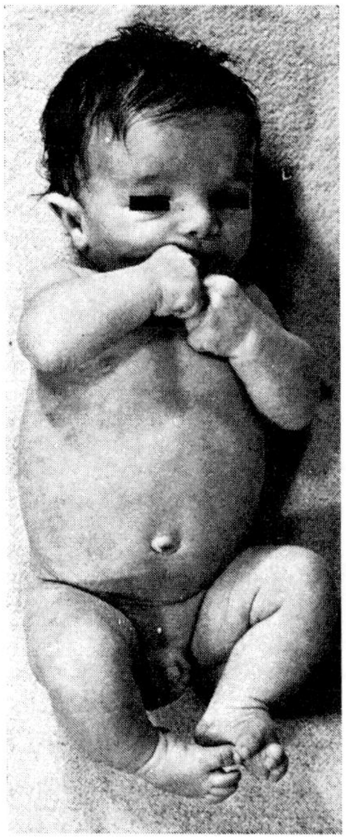

Fig. 3-30. Congenital spondyloepiphyseal dysplasia. This growth defect involves the trunk and extremities.

neck of the femur, since they not only are poorly ossified, sometimes there is delayed appearance, and there is often no ossification center for the femoral head. The neck is hypoplastic with irregular contours, and is sometimes fragmented and has a tendency to dislocate. Other epiphyses are generally less involved, but this varies. The metaphysis at the knee, along with those at the distal end of the forearm, are often irregular. The metaphysis of the long bones may be short, especially in the femur and humerus, and occasionally show incurving. Retarded maturation of the carpal and tarsal elements is normally recognized, however, the bones of the hands and feet are usually not significantly affected aside from the presence of extra metacarpal epiphyses. Occasionally, there may be an increased angle at the base of the skull and the apophysis of the dens may be poorly ossified.

Congenital spondyloepiphyseal dysplasia is inherited as a dominant. There have been observations among brothers and sisters, however, which makes genetic heterogeneity of this disorder likely.

At birth there is no reason to confuse this disorder with the Kniest syndrome, which we will now discuss. With respect to Morquio's disease, the manifestation of clinical symptoms leads to a later discovery. There is no noticeable loss of height in the vertebral bodies (p. 240).

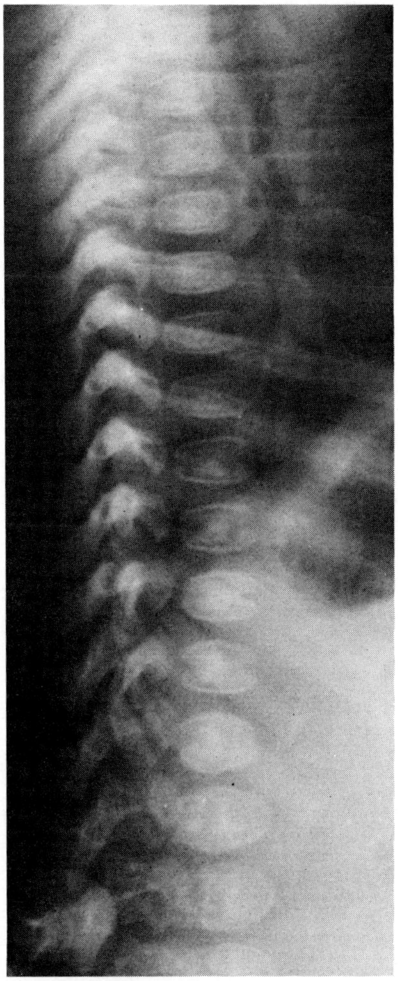

Fig. 3-31. Congenital spondyloepiphyseal dysplasia in a 2-month-old baby. Note the ovoid or slightly trapezoid form of the vertebral bodies.

Some spondyloepiphyseal dysplasias may be recognized at birth, when a radiographic study leads to an unusual early diagnosis or when we are dealing with a family known to be affected although they are generally recognized much later. Still, there are unquestionable, probably autonomous conditions recognizable at birth, which we will have to study further. We have followed such a patient and similar observations have been made by others (Kozlowski et al.).

THE KNIEST SYNDROME

This disorder can be recognized at birth because of its short stature, shortened spine and extremities, together with, on occasion, an already noticeable enlarge-

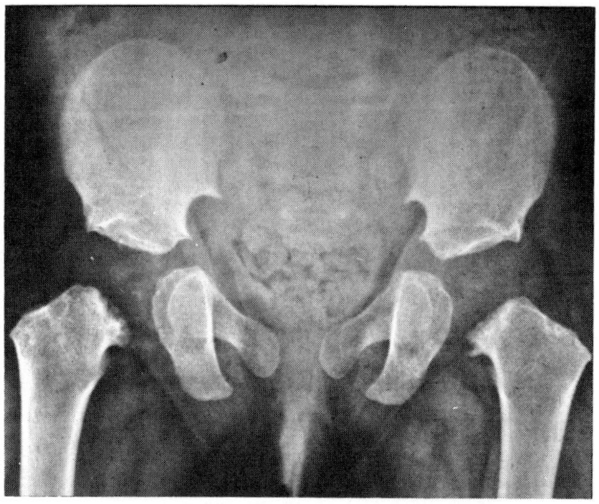

Fig. 3-32. Congenital spondyloepiphyseal dysplasia in a 6-month-old boy. There is delayed ossification of the ischiopubic segments.

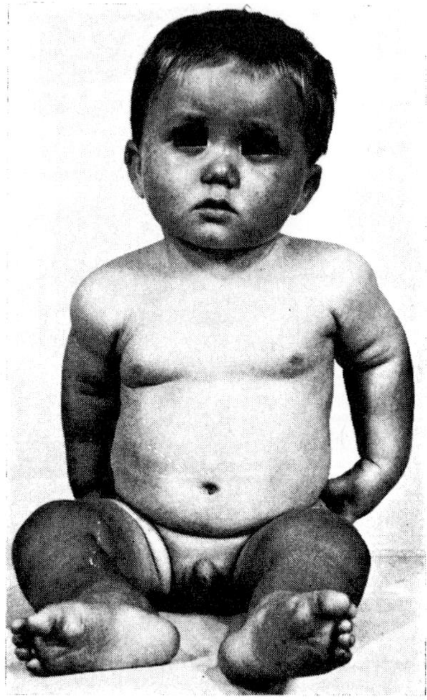

Fig. 3-33. This child has Kniest's disease. Note the characteristic facial appearance with hypertelorism and the absence of the root of the nose.

ment of the knees. Later a dorsal kyphosis will manifest itself and deviation of the lower leg external rotation with pes valgus will become apparent. The joints are unusually prominent and the fingers assume a fusiform appearance. There is a more or less dramatic limitation of joint movements. The face is typically rounded with a lack of growth at the nasal bridge. There may occasionally be a cleft palate (Fig. 3-33), and myopia and deafness are frequently noted. The definitive adult height is approximately 1.35 m or less.

Through radiographic study this disorder can be noted at birth due to the shortness of the extremity, the slight irregularity of the metaphyses, and, in particular, to the already reduced height of the vertebral bodies, some of which have a small anterior wedge (Fig. 3-34). The pelvis is somewhat square with slightly oblique acetabular roofs. Occasionally, one may note a dislocated hip. There will be abnormal epiphyseal findings appearing later, with the distal femoral and the upper tibial epiphyses undergoing excessive development, while there is either absence or smallness along with fragmentation of the femoral head. The upper femoral metaphysis may look like a saucer especially at its medial portion (Fig. 3-35). The hand often has extra phalangeal epiphyses. The anteroposterior size of different vertebrae may be too large, with irregular end plates and a mild degree of wedging of one or two bodies in the dorso-lumbar region (Fig. 3-36). All skeletal elements are excessively transparent. When growth stops there may be considerable deviation of the extremities together with marked epiphyseal changes, which, in particular, affect the femoral head. The spinal changes are much less progressive, however, than those in metatropic dwarfism.

Genetic transmission appears to be dominant. These patients will often require multiple orthopedic corrections for the abnormal relationship between the lower extremities. The spinal posture should be carefully supervised.

In recent studies performed with V. R. Stanescu we were able to demonstrate that there were inclusions within the endoplasmatic reticulum of chondrocytes. Microchemical analysis has revealed an anomaly of the proteoglycans of cartilage.

The Kniest syndrome has been consistently confused with congenital spondyloepiphyseal dysplasia. At birth one should be able to avoid this error by noting the entirely different appearance of the spine and the pelvis, where the deficient ossification is much more dramatic in the latter condition. It should be possible to recognize the Kniest syndrome, at a later time, because of the unusually dramatic development of certain epiphyses. Metatropic dwarfism has a narrow thorax, and a much more significant loss of height in the vertebral bodies which are visible at birth in combination with marked deformity of the metaphyses of the long bones. Later there is more marked involve-

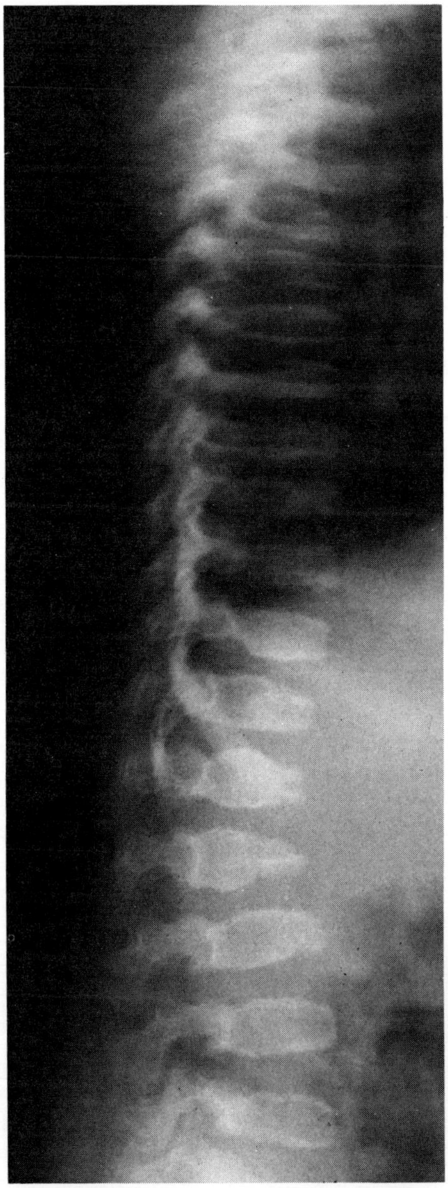

Fig. 3-34. Kniest's disease in a 3-month-old baby. The vertebral bodies have a reduced height and already appear to have an anterior tongue-like appearance.

ment of the spine, whereas, the development of the head of the femur is far less disturbed.

DYSPLASIAS RECOGNIZED FOR REASONS OTHER THAN SHORT STATURE

Under this heading we shall discuss three disorders: chondroectodermal dysplasia, most frequently recognized because of polydactyly, asphyxiating thoracic dysplasia with its impressive narrow appearance of the thorax, and cleidocranial dysplasia discovered be-

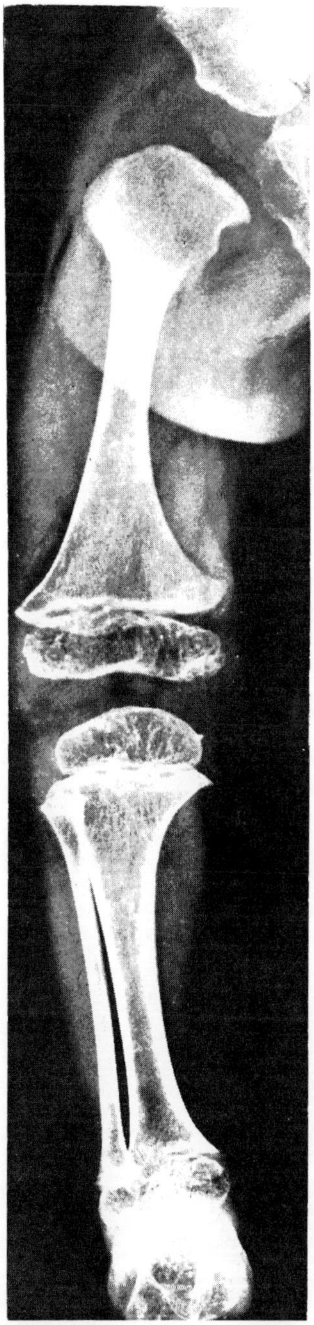

Fig. 3-35. Kniest's disease in a 2-year-old child. Note the markedly widened metaphyses, especially in the upper femoral region, with a poorly formed femoral head. This is in strong contrast to the size of the epiphyses at the knee.

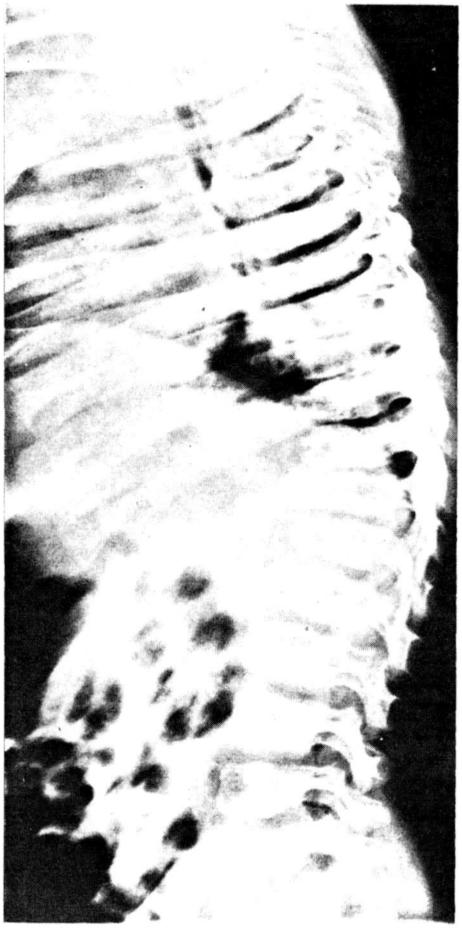

Fig. 3-36. Kniest's disease in a 2-year-old boy. Note the reduced height of the vertebral bodies and the iregularities of the anterior portion and the endplates.

cause of defective ossification of the skull or clavicular anomalies.

CHONDROECTODERMAL DYSPLASIA (ELLIS-VAN CREVELD SYNDROME)

Recognized as an individual disease in 1940, this syndrome had been seen earlier, but had been considered as an atypical form of achondroplasia (Mouchet, 1910).

Clinical Findings

Chondroectodermal dysplasia is a combination of disturbed enchondral growth and polydactyly, ectodermal anomalies of the nails and teeth, and a congenital heart defect present in two-thirds of all patients.

The disorder can easily be recognized at birth, since polydactyly is rarely overlooked. A careful study will then reveal the presence of further findings of this disease. Polydactyly is limited to the hands since the toes are less frequently involved. The exact type varies, and generally the malformed extra finger is on the ulnar side. Occasionally, there is only a minimal duplication. A mild degree of disproportion between the length of the extremities and the spine are combined with polydactyly. Changes in the thorax often appear similar to changes seen in asphyxiating thoracic dysplasia. The micromelia, present at birth in a mild form, will become progressively more severe and will involve, in particular, the middle and distal segments. The nails are small, irregular, often concave and malformed and are of poor quality. Changes can be seen which also involve the hands and feet. The hair is only rarely involved, although there have been several observations of thin hair. The premature eruption of teeth at birth, or during the first few months, is frequently noted with the later dental growth and appearance being irregular. Teeth may be malformed, small, widely spaced, or totally absent. At times one will see the fusion of two teeth. Teeth may be lost prematurally. The upper lip is narrow, sometimes with a gingival band or the absence of the gingivolabial groove. There is occasionally an outline of a harelip.

Congenital heart lesions vary. Primarily seen are atrial and ventricular septal defects. A single atrium has been reported several times. Other somewhat unusual further anomalies have also been described (hypospadia, vaginal atresia . . .). Mental retardation is not usually seen in this disorder.

The course of chondroectodermal dysplasia in patients varies. Some will not survive birth, and others may die within the first few weeks. Death is usually the result of the presence of severe heart lesions, although it may also be due to respiratory problems prompted by the narrow thorax, and possibly also, as suggested by Moore's study, from anomalies of the bronchial cartilage. One of our patients died from renal failure and tubular anomalies which have also been described by Blackburn. Surviving patients will eventually attain a height somewhat above achondroplasts, approximately 1.35 m. Their height displays a considerable degree of variation (McKusick).

Radiographic Findings

The long bones display a plump appearance at birth, particularly at the ends. Thus, the proximal end of the

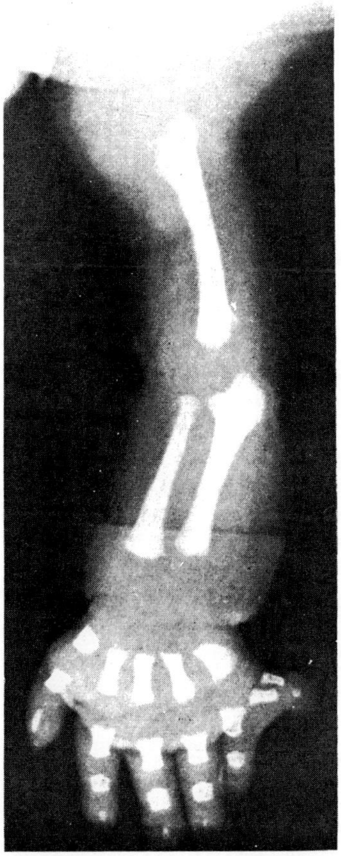

Fig. 3-37. Chondroectodermal dysplasia in a newborn. Notice the square appearance of the elements of the upper extremity, the small metaphyseal spur formation at the distal humerus, polydactyly, and narrow filiform appearance of the distal phylanges.

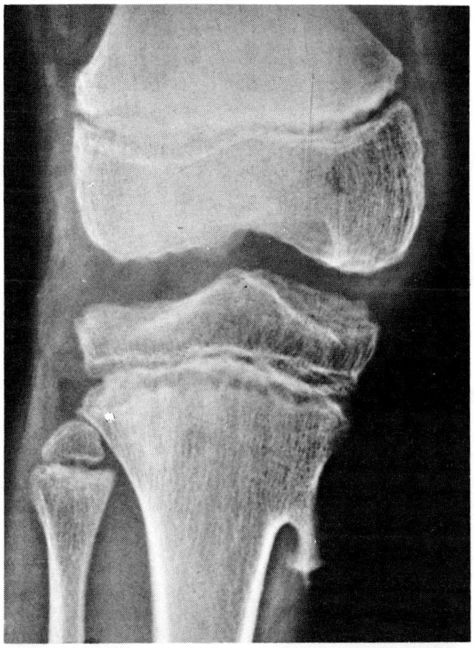

Fig. 3-38. Chondroectodermal dysplasia in a 7-year-old boy. Note the deformity of the tibial plateau and the small medial tibial exostosis.

tibia and the ulna assume a rather characteristic clubbed form (Fig. 3-37). The upper end of the humerus is large and oblique both distally and laterally. A small spur may be present at the metaphyseal end. When this is noted a lateral view should always be requested. The most pronounced shortening affects the middle segment, and in particular, of the lower extremities. The bones of the hand are plump, the extra metacarpals more or less malformed, and sometimes bifid. Proximal and middle phalanges are short, and often have an irregular metaphysis with slight concavity. The distal phalanges have a very characteristic filiform appearance.

The iliac bones are square and the acetabular roof has a very unusual appearance. It is horizontal with a medial convex socket with one spur on either side (Fig. 3-41). The ribs are often shortened with widened anterior ends. Contrary to this, there is an entirely normal skull and spine. During growth one can expect the appearance of further radiographic signs. The most characteristic one is the fusion of the os capitatum and hamatum which is occasionally associated with other malformed elements in the carpal region. This may involve the distal supernumerary bone and an asymmetric tibial plateau with flattening or hypoplasia of the lateral tibial plateau. This asymmetry is accompanied by a modeling defect of the upper tibial metaphysis and often by a small internal exostosis. The combination of these anomalies and the elective shortening of the middle segment of the lower extremity offers a very characteristic appearance and allows the well informed observer to establish the diagnosis of Ellis-Van Crefeld syndrome (Fig. 3-38). The widening of the ends of long bones may become more pronounced, especially at the proximal end of the ulna, and also to a minor degree, at the radius. Deformity of epiphyses and metaphyses of the phalanges result in a characteristic appearance as "cone-shaped epiphyses" (Fig. 3-39). This is most frequently present in the middle and distal phalanges. Those are proportionally much shorter than the proximal phalanges. The feet may show similar involvement as may the tarsal bones (lack of cuneiform bone). There is sometimes promi-

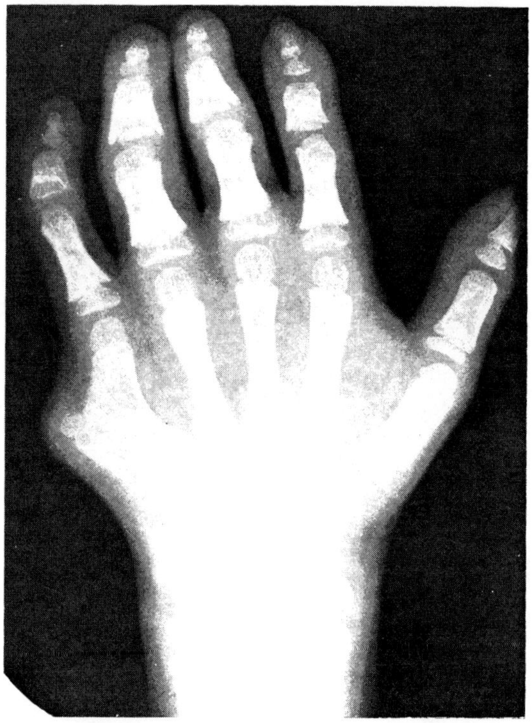

Fig. 3-39. A 7-year-old boy with chondroectodermal dysplasia. Notice fusion between capitate and hamate bones and the cone-shaped epiphyses. An extra finger has been surgically removed.

nent shortening of the extremities, very similar to the appearance of spondyloepiphyseal dysplasias or acrodysostosis (see p. 79). The skull and spine generally remain normal.

Genetic Data and Pathogenesis

A high degree of parental consanguinity and similar involvement of brothers and sisters strongly supports an autosomal recessive transmission. This disorder has been recognized by McKusick in the Amish community. Occasionally, minor anomalies have been noted in parents, and in particular, polydactyly. The interpretation of this finding is difficult.

The pathogenesis of this disorder is totally unknown. Study of the growth cartilage in its fatal forms shows that this structure is markedly disorganized. Hypertrophic cells are present without columnar arrangements. The ossification zone is extremely irregular and islands of cartilage may persist within the bony lamellae. The perichondral ring is abnormally long and in some areas it seems to be wider than usual. On the other hand, there is a lateral prolongation of cartilage towards the diaphysis alongside the periosteum. Within the latter there can be inclusions of cartilage which are recognizable at some distance from the growth cartilage.

Certain types of chondroectodermal dysplasia are fatal. In these patients the thorax is extremely narrow and radiographically the metaphyseal ends of the long bones are very irregular with prominent lateral spur formation (Le Marec et al.). This appearance is different from that of the form described by Saldino (see p. 36).

The absence of nails, together with the slenderness or lack of formation of the terminal phalanges, can be seen in infants born to mothers treated with hydantoin and in the Coffin-Siris syndrome combined with mental retardation. These conditions, however, are never confused with chondroectodermal dysplasia.

ASPHYXIATING THORACIC DYSPLASIA

Described by Jeune in 1954, this is a disorder with close similarities to the preceding condition, at least with respect to its radiographic appearance.

Clinical Findings

This disorder is not always recognized at birth. If the examination is not very thorough, it is possible to simply overlook the narrow thorax and the mild degree of shortening of the extremities. It is not surprising that respiratory problems of severe and recidivating character sometimes lead to a careful examination after a few weeks or months.

It is clinically impressive how very narrow and stiff the thorax remains during respiration (Fig. 3-40). Rare patients with extra fingers and dental anomalies are on record. The extremities are mildly shortened, but do not show significant morphologic changes. Signs of respiratory disturbances, such as dyspnea, retractions, and cyanosis are frequent.

The course is often fatal. In some patients, however, the involvement of the thorax is not as intense, increasing the chances of survival (Neimann). It appears that the risk of respiratory difficulties decreases with prolonged survival in spite of the fact that growth of the thorax remains abnormal. Another complication may be the development of renal failure. The mechanism of this complication is not consistent. There may be atrophy and tubular dilatation with significant interstitial fibrosis and infiltration by round cells (Herdman and Langer, Rabusson-Corvisard), or polycystic disease (Shokeir et al., Leclerc et al.).

It is needless to emphasize the serious prognosis of

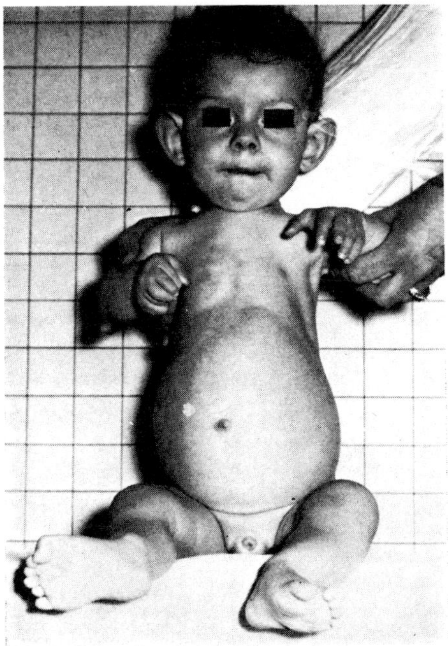

Fig. 3-40. Note the narrow thorax in this 9-month-old infant with asphyxiating thoracic dysplasia.

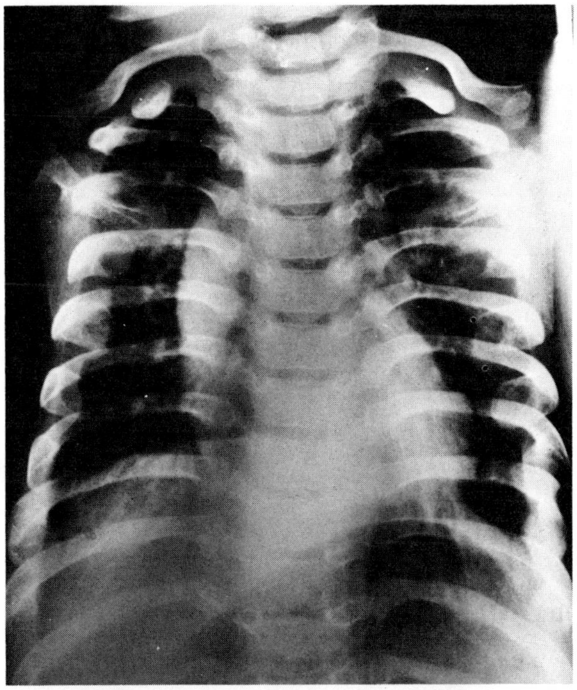

Fig. 3-41. Asphyxiating thoracic dysplasia in a 9-month-old infant. Notice the narrow cylindrical appearance of the thorax with short ribs.

this disease. In the majority of cases death is due to respiratory problems and occurs prior to the second year of life and even if there is survival there is the danger of renal failure.

Radiographic Findings

In the baby we find extreme shortening of the horizontal and coarse ribs with distal flaring (Fig. 3-41). The degree to which the ribs have been shortened is best seen on a lateral view. There is a slight irregularity of the metaphyses in the long bones along with a small peripheral spur. The abnormal findings of the iliac bones and the acetabular region are very similar to those already described for chondroectodermal dysplasia. This involves a middle protruberance with a spur on either side (Fig. 3-42). There are some patients, however, whose pelvic involvement is limited to a small acetabular angle and a square appearance of the iliac bones. In this situation it may be difficult to be certain about the diagnosis.

The appearance of the hand varies. Sometimes the phalanges have a coarse, square appearance and the metaphyses of metacarpals may be concave. The distal phalanges are not affected in this manner, but may have a median spur. Some patients show delayed ossification of the phalanges, particularly of the toes. On rare occasions entirely normal hands may be present.

The spine and skull are not affected. In the surviving patients we fail to find characteristic changes, for chondronectodermal dysplasia—the abnormal tibial plateau and the fusion of the hamate and capitate. The growth of the ribs is markedly delayed and the narrow thorax does not change in appearance. Metaphyseal changes of the long bones can be noted, particularly in the femoral neck. There is no coxa vara. The phalanges are quite often the seat of cone-shaped epiphyses.

Genetic Data, Pathogenesis, and Treatment

The disorder is familial and is transmitted by an autosomal recessive gene. Its pathogenetic mechanism is unknown. Biopsies of cartilage from ribs reveal an abnormal growth zone characterized by an obliquity of the costochondral junction and by anarchic arrangement of the cartilaginous columns which are of reduced height. Pulmonary hypoplasia has been reported with a major reduction in the number of alveoli and canals (Feingold et al.). In addition to renal anomalies there have been observations of changes in the liver parenchyma, dilatation and proliferation of biliary canals, and periportal fibrosis (Shokeir et al., Rabusson-Corvisard).

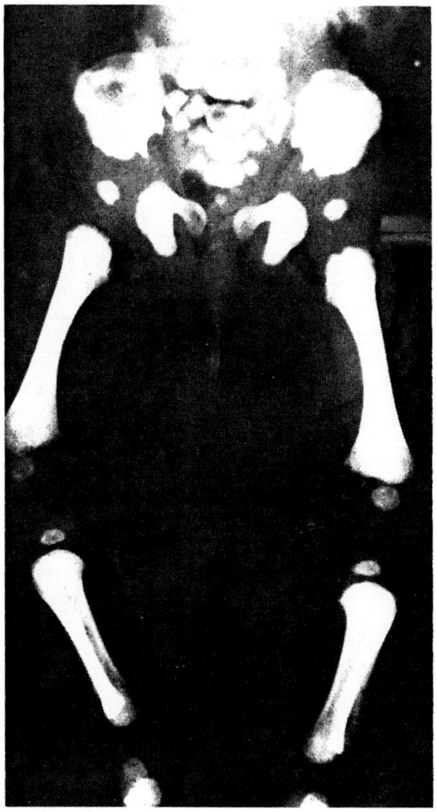

Fig. 3-42. This is a newborn patient with asphyxiating thoracic dysplasia. Notice the characteristic radiographic appearance of the iliac bones, which is similar to that seen in patients with chondroectodermal dysplasia, and also the irregular metaphyseal outline of the long bones. As a special finding, there is an unusually advanced and early ossification of both femoral heads.

Therapy will attempt to overcome airway and pulmonary infections and will be directed against respiratory failure. Antibiotics and oxygen will be combined with endotracheal aspiration and postural drainage. Alimentation should be at least by gavage feeding, and by gastrostomy in the most severe cases. These patients must be vaccinated against the flu, German measles, whooping cough and other infectious diseases. If such a patient survives the initial acute respiratory embarrassment, a surgical intervention aiming to increase the thoracic capacity may be discussed (Razzi et al., Barnes et al.).

There are obvious analogies between asphyxiating thoracic dysplasia and chondroectodermal dysplasia. In certain patients with dental anomalies or extra fingers, it may be difficult to arrive at the correct diagnosis. We have no doubt, though, that we are dealing here with two distinctly different diseases, due to separate genes, with a relatively close expressivity.

Some of the fatal forms of thoracic dysplasia should not be confused with thanatophoric dwarfism (see p. 33). There are a number of chondrodysplasias, achondroplasia or metatropic dwarfism, for example, with an abnormally narrow thorax. There should be no problem in distinguishing these from one another.

CLEIDOCRANIAL DYSPLASIA

This disorder was originally described in 1898 under the name of cleidocranial dysostosis by Pierre Marie and Sainton. Yet patients with this disorder had been seen earlier, most likely since 1765 (Martin). A number of other names have been proposed—mutational dysostosis (Rhinehart), osteodental dysostosis (Jackson), and pelvicocleidocranial dysplasia (Kaufmann). This disorder is the result of abnormal growth and not by our definition a dysostosis. We therefore prefer the name cleidocranial dysplasia.

Clinical Findings

The disorder can be recognized from birth, primarily because of the deficient ossification of the cranial vault. This is the case, in particular with families known to be affected. Often the diagnosis is delayed. The persistence of the anterior fontanelle associated with the abnormally shaped skull and foreheard frequently evokes a worried response from parents and their physician. In other cases recognition of the disorder may also follow an examination performed because of the individual's short stature, abnormal shoulder movements, walking difficulties or, dental anomalies. Rather exceptionally, discovery may be an unexpected one during a routine radiographic chest examination or when a woman develops obstetrical difficulties.

Physical examination reveals a brachycephalic skull with frontal bossing, occasionally separated by a somewhat noticeable medial vertical groove. Facial structures are small, the bridge of the nose is often deep seated, and the eyes seem to be somewhat protruding because of the recessed lower orbital rims (Fig. 3-43). The mandible displays prognathism, and besides a gothic arch, there is an anarchic arrangement of teeth. The primary dentition appears late, and is often incomplete with these teeth often persisting into adulthood. The definitive dentition is equally abnormal in its timing and development. The teeth are poorly aligned, of bad quality, and are small and malformed. The roof of the palate is highly arched.

The patient is usually not very disturbed by the abnormal movements which may possibly result from the absence of the clavicles, and may actually be the only

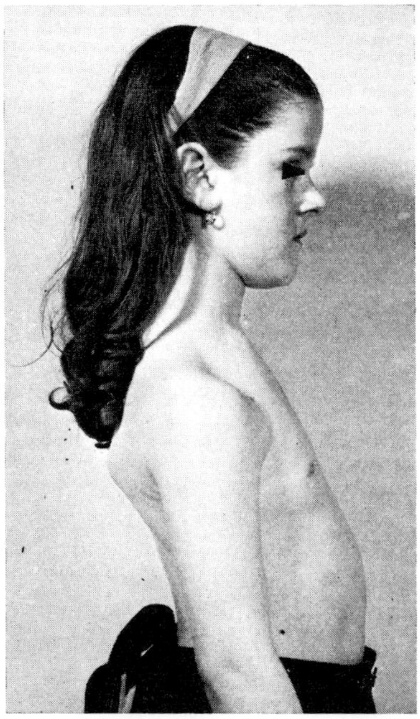

Fig. 3-43. Cleidocranial dysplasia. There is insufficient development of the facial structures and the normal contours of the shoulder have disappeared.

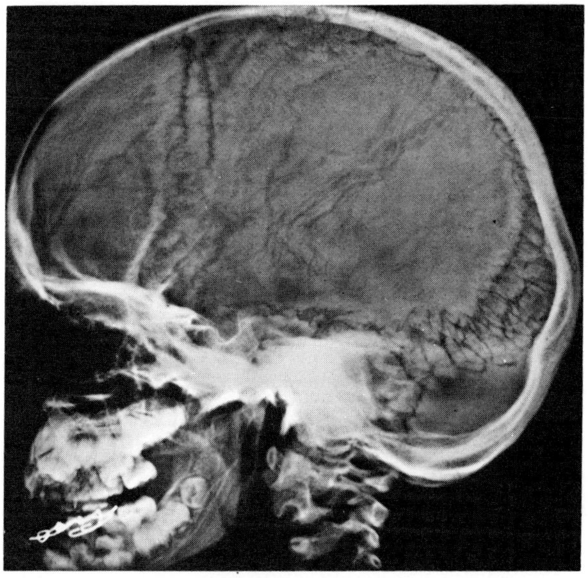

Fig. 3-44. Cleidocranial dysplasia in a 13-year-old boy. Note the large head with numerous wormian bones, the patent anterior fontanelle, and malaligned teeth.

functional manifestation of the disease. A careful physical examination reveals a shoulder of abnormally low position and prominence. Severe scoliosis and other spinal problems are not exceptional.

The extremities are only mildly affected. Genu valgum is seen with some regularity. Coxa vara may develop and can result in abnormal and painful walking. The fingers are often short and square with bulging fingernails, sometimes breaking easily and of poor quality. The shortness of the thumb is more marked than that of the other fingers.

The height is mildly affected, but these patients are not really dwarfed. These patients as a rule can be considered to have a normal mental status. There are some patients with a slight degree of mental retardation.

On the whole, we can consider this disorder to have a good prognosis, since the disturbance of growth is mild and the clavicular anomalies are hardly disturbing. Concern may be caused by the abnormal appearance which results from the craniofacial changes. The abnormal development of the pelvis leads in a number of affected women to dystocia. Complications are rarely seen with the exception of coxa vara. A recent study by Bach and collaborators reveals the possibility of several neurologic disturbances. If the etiology of such changes is still under discussion, we must seriously consider the possibility of spinal compression, secondary to the abnormal growth and form of the spine.

Radiographic Findings

The radiographic alterations present at birth and during infancy do not considerably differ from those which are present later in life. We would like to emphasize the degree of delayed skeletal maturation, which is more pronounced at an early age, though it may become less so later. This not only refers to the ossification of the skull, the clavicles and the pelvis, but also to the ossification of other skeletal areas, and in particular to the vertebral bodies which maintain the appearance of a newborn. Respiratory problems occasionally result from the shortness of the ribs.

In the older child, this can be noted by clinical findings, such as transverse enlargement, the persisting anterior fontanelle, frontal bossing and a median groove in between. Sutures remain wide, winding and a number of wormian bones are present in the occipital region which occasionally appear as a partial mosaic (Fig. 3-44). The body of the sphenoid is widened and shortened. Basilar impression is not exceptional, but this may only be simulated by an abnormal orientation on the foramen magnum. The posterior occipital synchondrosis may persist for as long as five years and a notch or even a defect of the posterior border of the foramen magnum can be recognized (Keats). Study of the facial structures often reveals insufficient maxillary

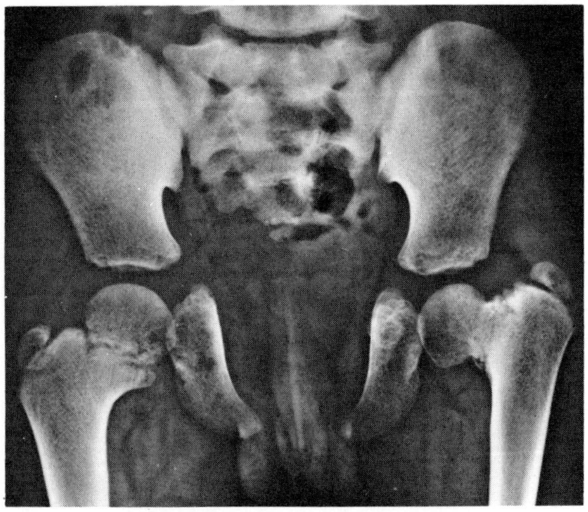

Fig. 3-45. Cleidocranial dysplasia in an 8-year-old boy. There is deficient ossification of the ischiopubic segments and coxa vara on the left.

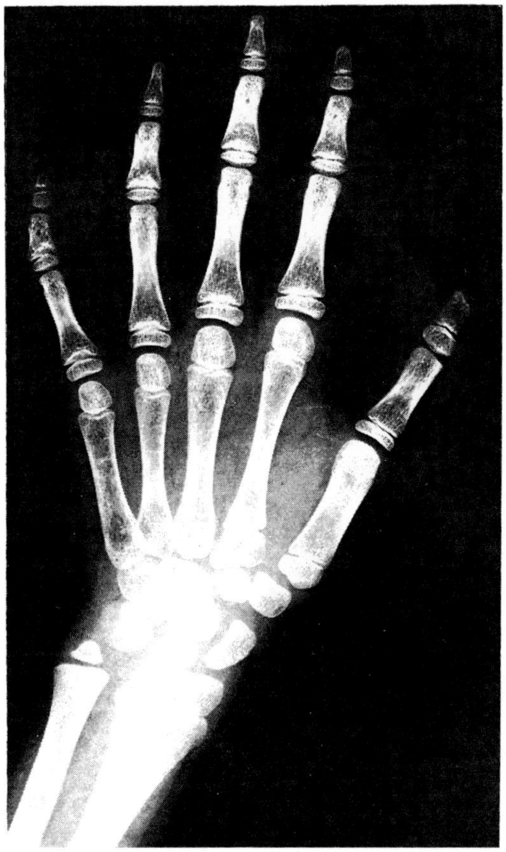

Fig. 3-46. Cleidocranial dysplasia in a 10-year-old girl. Note the large epiphyses of the terminal phalanges, the irregular metaphyses, and the mild degree of coneshaped epiphyses.

development. The mandibular angle may be increased with noticeable prognathism. Radiographs will confirm the presence of numerous dental anomalies along with a number of retained teeth.

The degree of clavicular involvement varies and is often asymmetric. Frequently there are one or two rudimentary stumps articulating with the sternum or acromion. Total absence is rarely seen more than once in 10 patients. The scapula is small with hypoplasia or bipartite acromion and a glenoid cavity.

Pelvic alterations have an equally high incidence and are quite characteristic. There is a marked delay of ossification of the pubis and ischio-pubic segments which results in a wide appearance of the symphysis pubis. The iliac wings are narrow. The pelvis itself is narrow and quite often asymmetric. Anomalies of the femoral neck, especially a coxa vara, can eventually lead to marked disturbances of leg function. The femoral head may be too large in relation to its neck (Fig. 3-45).

The biconvex aspect of vertebral bodies, a normal finding in the baby, persists for an abnormal length of time. Spina bifida, which results from a delayed fusion of the posterior arches and enlargement of synchondrosis between the body and the posterior arches, is seen with relative frequency. Finally some patients show the presence of supernumerary ossification centers. Wedged vertebrae may be responsible for an abnormal curvature, and this may result in a severe scoliosis.

The most characteristic changes of the upper extremity affect the hand. The slender metacarpals usually appear somewhat long, and they often have pseudo-epiphyses, particularly at the proximal end of the second metacarpal bone, which thereby assumes a conic appearance. The end phalanx of the fifth finger is shortened and the metaphysis of the middle phalanx is abnormally formed and looks like a "cone-shaped epiphysis." The end phalanges are coarse, massive, and triangular. Their epiphyses, larger than usual, are almost square. This is especially true of the thumb. The appearance of a pseudo-epiphysis is not unusual (Fig. 3-46). The foot is equally affected. Sometimes there is a mild degree of modeling in the metaphyseal region.

In the adolescent and adult symptoms will not be as defined. Aside from the clavicular anomalies, if present, there may be only a few remaining skeletal abnormalities. These may include a narrow pelvis, small iliac wings, an irregular symphysis, unusual length of the second metacarpal, shortening of several phalanges, and widening of the skull with midfrontal flattening.

In a younger child, radiographic studies will reveal a more extensive skeletal lesion than was suspected clinically. It must be emphasized that no single finding is constant, and that there are observations on record, where either the skull or the clavicles are entirely normal.

Genetic Data

Cleidocranial dysplasia is transmitted as a dominant disorder as Lasker has demonstrated. A number of cases seem to represent an isolated appearance, but before this can be accepted as a new mutation, one must carefully study the entire family. Such incomplete forms may only be accepted after a thorough skeletal survey has been obtained.

The pathogenesis of this disorder is unknown. As we have demonstrated, there is not only the problem of abnormal membranous bone formation as sometimes maintained, because of the dramatic involvement of the skull. Histologic studies of the growth zone in the case studied by Zellweger and collaborators revealed a mild degree of reduction in the growth zone with an increase in its ground substance. Periosteal ossification is also diminished. According to several authors following Rushton's observation there is only acellular cement present and a total lack of cellular cement (N. H. H. Smith).

There is no reason for surgical or orthopaedic intervention other than occasional measures directed against the coxa vara or scoliosis. Dental interventions, however, are frequently needed.

DYSPLASIAS RECOGNIZED DURING INFANCY AND ADOLESCENCE

In this chapter we shall discuss the spondylo-epiphyseo-metaphyseal dysplasias and the dyschondrosteosis of Léri and Weill.

THE SPONDYLO-EPIPHYSEO-METAPHYSEAL DYSPLASIAS

In this group of disorders disturbed growth can be recognized by abnormal radiographic findings, existing simultaneously or not, within the epiphyses of long bones, the adjacent metaphyses, in the hand, the foot, and the vertebral bodies. In the German literature these disorders have been grouped under the term "polytope enchondrale Dysostose," in the English literature as "osteochondrodystrophy" and in Italian as "osteodistrofia dell'acrescimento." Considerable controversy exists with respect to the classification of these disorders. A number of authors who are perplexed by their complexity simply group them together in a single descriptive category. We consider this to be a serious error, since the prognosis and development of these disorders are fundamentally different. Admittedly our present insight is still fragmentary. However, we feel that an attempt at a classification must be made, and we follow the one worked out by a group of European specialists.

Five groups of disorders will be successively dealt with. The first four usually have only mild involvement of the spine if at all, whereas the fifth is characterized by generalized platyspondyly. The first group refers to metaphyseal chondrodysplasias, radiographically recognized by irregularities of the metaphyseal outline immediately next to the growth cartilage, and by shortened long bones. The second group shows a prominent dysplasias in a number of epiphyses with elective involvement of their structure, while the vertebrae are only mildly affected by irregular end plates and maintaining practically a normal height. The third group refers to epiphyseo-metaphyseal dysplasias with an associated involvement of epiphyses and metaphyses. Such patients usually have micromelia. Involvement of the spine varies. The fourth group deals with acrodysplasias, particularly epiphyseo-metaphyseal or epiphyseal lesions localized in the extremities. Generalized platyspondylies are disorders where the height of all vertebral bodies is reduced in the presence of a mild, or somewhat more severe involvement, of the epiphyses or metaphyses. The latter may sometimes be absent. The symptomatology of these disorders varies. They all have in common a rather peculiar evolution, and only in unusual cases are they recognized at birth. This is in spite of the fact that they may eventually result in the most severe type of skeletal pathology. One disorder must be singled out from this group: congenital spondyloepiphyseal dysplasia is actually recognized from birth, thus we have discussed this disorder earlier. Other chondrodysplasias can show radiographic changes of the epiphyses and metaphyses, such as in diatrophic dwarfism or metatropic dwarfism. These have, however, other clinical and radiographic characteristics, which led to their individual definition. The Kashin-Beck disease is an endemic disorder with a characteristic geographic distribution in the Transbaikal region in Korea. Unanswered questions about its etiology and exact characteristics have led to its elimination from this study.

Some readers will be surprised at the relative simplicity of this chapter as we discuss the details. We have limited ourselves to the description of well defined disorders. Without any question there are other types of these dysplasias. It does not yet seem possible to accept an isolated description, or deal with a questionable entity. We will, however, mention some of those problems at the end of this chapter.

METAPHYSEAL CHONDRODYSPLASIAS

This term is preferred to the one created in 1934 by Jansen, who then spoke of "metaphyseal dystostosis." He thereby described a group of disorders with marked radiographic alterations of the metaphyses in long bones during growth without abnormal development of epiphyses.

If the disorder originally described by Jansen is a very rare one, this is not the case for the later described types. However, we can now distinguish the dominant type of Schmid, the autosomal recessive type (McKusick-cartilage hair hypoplasia), the Jansen type, and the metaphyseal dysplasias which have been observed to combine with the malabsorption syndrome with neutropenia and thymic lymphopenia.

Dominant Metaphyseal Chondrodysplasia of the Schmid Type

Clinical Study

This disease is usually recognized towards the second year because of a growth deficit or bowing of the lower extremities which is sometimes combined with a limp.

The disease can present with a mild degree of micromelia as the definitive adult height is around 1.40 m. Generally the length of the spine is normal, but the extremities are shortened. This shortening is sometimes more pronounced in the proximal segments. The pelvis is broad resulting from coxa vara and quite often there is bowing and varus deformity of the lower extremities. The feet are normal as is the skull and the facial structures (Fig. 3-47). There is no limitation in joint-movements with the single exception of abduction of the hip. The gait is waddling.

Radiographic Findings

Radiographic findings include metaphyseal changes and a local irregularity of the outline at the growth zone. This area may be uneven and serrated. The adjacent zone is abnormally structured with a clearer zone which is comparable to cartilaginous inclusions separated by darker zones. Contrary to this there is essentially normal form and structural development of the epiphyseal centers (Fig. 3-48). The diaphyses are short and broad at the extremities. The metaphyses sometimes widen abruptly, especially at the lower end of the femur.

The Schmid type of lesions are seen principally at the metaphyses of the femur as well as at the proximal metaphyses of the humerus and tibia. The lower end of radius and ulna along with tibia and fibula are also often involved and even the ribs may be affected. Contrary to this there is usually no involvement of the hands and feet nor of the spine and skull. In the area of the hip the metaphyseal lesions can lead to a short femoral neck and coxa valga. Sometimes scoliosis appears towards adolescence.

The metephyseal irregularities will disappear completely after the growth zone closes. This can happen early. Once this stage is reached it is very difficult to establish the diagnosis. The presence of coxa vara associated with short and broad long bones is suggestive of this disorder.

Genetic Data

The Schmid type is transmitted by autosomal dominant inheritance and familial studies are very important to the diagnosis. The discovery of an affected child may actually be the only reliable way to confirm the diagnosis in an affected adult.

There are a number of bilateral observations of coxa vara with similar radiographic appearance to the Schmid type. This is in spite of the fact that no other metaphyseal anomalies can be recognized. It is probably a wise idea to group them with the type Schmid, possible as a variant of minor expressivity.

Pathology and Pathogenesis

Histologic study of growth cartilage up until the present has not revealed any specific findings for metaphyseal chondrodysplasia and further study of this problem is needed. The columns are reduced in height and cellular clusters, more or less elongated, seem to lose their axial orientation. Cartilaginous islands persist right next to the zone of transitional calcification. The line of ossification is irregular. Sometimes cartilaginous bands of variable dimension are found within the metaphysis. The cortical bone, the spongiosa and the epiphyses are all normal.

Cooper and his collaborators emphasize that they have noted dilatation of the endoplasmatic reticulum by ultrastructural study of chondrocytes of the iliac crest. We conclude that this observation in spite of

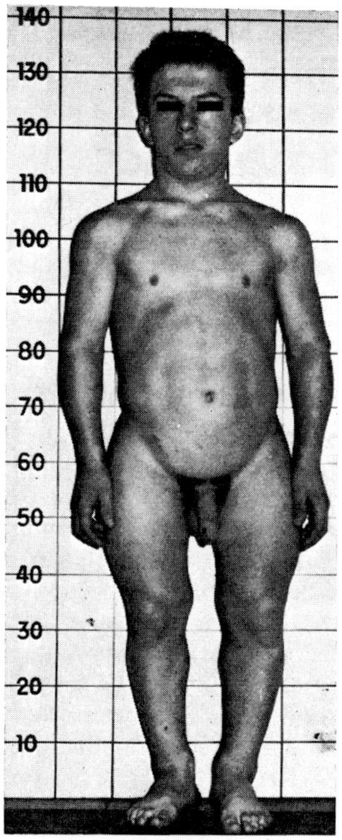

Fig. 3-47. Metaphyseal dysostosis type Schmid with micromelia and without facial alterations.

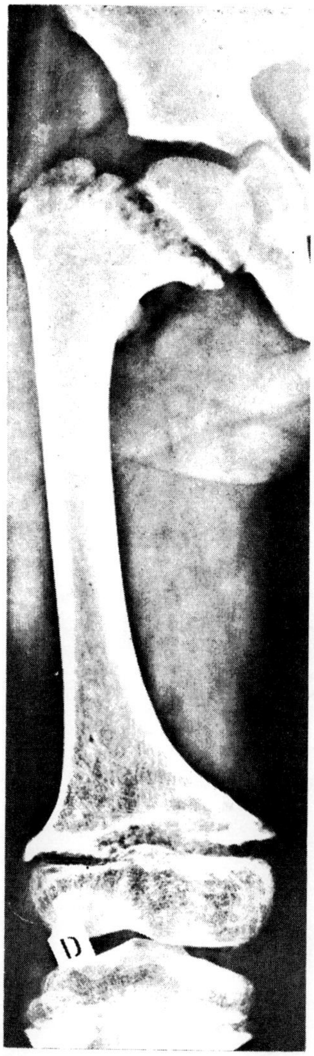

Fig. 3-48. Metaphyseal dysostosis type Schmid in a 12-year-old boy. There is coxa vara and irregularity of metaphyseal ends.

vague findings involving the vertebral bodies, should be grouped with the Schmid type rather than with the spondylometaphyseal dysplasias. The specificity of the described findings needs to be further confirmed.

The pathology of this disorder and those that we will subsequently discuss is still unknown. However, we will see that a disturbed metabolism of phosphorus and calcium appears to play a role in the Jansen type.

Confusion of these patients with a vitamin D resistant form of rickets must be avoided, since the intake of high doses of vitamin D is ineffective, unnecessary, and usually poorly tolerated in patients with metaphyseal chondrodysplasia. There are never abnormal findings of the bony stroma and the characteristic diaphyseal bowing of rickets is missing.

Autosomal Recessive Metaphyseal Chondrodysplasia

This type is relatively similar to the one just described, but the metaphyseal lesions are almost totally nonexistent in the proximal metaphyses of the femur and humerus, while there is marked involvement of bones of the hands and feet. This disorder is usually recognized towards the second year because of growth retardation. Micromelic dwarfism is accompanied by moderately shortened extremities, however, there is no pelvic widening. Radiographically there is similarity with the lesions of the preceding type, but their distribution is entirely different.

The distal femoral metaphysis and the proximal tibial metaphysis are most prominently involved by an irregularity in outline and structure as we have just described (Fig. 3-49). The distal epiphyses of the radius and tibia usually show mild involvement. The ac-

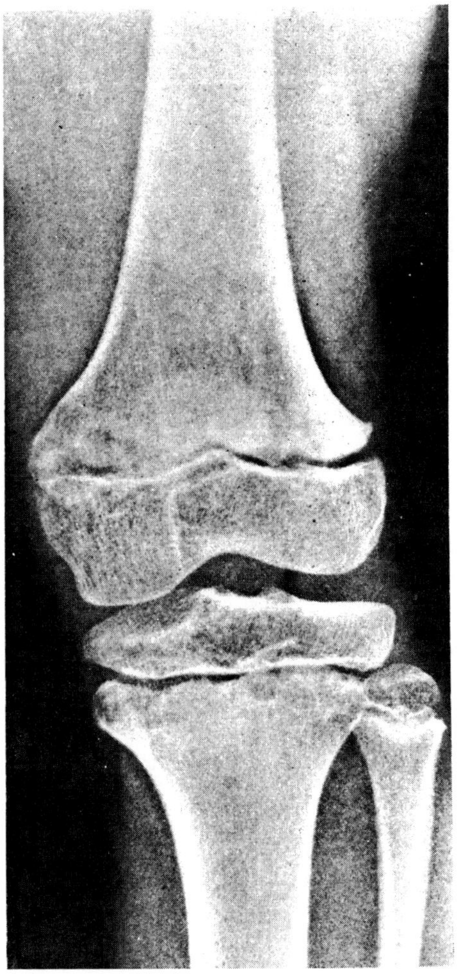

Fig. 3-49. Metaphyseal dysostosis of an autosomal recessive type, in an 11-year-old girl. Note the marked involvement of the metaphyses of the bones of the knee.

tively growing metaphyses of the metacarpals, the metatarsals, and the phalanges are regularly involved. This is in contrast to the Schmid type. Their border is irregular, wavy, and the diaphyses are somewhat short and plump. The proximal femoral metaphysis is normal in appearance. This area can sometimes be mildly abnormal, however, coxa vara is never seen.

Patients with the autosomal recessive type frequently have sparse, thin hair which is usually blonde. McKusick has carefully studied this disease in the Amish and has proposed the term "cartilage hair hypoplasia." This disorder is not rare and occurs regularly all over the world (Fig. 3-50). Occasionally there is abnormal intestinal absorption, an abnormal sensitivity to viral infections (McKusick), or a Blackfan-Diamond anemia (Sacrez et al., Lhirondel et

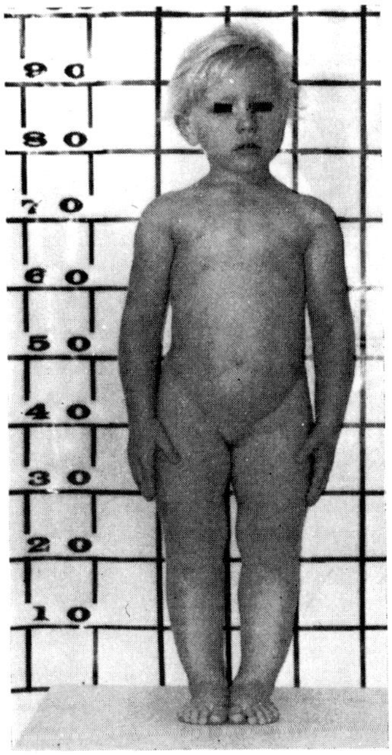

Fig. 3-50. Metaphyseal dysostosis, of autosomal recessive type with scarce hair.

al.). In all likelihood there is another variety of metaphyseal chondrodysplasia, probably due to another recessive gene, not accompanied by anomalies of ectodermal appendages, but with an identical radiographic appearance. On the other hand, Spahr has described a recessive form very similar to the dominant Schmid type.

The Jansen Type

This exceedingly rare disorder can generally be recognized from birth on, because of growth disturbances, an abnormal walk, or incurving of the extremities. Dwarfism is severe and electively involves the extremities, visibly deformed by epiphyseal prominence, which may be palpable.

On radiographs there is generalized and unusually severe metaphyseal involvement (Fig. 3-51). All metaphyses are considerably widened, with extremely irregular structure and unequally calcified areas which alternate with hyperlucent zones. The distal portions of the extremities are as involved as the long bones. The diaphyses are short and massive. Sometimes there is craniosynostosis (Gram). After closure of the growth zone, clubbing of the metaphysis persists with increased radiolucency.

Because hypercalcemia has been observed in several of these patients, there is a suggestion of abnormal metabolism of phosphorus and calcium in this type. The cases presently on record have been all boys and in one family two generations have been involved. This suggests a dominant transmission.

Besides the Jansen type we should mention certain recessive observations showing metaphyseal lesions of some severity with clear deep cone-shaped zones within the metaphyses (Vaandrager). Sometimes there is a slight reduction in vertebral height (Pena, Kozlowski). Rimoin has described yet another recessive type which manifests severe micromelia and marked shortening of the hands and feet. These skeletal lesions are associated with deafness and mental retardation.

Metaphyseal Anomalies Associated With Malabsorption With or Without Neutropenia or With Lymphopenia and Thymic Aplasia

Within the last few years there has been considerable interest in the association of radiographic metaphyseal changes accompanied by growth disturbances which are secondary to pancreatic insufficiency with or without neutropenia. Metaphyseal changes electively touch the proximal ends of the femur in spite of the fact that others may also be involved, for example, the knee or ribs (Burke). The severity of the lesions varies (coxa vara with severe deformity of the neck or simply irregularities of the metaphysis itself).

Metaphyseal lesions may also be seen in thymic aplasia with lymphopenia. In these cases there may be metaphyseal irregularities which usually present very early, and possibly involve all metaphyses of the long bones and ribs. Sometimes there is abnormal pelvic development similar to the changes seen in asphyxiating thoracic dysplasia or chondroectodermal dysplasia. The height of vertebral bodies may even be affected.

We will consider the appearance of spondylometaphyseal chondrodysplasias when discussing platyspondyly (see p. 82) associating metaphyseal changes with a reduction of vertebral height.

MULTIPLE EPIPHYSEAL DYSPLASIAS

This disorder is characterized by radiographic epiphyseal changes in the presence of normal metaphyses. Spinal involvement is not always present. Affected patients show irregular vertebral end plates without any significant loss of vertebral height.

In this chapter we present a discussion of dominant multiple epiphyseal dysplasia and its variants, in particular the localized types and hereditary arthroophthalmopathy.

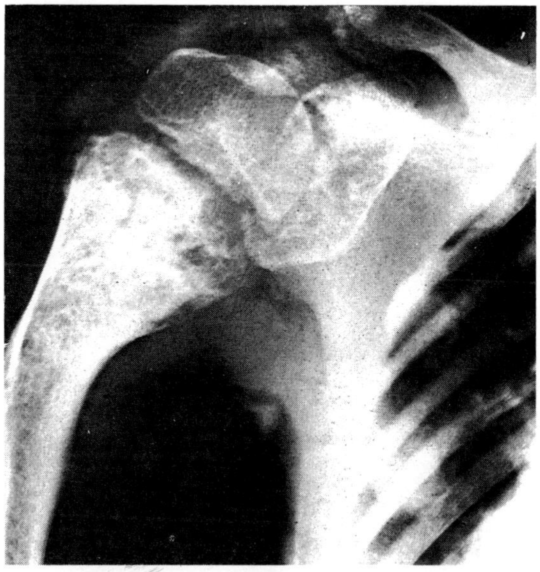

Fig. 3-51. Metaphyseal dysostosis type Jansen. Note the marked metaphyseal irregularities. (Courtesy of S. Weil)

The separation of this disorder from achondroplasia goes back to the description by Barrington Ward in 1912. It was further delineated and characterized by the publications of Müller, Fairbank, Ribbing, Clément, Turpin, and Coste. Contrary to what the name implies, there is frequently spinal involvement. This, however, can only be recognized on radiographs. The French term "polyosteochondrite" proposed by Turpin and Coste has also been used. For detailed description we refer to the most frequently seen dominant type described by Fairbank.

Clinical Findings

Multiple epiphyseal dysplasia is recognized at varying ages, however, most frequently between the second and tenth year. At times, it is detected in adulthood because of arthrosis development. In other cases an infant will have a noticeable waddling gait. Patients with this disease most frequently complain because of altered joint function which may take the form of a disturbed gait, movement limitation, or joint pain. These may become more accentuated during growth.

At physical examination a mild degree of shortening will be found. Adults reach a height of approximately 1.50 m. The trunk is normal, but the extremities are somewhat shortened. The hands and feet are characteristically coarse (Fig. 3-52). Sometimes patients have varus deformity of the lower extremity or, in con-

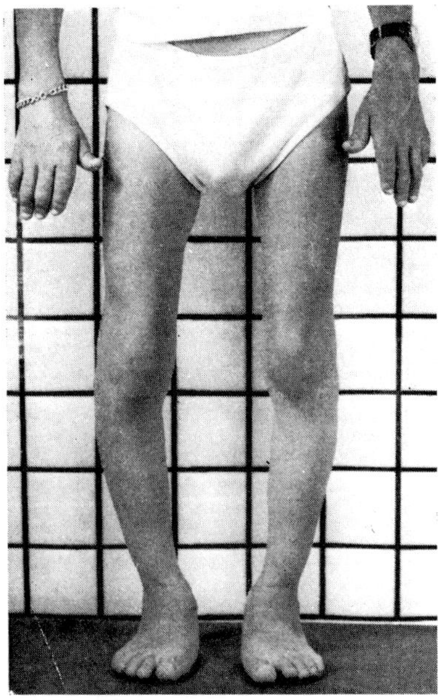

Fig. 3-52. Multiple epiphyseal dysplasia. Note the mild degree of knee deformity and the relative shortness of the hand.

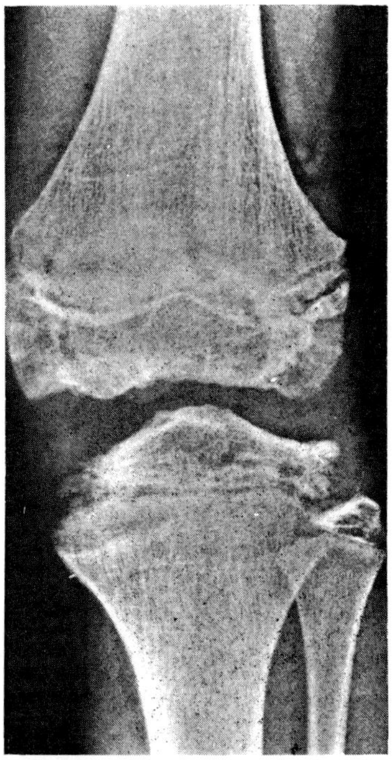

Fig. 3-53. Multiple epiphyseal dysplasia in a 15-year-old boy. Note the abnormal shape and structure of all epiphyses.

trast to this, a genu valgum. The skull and face are not involved. Studies of joint function reveal a limitation of motion in the hip, the shoulder, and frequently the elbow or knees. There are no visceral, mental, or ocular anomalies.

The most important complication of multiple epiphyseal dysplasia in the adult is the development of arthrosis, especially an early and severe hip involvement. This is the factor determining the severity of this disorder requiring proper attention, when decisions as to a professional career have to be made.

In rare instances inflammatory articular lesions were noted during the course of this disease (Briex-Corvol, Kahn et al.). Such attacks seem to occur mainly in adults affected by articular chondromes (Bouret et al.). All tests for chronic progressive polyarthritis are negative and there is no accelerated sedimentation rate. It is still difficult to determine the true nature of these findings which sometimes leads to the descriptive term *chondrodysplastic rheumatism*. This is not seen in children.

Pediatric patients often present with osteochondritis as a complication of the disease. This diagnosis can be difficult to establish. Onset of pain, a limp, and radiographic studies will confirm this finding. We have, on occasion, been able to recognize several patients with osteochondritis of the hips which we feel justifies the same management as a normal child.

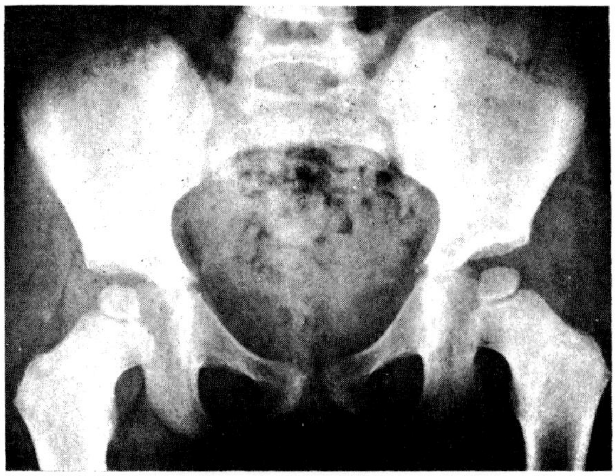

Fig. 3-54. Multiple epiphyseal dysplasia in a 5-year-old girl. Note the small and abnormally shaped femoral heads.

Radiographic Findings

Due to the inability of young infants to express themselves, these lesions will remain unnoticed since radiographs are not routinely taken. If available, radiographs will reveal slight irregularity and delayed appearance of the epiphyseal centers.

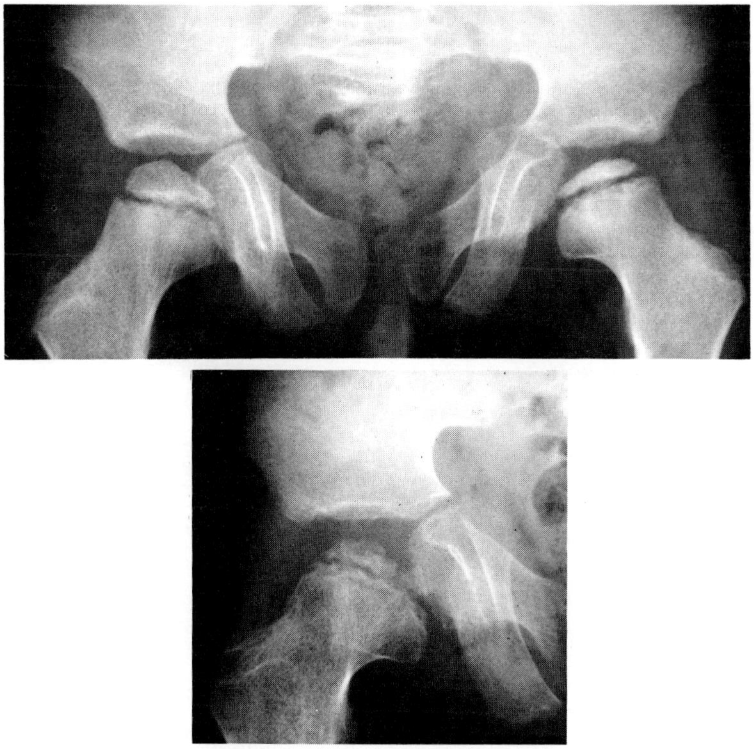

Fig. 3-55. Multiple epiphyseal dysplasia with osteochondritis of the right femoral head of a 6-year-old boy. Films obtained at 5-month intervals reveal the progressive nature of the disorder.

Most characteristic alterations can be recognized during the second year. They predominantly affect the epiphyses of long bones giving them an irregular form. Frequently they are small with an ill-defined outline. Furthermore, they are not of homogeneous structure (Fig. 3-53). There is, at times, fragmentation of the ossification center. In certain patients this appearance is very similar to that of osteochondritis dissecans. The age at which the ossification center is first recognized frequently is markedly delayed. All epiphyses may be affected. The femoral head of young patients is rounded and disproportional in comparison with its neck. It may occupy only the medial third (Fig. 3-54). Eventually there will be flattening and deformation. The neck itself may remain short and wide. The distal inferior and medial articular surface of the tibia is frequently oblique.

If there is marked asymmetry in the development of the femoral heads with a dramatic flattening on one side, possibly combined with sclerosis, this may indicate the presence of a complicating osteochondritis (Fig. 3-55). The metaphyseal zone adjacent to the epiphyses is normal with the possible exception of an occasional mild irregularity in the metaphyseal line. The hands are usually short and broad with clear metaphyseal lines. The morphology of the diaphyses in the long bones is essentially normal. The carpal and tarsal bones, however, are insufficiently and irregularly developed (Fig. 3-56). The sockets may be uneven, enlarged, and shallow.

In the great majority of patients one may find only mildly irregular end plates. Sometimes this is combined with intraspongious herniation. Changes are primarily localized in the lower thoracic or lumbar area. The facial structures and the occipito-cervical region are normal.

In the adolescent and adult, we note persistence of the deformities of the epiphyses and again would like to emphasize the precocious nature and severity of secondary arthroses which electively affect the hips. Free intraarticular bodies are present in unusually high incidence in most of the spondyloepiphyseal dysplasias, especially in multiple epiphyseal dysplasia. They are frequently found in several joints and their size is considerably larger than those usually recognized in synovial chondroarthrosis.

Pathologic Findings and Pathogenesis

The arrangement of the growth cartilage is markedly disturbed. There are only a few clusters of cells with a tendency to columnar arrangement. The zone of provi-

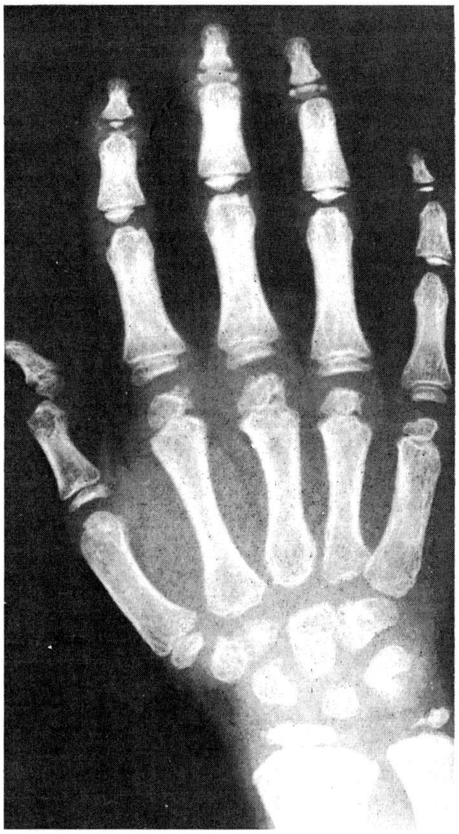

Fig. 3-56. Multiple epiphyseal dysplasia in a 10-year-old girl. There is marked anomaly in the shape of the carpal bones and of the distal epiphyses of the radius and ulna.

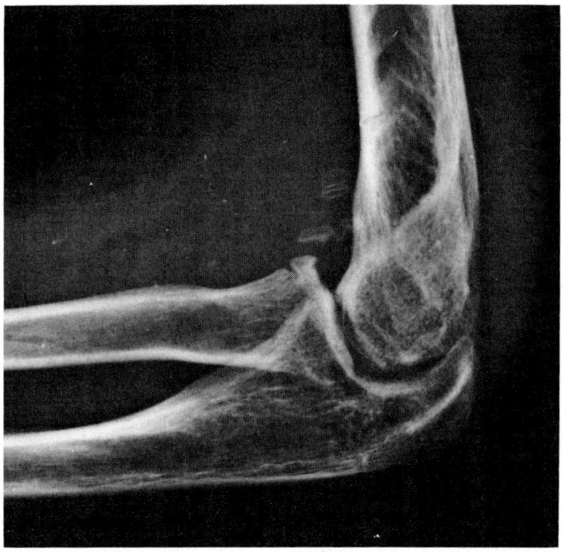

Fig. 3-57. Multiple epiphyseal dysplasia in a 15-year-old boy with elective involvement of the elbow with local osteochondromas.

sional calcification is irregular and ill defined. Vascularization appears to be normal, but the newly formed spongiosa is irregularly arranged and poorly calcified. Within the cartilage there may be fibrous strands or local areas of degeneration and necrosis.

The pathogenetic basis of this disorder is unknown. Several times we have seen infants with an elevated excretion of chondroitin-4 or chondroitin-6 sulfate, but we are unaware of the actual meaning of this inconsistent finding. Ultrastructural studies of chondrocytes in the dominant form of multiple epiphyseal dysplasia have revealed inclusions within the endoplasmatic reticulum which have an appearance quite similar to those seen in pseudo-achondroplasia. At variance with this we have recently noted, upon studying two patients with a probably recessive form, abnormal inclusions of lysosomal characteristics which may possibly contain a glycoprotein (R. Stanescu).

Genetic Data and Clinical Types

Multiple epiphyseal dysplasia is primarily transmitted as an autosomal dominant disorder. Aside from this type, there is also a recessive one. This is clearly a rarer disorder. It is clinically and radiographically quite similar and is thus hard to differentiate. The femoral head appears to be flatter and more fragmented in the young infant. The irregularities at the metaphyseal ends of the phalanges and metacarpals are not present, but cone-shaped epiphyses are noted.

In other patients with multiple epiphyseal dysplasia only certain epiphyses may be involved. Thus, a number of authors refer to families with a dominant involvement of both hips (Kehl, Brill, Monty). This is an isolated dysplasia in most of the affected patients, however, there may be an occasional situation where other epiphyses are also involved. Occasionally the femoral heads are spared in the presence of marked involvement of the distal femoral, tibial, and other epiphyses. We will discuss later that in the acrodysplasias only the most distal epiphyses of the hands and feet are involved.

We have studied other variants of this disease which involve the elbow and present at approximately 14 years of age by local pain and movement limitation. Radiographic findings include a deformed radial head and olecranon. In addition, emphasis is placed on the high incidence of osteochondromas, appearing secondarily at the elbow, usually quite rapidly (Fig. 3-57). In some instances, there may be involvement of vertebral bodies or of other epiphyses, especially at the knee, where similar findings of osteochondritis dissecans can be noted.

Special mention must be given to hereditary

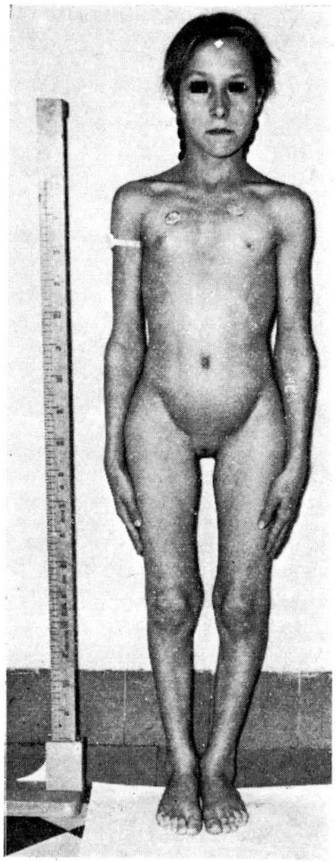

Fig. 3-58. Dysplasia involving primarily the spine. Note the relatively short trunk.

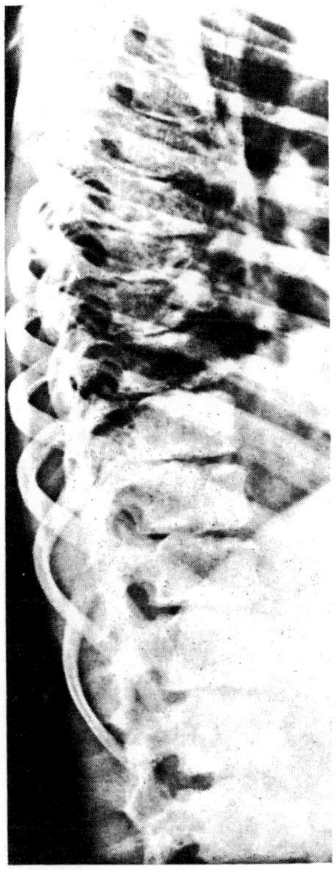

Fig. 3-59. Dysplasia involving primarily the spine in a 12-year-old girl.

arthroophthalmopathy, described by Stickler. This dominant disorder is most frequently recognized because of the presenting painful joints and a stiffness after exercise. Clinically, one finds swelling in the joints of the extremities. These changes may occur in the form of local exacerbations and thus simulate polyarthritis. A ligamentous hyperlaxity can occasionally be noted. Severe myopia and retinal detachment accompany the skeletal changes. Radiographically one can note slender diaphyses and narrow ribs. In contrast to this, the metaphyses are widened. The femoral neck is plump and poorly shaped. The epiphyses are slightly irregular or deformed and may occasionally be flat. This epiphyseal involvement usually is rather discrete or localized. The spine may be more severely involved by irregular end plates and a slight reduction of the vertebral height. Occasionally there even may be wedging. Dominant transmission has been noted.

This is not the only spondyloepiphyseal dysplasia associated with myopia. We must also note the recessive type described by Pfeiffer, which is combined with perception deafness and congenital spondyloepiphyseal dysplasia (see p. 54).

A further variant also with dominant transmission is the disorder which electively affects the spine and femoral heads. Its exact nature needs to be more precisely defined, however, because of a lack of true platyspondyly it is our thought that it belongs in this category. The disease is noted at the same age as multiple epiphyseal dysplasia and manifests by shortening of the trunk and by an antero-posterior enlargement of the thorax. All the changes are somewhat mild in nature and the extremities are not dramatically abnormal. Occasionally mild genu valgum may be present (Fig. 3-58).

Radiographic examination usually reveals extensive involvement of the spine, which practically affects all the thoracic and lumbar vertebrae. The end plates are irregular, wavy, and show intraspongious herniation. All these findings can be recognized on lateral views. Vertebral body height is only minimally affected. There may, however, be a slight wedging of one or two bodies (Fig. 3-59). The epiphyseal alterations are best noted at the level of the femoral head. Hands and feet are usually normal. As is true of the preceding forms of hip arthrosis, this will have to be strongly considered in the functional prognosis.

A poorly resolved problem is formed by excessive epiphyseal development in children with a growth deficit. We have seen several rare examples of this.

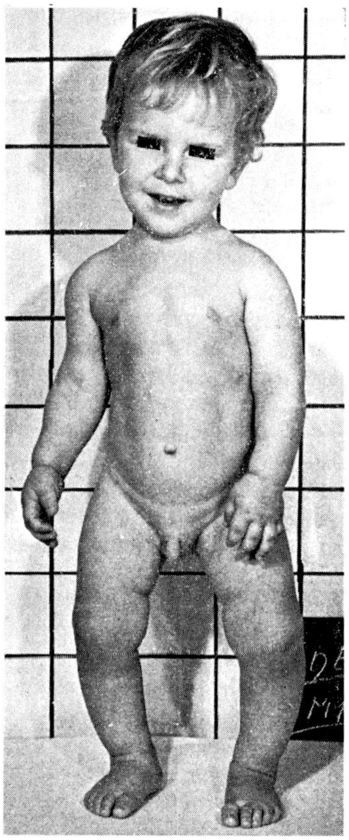

Fig. 3-60. Pseudo-achondroplasia. The shortening of the hands is particularly striking. There is no abnormal facial configuration.

Gorlin and his collaborators have published such an observation as "mega-epiphyses" in a child with homocystinuria presenting with other anomalies of skeletal growth, and especially a platyspondyly.

To close this chapter on disorders of multiple epiphyseal involvement, we emphasize the possible danger of confusing multiple epiphyseal dysplasias with hypothyreosis. This happens, in particular, to patients with ectopic location of the thyroid. Such an error would be particularly serious because of the need to offer proper therapy in hypothyroidism. This disorder must be seriously considered if the bone age is markedly retarded in the presence of fragmented epiphyses (see p. 204). If in doubt, one should never hesitate to request a plasma iodine determination.

THE EPIPHYSEOMETAPHYSEAL DYSPLASIAS

These disorders refer to the combination of radiographically recognizable changes of the epiphyses and adjacent metaphyses. The best known dysplasia is the pseudo-achondroplastic type. Its discussion is followed by a short review of othe variants.

Pseudo-Achondroplastic Dysplasia

As the name implies, this disorder has for a long time been confused with achondroplasia because of its marked micromelia. Its clinical and radiographic characteristics justify its individual nature and separation from other epiphyseo-metaphyseal dysplasias.

Clinical Findings

As a rule this disorder is recognized during the second year of life because of growth failure and walking difficulties.

The appearance is similar to achondroplasia as there is micromelic dwarfism, occasionally with rhizomelic predominance, combined with an exaggerated lumbar lordosis. Often we find discrete incurving and varus of the lower extremity, however, there are some definite findings that aid in separating the conditions on clinical grounds. Aside from the belated manifestation, one must insist on the shortness of the hands and feet, which is much more marked than that in achondroplasia. The craniofacial structures are always normal in appearance (Fig. 3-60). During further development there is marked growth failure. The hands have an unusually broad appearance and the sausage-like fingers have short nails. The gait is waddling and at times there is a discrepancy between the laxity of the hands and the limitation in movement of the more proximal joints.

There is a particularly serious prognosis since the definitive height is close to 1.10 m. In addition, there may be defective epiphyseal development resulting in early arthrosis, which may further complicate the course of the disease.

Radiographic Findings

In the very young patient there are only mild changes and slight alterations of both the epiphyses and the metaphyses may be completely overlooked by the uninitiated.

When the disorder is recognized, there is already a mild degree of diaphyseal coarseness in the long bone and an even more irregular metaphyseal line which is serrated and widened laterally by spurs. The carpal and tarsal centers and the epiphyses are too small in contrast to the enlarged metaphyses. Occasionally, an epiphysis inserts itself into a medial depression of the metaphysis, in particular, at the lower end of the femur

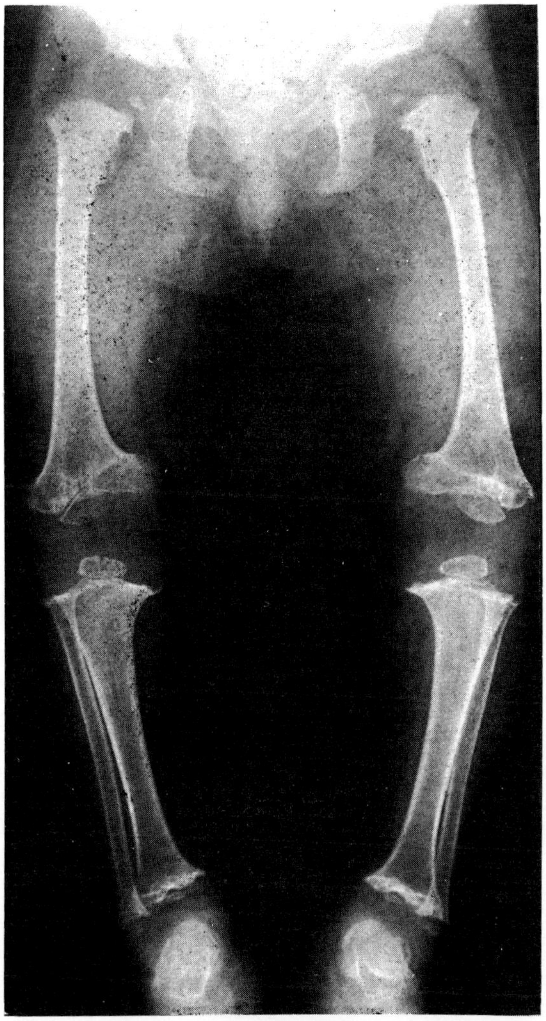

Fig. 3-61. Pseudo-achondroplasia in a 3½-year-old boy. There are marked metaphyseal alterations.

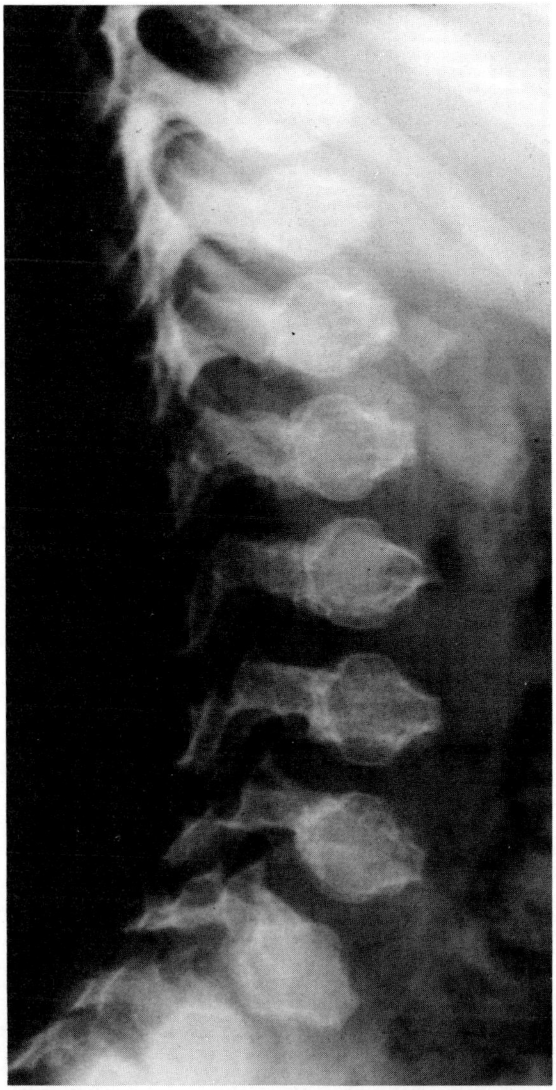

Fig. 3-62. Pseudo-achondroplasia in a 3-year-old girl. Note the marked deformity of the vertebral bodies with an anterior tonguelike protrusion.

(Fig. 3-61). The bones of the hands are especially short and coarse with a very irregular metaphyseal border. The pelvis is only minimally affected and one of the key findings is that the acetabular roof is not horizontal as in achondroplasia.

On lateral films the vertebrae are ovoid in appearance, primarily in the lumbar region. Their height is normal, but there may be an increase in their AP diameter by an anterior rectangular extension or by a slight beak, located in the midportion of the anterior border of the individual body and extending over roughly one-third of the vertebral height (Fig. 3-62). The pedicles are of normal dimension and on the AP view there is no reduction of the interpedicular distance of the inferior lumbar vertebrae. The skull and the suboxipital region are normal.

During growth the epiphyseal changes progress considerably. This is true also of the shortened and coarse appearance of the long bones, where there is only a slight accentuation of the epiphyseal and metaphyseal changes. In the adolescent and adult we find shortened long bones and the bony elements of the hands are coarse in appearance with almost square phalanges. The development and alterations of the epiphyses are such that even after closure of the growth line, they maintain diagnostic characteristics. The described alterations of the vertebral bodies during infancy and childhood will also disappear, and eventually there will be only a mild degree of wedging.

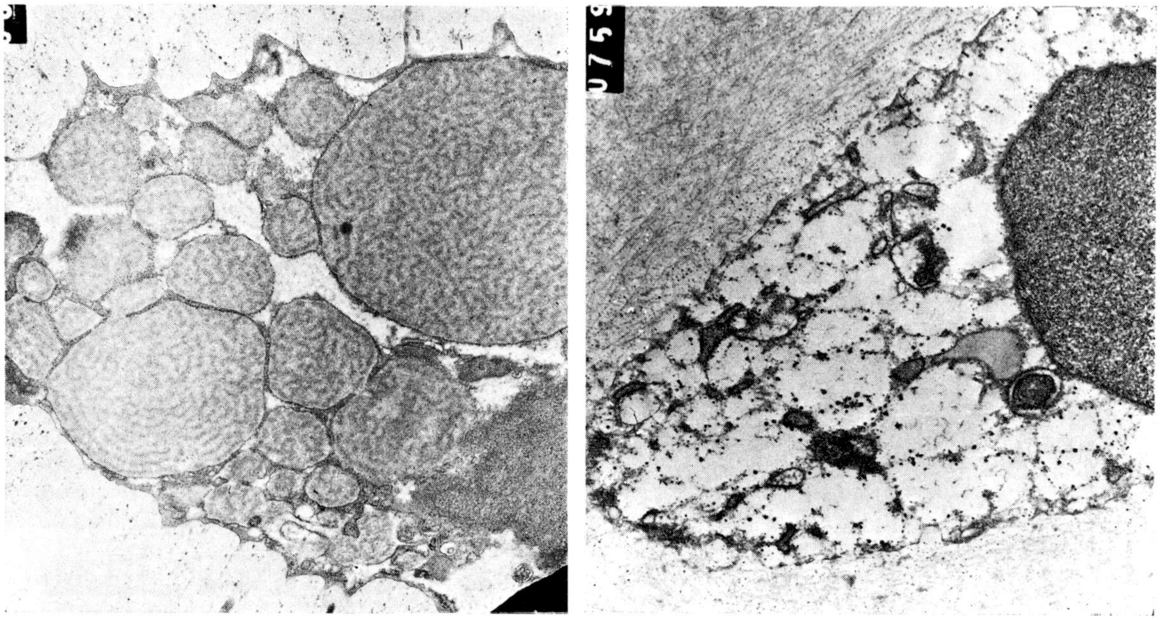

Fig. 3-63. Ultrastructural study of chondrocytes in pseudo-achondroplasia (*left*), and a variant of multiple epiphyseal dysplasia (*right*). Inclusions within the endoplasmatic reticulum are seen in pseudo-achondroplasia and vacuoles which probably contain glycoprotein are present in multiple epiphyseal dysplasia. (Courtesy R. Stanescu)

Genetic Data and Clinical Types

The pseudo-achondroplastic type appears to follow an autosomal recessive as well as a more frequent dominant transmission. In spite of its well defined clinical and radiographic characteristics, this is a heterogeneous disorder and there are ways to distinguish it into four different types. We do not feel that it is convenient to maintain these subdivisions.

Electronmicroscopic study reveals that there are abnormal inclusions within the endoplasmatic reticulum of chondrocytes (Fig. 3-63), within the growth cartilage. This finding suggests the presence of a protein accumulation, the nature of which is unclear (Cooper et al.). On the other hand, study of proteoglycans of cartilage by acylamid-agarose electrophoresis reveals abnormal migration (Stanescu and Maroteaux). It appears then, at least probable, that this disorder is due to abnormal proteoglycans.

Epiphyseometaphyseal Dysplasias

Besides pseudo-achondroplasia there are several epiphyseometaphyseal dysplasias with only mild spinal involvement as in multiple epiphyseal dysplasias from which they do not differ markedly. However, there may be a more marked growth deficit due to the shortening of the long bones, which further affects the prognosis. Predominant distal shortening and limitations in joint mobility are common to both disorders.

Radiographic Findings

Aside from the epiphyseal lesions there are abnormal findings involving the immediately adjacent metaphyses. Their border is serrated and fringed with the immediately adjacent zone above of uneven radiolucency. The diaphyses are short and coarse. Metacarpals and phalanges are also involved and may occasionally be very short and broad.

In adulthood, after closure of the growth lines takes place, the metaphyseal anomalies will disappear. All that will remain is the short and massive appearance of the diaphyses combined with epiphyseal deformity.

The transmission is dominant, but in all likelihood there are also some autosomal recessive types.

Occasionally, there are metaphyseal lesions, primarily of the hands and feet, that Silverskiöld described as the "peripheral" type in 1926. Such patients have massively appearing hands and feet with typically eliptic nails. During infancy the metaphysis of the metacarpals is very irregular (Fig. 3-64). All of these bones in the adult remain very short and broad. However, these patients do not suffer any significant loss in height. Transmission is autosomal dominant.

The disorder described by Léri under the name of *pleonosteosis* most likely refers to similar changes. We have been able to confirm this by a careful study of the documents of Léri's second patient and the subsequent follow-up.

It should be added that epiphyseo-metaphyseal changes can also be seen in other syndromes. For instance, in the Sjögren-Larsson syndrome which is characterized by dwarfism, growth retardation, ichthyosis, and pyramidal symptomatology (Ozonoff and Ogden).

Finally, a localized disorder of the tibia, Blount's disease can be listed with the epiphyseo-metaphyseal dysplasias. Most frequently this disorder is recognized between the ages of one and three years because of marked tibial incurving. About half of the patients have bilateral involvement. At the onset of this disease, radiographic findings are an abnormal appearance of the proximal tibial growth line in its mid-portion. In addition, there will soon follow a defect of the underlying metaphysis as well as a flattened and irregular outline of the adjacent epiphysis (see Fig. 12-6, p. 355). Besides this early form there is a somewhat belated disorder with a different radiographic appearance. Slight internal flattening of the proximal tibial center, together with an irregular outline of the proximal and medial portion of the growth cartilage, are combined with a narrowed medial portion and the formation of a bridge between the epiphysis and the metaphysis (Langensköld and Riska). This finding was documented by tomography. Treatment by early osteotomy is mandatory. Actually, mechanical factors seem to play a major role in the development of this anomaly with the radiographic appearance being a simple incurving of the varus position in the lower extremity (Langenskiöld and Riska). However, the recognition of several familial cases of this disorder strongly suggests the presence of a genetic factor.

THE ACRODYSPLASIAS

In this group epiphyseal or metaphyseal involvement is limited to the hands and feet. We will successively investigate the pure forms of this disorder. They are Thieman's disease, the epiphyseo-metaphyseal type of Brailsford, the tricho-rhino-phalangeal syndrome, and acrodysostosis (acrodysplasia with a facial anomaly).

Thiemann's Disease

Thiemann's disease, a very unusual disorder, is recognized during adolescence and is seen almost

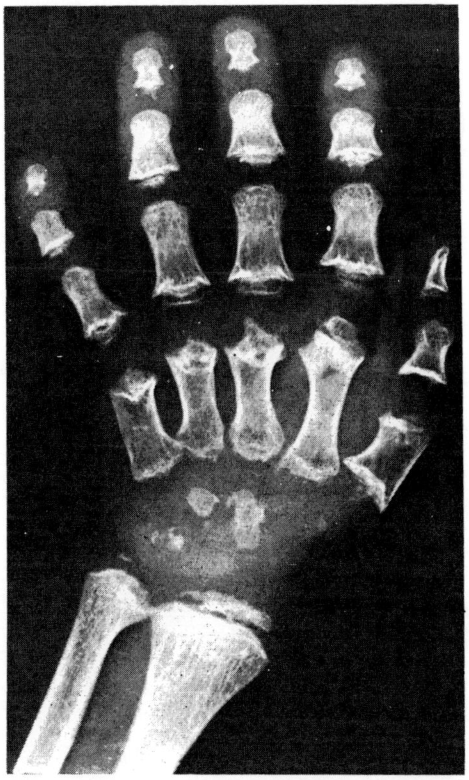

Fig. 3-64. Multiple epiphyseal dysplasia with elective involvement of the hands in a 12-year-old boy. Note the marked degree of metaphyseal alterations.

exclusively in boys. This is due to a more or less painful swelling of one of the interphalangeal joints and local limitation of flexion. The middle finger is primarily involved, often on both sides.

X-ray study reveals that the epiphyses of the affected fingers are thin, sometimes deformed, and assume a biconcave shape which look like "whiskers." They are sometimes fragmented with a median hyperlucency. Frequently, there is local condensation. In the pure form of this disease there is elective involvement of the epiphyses without any recognizable pathology of the metaphysis other than slight widening. There is no cone formation. Bone formation in the fingers is practically normal.

Several pedigrees have helped to confirm the dominant transmission of Thiemann's disease.

Brailsford's Disease (Peripheral Dysostosis)

This disorder is generally recognized early. Swelling of joints, limitation of motion, and axial deviation of one or several phalanges will bring the patient to the

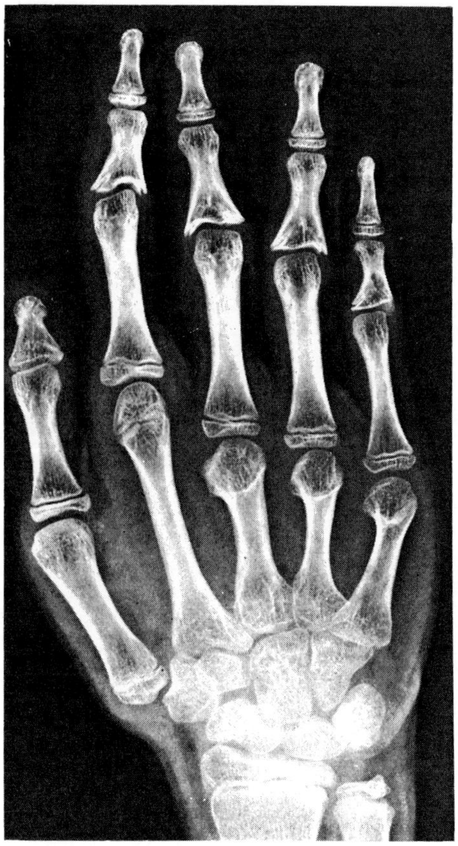

Fig. 3-65. Acrodysplasia with epiphyseometaphyseal involvement in a 13-year-old girl. (Courtesy of G. Fontaine)

physician's attention. The height of such patients is usually below average.

Radiographic investigation reveals that the epiphyses of the phalanges are deformed and are of irregular structure or density. Frequently there are cone-shaped epiphyses. The adjacent metaphyseal line is often widened and slightly irregular and may be somewhat concave or V shaped. Into this central portion there will be an insertion of a prolongation of the epiphysis. Its density may be somewhat increased and the size of the growth cartilage markedly reduced until sometimes it is no longer visible. Lateral deviation of the phalanges is frequently the result of asymmetrical involvement and brachyphylangy is generally present. The middle phalanges of fingers II-V are primarily involved, in particular, the midfinger (Fig. 3-65). In addition to this we note that the involvement of certain phalanges may be exclusively epiphyseal without any pathology of the metaphysis. In some cases there may be involvement of the femoral epiphyses along with the pathology of the hands. However, it appears to us

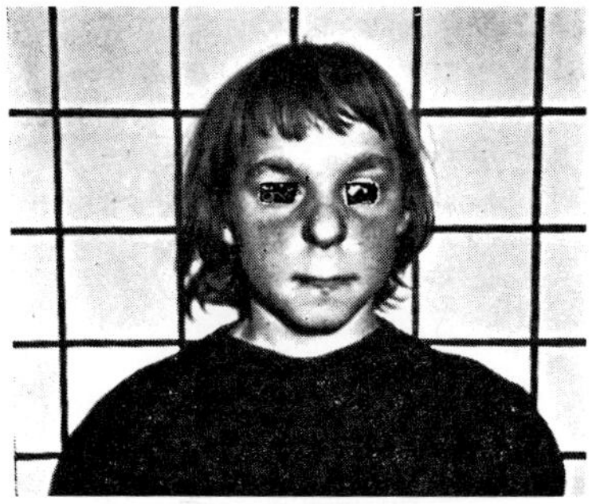

Fig. 3-66. Trichorhinophalangeal syndrome. (Courtesy of G. Fontaine)

that such cases should be diagnosed under the general term of multiple epiphyseal dysplasias.

The transmission of this type is most frequently dominant, but there are several observations on record which suggest the possibility of a recessive form.

Aside from their appearance knowledge of the cone-shaped epiphyses is important, as they can occur in entirely normal individuals. According to Giedion, who has studied this problem in detail, there are 7.5 per cent among girls and 1.6 per cent among boys. There are numerous variants, but it appears that the middle phalanx of the ring finger and the distal phalanx of the thumb can be electively involved. Symmetrical and often individual lesions can be seen.

Saldino and Mainzer have published a report of a brother and a sister with severe renal disease—nephronophthisis—cerebral ataxia retinitis pigmentosa and epiphyseometaphyseal pathology of the phalanges. In both patients the femoral heads were small.

The Tricho-Rhino-Phalangeal Syndrome

Described by Giedion this syndrome combines the changes which affect the face and hair with epiphyseometaphyseal involvement of the distal part of the extremities. These are similar to Brailsford's type, which may be its incompletely expressed form. The nose is broad and "pear shaped," giving the face of affected patients a characteristic appearance. Their hair is sparse (Fig. 3-66). Transmission is dominant and there are also several observations which suggest the existence of an autosomal recessive type. Another similar syndrome, occasionally called tricho-rhino-phalangeal syndrome type II combines identical involvement of the phalanges with abnormal hair and a peculiar facial appearance with a more prominent nose, large protruding ears, and micrognathia. Microcephaly, mental retardation, and the presence of multiple exostoses

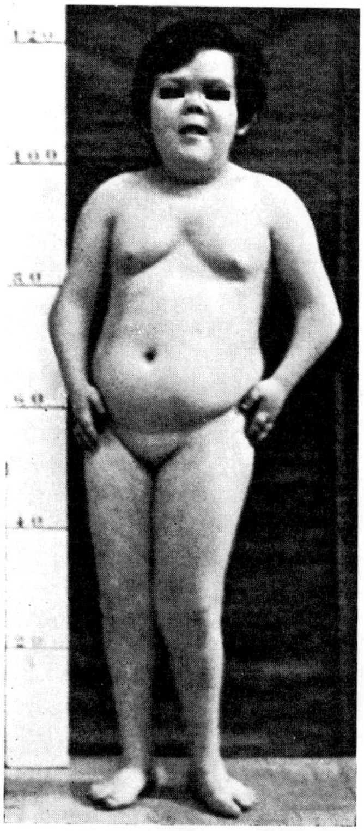

Fig. 3-67. Characteristic changes of the face in acrodysostosis. (Courtesy of G. Malamut)

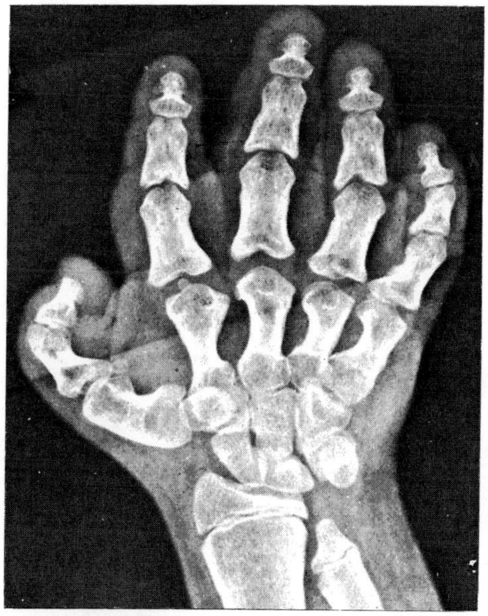

Fig. 3-68. Acrodysostosis in a 15-year-old girl. Note the extreme shortening of all the bones of the hand.

offer full confirmation that this type is an entity by itself. There may also be laxity of ligaments and skin.

Acrodysostosis (Acrodysplasia With Facial Changes)

This disorder is characterized by extremely short hands and feet along with abnormal facial features. Mental retardation and obesity are frequently combined.

Clinically, aside from the fingers, shortening involves the metacarpals and metatarsals. The fingers are short, broad, and are sausage-like in appearance. The face typically shows marked widening of the nasal bridge, while the nose itself is short and recessed. The lower teeth are markedly prominent and the mouth is usually held open. All patients are of short stature, but to varying degrees (Fig. 3-67).

Radiographically there is an impressive shortness of the massively wide bones of the hands and feet (Fig. 3-68). The epiphyses of the metacarpals and phalanges are often not visible and the metaphysis at the base of the phalanges may have the appearance of an open V. There may be cone-shaped epiphyses. The first metatarsal is especially prominent. There may be some mild changes involving the long bones: a discreet modeling defect of the metaphysis of the femur and the tibia, a medial exostosis at the proximal end of the tibia, and distal radial obliquity. The vertebrae may be small and the pedicles short. The mandibular angle is abnormally open.

All cases on record so far have occurred as isolated observations in normal families. This disease has been described by some as pseudo-pseudo-hypoparathyroidism. The clinical and radiographic findings that are typical for this disorder support the tendency to isolate it from the classical form of pseudo-pseudo-hypoparathyroidism (see page 208).

THE GENERALIZED PLATYSPONDYLIES

The term generalized platyspondyly refers to dysplasias where all the vertebral bodies are widened and have a loss of height. The flattened vertebral bodies are often associated with an anterior tongue-like deformity that can be well visualized on lateral films. Sometimes there is a protrusion like "a donkey's back" at the posterior aspect of a vertebra, while in other instances the end plates remain parallel.

We can distinguish three different groups of platyspondylies. In the first there is practically exclusive

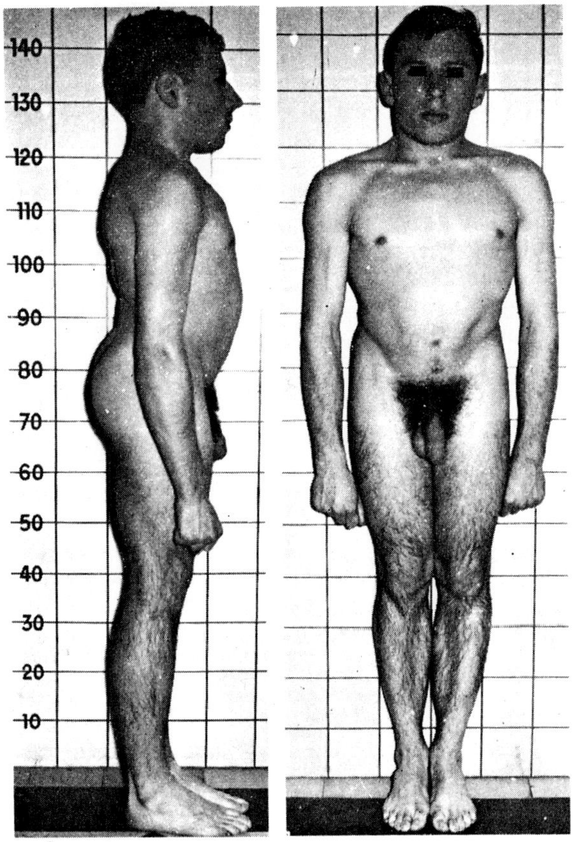

Fig. 3-69. Spondyloepiphyseal dysplasia tarda. Shortness of the trunk without involvement of the extremities.

spinal involvement and either mild or nonexistent peripheral skeletal lesions. The most well defined of these disorders is spondyloepiphyseal dysplasia tarda. In this group with late onset we find metaphyseal changes together with platyspondyly. This refers to the different spondylometaphyseal dysplasias. Finally, there is a third group with more or less generalized lesions affecting the epiphyses or metaphyses. Typical for this group is Morquio's disease. These disorders are discussed in the chapter on mucopolysaccharidoses (see p. 240).

Isolated Platyspondylies or Those Combined With Mild Epiphyseal Pathology

We will now investigate the two different disorders of recessive sex-linked spondyloepiphyseal dysplasia tarda and brachyolmy.

Spondyloepiphyseal Dysplasia Tarda

The characteristics of this disorder have been recognized since 1957. Prior to this it was constantly confused with Morquio's disease. The name given to this disorder reflects on its discovery only in the big child, sometimes in the adolescent, and even in the adult.

Clinical Findings

Spondyloepiphyseal dysplasia tarda is rarely recognized before the tenth year. It is usually not until then that the affected growth of the trunk will disturb the parents who will bring the patient to our attention. It is not at all exceptional for the disorder to go completely unnoticed for a much longer period of time. Its presence is sometimes only discovered when the adult develops arthrosis of the hips.

The growth disturbance is mild and adults reach a height of approximately 1.45 or 1.50 m. The disturbance is limited exclusively to the trunk which is increased in diameter. The sternum protrudes, the neck is short, and the head seems to rest on the shoulders. The skull and the face, however, are normal (Fig. 3-69). The extremities do not show any abnormal findings with the possible exception of an occasional mild limitation of hip movement. This finding is primarily limited to adults after the onset of arthrosis.

No visceral, ocular, or metabolic anomalies can be demonstrated. The prognosis is relatively good since growth is only mildly disturbed and the incidence of arthrosis of the hip is the principle lesion to be considered.

Radiographic Findings

In the young patient the only finding present is the ovoid appearance of the vertebral bodies, the exact nature of which is difficult to ascertain. The abnormal findings become progressively more defined and towards the age of 6 to 8 years there may already be the final characteristic appearance.

In the large child or adolescent we note on an AP spinal film generalized flattening of all vertebral bodies. Sometimes these changes are more marked in the thoracic region. The vertebral bodies may appear to protrude somewhat in their middle portion and the lateral appearance of the intervertebral space may be enlarged.

On the lateral view, this space is obscured in its posterior region by the deformity of the vertebra. This finding is particularly noticeable in the lumbar region (Fig. 3-70).

In the adult the radiographic appearance may simu-

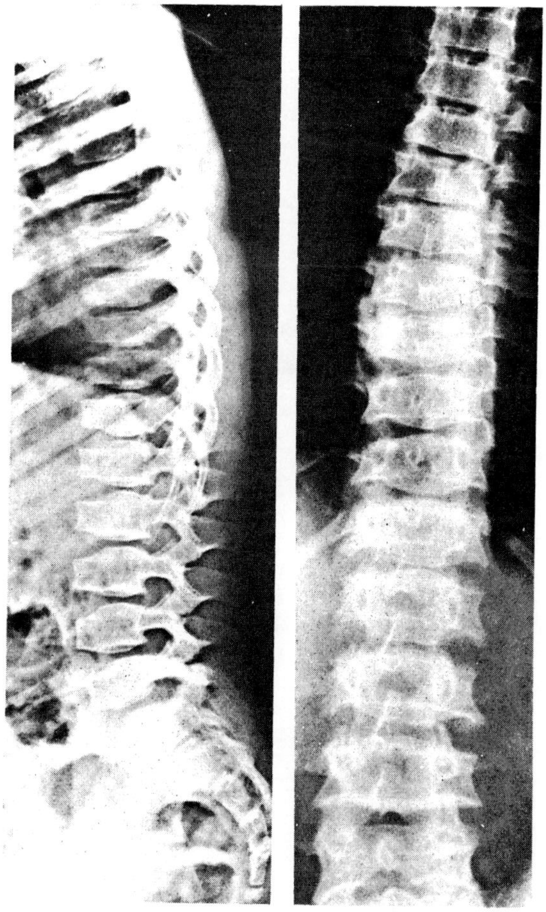

Fig. 3-70. Spondyloepiphyseal dysplasia tarda in a 12-year-old boy with deformity of the middle and posterior portion of the vertebral bodies.

late calcifications of the intervertebral disk and may appear similar to ochronosis. Tomographic studies, however, reveal that there is no calcification of the disks and that these findings are only the result of vertebral deformities. In some patients complete fusion of vertebral bodies has taken place (Barber).

Besides the spinal involvement there is pelvic smallness with occasional irregularities of the iliac crests and the ischial tuberosity. The proximal end of the femur may also be abnormal with a small, deformed head and a short neck (Fig. 3-71). Further epiphyses are only exceptionally involved.

Genetic Data

Spondyloepiphyseal dysplasia tarda has been identified as a distinct disorder because of its mode of

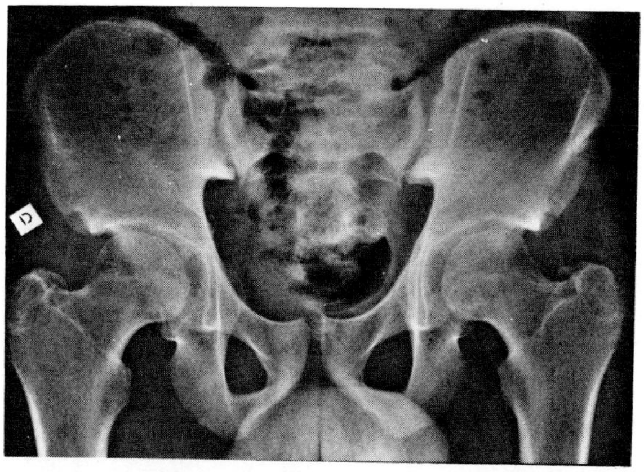

Fig. 3-71. Spondyloepiphyseal dysplasia tarda in a 12-year-old boy. The pelvis is reduced in size and there is mild deformity of the femoral head.

transmission. This is a sex-linked recessive disease, seen only in boys, and is transmitted by their mothers who are apparently healthy carriers.

The exact pathology of this disorder is still unknown. All attempts to demonstrate a disturbance of the acid mucopolysaccharide metabolism have been negative.

Brachyolmy

This skeletal dysplasia is recognized because of an impressive shortening of the trunk (Maroteaux et al.). The age of the patient at discovery of the disorder varies, but it is usually earlier than in spondyloepiphyseal dysplasia tarda. The extremities are normal, although they may be somewhat short and plump.

On radiographs we note a markedly reduced vertebral height with transverse widening (Fig. 3-72). On the lateral view the vertebral bodies appear slightly oval in younger patients, eventually with AP growth appearing too long, sometimes concave with irregular end plates. The bones of the limbs are somewhat plump and may show excessive radiolucency as those of the spine. The metaphyses are abnormal. The epiphyses are normal with the exception of a rare mild hip involvement.

This is an autosomal recessive disorder. However, the existence of a dominant type of very similar appearance is likely.

Elimination of chondroitin-6-sulfate, mildly sulfated, has been described in this disease by Mourao and collaborators. At this moment it is not possible to fully appreciate the significance of this finding.

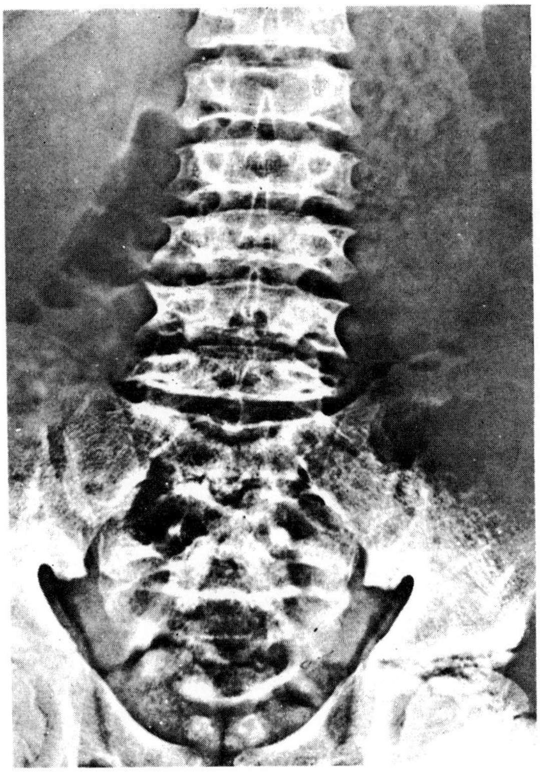

Fig. 3-72. Brachyolmy in a 16-year-old boy. Note the generalized platyspondyly.

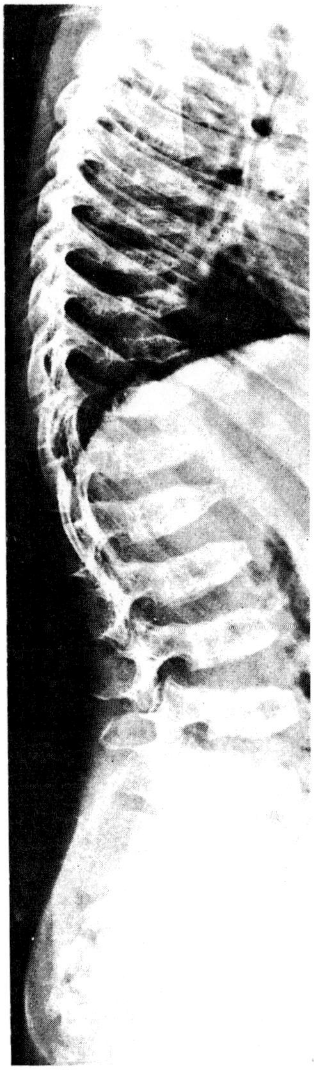

Fig. 3-73. Spondylometaphyseal dysplasia in a 5-year-old girl. There is generalized platyspondyly with tonguelike protrusion of the vertebral bodies.

Platyspondyly With Metaphyseal Involvement

The spondylometaphyseal dysplasia of Kozlowski was isolated in 1967 under the name "spondylometaphyseal dysostosis." This disorder is recognized towards the second year of life. Discovery may result most frequently from the recognition of delayed growth, but also from an investigation for an abnormal gait.

Clinically one sees a marked lack of growth affecting primarily the trunk which has a slightly protruding sternum. The limbs are only mildly affected aside from a moderate degree of shortening of the hand or a slight incurving of the lower extremity. A mild degree of limitation of movement may be noted affecting mainly the hips, and there may be a waddling gait. In the adult the definitive height is close to 1.40 m and the prognosis is much less serious than that in Morquio's disease, with which this disorder has been frequently confused.

Radiographically there is reduced height and widening of all vertebral bodies. On the AP view they markedly extend beyond the pedicles, and on the lateral view there is a tongue-like anterior extension (Fig. 3-73). Occasionally scoliosis is seen. The metaphyseal lesions are limited to the upper femoral metaphysis. The trochanteric region is irregularly structured. The neck is short in varus deformity and the acetabular roof is horizontal. Iliac wing height is reduced. Radiographic appearance is quite characteristic and it should be possible to reliably establish the diagnosis on a film of the pelvis showing both hips and proximal femora

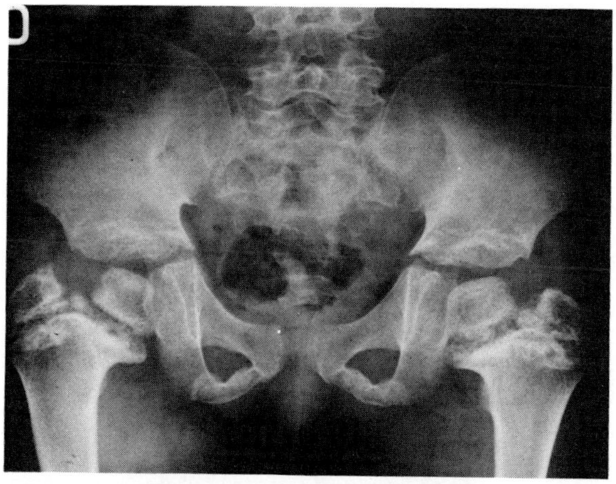

Fig. 3-74. Spondylometaphyseal dysplasia in a 7-year-old girl. Note the marked metaphyseal changes of the femoral neck and of the greater trochanter. The acetabular roof is almost horizontal.

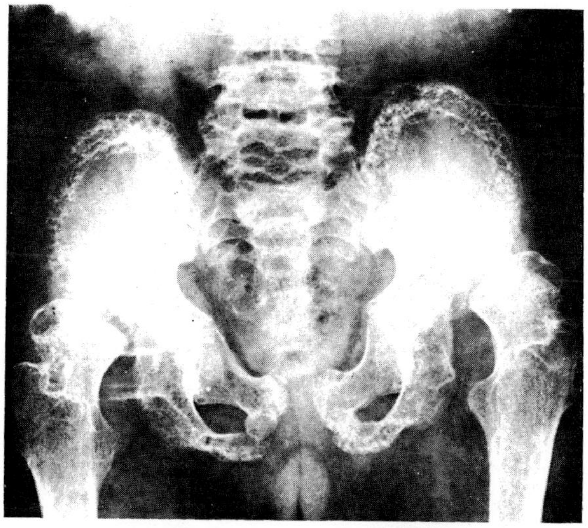

Fig. 3-75. Dyggve syndrome in a 16-year-old boy. Notice the scalloped, lacy appearance at the periphery of the iliac wings. (Courtesy of J. Naffah)

(Fig. 3-74). Other metaphyses are generally minimally involved, but the development of the carpal and tarsal bones is frequently retarded. Occasionally there may be broadening of the diaphyses of long bones.

Spondylometaphyseal dysostosis is transmitted as an autosomal dominant.

Other Types of Spondylometaphyseal Dysplasia

Besides the preceding disorder there are several rarer varieties of spondylometaphyseal dysplasia, in particular, those described by Schmitt and Sutcliffe. In these cases metaphyseal alterations are limited to the femoral neck and are accompanied by severe coxa vara. However, other metaphyses, such as the shoulder or knee, may also be involved. The vertebral bodies have an ovoid appearance with the beginning of anterior tongue formation. In the observation of Murdock and Walker there was a considerable increase in the height of the vertebral bodies without dramatic changes of form.

Wiedemann and Spranger have published on a patient, who, at the onset of disease, presented with a vertical fissure of the vertebral body. This is clearly visible on a lateral film of the spine. Eventually there is fusion of the anterior and posterior ossification center and the vertebra then has the appearance of butterfly wings. The height of the vertebral bodies is only minimally affected. No metaphyseal involvement of the hands or feet has been noted. The regressive evolution, without marked deficiency of growth as described by Wiedemann, does not appear to coincide with a personal observation in a patient followed and studied with M. Alizon.

Platyspondylies With Generalized Epiphyseometaphyseal Involvement

The best known disorder of this group is Morquio's disease, discussed with the mucosaccharidoses (see p. 240). We would just like to remind ourselves that in order to fully establish this diagnosis, one cannot rely only on recognizing generalized platyspondyly and epiphyseal lesions. The anterior hypoplasia of a vertebral body in the lower thoracic or lumbar region, coxa valga, distal radial, and ulnar obliquity, and a conic aspect of the possible metacarpalia are included in the spectrum of signs which confirm the diagnosis of Morquio's disease.

Besides this disorder there are a number of others which manifest generalized platyspondyly. Some of them also have a mild degree of keratan-sulfate elimination – Pseudo-Morquio Type I. This disorder will be fully discussed in the chapter on mucopolysaccharidoses.

A further type has been described by Dyggve and collaborators. Clinically the patients do not only show dwarfism with a very short trunk, but also mental retardation. The limbs, however, are only minimally affected.

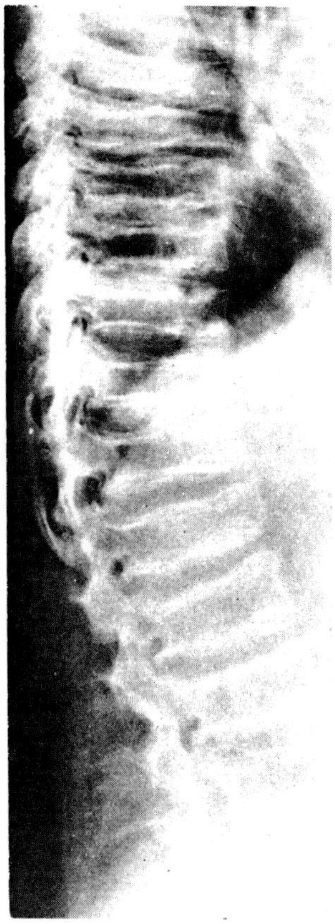

Fig. 3-76. Pseudo-Morquio disease Type II in a 16-year-old girl. The generalized platyspondyly is entirely different from that seen in Morquio's disease.

Radiographically platyspondyly is frequently accompanied by unequal end plates which gives the appearance, in the lateral view, of a double convexity—"camel humps." Emphasis must also be placed on the very unusual pelvic appearance. The iliac wings are rather narrow and the acetabula are shallow. The femoral heads appear to be located above the lateral border of the neck, which may be confused with the growth cartilage. Often there is subluxation in the larger child. The most striking finding, however, is the markedly irregular border of the iliac wings, along with the ischiopubic segments which appear as a scalloped or lacelike border (Fig. 3-75). The bones of the hands are somewhat broad without metacarpal alterations.

Transmission of this disorder is autosomal recessive. We have not been able to find an abnormal excretion of mucopolysaccharides in the urine. The cornea is normal.

There are further types of generalized platyspondyly which belong to this group. One is a dominant disorder manifesting in the adolescent, which has rather characteristically multilayered appearing end plates involving practically all the vertebral bodies—Pseudo-Morquio type II (Fig. 3-76).

COMPLEX SPONDYLO-EPIPHYSEO-METAPHYSEAL DYSPLASIAS

Before closing this chapter we find it necessary to add a number of dysplasias, which we have not been able to properly place within the defined groups. Such disorders are certainly not unusual. Localization of epiphyseal and metaphyseal involvement varies from one patient to the next and there is sometimes considerable spinal involvement. Because of its heterogeneity, it is as yet impossible to offer a precise definition.

The outward appearance of such patients varies. Some will have marked shortening of the extremities, while others may only have mild involvement. The peripheral portion of the extremities may be normal, but in some there is marked shortening and widened fingers. Patients in this group usually have a short trunk. In an occasional patient, however, this finding may be less dramatic and marked micromelia will be the prominent feature. In all cases the skull and face are normal (Fig. 3-77). It is very difficult to offer a prognosis for these varying types. One must always keep in mind that the degree of metaphyseal involvement and distribution together with progressive spinal involvement and the loss of vertebral body height are all key factors for the prognosis. Manifestation of these disorders is by severe dwarfism and a very conservative functional prognosis is in place, particularly if there is marked involvement of the hips.

Radiographic investigation reveals markedly differing lesions of the spine. Quite frequently there is loss of vertebral body height with irregular end plates. On lateral views several bodies may show a mild degree of wedging, most frequently in the thoracic region. An unusual patient may show fragmentation. Scoliosis or kyphoscoliosis may be associated with these anomalies (Fig. 3-78).

Peripheral bone involvement also varies. Usually we note generalized involvement. The femoral head is almost always the most severely involved. Hands and feet are more often not affected, but this is not constant. The skull and the suboccipital region are normal.

Certain patients in this group have already been individualized with a correct diagnosis attached to their disorder. This for example is the case in diastrophic dwarfism, metatropic dwarfism, and the Kniest syndrome, which have already been discussed in the

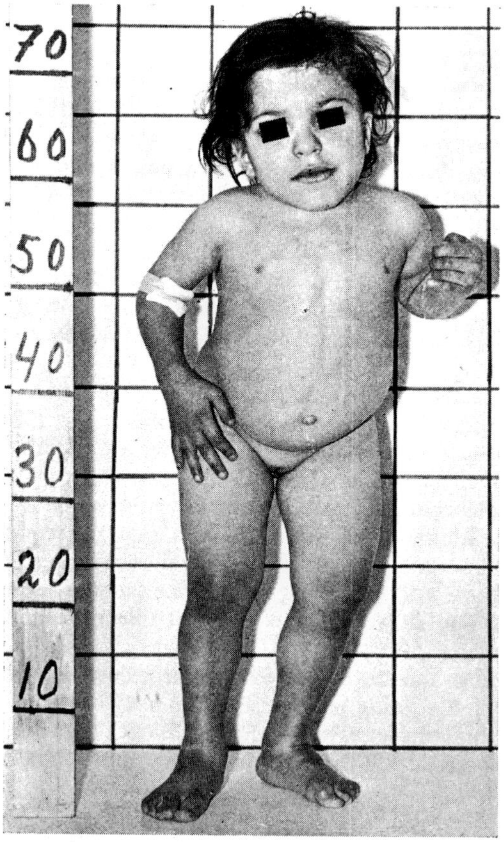

Fig. 3-77. Complex type of spondyloepiphyseal dysplasia in a 5-year-old girl. Note the extreme shortness and deformity of the trunk.

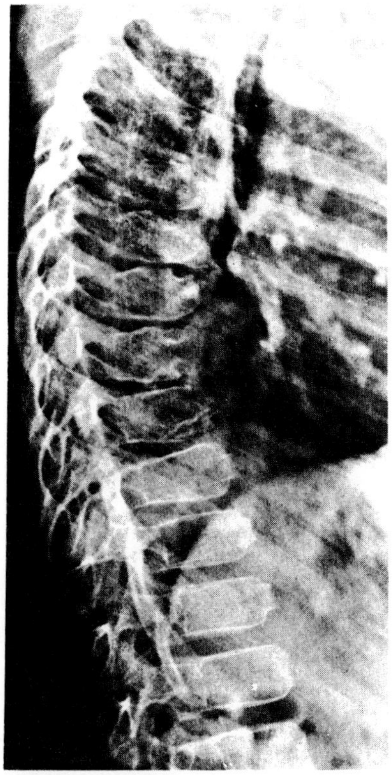

Fig. 3-78. Complex type of spondyloepiphyseal dysplasia in a 9-year-old girl. Notice the reduced height of vertebral bodies with a more marked deformity of the upper and middle thoracic region.

chapter on dysplasias (see p. 37). Similarly parastremmatic dwarfism has been defined as a special type by Langer et al. This is a severe dwarfing disorder with kyphoscoliosis, articular stiffness, and deviation of the extremities from their normal axis. On radiographic study this disorder is characterized by excessive radiolucency of the metaphyses, epiphyses, and of the vertebral bodies. The structure and outline of the metaphyses is irregular and in some places unusually dense. This appearance can also be noted by following the contours of the pelvis. The iliac wings are small. Marked deformity will be noted in practically all the epiphyses and vertebral bodies with reduced height and sometimes with a biconcave shape. The disorder is transmitted as a dominant (Rask).

Further clinical and radiographic studies will, in all likelihood, lead to the definition of other disorders belonging to this group. However, we are of the opinion that other methods of study will probably be more helpful in a more precise classification (histochemical, ultrastructural, microchemical studies of the growth cartilage, etc.).

Therapy

Aside from Morquio's disease, which can definitely be considered as one of the mucopolysaccharidoses, we must admit that our ignorance with respect to the pathogenesis of these dysplasias is vast. For this reason there is no rational medical therapy for spondyloepiphyseal dysplasias, and until quite recently, it was generally accepted not to consider any corrective orthopedic interventions for patients whose growth was not terminated. We feel that this attitude must be changed. In disorders where considerable deformity of the extremities results in a disturbed gait or an abnormal function of a joint, one should not hesitate to proceed with surgical corrections during childhood. Such interventions are particularly needed in several disorders of the hip in order to counteract threatening dislocation or subluxation of the femoral head which may cause irreversible damage. Pelvic osteotomy or a varisation osteotomy of the femoral neck along with other measures are indicated.

Scoliosis or kyphoscoliosis evidently requires con-

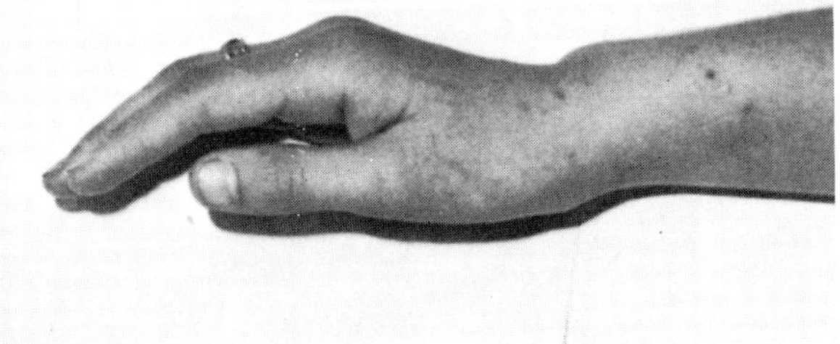

Fig. 3-79. Dyschondrosteosis. Characteristic deformity of the forearm.

sequent treatment long before growth is over. In a number of patients with lordosis and pelvic tilting, pelvic osteotomy could be considered.

Occasionally, it may be wise to perform tenotomy, in order to vastly improve articular function. This may lead to good results in an attempt to avoid an irreducible flexion deformity of the hip or knee. Together with methods of reeducation this can achieve considerable functional improvement.

Exercise on a bicycle or in a swimming pool should be recommended to these patients. However, violent sports and prolonged exertion such as walks should be avoided. They could have devastating effects. Advice in making the proper professional choice is also indispensable. Professions or jobs exposing the patient to repeated or occasional trauma should obviously be avoided, as should occupations requiring one to assume a constant upright position.

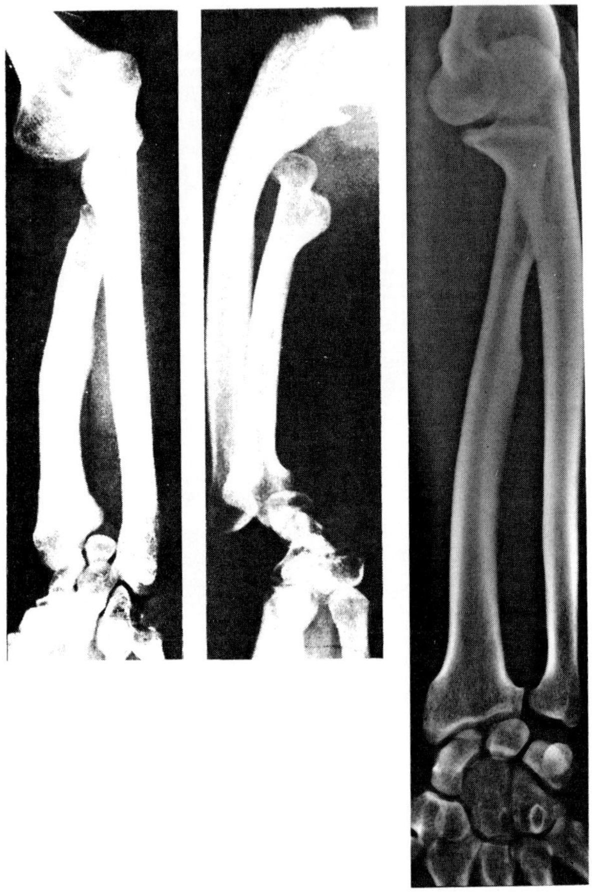

Fig. 3-80. Dyschondrosteosis in a 15-year-old girl and in her mother. Note the variability in the expression of this disorder.

DYSCHONDROSTEOSIS

This disease was first described by Léri and Jean Weill in the year 1929. Overlooked for many years, this disorder has been the topic of many recent publications. This is an expression of its relatively frequent occurrance.

Clinical Findings

This disorder is usually first recognized in the growing child or during adolescence. Slowness of growth and deformity of the forearm are the reason for the discovery. In the most severely affected patient there may be an earlier recognition of growth retardation. Usually there is a moderate degree of reduced height, which results from shortened extremities which electively involve the middle segment along with the forearm and lower leg (Fig. 3-79).

Abnormal development of the forearm similar to that seen in Madelung's deformity is associated with the growth deficit. The distal end of the ulna is dislocated posteriorly and assumes a characteristic position. This dislocation can be reduced by pressing the ulna upwards but upon release the dislocation will immediately reappear. The radius is slightly curved. Movements at the wrist are limited, especially extension and supination, which is only feasible by rotation of the humerus and displacement of the shoulder posteriorly. The lower extremity may be affected by genu varum. The skull, the face, and the trunk are practically normal. The prognosis is good. The definitive height is around 1.45 m in women and 1.55 m in men. On the whole, the deformity of the forearm will not be very disturbing.

Radiographic Findings

The principle changes are those of the bones in the forearm. Besides being short they are significantly altered (Fig. 3-80). The radius is curved in its frontal plane. This deformity is well visualized on AP views, as is the increased space between the two bones of the forearm and the accentuated interosseous radial crista. The ulnar curvature is sagittal and is seen on lateral films. The radial head is frequently flattened, sometimes hypoplastic, and the radiohumeral articular line is noticeably large. Thc distal end of the radius is oblique distally and laterally because of the curve of its diaphysis. Generally the olecranon is not involved. This structure may appear to be somewhat more massive than usual. The distal end of the ulna which is dislocated posteriorly may be more or less hypoplastic such as in observation No. 2 of Léri. The carpal region is altered in its relationship and instead of being arranged in a rounded curve, there is a gothic arch. The most proximal bone is the semilunar which is located in the space between the unusually widely separated distal ends of the radius and ulna. The arrangement of the second row of carpal bones is also abnormal. The trapezium and the trapezoid are displaced in a volar direction and may be seen in the lateral view.

Outside of the local shortening there are only minimal changes involving the lower half of the legs. However, there may be an exostosis or a modeling defect in the medial region of the proximal tibial end. The head of the humerus may show a mild "hatchet-like" deformity.

Genetic Data and Treatment

Dominant transmission of dyschondrosteosis has been proven by a large number of pedigrees. The disease seems to occur with a higher incidence in females. This may be the result of the fact that the disorder often remains unrecognized in men. The moderate growth deficit may be more readily noted in women who, on the average, reach a height of 1.45 m, while the men will grow to 1.55 m. The deformity of the forearm is usually less noticeable in men because of muscular development and a lesser esthetic concern.

The relationship between Madelung's deformity and dyschondrosteosis has been the subject of much discussion. Not one criterium proposed to distinguish the two disorders can stand up to a careful and critical review. This is due to the fact that in one and the same family there may be individuals with a mild deformity of the forearm exactly fitting the description of Madelung's deformity, whereas others may show considerable shortening and hypoplasia of the proximal radial end. We therefore conclude that this is one and the same disease. Léri and Jean Weill have demonstrated that the lesion of the forearm described by Madelung is not an isolated deformity, but an integral element of a chondrodysplasia with a very complex nature, the mechanism of which remains unsolved.

The diagnostic problems of these mesomelic disorders are not yet completely clarified. Silverman, for example, reports observing a woman with dyschondrosteosis with two sons suffering from severe mesomelic dwarfism, somewhat similar to the type described by Langer (see p. 52). We have made this same observation in one family. It appears then that a gene with variable manifestation may be causing the changes.

Most of the time there is no reason to actively treat dyschondrosteosis. However, in an exceptional patient the degree of the forearm's deformity may be so severe, that due to functional disturbance and compelling esthetic reasons, one may suggest radial osteotomy in an attempt to counteract bowing occasionally combined with a resection of the ulnar head.

Part 2: Osteochondrodysplasias With Anarchic Development of Cartilaginous or Fibrous Tissue

Two large groups must be distinguished depending on whether the anarchic proliferation involves cartilage or fibrous tissue.

DISORDERS INVOLVING ANARCHIC GROWTH OF CARTILAGE

The abnormal growth of cartilage may be localized to the epiphyses of the carpal bones or to the metaphyses of the long bones.

A disorder belonging to the first group known as dysplasia epiphysealis hemimelica or tarsomegaly, as its name implies, affects the epiphysis of only one portion of the lower extremity. In the second group of disorders cartilaginous tissue may develop within bone and thus leads either to the formation of chondromas or to the proliferation of exostoses at its periphery.

The disorders which involve the proliferation of fibrous tissue have been intensively studied and discussed. Certain authors have confused them, while others have distinguished three different disorders: multiple cartilaginous exostoses, Ollier's dyschondroplasia and multiple chondromatosis. The individual distinction of the latter two disorders is based on erroneous genetic arguments which result from a confusion between chondromatosis and certain observations of dominant multiple cartilaginous exostoses. This argument may be limited by simply distinguishing between the two diseases: multiple cartilaginous exostoses with a dominant transmission and Ollier's dyschondroplasia or multiple chondromatosis which is never familial.

HEMIMELIC EPIPHYSEAL DYSPLASIA

Mouchet and Belot originally defined this disorder in 1926 as tarsomegaly. It has been proposed by Fairbank to call it hemimelic epiphyseal dysplasia, which appears to be more exact. Contrary to the disorders we have described up until this point which affect the skeleton or certain other bones in a symmetric fashion, this disorder involves only the epiphyses or the bones of the tarsus of one leg. Involvement of the upper extremity is extremely rare.

Clinical Findings

Although this disease is recognized at various ages, it is most commonly noted during the first few years of life because of a foot or knee deformity, a limp, or a painful gait.

Physical examination reveals a median or lateral swelling of the knee or tibiotarsal joint. During palpation a firm or slightly elastic consistency can be noted. The skin over this tumor is of normal color and appearance. Sometimes there is a deformity of the leg or foot in the form of genu valgum or pes planus and valgus, but generally there are no major changes and there is only minimal loss of length in the involved leg. Movements of involved joints are limited. During the early years there are numerous local findings which become stabilized with time.

Radiographic Findings

Excessive growth of the involved epiphyses characterizes this disorder. Development occurs unilaterally and is most frequently accompanied by fragmentation. Ossification seems to proceed from multiple centers. These irregular centers will sometimes fuse into a single mass of unequal structure, appearing to partially incorporate the epiphysis. The adjacent metaphysis is usually normal.

The astragalus is the most commonly involved bone in the foot. Less frequently involved are the scaphoid, the first cuneiform, and as has been well recognized by Fèvre and Rigault, the distal epiphyses of the fibula and tibia (Fig. 3-81). Another localization is the medial condyle of the femur. Here the local lesions will develop medially and posteriorly. The upper tibial epiphysis is sometimes deformed, however, the femoral head or the acetabulum are rarely involved (Fairbank, Bianchi and Frassi, Theodorou and Lanitis). Frequently seen is the simultaneous involvement of several epiphyses, especially those of the foot and knee.

Most unusual are lesions of the upper extremity. Fairbank has seen only one patient with involvement of the trapezoid and first metacarpal, and one with involvement of the distal ulnar epiphysis.

Genetic Data, Pathology, and Treatment

Always an isolated disorder, hemimelic epiphyseal dysplasia appears to predominantly affect boys. Histology reveals the presence of cartilaginous tissue with hypertrophic zones and ossified islands. This ossification is enchondral.

The pathogenetic mechanism of this disease is still unknown. Fairbank assumes that the initial disturbance probably occurs at about the fifth fetal week. The only form of treatment available is surgery. Attempts should be made to remove all abnormal osteocartilaginous material. It is occasionally necessary to perform an osteotomy. Patients experiencing severe pain or a very marked deformity must be considered for this form of treatment.

MULTIPLE CARTILAGINOUS EXOSTOSES

This chondrodysplasia was already recognized at the beginning of the 19th century and has been under frequent study. Many publications have been devoted to its discussion and a number of different names have been proposed for it: osteogenic disorder, diaphyseal aclasis, maladie exostosante, and hereditary deforming chondrodysplasia.

Clinical Findings

The disorder is rarely noted before the third year of life and in some cases it is much later. Frequently the advice of a physician is sought because of a growth close to a joint, usually the knee, or because of a deformity of the scapula or a rib. Other conditions first noted can be a deviation from the normal axis of one extremity—genu valgum or bowing of the forearm, a growth deficit, or an unusual situation where the complication is due to nerve or vascular compression.

The most characteristic finding during physical ex-

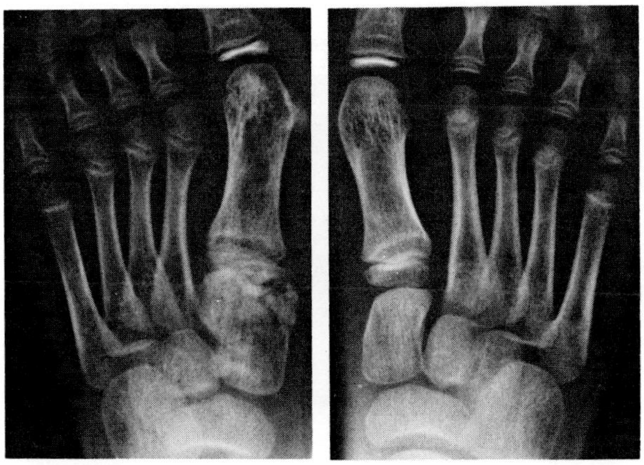

Fig. 3-81. Dysplasia epiphysealis hemimelica in a 4-year-old boy. There is excessive development of tarsal bones with abnormal shape and fragmented characteristics. (Courtesy of C. Fauré)

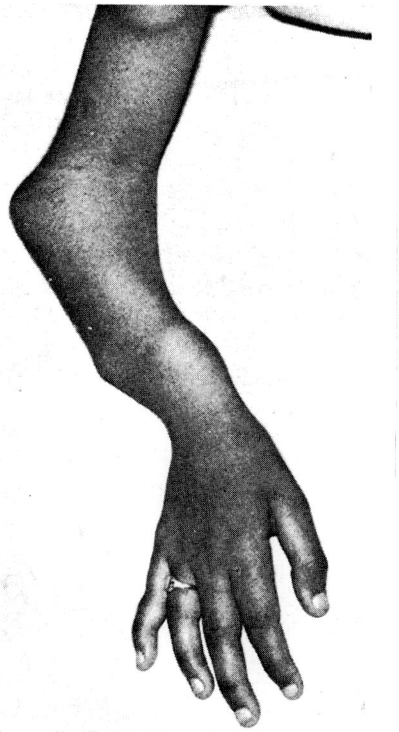

Fig. 3-82. Multiple cartilaginous exostoses. Ulnar deviation of the hand, dislocation of the radial head, and local tumors at the ends of the long bones.

amination will be the presence of hard, smooth, firmly attached immobile tumors, located in the metaphyseal region of the long bones, the scapulae, the pelvis, or ribs. There may be limited movement of the nearby joint. Quite frequently there is an easily recognized deformity of the forearm and the wrist, which is secondary to the shortened ulna. This results in a lateral deviation of the hand, referred to as "bayonette hand" (Fig. 3-82). Subsequent to the dislocation of the radial head limitation in wrist movement can be seen in some patients. Some fingers may be shortened due to metacarpal shortening. Genu valgum is not uncommon. Valgus deformity of the foot may result from a shortened fibula. As a rule, patients suffering from this disorder are short. However, this disorder does not generally result in true dwarfism. The prognosis of multiple cartilaginous exostosis can be considered on the whole to be favorable. Under average circumstances a normal life can be predicted. Still, the presence of the exostoses can result in a number of complications, most especially the compression of nerves and vessels. The vast majority of such complications occur in the adult and because of the nature of this text we will avoid further description. The disorder may also lead to obstetrical complications or medullary compression (Vinstein and Franken, Signargout), but the majority of these complications are quite rare.

Malignant degeneration is most unusual during childhood and its incidence in the adult is reported at varying levels. Jaffe indicates 11 per cent to be his clinical experience, but this number seems to be much too high. However, we must not overlook this danger. If suddenly an exostosis exhibits rapid growth and development, this possibility must be seriously investigated. The most frequently occurring locations are the femur, pelvis, and humerus.

Radiographic Findings

In the newborn and infant and prior to the appearance of clinical findings, it is very difficult to establish this diagnosis. Occasionally, slight irregularities seen in the diaphyseal cortical bone may lead to the suspicion of such a lesion (Fig. 3-83). Later typical exostoses will develop, but their number in a young child may still be limited. This does not mean that such a patient is suffering from a milder form of this disorder, because many other exostoses will progressively appear and become visible later. Their total number varies from one patient to another. The range may be from just a few to several dozen. The radiographic appearance is that of bony exostoses, originating from and deforming the metaphyses of the long bones, the scapulae, the pelvis, and ribs. Involvement of the spine (vertebrae) or skull is exceptional. The morphology of the exostoses is different depending on their location. Those at the distal end of the femur are pediculated

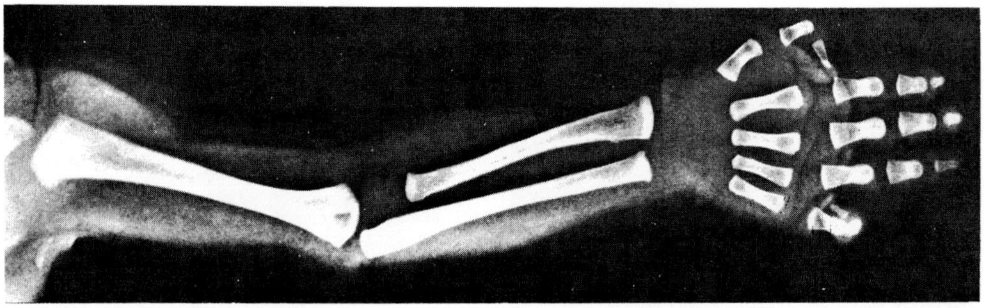

Fig. 3-83. The discrete irregularities of the medial cortex of the left radius are the earliest local change due to an exostosis. Boy 1 month of age.

and directed upwards, resembling a coat hanger or a horn. At the tibia the direction is reversed (Fig. 3-84). The exostoses of the fibula are sessile, as are those of the proximal humerus, where the location of the exostoses is usually at the medial surface where the upper and middle thirds meet. They may sometimes be accompanied by small pediculated lateral exostoses. Involvement of the metacarpals and phalanges is frequently seen, but the exostoses are small and do not markedly deform the fingers. They are somewhat comparable to chondromas. Location at the distal end of the ulna is usually combined with considerable shortening. This ulnar shortening explains the deviation of the hand and the deformity of the forearm, which were first mentioned by Kienböck. Besides the incurving of the diaphysis there is also dislocation of the radial head (Fig. 3-85).

Growth disturbances resulting from shortened long bones vary depending on the degree and local involvement. They are the second important element for the diagnosis of this disorder. The metaphyseal region is often irregularly formed and may appear cylindrical. This finding may be best seen at the distal end of the femur and at the proximal end of the tibia. A widened and shortened femoral neck is often seen (Fig. 3-86). The longitudinal growth of the bones is somewhat disturbed, which explains the deformities seen as they affect the forearm and at times the lower leg. The most serious involvement affects the ulna and fibula. Shortening of one or several metacarpals is also frequently present (Fig. 3-87).

Radiographic study may also reveal structural irregularities of the metaphyses and the localization of a chondroma in the center of the bone.

The following are potential danger signals for malignant degeneration: rapid increase in the size of an exostosis or an irregular or multilobulated structure, isolated areas of calcification, and local budding with vague lateral contours.

Genetic Data

Dominant transmission of multiple cartilaginous exostoses has been reliably proven. There is a higher incidence in males who make up 70 per cent of all involved patients. However, there are certain families who transmit this disorder by apparently healthy women, and only in an exceptional situation by healthy males. This fact has not yet been fully explained, and certain authors, for example, H. Harris have voiced the hypothesis that a modifying gene may be limiting the manifestation of the disorder in females.

Another dominant disorder similar to multiple cartilaginous exostoses is metachondromatosis. It must be clearly defined and can be properly identified by the location of the lesions, their appearance, and evolution. Hands and feet are almost electively involved, but there are rare juxtaarticular localizations with equally unusual characteristics. There are, besides the appearance of exostoses, irregularly calcified lesions which are sometimes separated from the bone by, most likely, a cartilaginous radiolucent band (Fig. 3-88). Furthermore, it is possible that these different anomalies may undergo changes and involution and, actually may almost completely disappear. The manifestations of the gene appear to be quite irregular.

Pathology

Histologic investigations of the exostoses demonstrate that they are formed by a peripheral mass of cartilage around a central ossification. This ossification is enchondral in nature and certain authors have noted the presence of different developmental stages analogous to those described for normal growth cartilage (Jaffe). An exostosis may contain a medullary cavity which may communicate with that of the bone itself. At its surface the periosteum is in continuity with that of the neighboring metaphysis. A serous

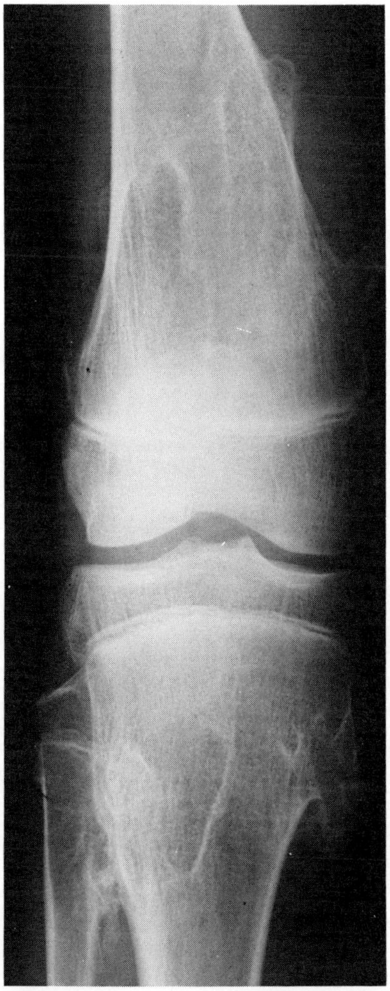

Fig. 3-84. Multiple cartilaginous exostoses in a 13-year-old boy. Note the marked defect of tibial modeling and the metaphyseal lucencies which is the result of overlying exostoses.

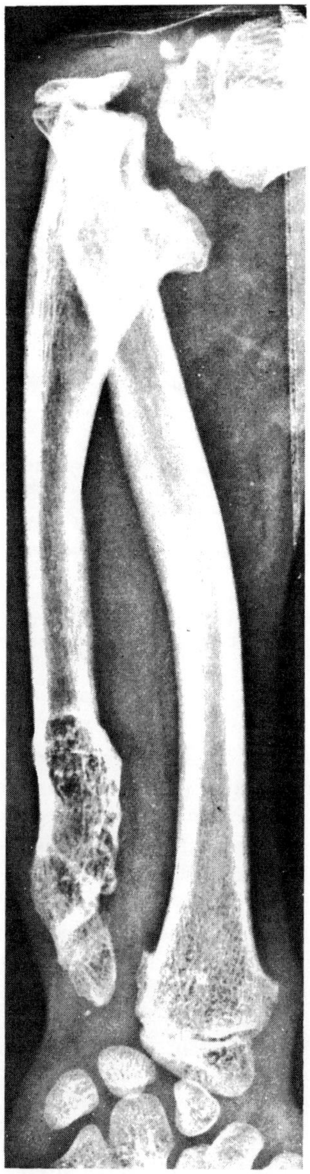

Fig. 3-85. Multiple cartilaginous exostoses in an 11-year-old boy. There is marked shortening of the ulna resulting in subluxation of the radial head.

bursa often covers such an exostosis and isolates it from the neighboring tissues. Aside from the histologic appearance of the exostosis Leveuf has insisted on cortical alterations near the malformed metaphyses, even in the absence of exostoses in the region of the lower extremity of the femur and the upper region of the tibia. The cortex would be only poorly developed and would contain cartilaginous inclusions. The ossification notch would simply be displaced beyond the abnormal metaphyseal region.

Study of the growth cartilage does not reveal any strikingly abnormal findings in its midportion. However, in the periphery immediately next to the exostosis there are oblique columns which have the tendency to become horizontally arranged. It is possible that this anomaly does have a direct relationship with abnormal ossification.

Physiopathology

A number of studies have been conducted in horses (Morgan), dogs (Chester), and cats (Pool and Car-

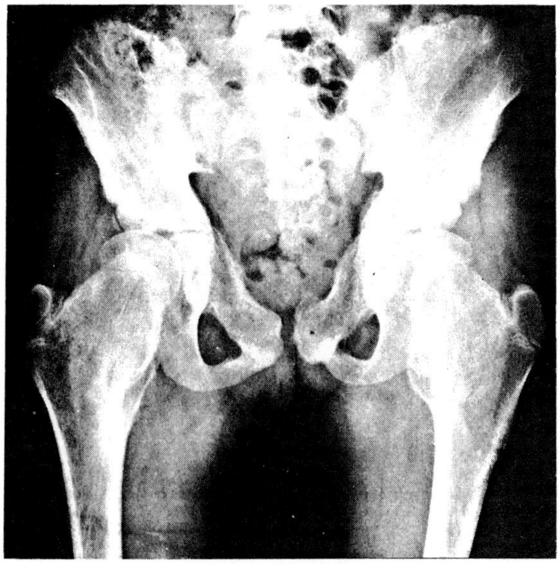

Fig. 3-86. Multiple cartilaginous exostoses in a 12-year-old girl. There is marked widening of the femoral necks and characteristic involvement of both iliac and pubic bones.

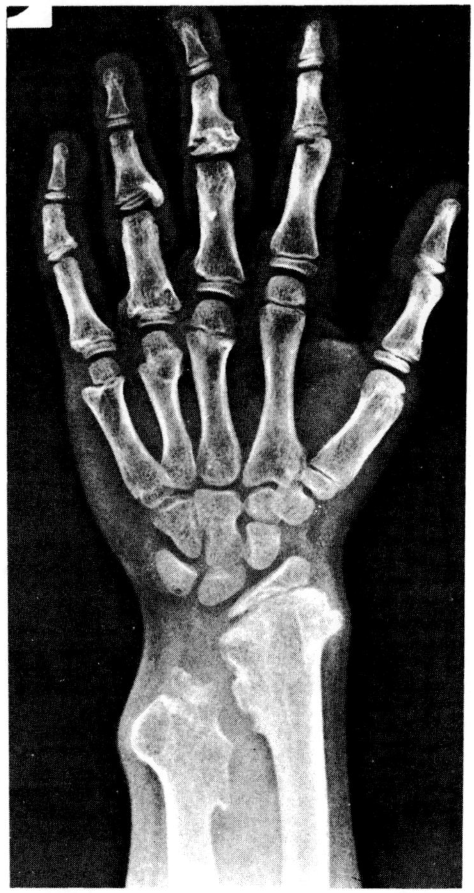

Fig. 3-87. Multiple cartilaginous exostoses in a 10-year-old girl. Note phalangeal exostoses with shortening of the 4th and 5th metacarpals and deviation of the distal end of the ulna.

rig) with the aim of clarifying pathogenetic mechanisms. Several hypotheses have been developed. They can be divided into two groups depending on whether they refer to the origin of the anomaly within the growth cartilage or within the periosteum.

According to Virchow, the pathology results from anarchic cellular proliferation in a lateral direction from the growth cartilage instead of in its usual longitudinal manner. Langenskiöld believes that undifferentiated cells of the growth zones form chondroblasts and cartilage, instead of forming osteoblasts which would lead to the growth of the periosteum. Keith thinks that the initial disturbance resides in an insufficiency of the periosteal barrier. The cortical anomaly according to Leveuf is accompanied by ectopic ossification to which he attributes an essential role for growth, while Müller maintains that the exostoses result from cartilaginous islands which are formed from the osteogenic layer of the periosteum.

Without negating the existence of periosteal anomalies in multiple cartilaginous exostoses these do not explain the growth deficit of the involved bones which are so frequently seen in this disorder and preferentially affect, to a very marked degree, a limited number of bones. They are the ulna, the fibula, and the metacarpalia. Lacroix has freely transplanted growth cartilage, cleaned of its periosteum, under the fascia of a rabbit's kidney demonstrating that growth continues according to its physiologic axis and that the transplant was capable of regenerating a ring which limited its peripheral growth. In multiple cartilaginous exostoses it appears most likely that we are dealing with a very early disturbance of bone formation. Due to our limited knowledge no further insight can be given.

Treatment

Treatment is limited to the removal of exostoses and to surgical correction of resulting deformities. Intervention is indicated when the volume or position of an exostosis leads to a dangerous or esthetically unacceptable condition. Such interventions should be undertaken towards the end of growth with the exception of the patient who suffers from significant functional difficulties or in whom a dangerous complication is imminent. The following conditions offer clear indications for orthopeadic surgery: if the femoral neck threatens to push the femoral head out of the socket, if

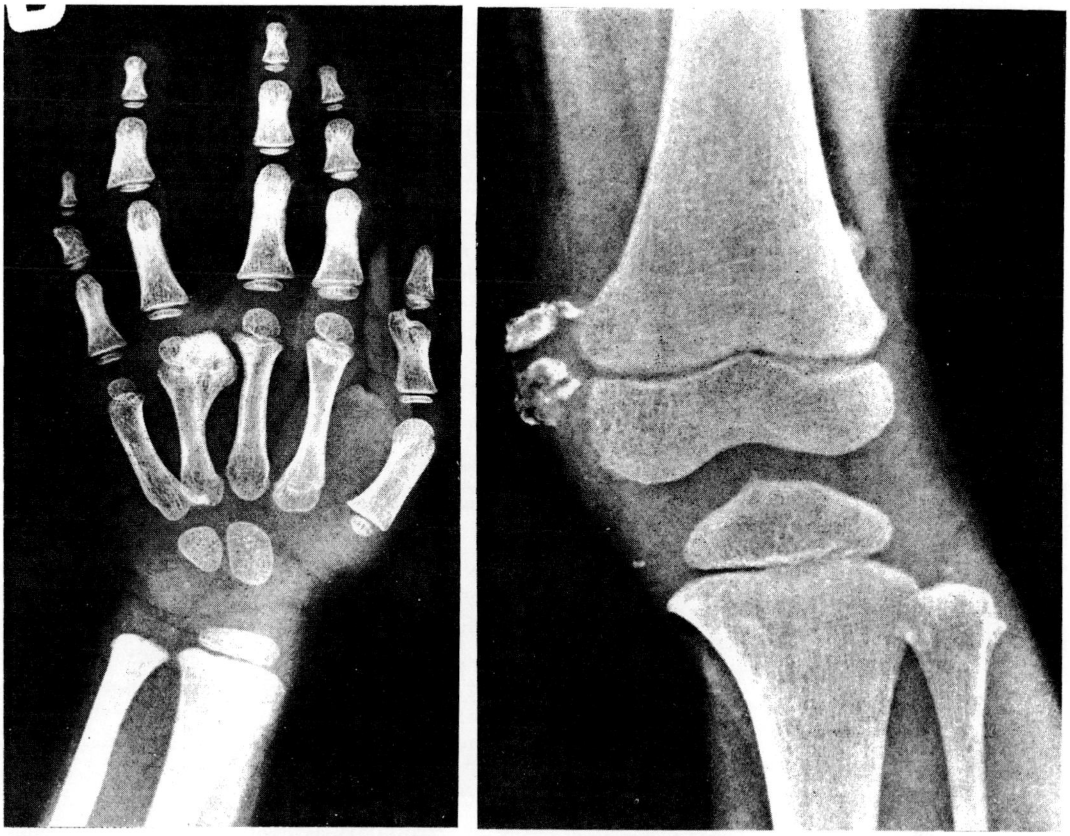

Fig. 3-88. Metachondromatosis in a 4-year-old boy. There is elective involvement of the hand and local soft tissue calcifications with an appearance clearly distinguishable from exostoses.

a hooklike exostosis of the humerus threatens to compress the adjacent nerves and vessels, or if an exostosis at the distal tibia threatens to push the tibia and fibula apart. If local malignant degeneration is suspected, a simple local excision is recommended, followed by a detailed histologic study. Only when a malignancy can be histologically proven, should more aggressive surgery be undertaken.

DYSCHONDROPLASIA (MULTIPLE SKELETAL CHONDROMATOSIS)

Multiple skeletal chondromatosis, mainly involving the extremities, has been known for a long time. Credit must be given, however, to Ollier, who in 1899 emphasized the peculiar topographic characteristics of this disorder with unilateral predominance. Certain authors have tried to isolate these forms as Ollier's disease, but this does not appear justified. Ollier did insist on one of the basic characteristics of this disorder by describing and emphasizing its asymmetry and the irregular localization of chondromas in dyschondroplasia.

In 1881 Maffucci described the combination of chondromas and multiple angiomas in a single patient, a combination noted later by a number of authors. This disorder is now generally known as Maffucci's syndrome.

Clinical Findings

The disorder is most frequently recognized after the second year of life because of a shortened leg which leads to a mild limp or the swelling of a finger or toe.

During physical examination there may be visible chondromas involving the extremities. These tumors are somewhat elastic and seem to be strongly attached to the phalanges or metacarpals (Fig. 3-89). Palpation of the long bones may reveal swelling in the metaphyseal regions. The shortened involved bones are frequently the only early manifestation of the disorder. Its distribution is entirely asymmetrical and,

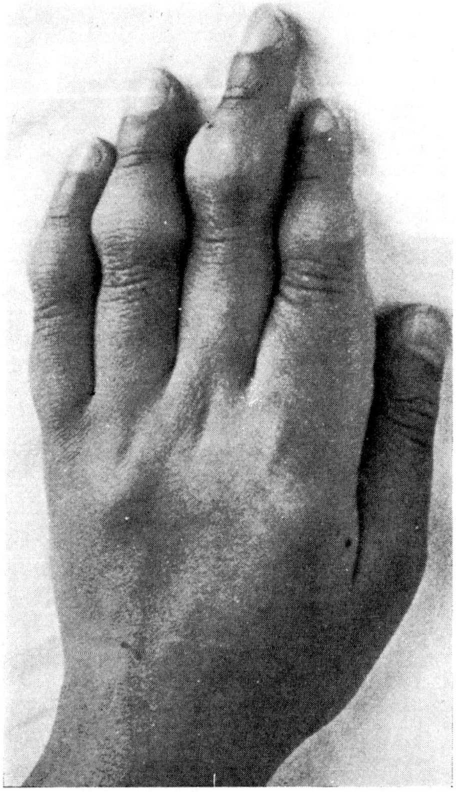

Fig. 3-89. Multiple chondromatosis with phalangeal deformities. Girl 10 years of age.

as localization of the incurving chondromas or deviation of long bones, is often associated with growth disturbance. Neighboring joints have limited motility. The deformity of the forearm is one of the most striking involvements and is comparable to that seen in multiple cartilaginous exostoses. The trunk is hardly ever involved. There may be several rib chondromas or a scoliosis secondary to pelvic tilting. The skull is usually normal.

The prognosis of dyschondroplasia is more serious than that of multiple cartilaginous exostoses because its effect on growth can be dramatic and its asymmetry can result in severe morphologic disturbances. However, certain generalized forms may occasionally modify growth very little, while others more localized in nature result in serious deformity. From these observations we must conclude that it can be exceedingly difficult to offer a precise prognosis in young patients. An early effect on growth must always lead to a most careful evaluation and guidance. Nerve compression is rarely seen, but malignant degeneration seems to occur with about the same incidence as in the preceding disorder.

Radiographic Findings

Contrary to the situation described in multiple cartilaginous exostoses which present with only minimal radiologic findings at birth, chondromatosis manifests itself quite clearly by the presence of findings similar to those seen later during infancy. The most characteristic lesion of the hand is the presence of multiple chondromas, a clear and homogeneous local lesion with fine oval or elongated borders in parallel arrangement to the longitudinal axis of the bone. Sometimes there is slight trabeculation visible along with dark streaks of opacification which indicate calcification. These chondromas are generally grouped as a polycyclic mass which leads to swelling in the metaphyseal region. Others have columnar arrangement. When they are located at the periphery of the bone, they are visible as a characteristic notch since they are separated from the neighboring tissues by the fibrous periosteum, which is radiographically invisible. Chondromas are localized electively in the metaphyseal region of the long bones and the hands and feet. Initially close to the growth zone, they will subsequently migrate towards the diaphysis (Fig. 3-91). This displacement can be followed on successive films. Still, it is not unusual for a chondroma to be located in the center of a diaphysis. The evaluation of such an image would be very difficult were it not for the presence of other lesions of typical characteristics and location. Phalangeal chondromas sometimes lead to considerable deformity and may completely invade the bone, leaving it unrecognizable.

There is frequent involvement of the scapula and pelvis. The vertebral bodies and the base of the skull are rarely involved with the cranial vault not being involved at all. We would like to insist on the totally irregular distribution of the chondromas. These are sometimes localized to one segment of an extremity or to one side of the body (Fig. 3-90). Quite frequently, however, one or more chondromas are present on the opposite side, usually involving the bones of the hand. In the presence of generalized involvement, one side is the seat of more lesions than the other. There is hardly ever simultaneous involvement of all metacarpals and phalanges in the hand. Several of these are generally normal.

The effect of chondromas on growth is usually much more serious than that of exostoses. The diaphyses of involved bones is short and broad occasionally with bowing close to the metaphysis. Ulnar shortening is usually much more dramatic than the radial changes. The fingers are of uneven length. The epiphyses may be normal, but occasionally they are irregular in form or structure.

The uneven distribution and development of the

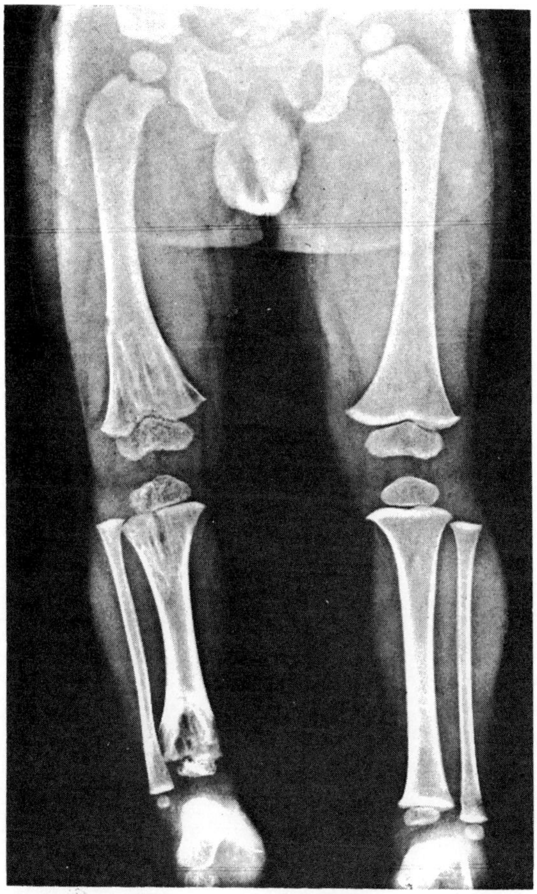

Fig. 3-90. Unilateral chondromatosis in a 18-month-old boy. Note the involvement of the shortened right leg in addition to the metaphyseal location of enchondromata a small lateral notch in the lower femur resulting from a local chondroma.

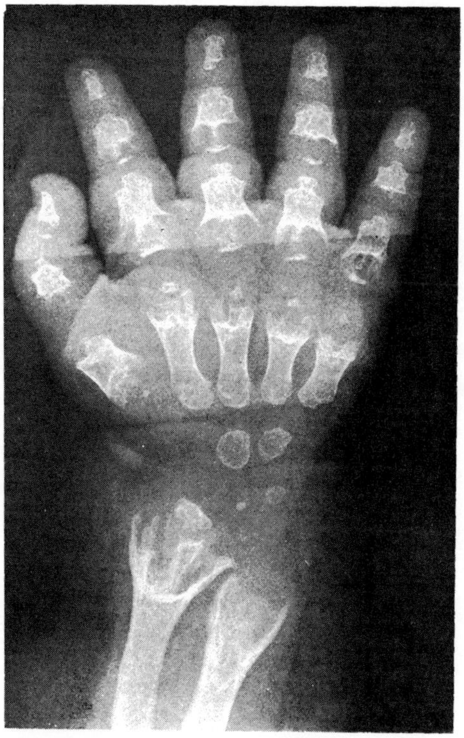

Fig. 3-91. A 1-year-old girl affected by a particularly severe and precocious form of multiple chondromatosis.

chondromas explains the similarly uneven growth disturbance of different regions. We can thus understand the considerable differences seen in the total length of the extremities.

The radiographic study may also reveal a fracture which is quite unusual in chondromatosis, or the presence of phleboliths in the Maffuci syndrome. As in multiple cartilaginous exostoses these findings will help one to recognize malignant degeneration (Fig. 3-92).

Genetic Data

Several publications have reported on familial cases of chondromatosis. Critical analysis shows that this is either in reference to patients with clearly different diseases, or to questionable observations where the history was not clarified by radiographs. However, information is given that there were deformities of the toes and fingers in a brother of one of such patients, an uncle or a grandfather. Multiple chondromatosis of the skeleton is not a familial disorder and there is no evidence to qualify it as a genetically transmitted disease.

The systemic distribution and nature of the bony lesions are arguments which favor its being a constitutional bony tissue disorder and not an embryopathy or an acquired disorder. Does this disorder then result from a somatic mutation or from yet another genetic factor? We do not yet know this answer.

Clinical Types

Certain authors distinguish two separate disorders in this group: chondromatosis and multiple chondromatosis more often called Ollier's disease. In the first of these, men are primarily affected by bony lesions generally of the extremities. Only rarely is there development of calcification and this has only a weak influence on growth. This disorder is frequently transmitted as a dominant. Ollier's disease is seen with a higher incidence in females and does not have familial characteristics. Furthermore, its topographic distribution is frequently bilateral. The individual lesion has a ten-

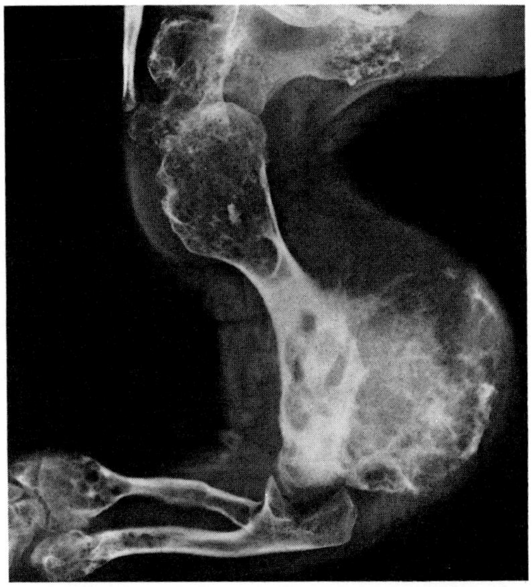

Fig. 3-92. Malignant degeneration of a chondroma in the humerus of a young adult. (Courtesy of M. Fèvre)

dency to become calcified and the effect on growth is considerable.

None of the proposed criteria in support of this distinction can stand up to a critical evaluation. Sex distribution is identical. Dominant transmission is never seen and practically all intermediary degrees of involvement between strictly unilateral and generalized distribution of more or less asymmetrical characteristics occur. The effect on growth can result in more severe deficits in unilateral distribution as compared to the generalized form, which is apparently more severe in nature, but these criteria alone can not serve as a base to distinguish between the two types.

There is only one special group which can be defined and that is multiple chondromatosis of the hand. This actually does seem to occur with a higher incidence in males, which aids in its differentiation from other types of chondromatosis.

MAFFUCCI'S SYNDROME

The combination of angiomas and chondromatosis was originally described by Maffucci in 1881. Since then there have been many publications that support the thought that this is not just a coincidental association. The skeletal findings are those which we have just described. The association with angiomas can be seen in a unilateral as well as a generalized distribution. It may be important to note that the bony lesions are frequently progressive, leading in some patients to monstrous deformities. There is a very high incidence of malignant degeneration.

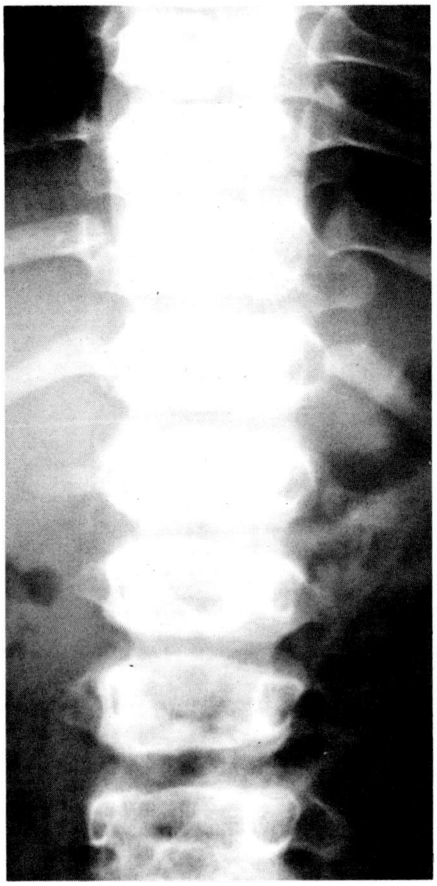

Fig. 3-93. An excessive development of vertebral bodies and their pedicles in a 4-year-old girl.

Vascular lesions are, on the whole, hemangiomas, and are frequently accompanied by phleboliths which are visible on radiographs, but the distribution of the vascular lesions and of the equally anarchic chondromas is not superimposable. Thus, certain types of unilateral bony involvement or those with a marked unilateral predominance may be combined with generalized angiomas. Similarly, there may be a restriction of angiomas to the lower extremities in the presence of generalized bone lesions.

The prognosis in Maffucci's syndrome must be much more guarded than that of a case of isolated chondromatosis because of the marked tendency towards progression and malignant degeneration. The coexistence of other tumors, especially of the ovaries, has been repeatedly noted (teratoma or thecoma of the ovary and lymphangioma). A secreting tumor of the ovary has been reported in Ollier's disease (Grenet et al.).

Besides the Maffucci syndrome, there are other syndromes which associate chondromas and cutaneous and several other malformations. One such combination, described by Granges, involves hypertrophy of the vertebral bodies and periarticular calcifications. We have studied a similar case with identical spinal involvement, but without chondromas (Fig. 3-93).

Pathology and Pathogenesis

Histologic testing confirms the cartilaginous nature of these lesions. The cartilage is arranged in islands with markedly dense cells and are separated by matrix strands of few cells. Occasionally, there may be calcified areas, sometimes with local points of early ossification.

A number of hypotheses have been formulated in an attempt to understand the origin of dyschondroplasia. A number of authors feel that the chondromas develop from growth cartilage, in the human disorder where they believe to have documented this by successive radiographic studies during growth or by experimental animal studies. Langenskiöld working in rabbits after irradiation of growth cartilage has produced chondromas. He believes that they originate from undifferentiated cells of the growth zone. It still appears difficult to accept that certain chondromas localized in the center of a diaphysis originate from the growth cartilage. Thus, a number of questions are still open. Bentzon, after injecting alcohol into the sympathicus, has been able to induce chondroma formation of a phalanx in the rabbit. Dahl believes that in dyschondroplasia there is a defect in the destruction of cartilaginous cells which normally preceeds ossification. He feels that this defect is secondary to a functional disturbance of the capillary endothelial cells and attributes the cells of Bentzon's experiments to a neurotrophic alteration of the endothelial system.

The presence of angiomas in the Maffucci syndrome could possibly add support to these vascular theories. Still, the development of chondromas and angiomas is in no way parallel, and it is quite difficult to accept an interaction between those two series of facts and to understand the obvious disorder of localization of bony, as well as cutaneous, lesions.

Treatment

Treatment is essentially surgical. Orthopedic corrections must be considered in serious incurving or extremity deviations. Leg elongation can be considered after the age of 8 and may possibly be repeated later. Surgical attempts directed against chondromas—removal and grafting—seemingly lead to disappointing results and numerous lesions limit interventions in dyschondroplasia. An intervention should only be considered if there is significant deformity or in the presence of a severe functional disturbance. The questions raised by the possibility of malignant degeneration does present a difficult problem. The same facts pertain here as were discussed for multiple cartilaginous exostoses.

DISORDERS WITH ABNORMAL FIBROUS TISSUE PROLIFERATION (FIBROUS DYSPLASIA)

Fibrous dysplasia offers certain analogies with multiple chondromatosis of the skeleton, because of the existing asymmetry and the irregular distribution of the bony lesions which sometimes involve only a single bone, and by the occasional presence of multiple geodes. For a long time this disease was confused with osteitis fibrosa cystica of Von Recklinghausen, the parathyroid origin of which was demonstrated 35 years later. This was well documented following the work of Hunter and Turnbull, and of Lièvre, Jaffe and Lichtenstein. However, it was Albright who insisted on the association between fibrous dysplasia and precocious puberty with skin pigmentations.

Clinical Findings

The disease is discovered at various ages, but usually during adolescence. A malformed leg or its functional consequences will lead to studies revealing bony lesions. Involvement of the leg may be noted earlier because of a disturbed gait. Other patients may present with a tumor of the skull or face (Fig. 3-94 *A*). More frequently, fibrous dysplasia is noted subsequent to a fracture. This may be the result of only minimal, trivial trauma. Recurrence is frequent, either within the same bone or in another location. Finally, the patient may present because of dull pains located within the femur or tibia and which increase under local pressure. Physical examination may show deformity of the involved extremity by incurving or swelling. The femur is often held in a typically abducted position or there may be a tibia recurvata. Unequal leg lengths are not unusual by elongation of the involved side. If the face is affected there may be leontiasis ossea, usually asymmetrically. Cranial nerve compression, especially of the optic tract, can be the result of cranial base condensation.

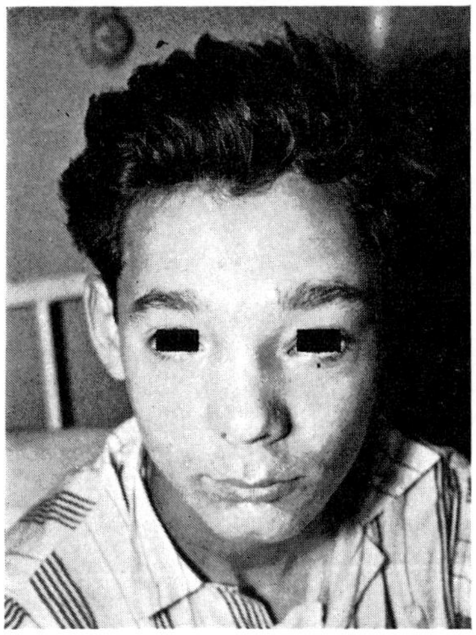

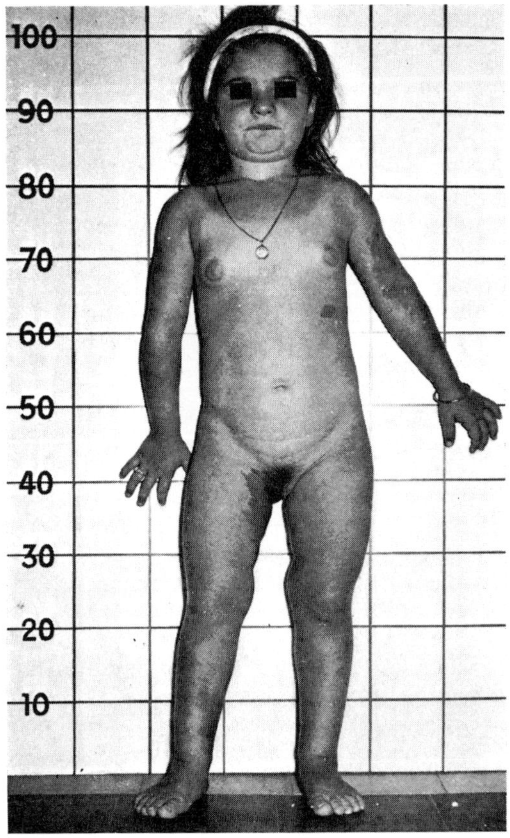

Fig. 3-94. (*Left*) Fibrous dysplasia. Note the facial dysproportions and the prominent forehead. (*Right*) Note the cafe au lait spots on the inner surface of the right thigh and the left upper leg. Precocious development of secondary sexual characteristics in a 3-year-old girl. (Courtesy of R. Rappaport)

Palpation may reveal a tumor in easy to palpate areas, such as the clavicles, the ribs, the mandibles, and the cranial vault. Limitation of motion in the neighboring joint may accompany the bony lesion and vertebral involvement can result. There are several observations on record of elevated alkaline phosphatases.

The prognosis of fibrous dysplasia is relatively good, if there is only one extremity involved. Usually there is only a mild effect of this disorder on growth. However, local deformities or repeated fractures may be somewhat more serious.

Involvement of the spine and skull are more worrisome. Spinal involvement may lead to serious vertebral pathology, and occasionally may lead to medullary compression and paraplegia. Involvement of the base of the skull should always be a danger sign because of the possibility of cranial nerve compression, especially of the optic tract, the most frequently seen complication. Facial disfigurement may cause serious problems. Malignant degeneration occurs more rarely than in Ollier's disease. This possibility should however not be overlooked. Radiotherapy previously applied may have contributed to its formation.

Radiographic Findings

Involvement may concern both the long bones and the skull. In long bones the diagnostic feature is a fibroma corresponding to a chondroma of Ollier's disease. There is a clear, rounded or polycyclic zone in which the normal bony structure disappears (Fig. 3-95). The geodes are located electively in diaphyses, in contrast to the chondromas. They may, however, invade the metaphyses, in particular, at the femoral neck. If their borders are defined, the size varies and has a tendency to combine and invade a large part of the affected bone. The diaphysis is often wide and loses its normal modeling changing to a cylindrical form. The cortex is thin and somewhat dense. Bowing is often noted. This combination of bony defects, abnormal tubulation, and bowing most frequently affects the femur in a characteristic way (Fig. 3-96). If other areas are affected, the diaphysis is widened or "blown

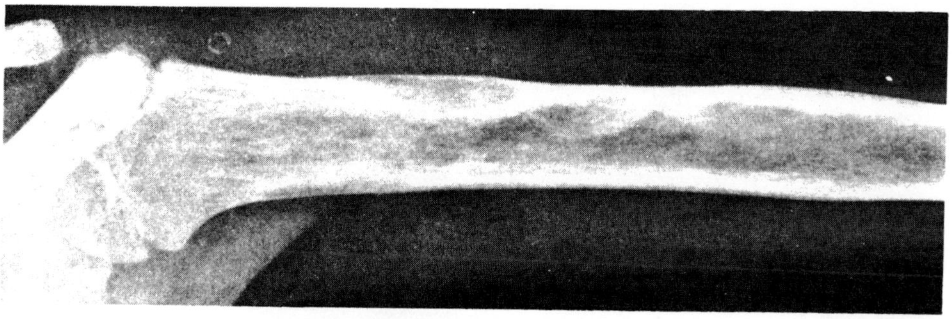

Fig. 3-95. Fibrous dysplasia in an 8-year-old girl. Notice the cylindrical appearance of the humerus with its clear zones where the bony structure has disappeared.

up." For an example note the fibula in (Fig. 3-97). As in Ollier's disease there will be a considerable asymmetrical distribution. Involvement of the long bones is the rule but any bone may be affected. This includes the ribs, pelvis, and scapula. Hands and feet are not spared but fingers usually are not deformed.

Skull lesions have been studied extensively by Leeds and Seaman. The additional finding of sclerosis at its base may also involve the sphenoid wings, and there may be growth within the vault occasionally appearing like "cotton balls." This is similar to Paget's disease (Fig. 3-98). It is not unusual to find a sclerotic and asymmetric involvement at the base of the skull or of the face. These changes have led to a confusion with melorheostosis. The latter condition sometimes shows small areas of rounded densities within the cranial vault. There may also be cystic changes involving the parietal bones and more rarely the frontal or temporal bones. There may also be widening and prominence of the external table with a small peripheral surrounding density.

Clinical Findings

Anomalies of pigmentation combined with precocious puberty and hypoplasia of bones are the essential features of Albright's disease (Fig. 3-94*B*). "Café au lait" lesions of the skin are of various sizes and their distribution is without any direct relationship to the localization of the skeletal involvement. Precocious puberty is almost exclusively seen in females, whereas advanced bone age, early closure of growth zones, and growth deficit may be noted in both sexes.

No detailed discussion of isolated bone fibromas is attempted here. During normal growth localized fibromas are occasionally seen and they are described under the term cortical defects (see p. 373).

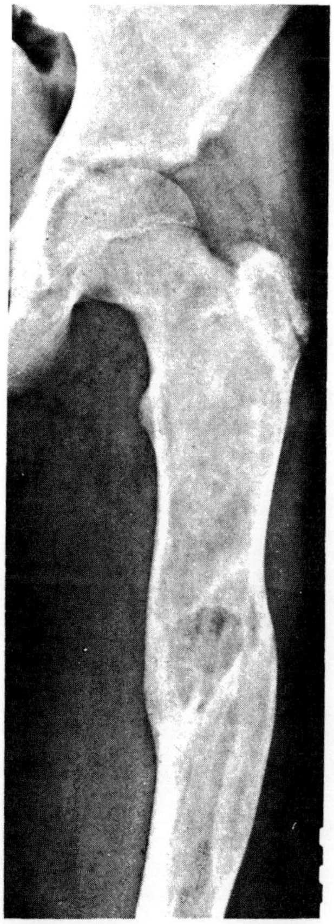

Fig. 3-96. Fibrous dysplasia in a 13-year-old boy. Besides the clear zones within the femur there is also marked deformity resulting from a healed pathological fracture.

Pathology and Pathogenesis

In long bones normal bone tissue is replaced by fibrous tissue with irregularly arranged bony trabeculae.

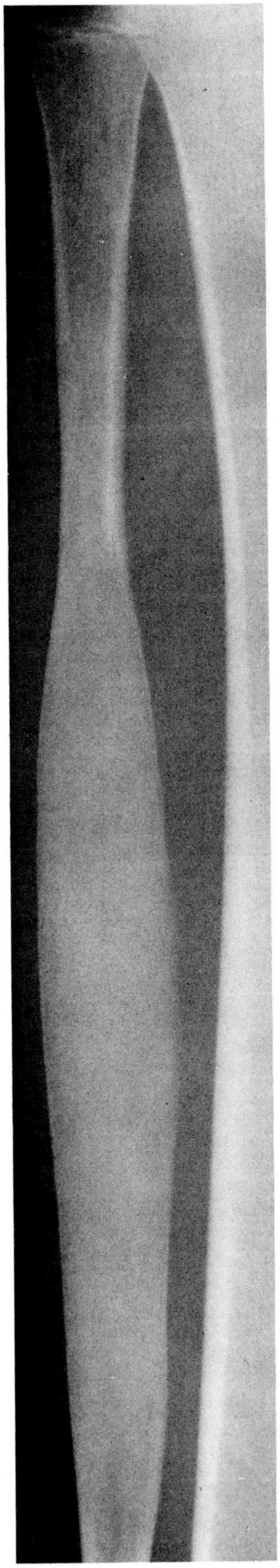

Fig. 3-97. Fibrous dysplasia in an 11-year-old girl. There is marked widening over most of the diaphysis of the fibula.

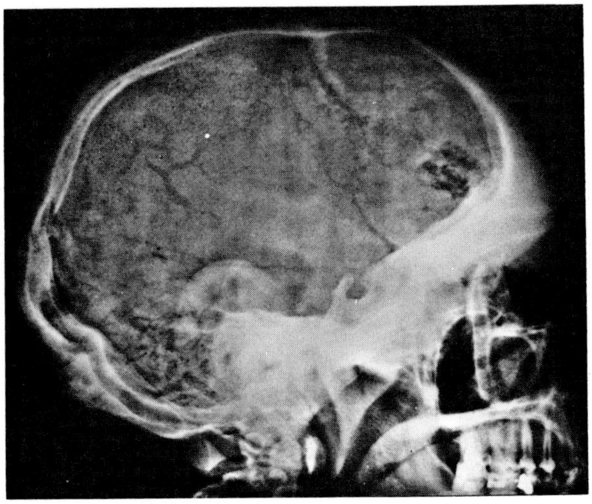

Fig. 3-98. Fibrous dysplasia in a 19-year-old boy. Note the markedly dense base of the skull with the cottony appearance of the vault.

Calcification is uneven and usually there are no osteoblasts. This type of involvement occurs most frequently in regions of abundant vascularization. Within the skull we find only nonspecific bony condensation. The pathogenesis of fibrous dysplasia is unknown as we do not have any insight into the mesenchymal anomaly which is at the base of the development of this fibrous material. The disease involves both sexes evenly. Only single cases are seen in a family and no genetic transmission is known.

In view of the appearance of precocious puberty in Albright's disease there is still too little known about its mechanism. It seems quite clear that this is not the result of the presence of the cranial lesions, nor is it secondary to a tumor. Hall speculates that it is due to an abnormal secretion of hypothalamic factors. Cushing's disease, or a hypophyseal adenoma, which is rarely seen in combination with fibrous dysplasia would be due to a similar mechanism.

Treatment

Treatment is directed against secondary deformity after fractures, and against the danger of recurrence using either bone grafts or synthetic material. Repeated fractures present a very real problem.

Involvement of the base of the skull requires careful neurologic follow-up with meticulous and repeated attention to the eye ground. Neurosurgical interventions must be considered in patients with nerve compression. The same is true with spinal involvement.

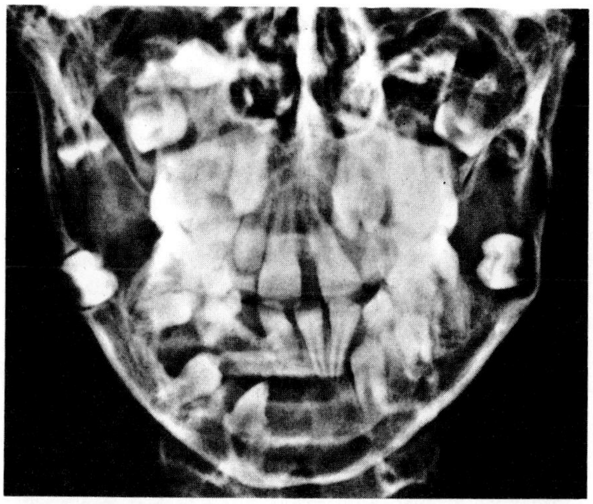

Fig. 3-99. Cherubism in a 10-year-old boy. There is prominent widening of the mandible with cyst formation at the angle.

OTHER DISORDERS WITH ABNORMAL FIBROUS TISSUE DEVELOPMENT

The two disorders which will be discussed here are cherubism and multiple fibromatosis.

CHERUBISM

This rather peculiar disorder described by Jones is clearly different from fibrous dysplasia. Cherubism results from an infiltration of fibrous tissue within the mandible. The clinical appearance is that of marked swelling of the cheeks appearing between the ages of 2 and 4 developing up until age 7. The disease then stabilizes until puberty, at which time the facial structure development leads to an apparent regression. Severe dental anomalies are present. Teeth may be totally absent and there may be early eruption.

Radiographically there is widening and deformity of the ramus. The angle of the mandible reveals invasion of multifocal geodic lesions which lead to a thinned inner and outer cortex. Involvement is always bilateral (Fig. 3-99).

Histologic study reveals the presence of fibrous tissue with large fusiform cells and even giant cells. Dominant autosomal transmission of this disorder is established and is characteristic of it.

MULTIPLE FIBROMATOSIS

This is a rare disorder affecting the newborn or very young infant. Due to the presence of very hard muscular tumors of various sizes, number and location this disorder is recognized within the first few days or weeks of life. This leads to a careful investigation and radiographic study.

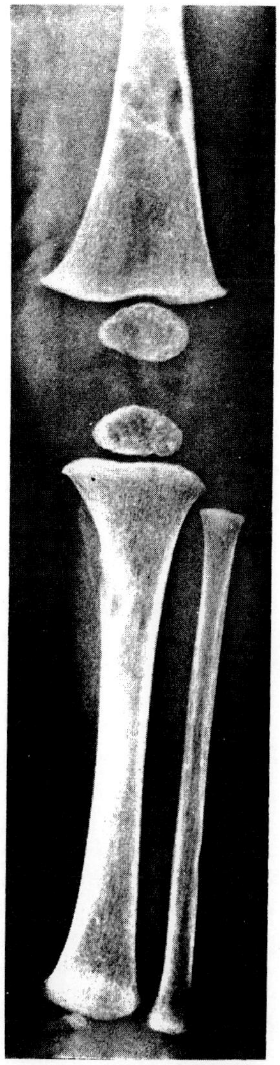

Fig. 3-100. Multiple fibromatosis of the skeleton. (Courtesy of C. Fauré)

Radiographs reveal the presence of well defined and clearly delineated areas of defects surrounded by a thin zone of peripheral condensation (Fig. 3-100). The lesions can be rounded or irregular and the size varies. Involvement may range from minimal hardly visible lesions to large defects extending practically across the entire bone. There may be dense bands within these lesions, usually located at the metaphyseal ends of long bones, vertebral bodies, the pelvis, ribs, or even in the skull.

The evolution of the disease is quite variable. Some patients show rapid fatal development with a clinical picture of respiratory failure. At autopsy a large number of intrapulmonary tumors and proliferation of the media of the pulmonary arterioles explain these events. Other patients experience a rapidly regressive development of their lesions and have a very good prognosis.

The etiology of this disease is mysterious but does not seem to be familial. Due to an occasional trend to form intestinal polyps, this disorder has been compared to the Gardner syndrome. Still, it is a clearly distinct entity of its own. Histologic study of the lesions demonstrates the presence of young fibroblasts, often of unusual size, with a nucleus containing nucleoli lacking malignant characteristics.

As to juvenile fibromatosis of the fingers, an unusual disease, no confusion seems possible. This is a disorder with an early onset, at birth or during the first years, and is limited to aponeuroses or nonskeletal tissues. There are fibromas involving the lateral surface of fingers, sometimes of the forearm, and also of the paravertebral region. Radiographically we can note areas of calcification, but no bony changes can be seen (Des Marchais et al.). The prognosis is good.

These different diseases, just as multiple chondromatosis, should not be confused with certain disseminated vascular tumors (see p. 392), and, in particular, with multiple osseous lymphangtiectasia (Sacrez et al., Sauvegrain et al.). Both of these disorders may be recognized during radiographic study for bowing. In others local lymphedema leads to a careful investigation. Radiographically we find small rounded or oval defects of somewhat unequal and unusually small size. These are almost exclusively localized to the metaphyses, and rarely in the diaphysis. The defects do not have dense borders and the affected bone does not show any morphologic changes, nor is there any periosteal reaction. Localization seems to be frequently in the legs, but practically all parts of the skeleton can be involved. This can be best appreciated when a contrast agent fills the defects after lymphangiography proving that indeed they are due to a malformation of the lymphatic system.

Part 3: Anomalies of Structural Density of the Diaphyseal Cortex or of Modeling

Under this title we will focus on four different sets of circumstances. First, we will discuss osteogenesis imperfecta and idiopathic juvenile osteoporosis, conditions with an unusually excessive skeletal radiolucency. Secondly, we will focus on disorders of abnormally dense bone. A third chapter will be devoted to anomalies of the diaphyseal cortex, and the last part to modeling defects.

DISORDERS WITH INCREASED SKELETAL RADIOLUCENCY

Several constitutional disorders may manifest increased radiolucency of bone. Some of these occur as the result of a disturbed phosphorus and calcium metabolism, such as vitamin D resistant rickets and hypophosphatasia, which will be studied in the second part of this book (see p. 218).

In other cases diseases are due to abnormally developed connective tissues which form the bone. We are thus faced with a true osteoporosis. This is the case in osteogenesis imperfecta in both the congenital and tarda types. It can also involve the adolescent by varying types of osteoporosis which have a rather poorly understood pathogenesis.

OSTEOGENESIS IMPERFECTA

Usually two different disorders are distinguished. The congenital type of Vrolik which is present at birth and osteopsathyrosis, or Lobstein's disease, which is discovered later. This is an artificial distinction, which is useful in practice and is the reason why we will successively study these two types of osteogenesis imperfecta, fully aware however, that there is no clear cut border between the two.

OSTEOGENESIS IMPERFECTA CONGENITA (VROLIK)

First described by Vrolik in 1849, Porak and Durante in a 1905 study, clearly defined the individual characteristics of congenital osteogenesis imperfecta identifying it separately from achondroplasia with which it had been previously confused.

Clinical Findings

In its most classic expression this disorder is sometimes recognized before birth. Poor fetal development and difficulties in palpating the skull may lead to an intrauterine radiographic study revealing abnormal ossification of the skull, the defective skeletal mineraliza-

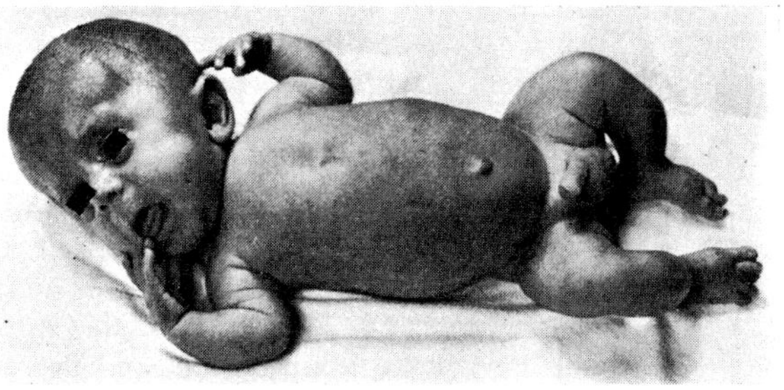

Fig. 3-101. Osteogenesis imperfecta congenita. There is severe bowing of the limbs as a result of fractures and a widened skull.

tion, and at times even shortened or fractured long bones. At birth, patients present with a combination of micromelia and softness of the skull. The extremities may be markedly shortened with deformity and bowing. An attempt to mobilize these can reveal crepitation or abnormal mobility. Hands and feet are hardly ever affected. However, they may show abnormal deviation due to the bowing of the lower legs simulating clubbed feet. The skull is large and soft. The sensation during palpation is similar to touching parchment. The forehead protrudes, and the bridge of the nose is flat like "an eagle's bill." Occasionally we have noted mandibular hypoplasia (Fig. 3-101).

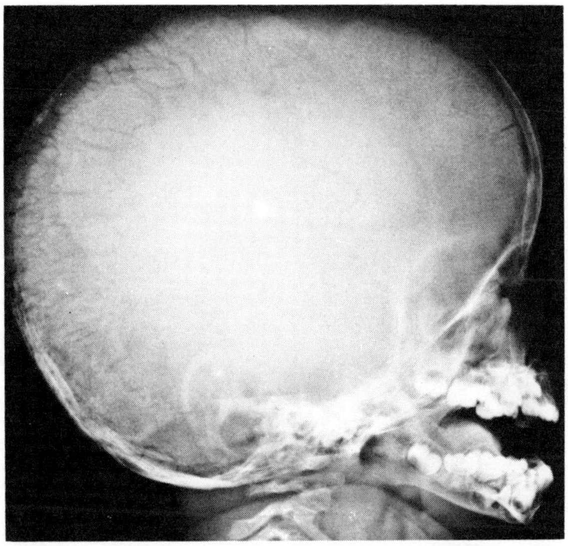

Fig. 3-102. Osteogenesis imperfecta congenita in a 3-week-old baby. Note the defective ossification of the cranial vault with its "mosaic" appearance.

Radiographic Findings

The cranial vault is poorly mineralized and ossification consists of numerous wormian bones. Later their presence leads to the "mosaic" appearance (Fig. 3-102). The long bones of the extremities are short and broad, curved and callus formation at several levels sometimes result in a wavy contour (Fig. 3-103). Aside from the areas of callus formation, there is an increased radiolucency of bone and a very thin cortex. The vertebral bodies are more or less flattened, and some are wedged which is most likely as the result of fractures. The ribs are often involved and have many callus areas. The thorax may be narrow and the iliac wings have a somewhat square appearance at times with the acetabula in a horizontal position. The pelvis is unusually radiolucent as are the scapulae.

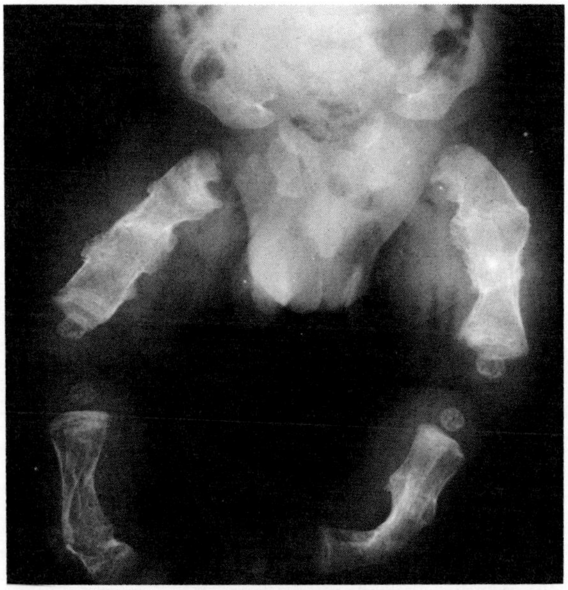

Fig. 3-103. Osteogenesis imperfecta congenita in a 2-week-old baby. Notice the plump and irregular appearance of all the long bones with their many areas of callus formation and the thin cortex.

Development, Clinical Types, and Genetic Data

Despite contrasting statements osteogenesis imperfecta congenita does not always lead to death. It is necessary to distinguish several types of varying severity. In some patients it is virtually impossible to count all of the fractures present. The bones assume the characteristic "bamboo" appearance. There is generalized platyspondyly, along with the pearshaped deformity of the thorax. The ribs have almost the same appearance as the long bones. This lesion is most likely to be fatal because of the extremely severe thoracic involvement and the resulting respiratory failure (Fig. 3-104).

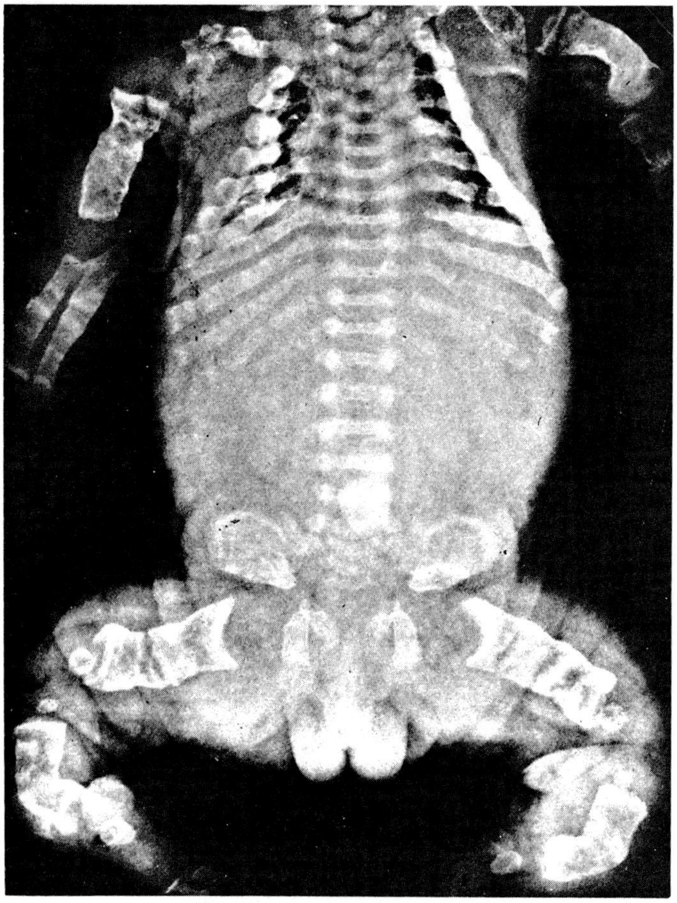

Fig. 3-104. Fatal type of osteogenesis imperfecta congenita.

In the type selected for our description we note a different evolution. These infants will generally survive but remain "fragile" and often die during the first years of life because of respiratory infection. Sometimes a hydrocephalus complicates the course. Growth failure in surviving infants is usually serious and by the time they reach 6 to 8 years of age these patients have hardly reached the development of a two-year-old. The lumbar fractures vary remarkably from one patient to another and it is not unusual that there is only a rare recurrence of fractures in spite of an apparently severe bony fragility present at birth.

It is quite interesting to follow these lesions radiographically. There is progressive ossification of the skull from wormian bones and the "mosaic" appearance develops. The long bones have a tendency to become very slender as in osteopsathyrosis. Spinal changes are often dramatic with the vertebral bodies undergoing a height loss. There is also a much less obvious type, where, for instance, bowing of the extremities may be limited to one site. Occasionally, there may be only a single fracture at birth, which leads to the recognition of this disorder. In this patient one of the key findings to investigate for is the presence of deficient ossification of the cranial vault, since the appearance of long bones may barely be affected (Fig. 3-105). Its development is much less severe and it has an excellent prognosis. It is comparable to osteopsathyrosis and is usually discovered at a later time.

The genetic aspects of Vrolik's disease have led to numerous discussions. The most severe types are seen in isolated instances and the most likely explanation is that they represent a dominant mutation. However, there are several cases, of brothers and sisters who suffered from this disorder but who have entirely normal parents. Occasionally, there is consanguinity as in the family studied by Kaplan and reinvestigated by Laplane with a pedigree suggesting autosomal recessive transmission. We do not, however, maintain that this type of transmission is specific for this severe variant.

In the less severe types dominant transmission can be verified by a study of several generations. In the following pages we will review this problem and the variable expressivity of the gene. Pathology and treatment

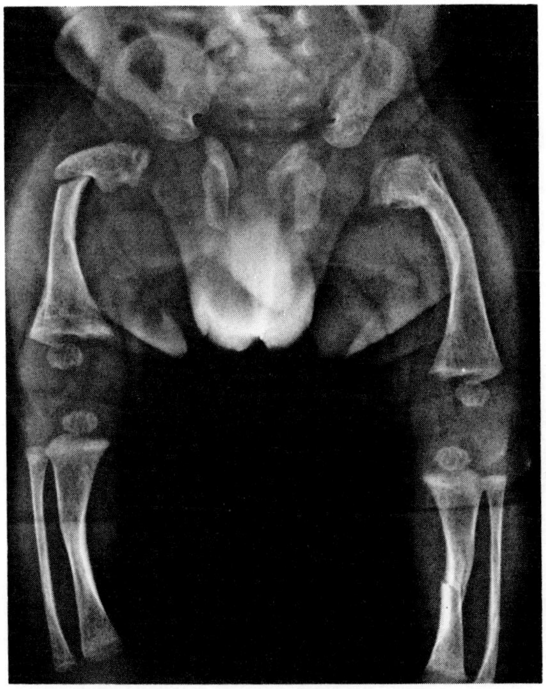

Fig. 3-105. Mild osteogenesis imperfecta congenita in a 3-week-old baby. Note that the bones do not have the plump appearance as in Fig. 3-103.

do not differ significantly from the congenita to the tarda type.

LOBSTEIN'S DISEASE (OSTEOPSATHYROSIS)

Discovery usually occurs at about the time when the child begins to walk, however it can be much later.

Clinical Findings

In the majority of patients the disease presents itself following a fracture which is either a repeat fracture or from minimal trauma. In rare instances it is because of a growth deficit, recidivating dislocations, or deformed extremities that medical help is sought.

Initially the diagnosis may be difficult to establish, since skeletal involvement can be mild and a radiographic examination is not always requested. The child must be carefully studied, in order to fully recognize the slight alterations of the skull, an occasional ligamentous hyperlaxity, or blue sclerae.

Bony changes are usually quite evident, giving away the diagnosis. Fractures, resulting from minimal or even unrecognized trauma, occur often. The legs, particularly, are prone but any bone of the arm as well as the spine may be affected.

Typically affected children are short, and have curved legs with lateral bowing of the femora and saber shins (Fig. 3-106). The trunk is short because of the reduced height of the vertebral bodies. The sternum protrudes giving the patient an appearance somewhat similar to Morquio's disease. The disease, when fully manifested, shows transverse widening of the skull. Palpation of the temporal region will reveal a rim. Bony deformity results from the fractures as well as from abnormal bone molding. This is responsible for the tibial curving, the platyspondyly, and the distortion of the pelvis and the skull. Muscular underdevelopment and hyperlaxity of joints are frequently noted. The latter may result in repeated sprains and dislocations.

In addition to skeletal and ligamentous involvement two other anomalies, blue sclerae and deafness, may meet the crtieria of van der Hoeve's triad. Blue sclerae result from a variable degree of excessive scleral transparence. Sometimes, this is very intense "porcelain blue," but at other times it is only minimally noticeable. Deafness is rarely found in the child as its onset usually occurs during adolescence or adulthood. Another important anomaly is the defective development of the teeth which are yellow and transparent in appearance. This "dentinogenesis imperfecta" is frequently noted in the primary dentition. Its characteristics are identical with those of the dominantly transmitted Capdepont disease.

It is often difficult to reliably predict the outcome and prognosis of osteogenesis imperfecta. Great restraint is required because of the unpredictable occurrence of further fractures, deformities, and defects in bone modeling. In these patients growth defects and deformities of the extremities and trunk may be very severe. If left to themselves they will become severely crippled. However, even in such severely affected patients, stabilization of the disease will occur after puberty resulting in a much lower incidence of fractures. This serves to emphasize the value of all preventive measures. There are also milder forms of this disorder which result in few fractures if any. Recurring sprains or dislocations may be the only manifestations aside from a broad skull, blue sclerae, or deafness. Not all of these findings are constantly present, and the disease may go unrecognized if the family history and careful skeletal radiographic investigation does not support the diagnosis.

Radiographic Findings

At the time of a first fracture, radiographic findings of the long bones may be very mild with only a slight degree of osteoporosis and minimal cortical thinning to aid in establishing the diagnosis. Quite often only

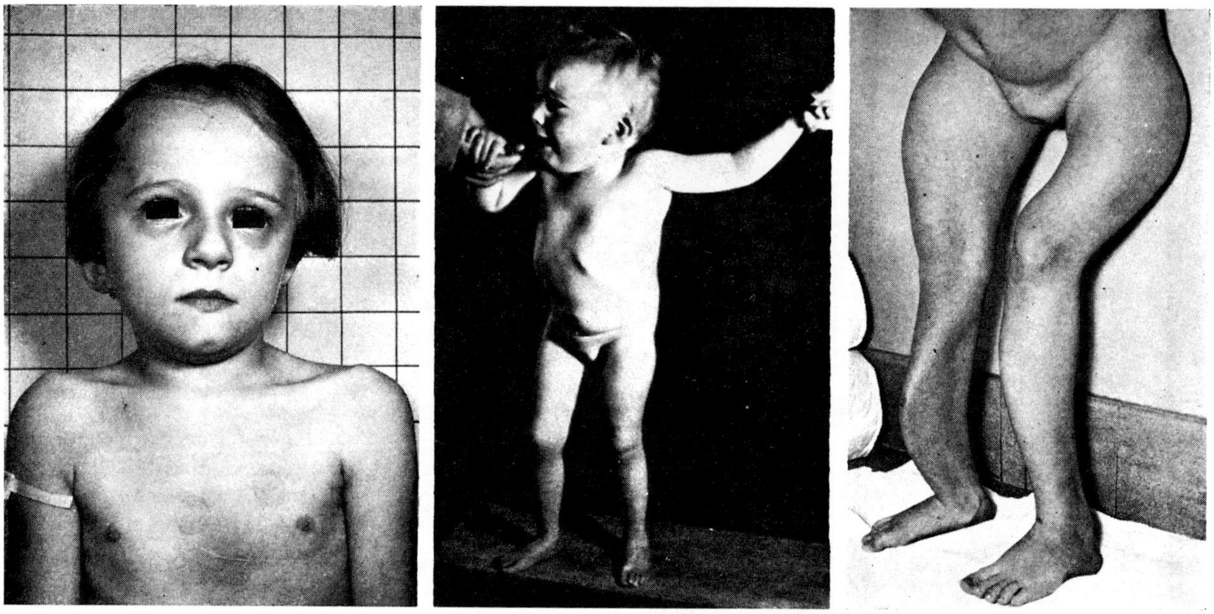

Fig. 3-106. Osteogenesis imperfecta tarda with marked widening of the skull, shortening of the trunk and deformity of the lower legs so that they are "sabershaped."

repeated fractures will confirm this. A complete study of the skeleton is needed once osteogenesis imperfecta is clinically suspected or suggested by local radiographic findings. A mild degree of vertebral osteoporosis with a loss of height and the typical "mosaic" appearance of the cranial vault are reliable signs when the diagnosis remains questionable.

The more severe types or advanced states of the disease may be revealed by the following findings: Increased radiolucency of long bones, an abnormally visible outline, wide meshing, and a thin cortex (Fig. 3-107). Cortical loss is not evident on the concave side of bowed or fractured areas. Fractures usually involve the midportion of the diaphysis and develop normal consolidation. The femur is most frequently involved. The upper extremities are rarely affected, although if they are it is generally the olecranon that will be fractured.

Bones are slender, in particular, the occasional "filiform" fibula. Diaphyseal bowing is seen regularly and may be the result of fractures, but often is due to abnormal skeletal molding. The anterior bowing of the tibia simulating a "saber shin" has the same origin.

Vertebral height is reduced and results in an occasional generalized biconcave appearance (Fig. 3-108). Individual vertebral bodies may be wedged, as the result of an overlooked fracture. Acetabular protrusion is not uncommon. The cranial vault is widened and increased in the AP diameter with regional depression where the occipital and parietal bones meet. In typical cases wormian bones are numerous, eventually resulting in a "mosaic" appearance. Finally, we must emphasize that the incidence of basilar impression in osteogenesis imperfecta is high and is present in about one-third of all patients (Fig. 3-109).

This is the clinical and radiographic appearance of the complete form of Lobstein's disease. However, we are quite often not dealing with the entire spectrum. Thus, there may be no involvement of the skull or spine in about one-third of all patients. Thinning of the cortex is not always evident, although it is sometimes due to the presence of marked callus. These facts should serve to emphasize the occasional difficulty encountered in the radiographic diagnostic approach.

Finally, we would like to note some of the appearances which result in possible errors. Beside being familiar with defective metaphyseal modeling (Fig. 3-110), epiphyseal irregularities, thickening of the skull —personally observed in one patient, and the double contour of vertebrae sometimes seen in young infants, it may be of key importance to become fully familiar with the different appearances of hypertrophic callus. There are patients with unusually excessive callus formation simulating a sarcoma (see Fig. 14-23, p. 391). Such lesions are entirely benign and never justify surgical intervention. Amputation would be a catastrophy. Patients affected in this manner usually have subluxation of the radial head and ossification of

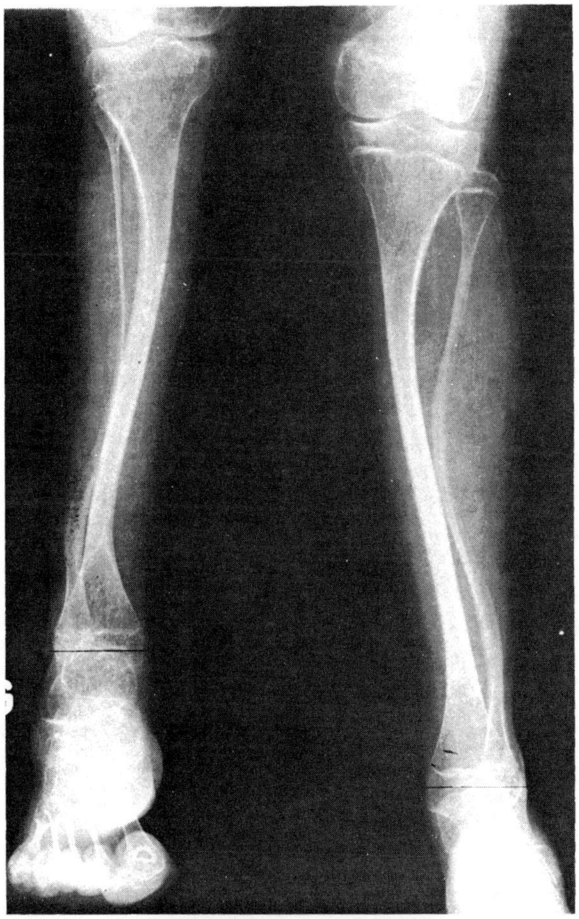

Fig. 3-107. Osteogenesis imperfecta tarda in a 15-year-old girl. Notice the slenderness and bowing of the long bones with a loss of bony structure.

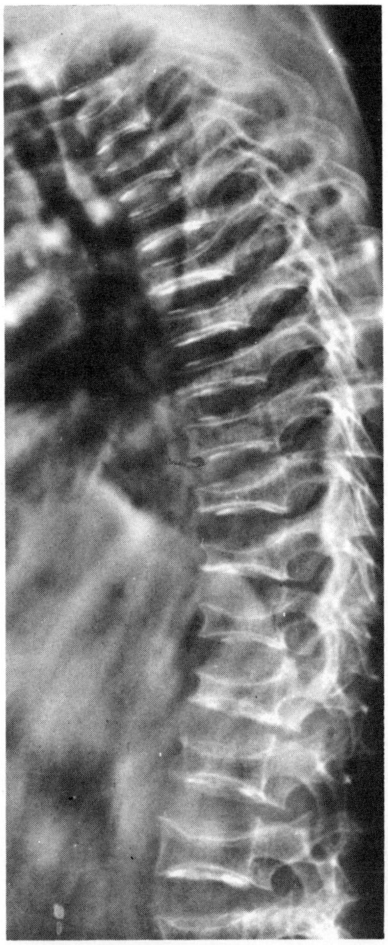

Fig. 3-108. Osteogenesis imperfecta tarda in a 9-year-old girl. Practically all of the vertebral bodies are of abnormal shape along with reduced height and increased radiolucency.

the interosseous membrane of the forearm. These findings can be of considerable value if one is in doubt (Fig. 3-111).

Genetic Data

There is unquestionably heterogeneity of osteogenesis imperfecta. Criteria presently used are insufficient for the recognition and definition of the different subtypes. Our approach to distinguish between the congenita and tarda types is actually a misleading approach to a much more complex reality.

Whichever the true situation may be osteogenesis imperfecta follows in a large number of observations a dominant transmission. There may be marked variability in the degree of manifestation of the gene in one family. Some individuals may only present with blue sclerae, and yet their offspring may suffer from fragile bones. Because of this, it is often difficult to reliably ascertain a recessive mode of transmission of the disease from pedigrees. This latter modality occurs rarely.

Pathology and Pathogenesis

In the old days investigators were particularly struck by alterations of the periosteum. Thus, they attached the name periosteal dysplasia to the congenital form of the disease. When examined microscopically, the cortex is only of minimal thickness. The growth cartilage is also, at times, involved. Occasionally, there is a slight irregularity which results in atypical columnar arrangement. This finding fully explains the severe growth disturbances of some patients who are not affected by fractures.

The most classic striking finding for this disorder is the anarchic arrangement of the collagen fibers of the

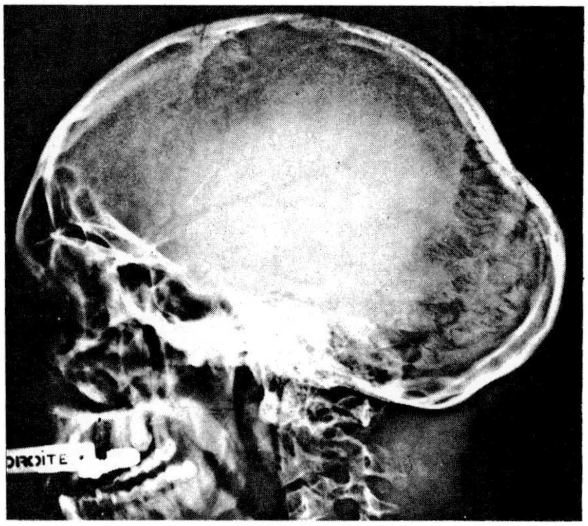

Fig. 3-109. Osteogenesis imperfecta tarda in a 18-year-old young man. The skull has a deformity similar to a "bun." The "mosaic" appearance is due to the presence of many wormian bones and basilar impression.

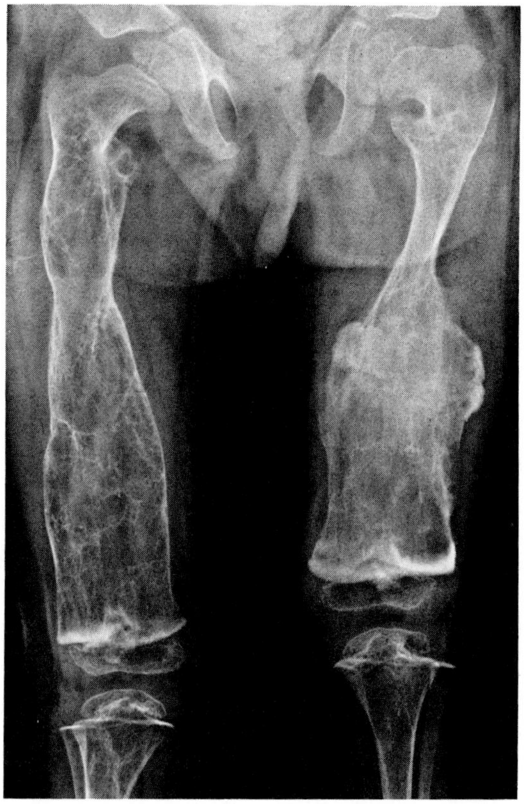

Fig. 3-110. Osteogenesis imperfecta in a 3-year-old girl. She also suffers from a severe modeling defect of the metaphyses. (Courtesy of J. Marie)

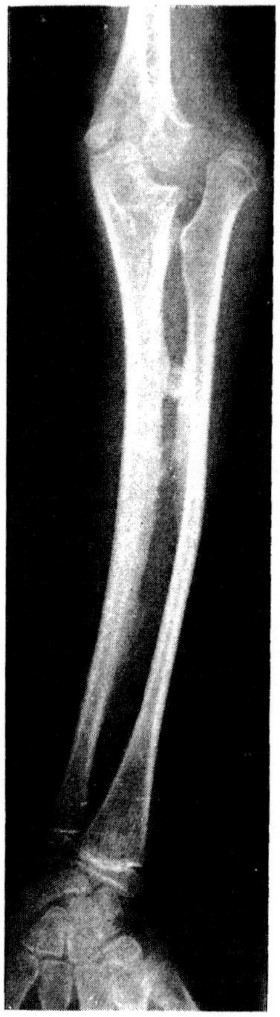

Fig. 3-111. Osteogenesis imperfecta with exuberant callus formation in a 13-year-old boy. There is dislocation of the radial head and ossification of the interosseus membrane.

osseous matrix. This has been documented in older studies (Engfeldt et al.) using polarized light. These studies reveal that the collagen fibers are thin, widely spaced, and irregularly distributed as they are in immature fetal bone. These findings have been fully confirmed by electron microscope study of the cornea as well as the bone. Both reveal a reduction in the diameter of fibers and abnormal striation (Lindenfelser et al., Blümcke et al., Haebara et al.) These alterations, however, are not constant.

Dynamic studies by tetracycline marking have confirmed that bone formation occurs more rapidly than normal (Jett, Villanueva, Ramser et al.).

The few examples of abnormal bony fragility in animals, especially in the dog (Calkins), and in sheep (Holmes), add very little to the understanding of human disease pathophysiology. Findings from anatomic studies in humans suggest that the primary defect is within the collagen. The weak content of glycosaminoglycans within the ground substance, reported by Blümcke, is probably only a secondary phenomenon. Collagen studies of cultured fibroblasts reveal an increase in the soluble fraction of the latter along with a decrease in the ratio of hydroxyprolin to prolin (Brown). Analysis of amino acids in collagen, studied by Bleckman, reveals an elevation of hydroxylysin. Eastoe has noted this elevation together with that of other amino acids, in particular, with a lipidophilic lateral chain. Solomons and Styner, on the other hand, insist on the inhibiting action of calcification which they have observed in vitro with the collagen of patients suffering from osteogenesis imperfecta. This effect would be inhibited by pyrophosphatase. These authors have found elevated concentrations of pyrophosphatase in the blood and urine of their patients. However, this finding has not been confirmed by others (Russell et al.).

The disparities between these findings may possibly be a reflection of the heterogeneity of this disease, as has already been suggested by the clinical and radiographic study. Thus, physiopathologic findings should be very cautiously interpreted.

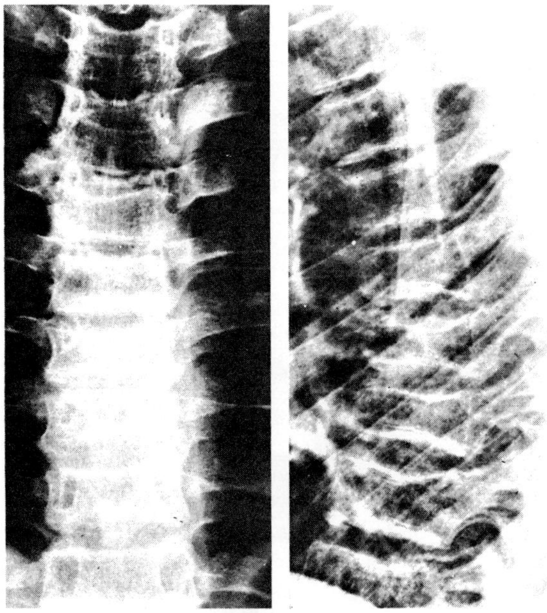

Fig. 3-112. Juvenile osteoporosis in a 15-year-old boy: the vertebral bodies are reduced in height and are biconcave in form. (Courtesy of S. Balsan)

Treatment

In spite of the fact that there is no decisive treatment one should not abandon these patients. We would like to emphasize the value of orthopedic surgery as others have done (Reichelt).

Initially, attention must be carefully directed to the handling of all fractures, possibly utilizing internal fixation, particularly when dealing with fractures of the leg. A frequent indication for the use of screwed plates or the pin insertion is the need for early mobilization. Diaphyseal bowing can be corrected by osteotomy and the insertion of an intramedullary nail. There are some who propose multiple osteotomies (Sofield and Millard). Such corrective interventions require great technical finesse because of the fragile quality of the bones. The second major requirement of therapy is directed towards the prevention of prolonged immobilization as this only increases the risks and aggravates osteoporosis. Therefore our attention must be directed against loss of muscle mass by active motion. The patient should resume normal activity and begin walking at the earliest possible moment after the fracture or the surgical management. Proposed therapeutic approaches using medication have turned out to be rather deceptive. If calcitonin appears to increase the retention of calcium (Castells et al.) it is still difficult to decide whether it really does have a positive effect. No positive effect can be attached at all to sodium fluoride (Albright et al.). The same must be said for anabolic steroids, although they may be tried in severely affected patients, where mobilization is attempted in addition to moderate doses of vitamin C and D. However, one should never expect too much from such treatment.

The use of magnesium oxide has been recommended on the basis of the previously mentioned observation by Solomons and Styner. This approach is still rather controversial. The selection of an appropriate career is very important. Competent help and sound council is needed as the future way of life may be critical. In one's approach to deafness it seems justified to attempt surgical correction. However, one should not overlook the difficulties encountered as a result of fragile bones and the local anatomic peculiarities of the stapes (Kosoy and Maddox).

IDIOPATHIC JUVENILE OSTEOPOROSIS

Besides osteogenesis imperfecta Dent and Friedman have defined juvenile osteoporosis as a distinct entity. Before establishing this diagnosis, however, one must be careful to eliminate the possibility of osteogenesis imperfecta, as this disorder can be quite deceptive, and may have an unusual late manifestation.

The discovery of juvenile osteoporosis, usually between the ages of 8 and 11, results from a fracture caused by minimal trauma or spinal pain. Sometimes this fracture may go unnoticed and recognition follows a radiographic study in response to persistent local pain or walking difficulties. Clinically, the most striking finding is a dorsolumbar kyphosis accompanied by a slight reduction in trunk height with sternal protrusion. Sometimes there is deformity of the extremities secondary to the fractures. The craniofacial structures, however, are normal. Calcium, phosphorus, and alkaline phosphatase levels are all normal, sometimes falling in the upper ranges of normal.

Radiographic investigation reveals marked generalized osteoporosis with diminution of cortical thickness in the long bones and a reduction in the cortico-diaphyseal ratio. Fractures are limited to the femur or tibia in the metaphyseal vicinity. Initially, they may be visible only as a narrow line at the border of the bone, but then result in bowing. Callus formation is normal and good consolidation will follow. Spinal involvement is very dramatic (Fig. 3-112). Vertebral bodies are reduced in height and have a classic biconcave appearance. It is not uncommon to note one or several wedged vertebrae. The radiolucency of all the vertebral bodies is abnormal and their outline is unusually well delineated. On the other hand, there are no modifications of the skull or cranial vault.

The evolution of this disorder varies. The prognosis is generally good. Because of this, it is quite difficult to evaluate the effectiveness of calcium, vitamin D, and anabolic steroids which are the recommended forms of therapy. Fractures should be immobilized for as short a period as possible, as we have discussed for osteogenesis imperfecta. The etiology of this disease is unknown and at this time no evidence supports familial transmission.

Microradiography reveals an increase of bone resorption (Jowsey and Johnson). Dent and Friedman believe that calcium malabsorption is one of the most characteristic findings of juvenile osteoporosis.

OTHER TYPES OF IDIOPATHIC OSTEOPOROSIS

Aside from the disorders mentioned there are other types of osteoporosis. This may lead to difficult problems in differential diagnosis from osteogenesis imperfecta (see p. 314). Among others is the autosomal recessive syndrome associating a pseudoglioma with generalized osteoporosis (Briard Guillemont and Frézal, Bianchine et al.).

Similarly, several authors have reported on a disorder characterized by a thin, fragile sclera and a cornea susceptible to rupture. This can be accompanied by fragilitas osseum (Arkin) and a number of other anomalies, in particular, dentinogenesis imperfecta. Autosomal recessive transmission seems probable (Stein et al., Hyams et al.). A number of metabolic lesions may result in osteoporosis, which also leads to confusion. For example, one disorder has been described (Malmquist et al.) under the term familial protein intolerance.

CONDENSING BONE DISEASES

These disorders can lead to markedly different radiographic changes. Sometimes there is a generalized abnormal bone structure as in osteopetrosis or pycnodysostosis, along with other findings such as alterations of the skull, mandible, and distal phalanges.

In osteopoikilosis we find only small punctate or striated condensations, while in melorheostosis there is an appearance of "candle guttering" (like flowing wax) which deforms the bony contours.

Certain disorders secondary to disturbed phosphorus and calcium metabolism may have more or less generalized skeletal condensations. Idiopathic hypercalcemia is an example of this group. They will be discussed later in this book (see p. 220).

OSTEOPETROSIS – ALBERS – SCHÖNBERG'S DISEASE

First described in 1904 by Albers-Schönberg, whose name is attached to it, this disease is frequently discovered during infancy, at least in its autosomal recessive form. This is the form we have selected for detailed description. Many publications have been devoted to its radiographic peculiarities, its hematologic, and, most recently, to its metabolic characteristics.

Clinical Findings

The precocious form of the disease is most frequently discovered during the first few months of life, because of disturbed general development. The infant is in poor general condition with pallor and fever. Abnormal visual findings, and in particular, unusual ocular movements may disturb the family. In rare instances, a fracture leads to medical attention.

Physical examination reveals a striking pallor of the skin. The infant is "aged" in appearance and has a sparse amount of hair. Purpura or ecchymoses are often noted. The skull may be larger than normal. Sometimes there is true hydrocephalus. The infant will not follow with the eyes, however, there is asynergic ocular motion, pupillary trembling, and frequent nystagmus. Examination of the eye ground will confirm early onset of optic atrophy. Teeth eruption occurs late and they are of poor quality resulting in early loss.

Abdominal palpation demonstrates hepatomegaly and splenomegaly, sometimes lymphadenopathy. The

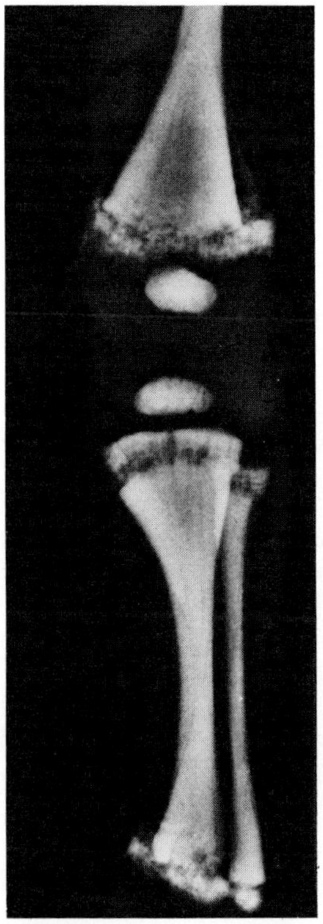

Fig. 3-113. Malignant form of osteopetrosis in a 5-month-old infant. Changes taking place at the metaphyseal ends are similar to those in rickets.

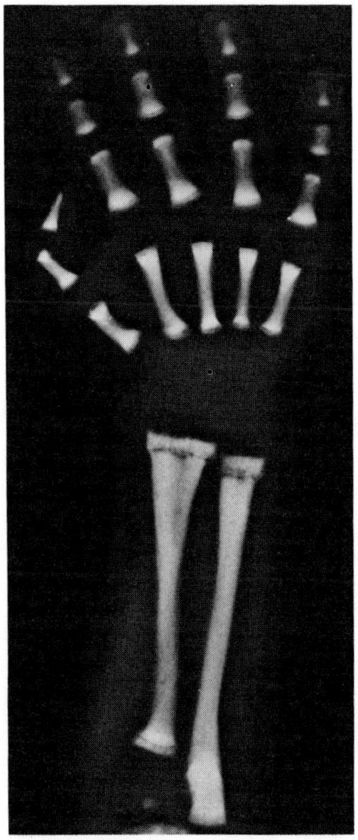

Fig. 3-114. Congenital osteopetrosis at 3 months. The dense "bone in bone" appearance of centers within the carpals and phalanges is still visible.

size of liver and spleen is variable, however, they may be very large. Mild bowing of the extremities is seen regularly. Inspection and palpation of the chest wall may reveal the presence of a rosary or a palpable costochondral prominence, as well as more marked metaphyseal widening.

The development of the precocious type of osteopetrosis is very serious. Blindness is usually total. Anemia and poor health are progressive, and there is a further growth deficit. Death generally occurs within the first few years of life.

Radiographic Findings

The diagnostic finding is the association of an unusual, generalized skeletal density, combined with a defect of metaphyseal modeling and "bone in bone" appearance.

The condensation is usually diffuse with the visible disappearance of the cortex and medullary canal (Fig. 3-113). In the very young infant cone-shaped condensation may be recognized, in particular, in the phalanges. The long axis of these cones is parallel to that of the bone and its base is located at the growing end. The metacarpals have the appearance of two cones facing one another by their tip, located in the center of the diaphysis (Fig. 3-114). In other instances, these condensations electively affect the metaphyseal region as a large dense zone. The more central diaphyseal area is somewhat less dense. Parallel striation of the growth cartilage may appear rapidly, resulting in an appearance of piled up plates. Occasionally, early longitudinal striation is noted (observation by Moretti).

The metaphyseal modeling defect can be relatively mild during the first weeks, but will become clearer later leading to the characteristic clubbed appearance. In addition, affected babies often show disturbed mineralization at the growing ends of the long bones similar to that seen in rickets (Fig. 3-113). The metaphyseal region is irregular, wavy and fringed and is combined with a loss of opacity in the immediately adjacent zone which has an uneven structure. This is in contrast with the extremely dense appearance of the rest of the diaphysis. A clear band below the cortical density may be recognized along with a transparent zone at the epiphyseal periphery.

The entire skeleton is affected by this condensation. The vertebrae sometimes look like a diabolo in the lateral view. The iliac bones occasionally show striation. Noteworthy findings may be found in the skull revealing a very dense base and an almost normal appearing vault. Later these structures may become more dense and may even develop a "hair on end" appearance. On AP films a particularly dense orbital rim in the maxillary region may be noted.

Hemotologic and Biochemical Studies

Anemia is severe in this form. The number of red blood cells falls between one and three million. We usually find anisocytosis, poikilocytosis, and polychromasia. The number of white blood cells varies. Frequently there is neutropenia. A low platelet count is often present. Bone marrow studies are particularly difficult due to the hard nature of the bone. The bone marrow is hypoplastic or even aplastic with all three cellular lines affected. Frequently there is a total absence of megacaryocytes. Anemia has been at the center of several controversies and we will return to these when we discuss pathogenesis.

In patients with lesions similar to rickets serum calcium is usually low as is phosphorus. Hyperphosphatasemia is a constant finding. These biologic anomalies may be noted when there are no radiographic signs of rickets. This may be because they have not yet established themselves or they have not yet manifested due to the marked delay of growth.

Genetic Data

The precocious type of osteopetrosis is transmitted as an autosomal recessive disorder. This has been conclusively shown by the study of a number of pedigrees with involved brothers and sisters along with increased parental consanguinity. We will emphasize later the clearly distinctive dominant form.

Pathology

The growth cartilage is normal and ossification seems to develop in the usual manner with normal penetration of the vessels into the degenerating cartilage. In the case of superimposed rickets, the line of ossification is irregular and large zones of osteoid tissue are present. Periosteal ossification is normal.

The most characteristic abnormal finding of this disease is the presence of chondroid tissue inclusions persisting within bony lamellae, while normally this tissue disappears during ossification. These islands will have a strong uptake of Alcian blue as evidence of the high content of acid mucopolysacchrides, just as in the normal cartilaginous matrix. They also have a strong tendency to fix calcium salts. Baruffaldi and Lojodice emphasize the tendency of the hematopoetic marrow to form fibrosis.

Pathogenesis

Numerous theories have been formed on the pathogenesis and it would be impossible to discuss all of them. As in achondroplasia there are many animal models, some of which are of only remote interest, as their mechanisms are entirely different. This is the case, for instance, in avian osteopetrosis which has a well proven viral origin. Osteopetrosis of the rabbit, of the lethal grey line of the mouse, and that of the bull are much closer to the human disorder (Brown and Dent). The second mentioned disease has been particularly well studied and it could be shown that parabiosis with a normal mouse could correct the defect. This suggests the possibility of a humoral factor (Walker). This same correction possibility has been noted in the "op" rat (Toyama et al.). These findings, however, do not allow us to conclude that the identical mechanisms are operative in human osteopetrosis, since we are aware of certain complexities of the sclerosing human diseases. It is highly unlikely that a single pathophysiologic mechanism is responsible for all of these disorders.

As we indicated earlier osteopetrosis is related to the persistence of abnormal chondroid tissue and its very active uptake of calcium. But no theory presently under discussion is capable of explaining this mechanism. A defect of osteoplastic resorption does not seem to be operative and would not explain the defect in the turnover of the body matrix. The same goes for a hypothetical disorder of phosphorus and calcium metabolism. In osteopetrosis there is an unquestionable elevation in the intestinal absorption of calcium with ensuing great difficulties in attempts to bring about a negative calcium balance. These patients face the risk of hypocalcemia. It is probable, however, that this metabolic disturbance is secondary to the avidity of the skeleton for calcium and is not the primary factor causing this disorder as (Dent et al.) has been suggested. The pathophysiology of the lesions similar to rickets is still unresolved and such changes may appear in spite of an adequate prophylactic intake of vitamins.

With respect to mechanisms which lead to anemia there are numerous speculations. The choking of bone marrow space secondary to skeletal condensation appears to be too simplistic a view. Studies with radioactive chromium have demonstrated that there is a significant reduction in the survival time of the red blood cells suggesting hemolysis. Presently the most popular hypothesis favors a mesenchymal disorder with a simultaneous effect on bone and its marrow. However, our level of understanding at this point does not enable us to explain this disease.

Clinical Types

Besides the precocious type we have described, there is another variant of osteopetrosis which manifests in approximately one-half of the cases which present after the age of 20. This disorder has frequently been confused with the cortical hyperostoses and it is still difficult to reliably define its limits and offer a precise description. A recent attempt at this has been undertaken by Segond.

A fracture is generally the precipitating factor which leads to radiographic study, thus resulting in the discovery of this disease. Sometimes there are bone or joint pains of varying origin (epiphyseolysis, post-traumatic dislocation, septic arthritis), or the involvement of cranial nerves (visual disturbances, facial palsy). Finally, accidental discovery of the disorder may result from a routine radiographic investigation of the entire family.

Even if one-third of the patients had at least one fracture, unusual bone fragility has only been noted in one-tenth of all patients observed. This may, on occasion, be rather severe. Johnston reported 33 fractures in one patient. Clinically there may be no other manifestations besides the sequelae of fractures. There may be mild craniofacial disproportion along with a large vault and hypertrophy of the frontal and parietal regions. Patients do have a tendency to develop caries.

This disorder often has a very good prognosis. Occasionally, the disease will not be recognized until a very late stage. This was the case in the mother of a patient described by Albers-Schönberg, whose diagnosis was only established at autopsy. Still, several complications can result.

A mild anemia may be found if a careful investigation is done. Cranial nerve compression with local osteitis or osteonecrosis of the mandible is the most feared complication. The optic nerve is frequently involved with a risk of blindness and there may also be lesions of the facial nerve. This lesion occurs with some regularity in certain families. Involvement of the acustic nerve is rarely seen.

Osteomyelitis occurs almost exclusively in the maxilla, and is secondary to dental infection. Necroses are also seen, as the result of compression in the shrunken dental canal. In earlier times a grave prognosis was attached to local maxillary infections and these sometimes lead to death.

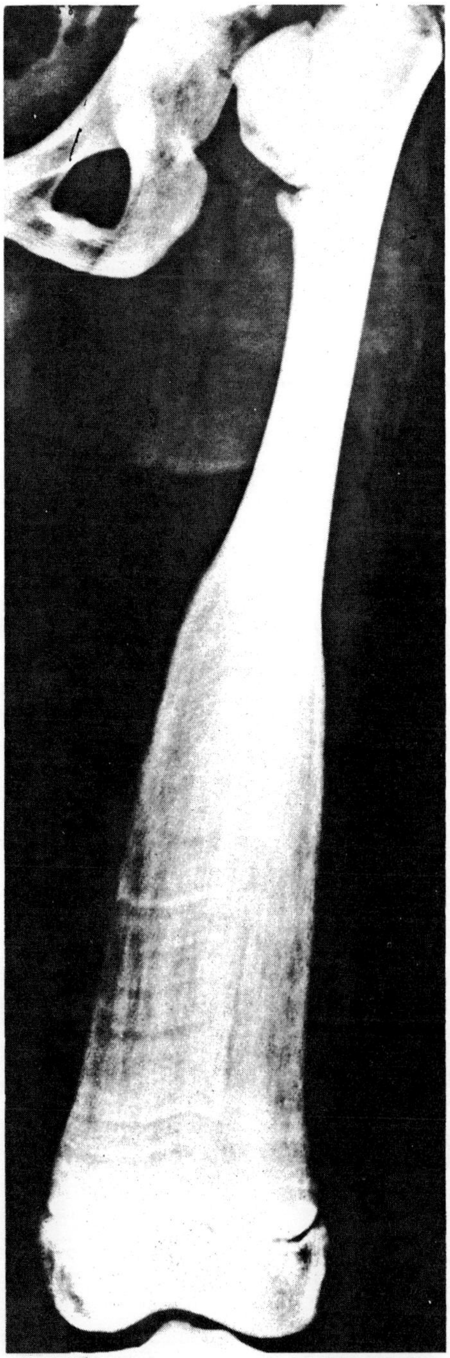

Fig. 3-115. Osteopetrosis, tarda type in a 12-year-old boy. Note the modeling defect, the longitudinal and transverse striation of the metaphyseal region, and the severe coxa vara.

Radiographic study reveals an unusually dense skeleton. In a typical case the appearance is that demonstrated by Albers-Schönberg of poor metaphyseal

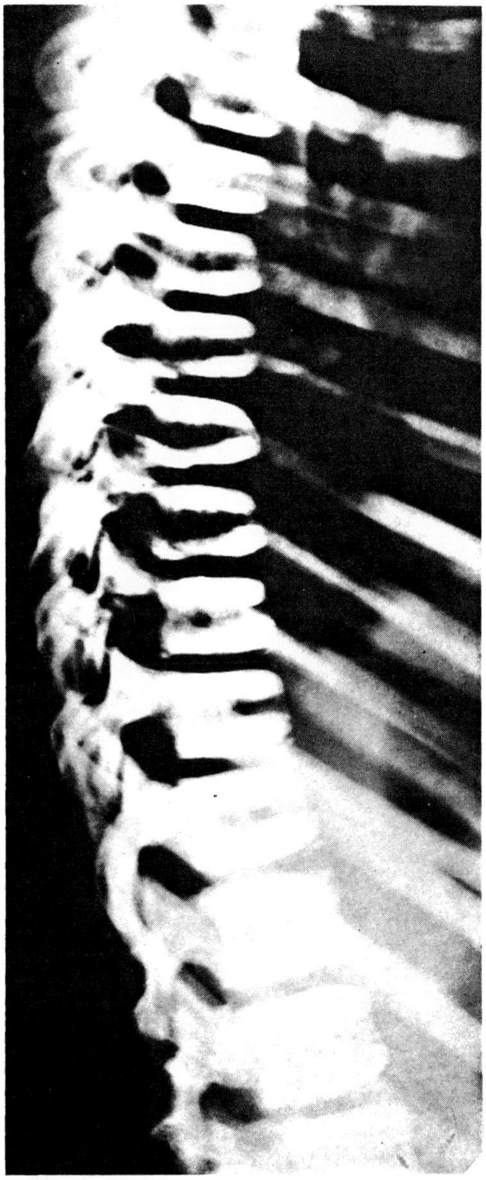

Fig. 3-116. Osteopetrosis, tarda type in a 12-year-old boy. The excessive density is limited to the upper and lower vertebral plateaus.

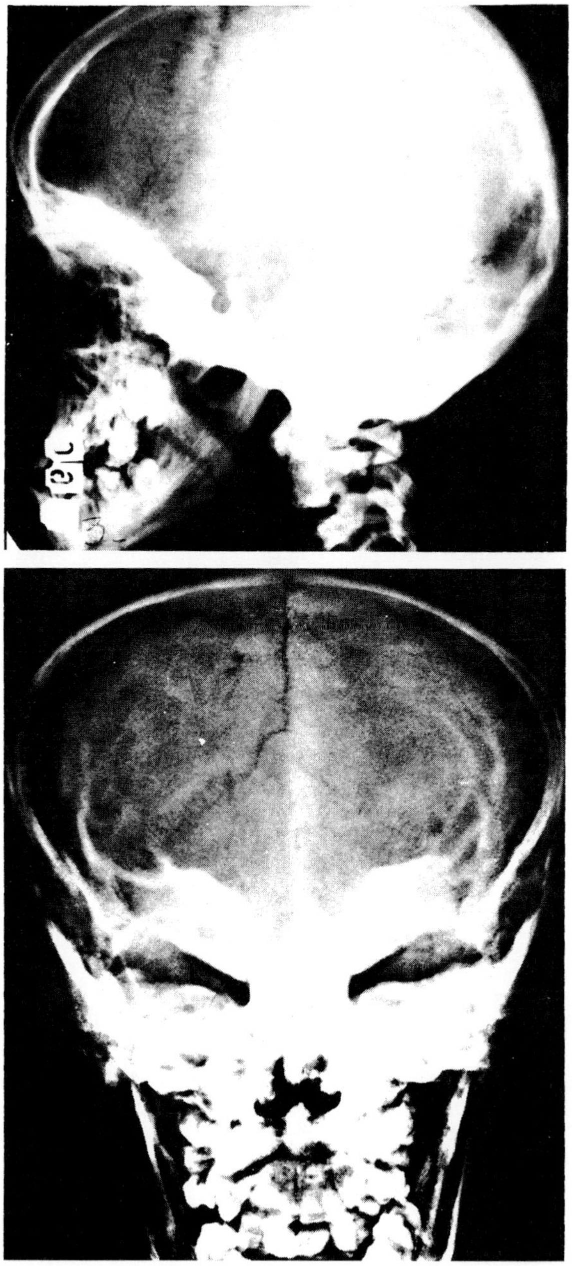

Fig. 3-117. Tarda type osteopetrosis in a 12-year-old boy. Very dense base of the skull and appearance like a "carnival mask" on this AP view.

modeling in the long bones which results in a clubbed appearance (Fig. 3-115). Transverse striation parallel to the growth cartilage outlines its shape. The medullary canal cannot be recognized. The bones of the hands and feet as well as the ribs and clavicles are all involved. In one-half of the cases, however, there is no association of skeletal condensation with a modeling defect or with bony striation. It is not possible to ascertain whether these actually are different features.

In the vertebrae there is a limitation to the unusually dense regional appearance immediately adjacent to the end plates, whereas the middle third does not show this finding. This alternating appearance of hyperlucent and very dense bands leads to an entirely characteristic spinal appearance (Fig. 3-116). The pelvis is also very dense, especially in the pubic and the acetabular region, as are the glenoid and coracoid apophyses of the scapula. The base of the skull is often equally involved. This helps to explain the narrowing of the nerve canals. There may be an unusually dense appearance of the sphenoid and the petrous bone. The sphenoid and maxillary sinuses may disappear and the apophyses of the clinoids may thicken. The vault is not as affected by disappearance of the diploe and the face on the whole is only mildly involved (Fig. 3-117).

Biochemical studies may show an elevation of acid phosphatases (Johnson et al.). However, this finding is not always present. Phosphorus and calcium metabolism is generally normal. Histologic study reveals the same basic changes as have been described for the precocious type, in particular, the presence of chondroid inclusions within the bony lamellae. A paucity in fibrils of the osseous matrix has been noted by several authors and could serve as an explanation for bone fragility.

Transmission is dominant, however, in certain rare families there can be variable or irregular genetic manifestation sparing one generation.

Diagnosis and Treatment

No treatment can slow down the development of osteopetrosis. Chelating agents or the use of parathormone have given disappointing results. Restricted calcium intake has led in one of Dent's patients to a diminished skeletal condensation and appears to have improved the prognosis of the disease. However, such a form of therapy is exceedingly difficult to implement rigorously. An outcome of studies done with J. Rey was the impression that no effect could be brought about in a patient suffering from the precocious form. This approach has the inherent danger of severe accidents due to hypocalcemia. Recently (Morrow et al.) it has been shown that intramuscular injections of heparin can provoke a drop of serum calcium and an increased calciuria. It is our thought that heparin may have a therapeutic effect, but verification of this is still needed.

In the majority of cases therapy will limit itself to the prevention, the recognition, and the limitation of complications. Transfusions are justified in order to counteract the existing anemia. Splenectomy may be an option in certain precocious types, however, its effect on anemia is inconstant. The fear of cranial nerve compression will justify regular careful study and follow-up of the eye ground. Local changes could very well result in surgical attempts to enlarge the optic foramen, at least in the benign forms of this disorder. Unfortunately this intervention is often undertaken when it is too late, and no longer fully effective. Prevention of dental infection is an absolute rule as previously the most feared complication which often

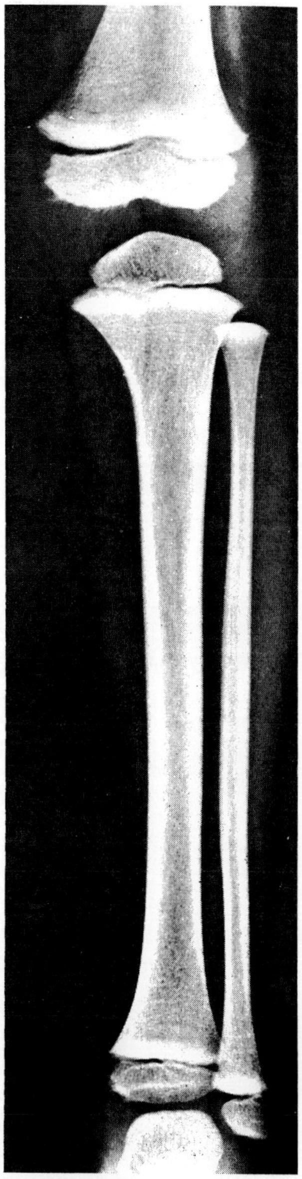

Fig. 3-118. Lead intoxication in a 5-year-old boy. Notice the dense metaphyseal lines. (Courtesy of J. Vialatte)

led to the death of a patient with the dominant type was subsequent osteitis of the maxilla.

During infancy osteopetrosis was frequently confused with a number of constitutional condensing skeletal disorders which will be described in the following pages, or with syndromes still undefined. An example is one described by Lichtenstein and Warson which is transmitted as a dominant disorder and is associated with looped hair and dental anomalies. Other disorders with skeletal condensation, such as osteomyelosclerosis, only rarely manifest themselves

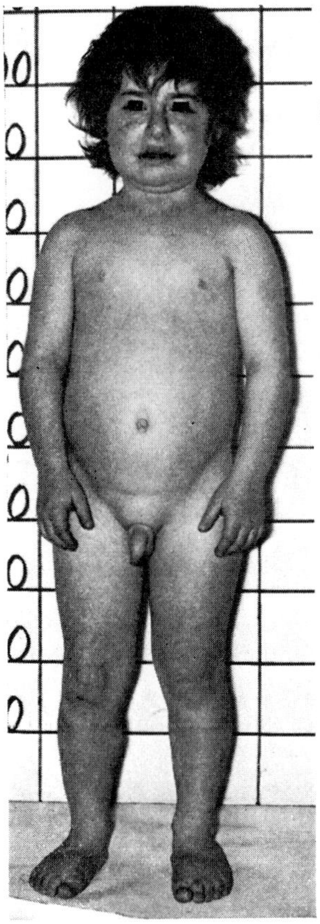

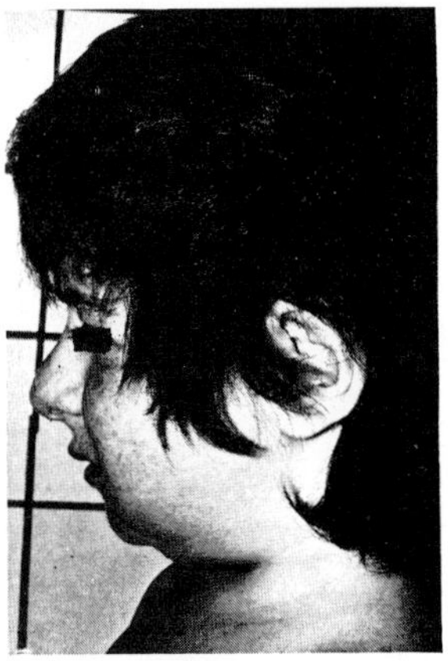

Fig. 3-119. Pycnodysostosis. This child is short in stature and has facial disproportion with a small receding chin.

early in life, leading to condensation as could be the case in the mastocytoses (see p. 300) or renal osteopathies. Fluorosis is hardly ever recognized in children.

If present, there is elective and even precocious spinal involvement, along with initial thickening of the vertebral outline. Eburnisation will then extend to the ribs and long bones and will be accompanied by sacral ligament calcification and by characteristic dental lesions.

Heavy metal poisoning, in particular lead, phosphorus, and bismuth, can be at the base of a mild metaphyseal modeling defect. However, there may only be dense transverse bands immediately adjacent to the growth cartilage. This is entirely different from the appearance of an osteopetrosis. If present, these findings would immediately require a careful study for the possible absorption or inhalation of heavy metals. This fact, however, can not be fully established in every patient and sometimes it remains impossible to clarify the origin of these dense bands (Fig. 3-118).

PYCNODYSOSTOSIS

Pycnodysostosis has recently been clearly defined as a separate entity from Albers-Schönberg disease with which it was previously confused.

Clinical Findings

The disease is recognized at various ages. During infancy it may be skull changes or a growth deficit that lead the parents to seek medical help. Sometimes it is only much later, even in adulthood that the disease is recognized. Medical aid may be sought because of a fracture or for a general physical workup.

Clinically, the symptoms of this disorder are shortness in stature with a varying degree of extremity involvement. The adult will reach a height between 1.35 m and 1.52 m. The hands and feet are short and broad and the nails may be malformed and brittle. Trunk length is normal. The skull appears larger with excessive frontal and occipital bossing. A wide open anterior fontanelle closes very late and the eyes are somewhat protruding often with blue sclerae. The mandible is hypoplastic and the teeth are frequently abnormally located with a tendency toward developing caries. All these changes result in a specific facial configuration and expression (Fig. 3-119). Fractures are part of the leading manifestations of pycnodysostosis. However their number is usually not elevated and there may not be any during infancy.

The prognosis of pycnodysostosis is much better than that of osteopetrosis. Anemia is seen rarely (Balthazar et al.) as is maxillary osteitis or cranial nerve compression. Abnormal growth and a moderate degree of bone fragility are the key problems of patients with this disorder. Those afflicted with this disorder had virtually a normal life. One of our patients did suffer from serious respiratory problems which were secondary to a narrowed upper airway aggravated by the lack of a mandibular angle.

Radiographic Study

Radiographic study reveals a generally dense skeleton without normal long bone striation. There is only a very mild, if any, metaphyseal modeling defect. The spine is uniformly involved and does not have alternating bands of dense and hyperlucent zones. Bones are somewhat short, especially in the hand. One of the key findings is a peculiar affection of the terminal phalanges of fingers and toes. Some of these are thin, whereas others have lost a varying segment of their distal portion (Fig. 3-120).

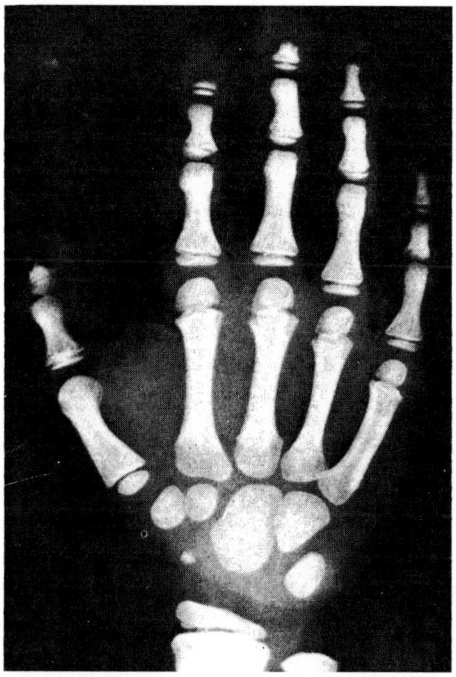

Fig. 3-120. Pycnodysostosis in a 7-year-old girl. Note the markedly dense skeletal appearance with a mild modeling defect and a lytic or central deformity of the distal phalanges.

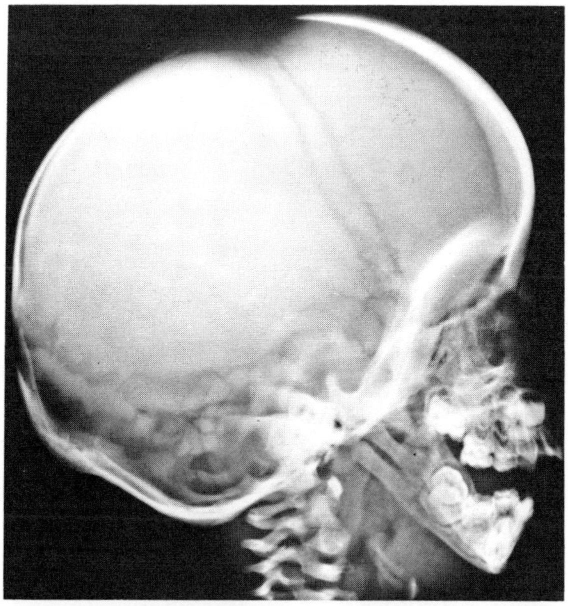

Fig. 3-121. Pycnodysostosis in a 7-year-old girl. There is persistent widening of the anterior fontanelle and cranial sutures, especially the lambda suture. There is no mandibular angle.

The base of the skull is slightly dense, as is the vault. The most significant local finding, however, is the considerable widening appearance of the sutures, especially the parietooccipital ones, combined with an open anterior fontanelle which may persist into adulthood. The mandible is poorly developed and the mandibular angle has disappeared to the point that the horizontal and vertical branches are seen as one line (Fig. 3-121).

Transmission follows the autosomal recessive mode. Deletion of the short arm of chromosome 22 (Elmore et al.) in a patient and several family members suggests the possibility that this gene might be localized on the short arm and may have manifested itself in the hemizygote state in this patient.

The pathogenesis of this disorder is still unknown. Studies of growth cartilage reveal striking abnormalities (Stanescu et al.). The structure is narrow and the columnar cartilage is replaced by cellular islands, while the primary trabeculae are short, thick, and irregular. There is intense metachromasia and an increase in hexosamine content. Ultrastructural study of chondrocytes demonstrates the presence of inclusions that are probably phospholipids. A dynamic study of tetracycline uptake leads to the conclusion that there is a slowing down of the formation and resorption of bone (Sarnsethsiri et al.). An increase in plasma calcitonin has also been reported (Baker et al.).

Stanescu and his collaborators have described an autosomal dominant disorder with clinical manifestations similar to those seen in pycnodysostosis. These are small stature, a brachycephalic skull with wide sutures, an open mandibular angle, and skeletal sclerosis. However, no fractures have been noted and there are no phalangeal alterations.

MELORHEOSTOSIS

The term melorheostosis was proposed by Léri and Johanny, who clearly defined this disorder in 1922. The authors noted the segmental localization and the peculiar appearance of the denser skeletal areas which reminded them of candle guttering (μελος = limb and ρεω = I flow, in greek). This diagnosis is hardly ever established during childhood and, therefore, it is difficult to recognize this disease. It is generally first noted in adulthood.

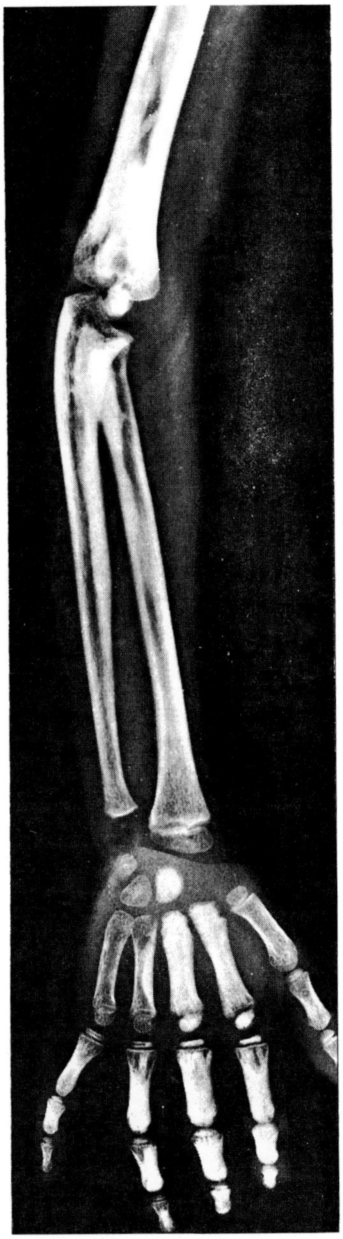

Fig. 3-122. Melorheostosis in a 6-year-old boy with a rather peculiar distribution of lesions. (Courtesy of D. Gosselin)

Clinical Findings

Attention is directed to a difference in the length of the affected extremity and which may cause local difficulty in walking as a secondary manifestation. In one-third of the patients local pain will lead to careful investigation.

Physical examination reveals a growth disturbance by relative lengthening of the involved limb. Occasionally there is also mild deformity, a genu valgum, or a slight articular limitation. An increase in finger size is rarely seen during childhood.

Generally the prognosis for this disorder is good, as its effect on the growth of the involved body parts is mild. Complications, in particular nerve compression, by bony hypertrophy is limited to the adult and even then, is quite rare.

Radiographic Findings

Radiographic study reveals that the diaphysis of long bones contains bands or spots of unusual density, which are usually arranged parallel to its axis (Fig. 3-122). Bones are widened to a moderate degree. The image of candle guttering is hardly ever seen in a young patient. Within the epiphyses we often recognize rounded dense spots. They are suggestive of osteopoikilosis, but are larger and are strictly localized within the epiphyses.

The localization of the bony lesions is highly unusual and chacracteristic. This has been previously emphasized by Léri. Exclusive involvement of a single limb is not always the case. There have been rare observations which demonstrated the involvement of both legs. In one patient all four extremities were involved (Müller-Alberti). However, this is the basic pattern in the great majority of observations. In an affected extremity all the bones are not involved although the distribution of the lesions is not haphazard. There is a rather peculiar continuity of involvement. For example, in melorheostosis of the radius, the two first metacarpals and their corresponding phalanges are abnormal or inversely the ulna and the metacarpals three-five. Upward continuity is not always maintained in an affected limb. For instance, there may be no involvement of the forearm. Sometimes only the epiphyses of certain bones are electively involved. In such a case the disease may manifest within the diaphysis at a later time (observation of Wallenstein).

Clinical Types, Pathogenesis, and Treatment

Melorheostosis is seen only in isolated patients and its etiology and transmission is totally unknown. Histologic study reveals that the areas of hyperostosis are due to very dense bone surrounded by loose trabeculae at their centers. Fibrocartilaginous islands are sometimes noted in intraarticular hyperostosis (Campbell). Peripheral ossification of the involved limb is very active, even in the adult. Several authors, follow-

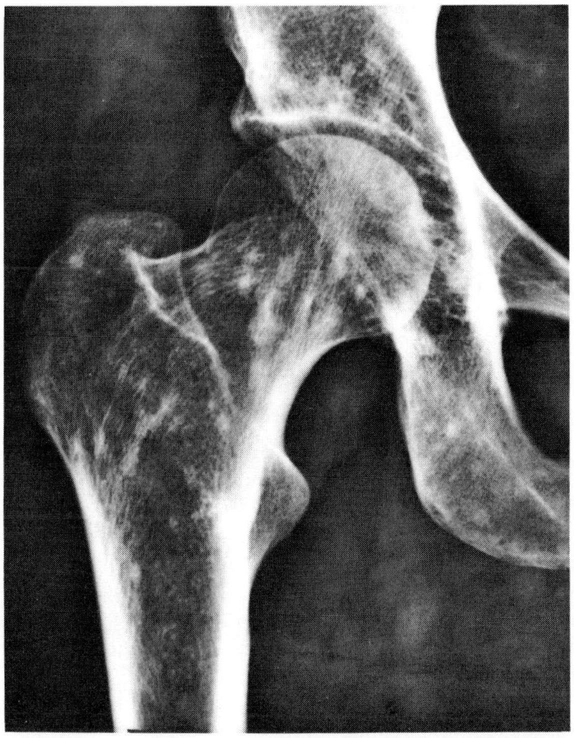

Fig. 3-123. Osteopoikilosis in a young woman. There are numerous round densities at the upper end of the femur and in the acetabulum and pubis.

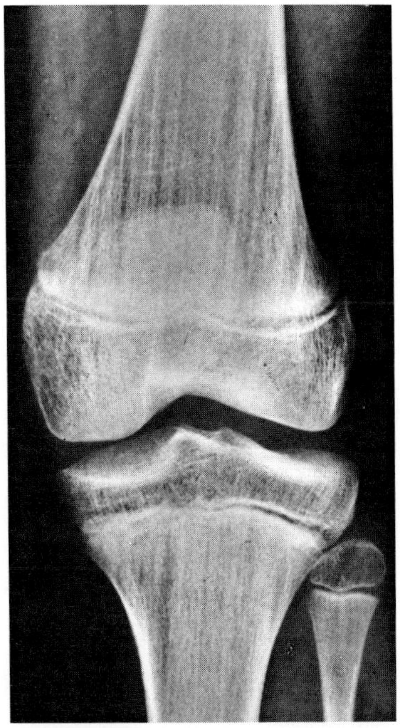

Fig. 3-124. Osteopathia striata in a 10-year-old girl. This girl also suffers from focal dermal hypoplasia.

ing Putti's idea, have suggested that the origin of this disease is vascular and they insist on the observation of inflammatory lesions followed by vascular obliteration (Morris). This interpretation, however, is still under discussion.

Melorheostosis can be associated with scleroderma circumscriptum and osteopoikilosis which was mentioned earlier. Sometimes only two of these elements may be present (Dume et al., Wagers et al., Abrahamson).

In melorheostosis an occasional orthopedic measure may be needed because of a deformity in an extremity, pain, or compression symptoms.

OSTEOPOIKILOSIS

This is not actually a disease, but rather an anatomic peculiarity with the majority of patients having no clinical manifestation whatsoever. Still, we must be aware that arthralgias or a painful extremity will sometimes focus attention on the skeleton, primarily in adulthood. There may also be associated cutaneous anomalies, generally lenticular dermatofibrosis, or more rarely, palmoplantar keratosis.

In the vast majority of patients, however, there will be a coincidental discovery of this condition at the time of a radiographic investigation which may be performed for a variety of reasons, revealing the unusual structure of the bones. Characteristically noted are opacities of oval or circular shape which are the size of a lentil. Individual lesions can join together and form a cockade appearance. There are numerous such spots, usually symmetrically distributed. Localization is mainly in the metaphyses and epiphyses of the long bones, the carpus, the tarsus, and the bones of the hand (Fig. 3-123). The pelvis and scapula are frequently involved. However, it is unusual for the patella, the ribs, or the spine to be involved. It is even more rare to have this finding in the skull.

Osteopoikilosis is transmitted as an autosomal dominant lesion. Its pathogenesis is unknown. Pathologic study demonstrates that the skeletal changes are composed of spongy tissue with abnormally thick and dense lamellae. Sometimes there is a central persisting medullary space occupied by osteoblasts and osteoclasts. Both are present in average numbers.

Under the name osteopathia striata another anomaly of bony structure has been described with the radiographic image of longitudinal striae in the metaphyses of the long bones (Fig. 3-124). The first description goes back to Voorhoeve in a patient with multiple cartilaginous exostoses. This combined with a metaphyseal modeling defect has also been described (Culver et al.), and with unusually dense appearing skull and ribs (Hurt, Bloor). In otherwise normal radiographic films we can sometimes recognize the suggestion of this finding. It is always difficult to fully ascertain its actual significance.

This radiographic "condition" is frequently noted in patients who suffer from the syndrome of focal dermal hypoplasia, which is most likely a sex-linked dominant disease. This syndrome, defined by Goltz, is recognized because of atrophy and pigmentation of the skin, papillomas of the mucus membranes, and by yellowish nodules which contain fatty accumulations that may herniate through the skin lesions. Anomalies of fingers may be present, for example, syndactyly between the second and third finger, polydactyly, or the absence of a finger. More complex malformations of the hand, clavicular aplasia, scoliosis, spina bifida, and sacral deviation have all been reported on occasion. Approximately one-half of the patients have dystrophic fingernails.

DIAPHYSEAL CORTICAL ABNORMALITIES OF LONG BONES

In view of the complex cortical pathology in the diaphysis, we will distinguish three major groups. In the first we will review diaphyseal dysplasia and craniodiaphyseal dysplasia, both of which display cortical thickening in the long bones of fusiform character. The second group combines two disorders whose cortex has a layered appearance—osteoectasia with hyperphosphatasemia—or which has an uneven thickness and borders—osteodysplastia. In the third we have put together those cortical hyperostoses whose cortex is thick but without a significantly abnormal shape or structure—endosteal hyperostosis and narrowing of the medullary canal.

Constitutional diseases affecting the cortex are usually not confused with posttraumatic hyperostoses. They occasionally involve several bones (see Fig. 11-14, p. 347).

FUSIFORM DIAPHYSEAL APPEARANCE

Two disorders to be considered in this first group are diaphyseal dysplasia with only minimal involvement of craniofacial structures, and craniodiaphyseal dysplasia with marked craniofacial changes.

DIAPHYSEAL DYSPLASIA—CAMURATI-ENGELMANN DISEASE

This disorder had already been noted by Cockayne in 1920 and it has been recognized as a distinct entity following the publications by Camurati in 1922 and Engelmann in 1929.

Clinical Findings

The disease is primarily noted during infancy or adolescence, but may remain unnoticed until a radiograph is obtained. These patients frequently complain about walking difficulties or painful legs. These pains vary in character and intensity. They are sometimes very severe after a long walk or during the night.

These patients are slender with long extremities and are underweight. There is often a disproportion between the trunk and the extremities, which appear to be too long (Fig. 3-125). The musculature of the limbs is underdeveloped and at times hardly any subcutaneous fat is present. Muscular strength is diminished. The tendon reflexes, however, are quite active. Flat feet and genu valgum have been noted, as has an exagerated lumbar lordosis. Pubertal onset is slow and the secondary sex characteristics are occasionally poorly developed. These patients often suffer from dental caries. They walk abnormally, hesitating and slightly waddling with a wide stance.

Laboratory investigations do not reveal any abnormalities. There may be an increased sedimentation rate and low hematocrit and hemoglobin have been often reported.

This disorder has very few complications and its prognosis is good.

Radiographic Findings

The diaphyses of long bones have a fusiform appearance which results from an enlarged cortex in its middle third (Fig. 3-126). The inner border of the cortex has an irregular outline and its proper recognition is often difficult. During development the lesion may extend towards the metaphyses. These may become cylindrical and loose their normal modeling. The outer surface of the bone is somewhat irregular and its medullary cavity tends to disappear. The epiphyses which are not involved in this sclerosing disorder may at times appear large and slightly deformed. On good films we can also recognize the poorly developed musculature. The lesions are generally distributed symmetrically, but not all long bones are always involved. The femur, the tibia, and the fibula are the primary sites of localization. The arms are less frequently affected, and the bones of the hand and feet

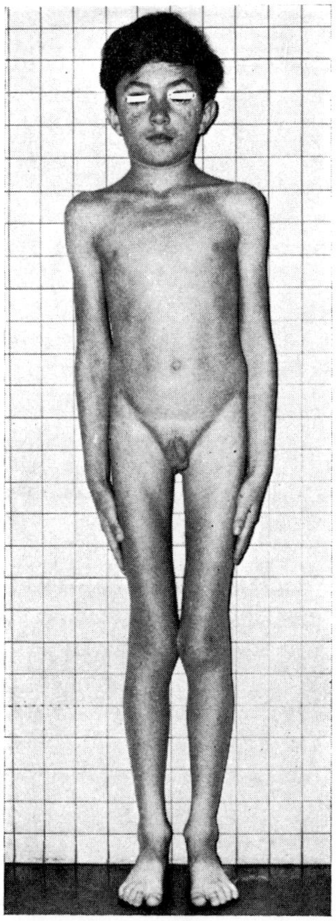

Fig. 3-125. Diaphyseal dysplasia with relative shortness of the trunk along with slender limbs.

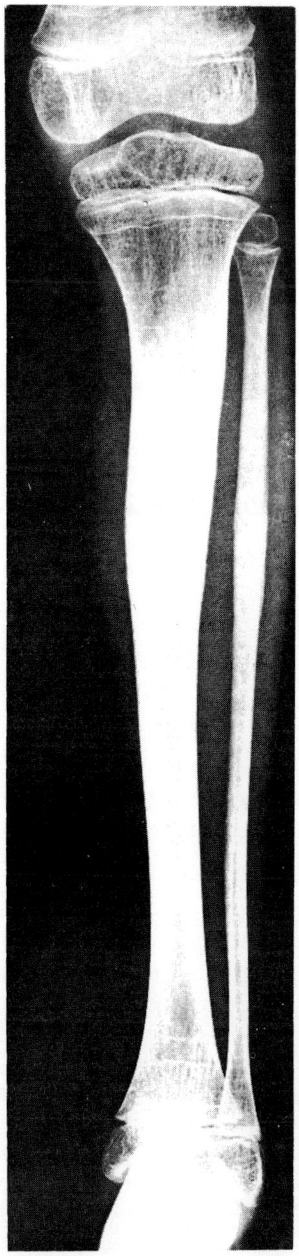

Fig. 3-126. Diaphyseal dysplasia in a 9-year-old boy. Note the spindle shaped appearance of the diaphyseal cortex.

are usually spared. The base of the skull and the vault has a mildly dense appearance.

Genetic Data, Pathology, and Pathogenesis

This disorder is transmitted as an autosomal dominant lesion. Both sexes are equally affected. The disease may be overlooked and a complete skeletal survey of the involved children's parents should always be obtained in order to find out if they suffer from an unrecognized form of the disease.

Pathology reveals cortical thickening with normal osteons. Osteoblastic activity often appears to be increased and there is new bone formation. Histologic studies produce a great variety of findings. Proliferation of the arterial media and intima has been reported several times and within the bone marrow interstitial fibrosis has been noted. The muscles are normal.

The pathogenesis of diaphyseal dysplasia remains a mystery. The abnormal findings that affect the arteries have led to the theory of a possible vascular etiology (Battaglia and Venturi). This disease should not be confused with muscular disorders, and in particular, the myopathies.

Treatment

No specific treatment is available. Attempts with corticosteroids have been made and possibly may

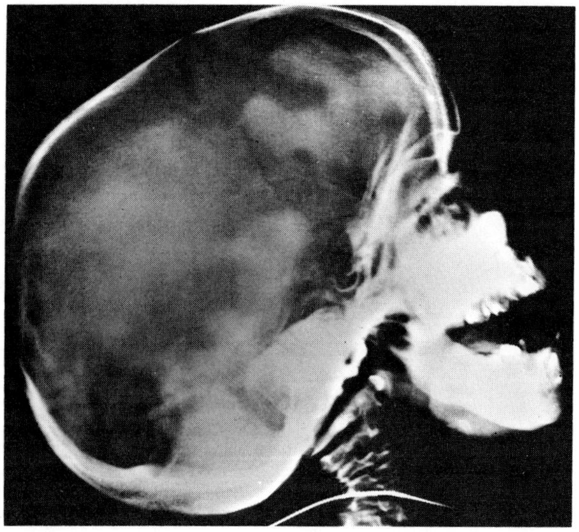

Fig. 3-127. Craniodiaphyseal dysplasia in a 6-year-old boy. Eburnization has led to the disappearance of most of the bony details. (Courtesy of J. C. Job)

have resulted in a reduced condensation. They should be used in patients who complain of severe pain. Clawsen and Loof have reported on a patient who improved considerably after corrective osteotomy. It is, however, difficult to arrive at a valid conclusion from one observation.

CRANIODIAPHYSEAL DYSPLASIA

Sometimes mistaken for Camurati-Engelmann disease this disorder must be clearly distinguished (Joseph et al.). Due to severe craniofacial involvement, the latter often leads to the recognition of the disorder and its degree is the key to the prognosis.

Carniodiaphyseal dysplasia may present clinically with an early, severe facial deformity called leontiasis ossea, which is characterized by thickening and distortion. The forehead is wide and high and we note hypertelorism, strabismus, exophthalmus, thickened nasal and maxillary bones, and a heavy set mandible. There is nasal obstruction and cranial nerve compression which may frequently lead to either blindness or deafness. Growth is usually markedly affected as is sexual maturation.

Radiographic investigation reveals a striking degree of hyperostosis of the skull, the facial structures, and the mandible (Fig. 3-127). The disorder is rapidly progressive and the bony contours eventually are lost in a homogeneous opacity. The long bones are cylindrical in appearance due to cortical thickening which involves mainly the inner compacta. The bones of the hands, the ribs, and the clavicles are involved (Fig. 3-128). The iliac wings are unusually dense in appearance as are the ischia and the posterior vertebral arches. A coxa valga results from a deformed femoral neck. Transmission follows an autosomal recessive mode.

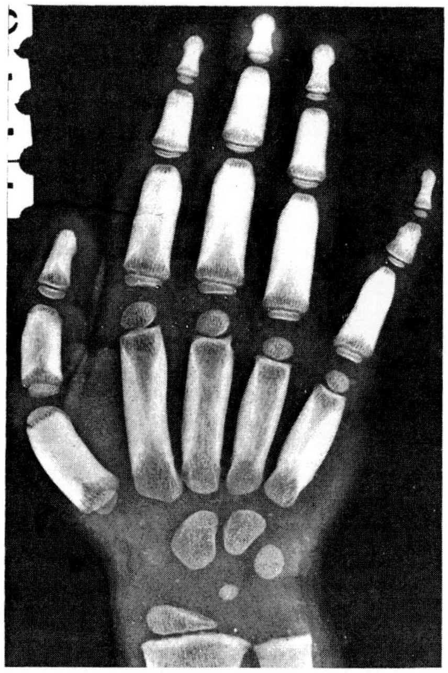

Fig. 3-128. Craniodiaphyseal dysplasia in a 5-year-old boy. The metacarpals and phalanges are not spared as in diaphyseal dysplasia. (Courtesy of J. C. Job)

IRREGULAR CORTICAL STRUCTURE

The second group consists of osteoectasia with hyperphosphatasia and osteodysplastia.

OSTEOECTASIA WITH HYPERPHOSPHATASIA

This disease is usually recognized towards the second year of life, although at times it may be later. The parents frequently will note a painful deformity of the extremities or walking difficulties. If a patient is severely affected, he may not be able to walk or remain in an upright position. Pathologic fractures are not uncommon.

Physical examination is striking, because of the markedly bowed and often widened extremities. The tibia may impress as a sabre shin. The hands and feet are relatively normal. Muscular development is defective. The trunk is rather short with sternal protrusion. The skull appears to be too large and tumors of the vault may be recognized by palpation. Intellectual development in these patients is normal, but there may be a loss of hearing or sight. Study of the eye ground can reveal angioid striae. Fever and anemia are not unusual and severe hypertension has been noted on occasion.

The most striking radiographic findings are those which involve the long bones and the skull. The bones of the extremities are massive and cylindrical in appearance. They are unusual in character because they are combined with a very active turnover in the cortical area, which appears divided into two or more layered structures. The bone is excessively transparent and has an irregular outline, at times with pseudocysts surrounded by a darker halo (Fig. 3-129). Frequently there is diaphyseal bowing and cortical widening with marked periosteal apposition. This finding has led to the earlier term "juvenile deforming hyperostosis" (Swoboda). The hand bones have the same cylindrical appearance with identical structural changes. The vertebrae, ribs, scapula, and the pelvis are all osteoporotic with uneven borders and abnormal striation. There may be reduction in height of vertebral bodies and scoliosis or kyphoscoliosis. Occasionally, a patient will have protrusio acetabuli.

The cranial findings are diagnostic. The diploe is markedly widened with a vague cotton-like structure containing dense islands. The inner table is normal, but the outer table is either thin or invisible. The facial bones are usually only mildly abnormal, but this need not always be the case (observation of Marshall). There are few teeth and the lamina dura may not be recognizable.

The most important biochemical abnormality is the dramatic elevation of alkaline phosphatase which may reach four to ten times normal, and may sometimes be even higher. Histologic study of the diaphysis reveals spongy tissue with wide meshes and an underdeveloped Haversian system. The spaces between the bony lamellae contain a rich, vascular, highly cellular, loose connective tissue. Huge osteoblasts are present and line the borders of the bony lamellae. There are many osteoclasts.

The late development of this disorder has not yet been completely clarified. Calcitonin has been successfully used to improve this condition (Whalen). The pathology seems to be due to delayed maturation of membranous bone with an accelerated metabolism of bony tissue. This disorder is similar to Paget's disease in the adult, but it occurs in a more generalized and symmetrical distribution.

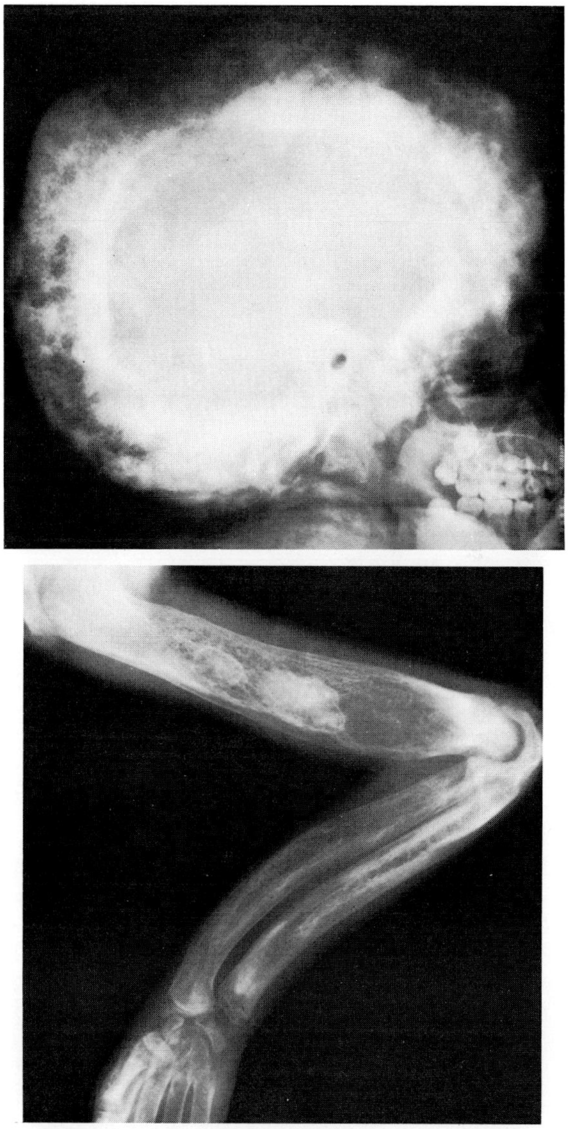

Fig. 3-129. Osteoectasia with hyperphosphatasemia in a 9-year-old boy. (Courtesy of J. Caffey)

OSTEODYSPLASTIA – MELNICK – NEEDLES SYNDROME

This rare disorder has recently been identified under the name of osteodysplastia. πλασσω = I shape, I

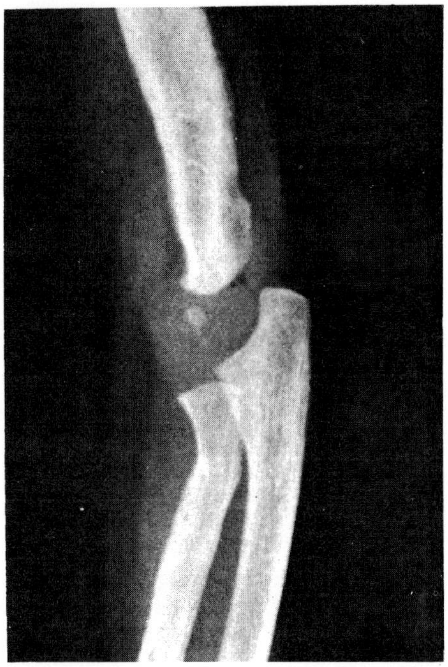

Fig. 3-130. Osteodysplastia, the Melnick-Needles syndrome, in a 1-year-old infant. Besides the uneven formation of the cortex there is a slight angulation of the upper end of the radius.

form. The bones are altered in form and contour. It is discovered at various ages and will come to attention because of an abnormal gait and bowing of the extremities. Occasionally, one may find a dislocated hip or delayed closure of the anterior fontanelle. The disorder does not seem to lead to a growth deficit. Clinically, the most characteristic findings are facial symptoms. These may include slight exophthalmus, protruding cheeks, a high and narrow forehead, prominent orbital rims, micrognathia, and malaligned teeth. The lower part of the thorax is decidedly narrow and there may be a discrete incurving of the distal thumb.

The radiographic findings will reveal the true nature of the disorder. The cortex of the long bones is unevenly thick and has irregular contours with multiple constrictions and a wavy border (Fig. 3-130). The diaphyses are slightly curved and show a metaphyseal modeling defect. This may be well visualized in the tibia. There is frequent diaphyseal angulation in the radius, with its tip being close to the bicipital ridges. The femoral necks are wide and somewhat deformed resulting in coxa valga. A dislocated hip is occasionally present. The ribs have an even cortical thickness and are wavy in appearance. The pelvis is triangular. The iliac wings have an unusually narrow supraacetabular portion and are in contrast to the much wider area above (Fig. 3-131). The anterior fontanelle closes late

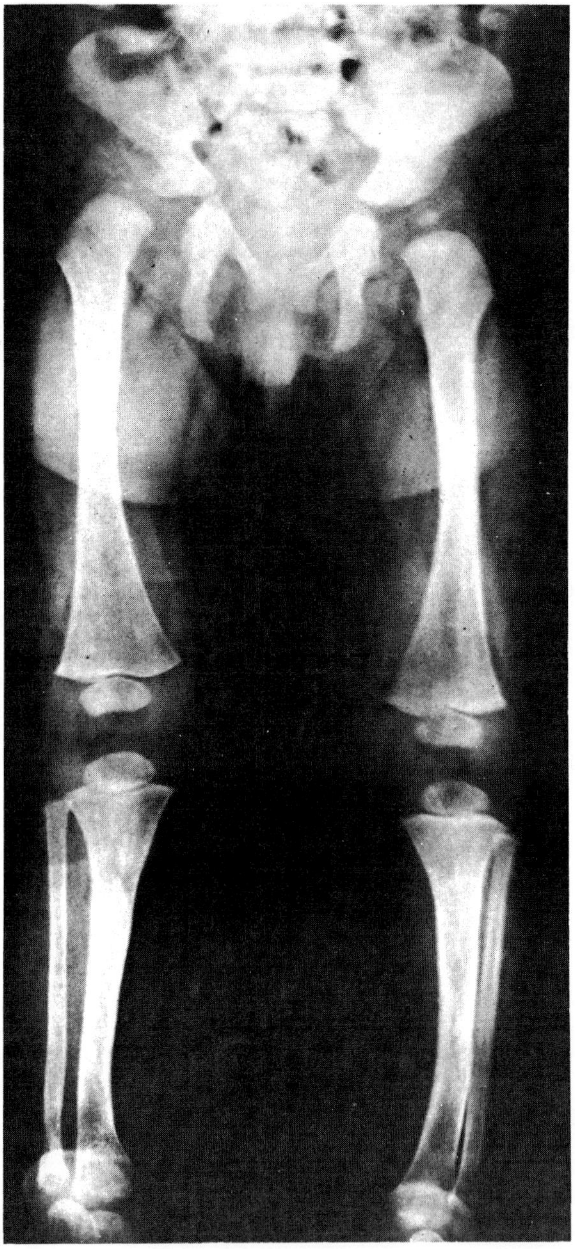

Fig. 3-131. Osteodysplastia in a 1-year-old infant. Notice the mild modeling defect of the metaphyses, the coxa valga, and the characteristic appearance of the iliac wings with an acute lateral tilt.

and the vault, particularly its frontal region, is abnormally thick in adulthood.

In spite of the fact that the uneven thickness and appearance of the cortical bones appears to be the most characteristic finding, it can also be argued that the metaphyseal deformity can lead to its being classified with the disorders of metaphyseal modeling. Thus,

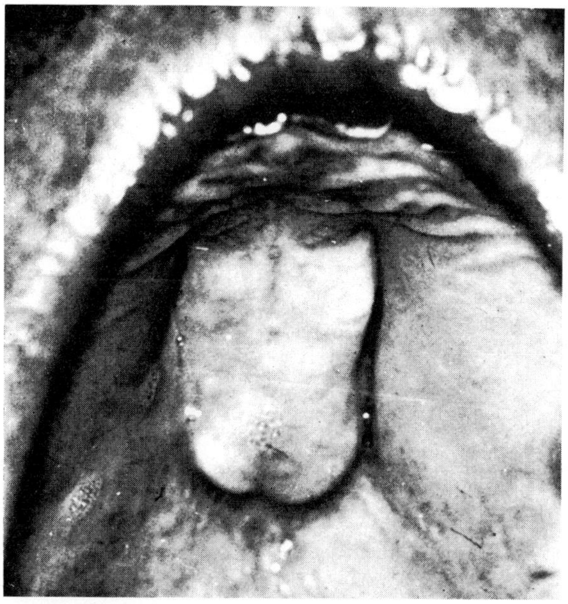

Fig. 3-132. Torus palatinus in a patient with endosteal hyperostosis. (Courtesy of J. Menkes)

Gorlin in 1969 under the title *frontametaphyseal dysplasia,* described a disorder that we consider only slightly different from osteodysplastia. Gorlin was struck by the very marked prominence of the orbital rims in his patient. This finding is not usually stressed as one of importance in the descriptions of osteodysplastia. When reporting on the above patient, no mention was made of rib anomalies, which are most characteristic. These were later noted (Holt et al.) in this patient. The pelvic alterations and the presence of coxa valga appear to be identical in both disorders. It is our opinion that we are dealing with a variable expression of one gene which is responsible for a more or less severe involvement of the skull.

REGULAR CORTICAL THICKENING

In the third group we will discuss endosteal hyperostosis and narrowing of the medullary canal.

ENDOSTEAL HYPEROSTOSIS (GENERALIZED CORTICAL HYPEROSTOSIS)

This is a heterogeneous group containing a dominant form which is seen during infancy and a recessive type which presents in the somewhat older child (Wilcot). However, it often manifests only in adulthood.

The dominant type is generally discovered accidentally, but can be occasionally suspected due to the presence of a torus palatinus. This refers to a painless tumor located at the top of the palate and which is covered by normal mucosa (Fig. 3-132). No cranial nerve compression has so far been noted.

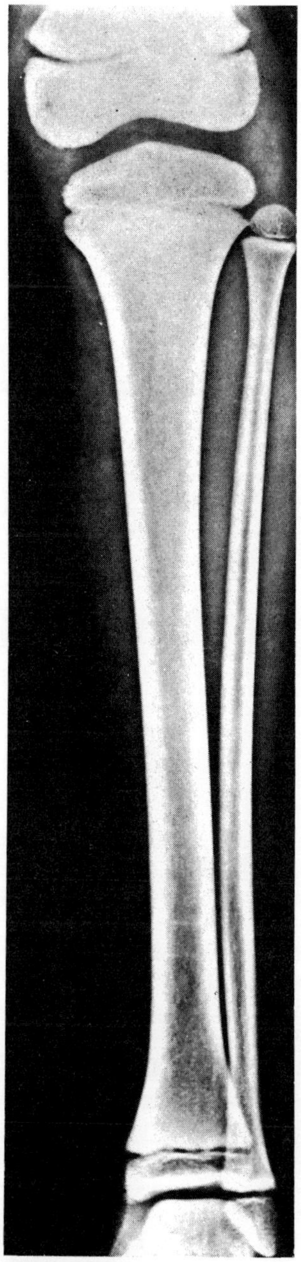

Fig. 3-133. Endosteal hyperostosis in a 7-year-old boy. (Courtesy of G. Fontaine)

Radiographic investigation demonstrates an unusually dense skeleton with cortical widening of the long bones, but without any morphologic alteration other than a smaller medullary canal (Fig. 3-133).

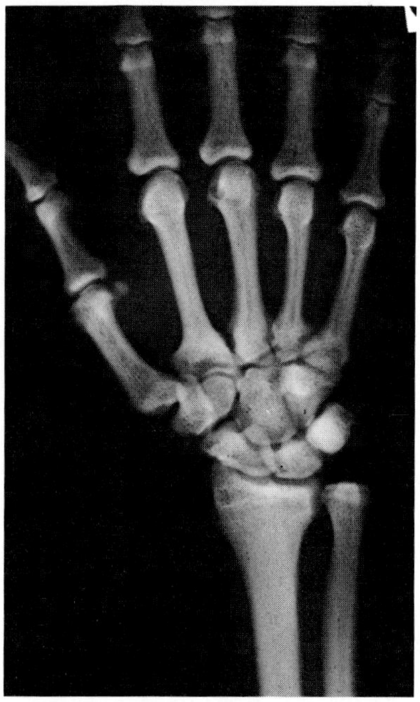

Fig. 3-134. Narrowing of the medullary cavities in a young adult. (Courtesy of J. Menkes)

Condensation of the skull begins at its base and slowly reaches the vault.

In the recessive type of van Buchem the most characteristic clinical finding appears to be the mandibular deformity with its anterior protrusion. This finding is most striking when present in the adult. Cranial nerve involvement may also be a complication. There are frequently elevated value for the alkaline phosphatases. In two patients examined by van Buchem there was an elevated value for thyrocalcitonin.

Radiographically there is marked thickening of the skull along with cortical alterations in the long bones. The mandible may be widened and instead of the mandibular angle there is just a mild curve. This disorder does have progressive characteristics.

NARROWING OF THE MEDULLARY CAVITY

A more detailed analysis and investigation of this disorder is still needed. Its dominant transmission seems established. Discovery is usually accidental at the occasion of a radiographic examination, possibly done because of a mild growth deficit. In the family studied by Kenny and Caffey findings were: delayed closure of the anterior fontanelle, tetanic seizures secondary to hypocalcemia, and early myopia. Contrary to endosteal hyperostosis this disease does not appear to be progressive. Thus, its prognosis appears good.

The most striking radiographic finding is the diaphyseal cortical thickening of the long bones without any widening of the involved diaphyses. The result is a very thin filiform appearance of the medullary canal. The bones of the hands and feet are involved, in particular, the metacarpals. The ribs are also involved (Fig. 3-134). As an inconstant finding there may be a densely appearing pelvis, spine, carpal and tarsal bones (Segond) but this is not a constant finding. Involvement of the skull is minimal. For example, there may be a slightly dense vault, or petrous bone, as well as the disappearance of the frontal sinus.

Sclerosteosis (Hansen) an autosomal recessive disorder should be mentioned here. This disorder presents with craniofacial disproportion and a high forehead, along with mandibular protrusion and syndactyly.

The radiographic findings, aside from the absence of, or triangular appearance of the index finger's middle phalanges, are cortical widening of the long bones and thickening of the base and vault of the skull. Cranial involvement often leads to compression of cranial nerves (facial palsy, deafness).

ANOMALIES OF METAPHYSEAL MODELING

In this group of disorders the most striking finding is clubbing of the metaphyseal ends of long bones. This is the result of a modeling defect, and a lack of normal resorption in the metaphyseal region (see p. 21).

Osteopetrosis was the first disorder in which the modeling defect was properly recognized. We have referred to it before. In this chapter we will study metaphyseal osteodysplasia which is known as Pyle's disease, craniometaphyseal dysplasia, several similar syndromes and occulodentodigital dysplasia.

Metaphyseal Osteodysplasia—Pyle's Disease

This disorder was first described in 1931 by Pyle, who noticed the unusual modeling defect at the metaphyseal ends of long bones. Cohn offered the first complete description of this disorder by insisting that the alterations of the skull were included.

Clinical Findings

The disorder is recognized at various ages, sometimes because of a mild deformity of the extremities or through radiographic examination. Occasionally there are joint pains and even a fracture can lead to its discovery.

Clinically, there will only be very mild alterations, such as genu valgum, a flat foot, or excessively long legs. The widened metaphyseal ends of the long bones may be palpated. Some patients do have a reduced muscular development, motion limitation of some joints, and in particular, the elbow. The involvement of the skull is not generally noted. There may be a slight degree of prognathism. Studies of the metabolism, the blood, and the bone marrow all have normal results in Pyle's disease.

Radiographic Findings

The most characteristic finding is the lack of metaphyseal region modeling in all the long bones. The classic appearance of the metaphyses are suggestive of Erlenmeyer flasks (Fig. 3-135). In this widened zone we can note a very thin cortex and sometimes an excessively radiolucent bone revealing transverse striation. On the other hand, there will be a much thicker cortex in the middle of the diaphysis and a reduction in the width of the medullary cavity. Slight diaphyseal bowing may accompany this modeling defect. The most frequently involved bones are the femur and tibia, but the long bones of the arms together with the metacarpals and phalanges may be similarly involved.

The shape of the ribs and clavicles can also be affected and scoliosis has been repeatedly noted. The pelvis may show an enlarged ischium and pubis. If the skull is involved, mild thickening of the vault and of the orbital rims can be noted. The mandibular angle may be increased. There is a total lack of pneumatization, therefore, no sinus or mastoid cells are recognizable. The facial bones and the maxilla may be involved. The teeth are often of poor quality.

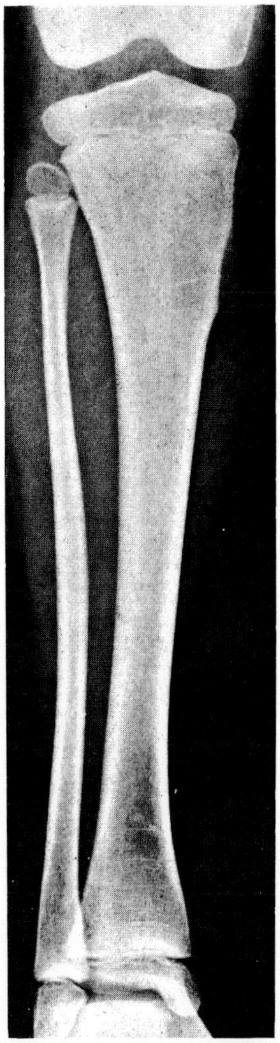

Fig. 3-135. Metaphyseal dysplasia in a 6-year-old girl. (Courtesy of P. Royer)

Genetic Data

Recessive transmission has been reliably proven on the basis of the observation of several brothers and sisters and parental consanguinity. We have also observed dominant transmission.

Pathology and Pathogenesis

Microscopic investigation confirms the abnormal condition of the metaphyseal region. Histologic studies reveal that the bone is poorly mineralized and that the cortex is thin and poorly defined. There is no specific lesion present. The essential finding is a modeling defect due to the lack of resorption at the metaphyseal end of the long bones during growth.

This metaphyseal modeling defect has been experimentally produced by x-rays (Rubin). Dichlormetylene diphosphonate has a similar effect, but while this metabolite has an inhibiting action on the dissolution of apatite crystals, there is no clear understanding of its elective effect on modeling resorption (Schenk et al.). The pathogenesis of Pyle's disease is totally unknown. This disorder does usually not require treatment because there is no cranial nerve compression.

Pyle's disease should not be confused with the other disorders of abnormal modeling. Without returning to a discussion of osteopetrosis, it should be mentioned that several storage diseases, for example, Gaucher's disease and lead poisoning, can result in a defective tubulation. The latter forms metaphyseal bands parallel to the growth cartilage.

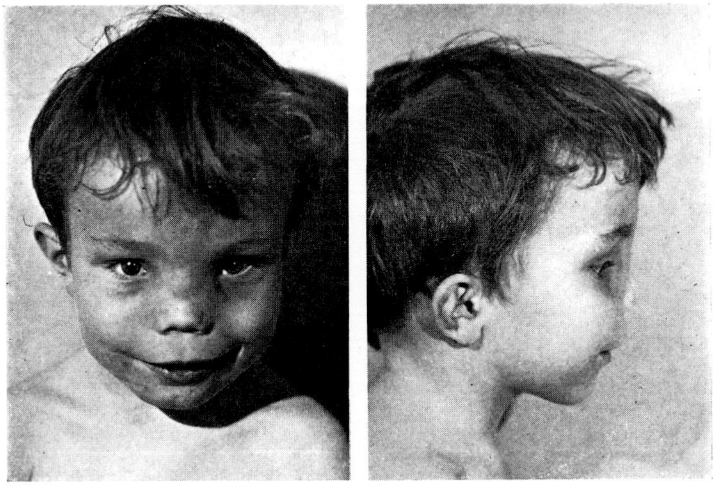

Fig. 3-136. Craniometaphyseal dysplasia with flattening and widening of the bridge of the nose. (Courtesy of Malpuech)

Carniometaphyseal Dysplasia

This disorder was recognized by Jackson in 1956. We will discuss the dominant form which is most frequently seen and which is often confused with the preceding disorder.

Clinical Findings

Patients usually present because of facial deformity. This is the most dramatic clinical finding. The base of the nose is markedly widened and thick, continuing straight up to the forehead. It may display a slight convexity. The lower third of the nares is not affected, but appears recessed and separated from the rest of the nose because of a bulge. Generally there is hypertelorism (Fig. 3-136). It is only an unusual patient who presents with eye problems, although there seems to be a high incidence of deafness.

Radiographic Findings

Hyperostosis is localized to the skull and face. Frontal and occipital bones are predominantly involved, as well as the mandible, on occasion. Pneumatization of the skull is affected and there are no visible mastoid cells (Fig. 3-137).

The long bones have the same modeling defect as were described for Pyle's disease, although to a slightly lower degree. The hands and feet are not spared. The spine and pelvis, however, are hardly ever involved. Transmission is dominant as has been demonstrated by several published pedigrees.

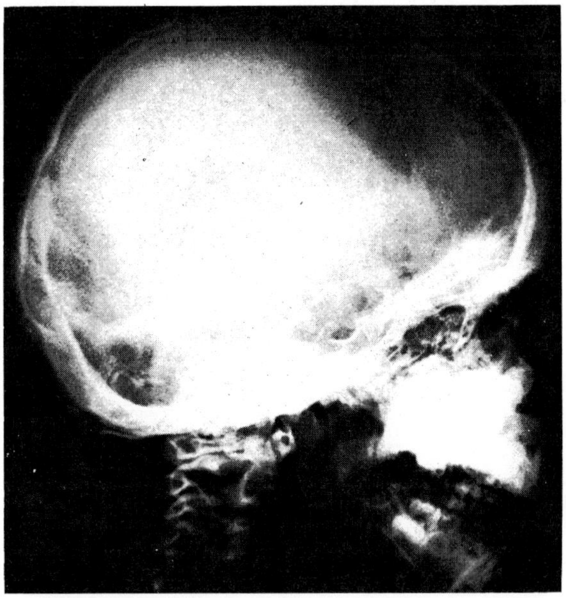

Fig. 3-137. Craniometaphyseal dysplasia with a markedly increased density of the base of the skull and the facial structures. (Courtesy of P. Guibaud)

In addition to this type there is also a recessive variant, somewhat similar, but with a more severe craniofacial deformity which is frequently complicated by cranial nerve compression, and in particular, the optic nerves (Lièvre and Fischgold). Neurosurgical intervention may be required for the complete manifestation of such compressions.

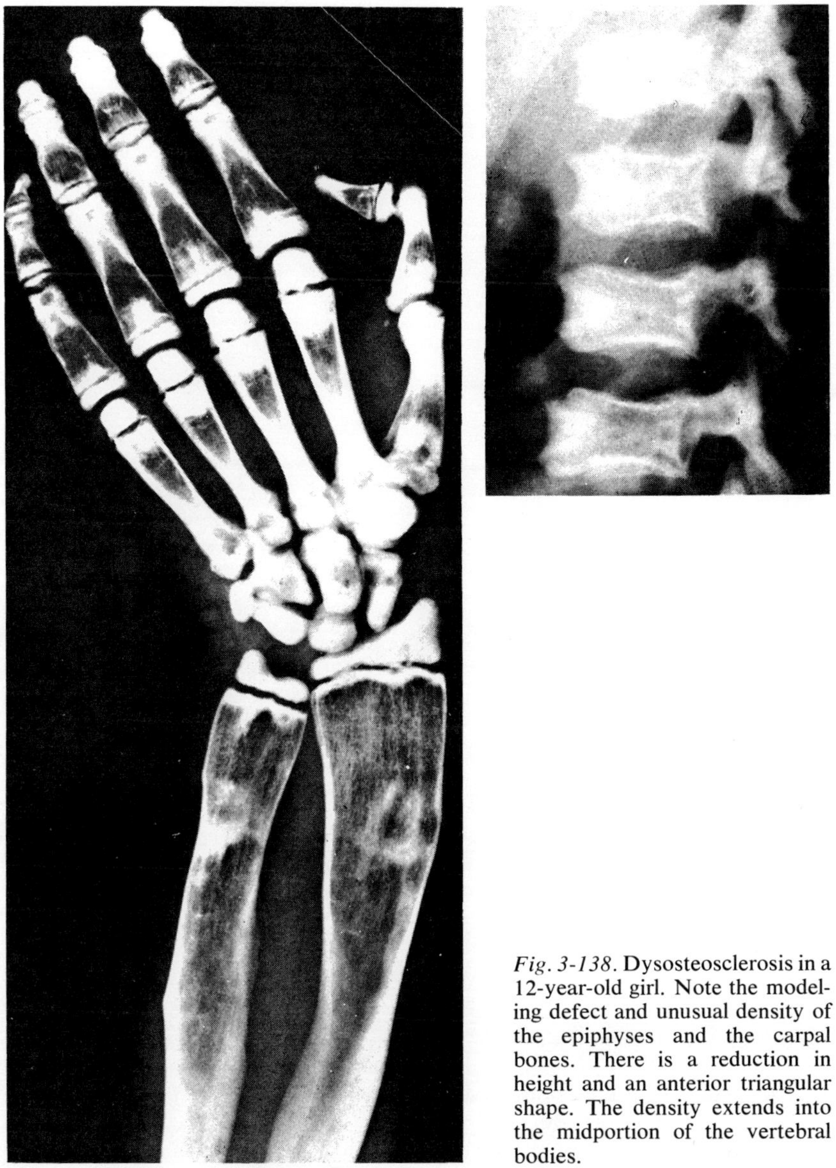

Fig. 3-138. Dysosteosclerosis in a 12-year-old girl. Note the modeling defect and unusual density of the epiphyses and the carpal bones. There is a reduction in height and an anterior triangular shape. The density extends into the midportion of the vertebral bodies.

Other Disorders of Metaphyseal Modeling

Other disorders affecting metaphyseal modeling can be clearly differentiated from Pyle's disease. We will focus on dysosteosclerosis and the Schwartz-Lelek syndrome. Frontometaphyseal dysplasia has already been mentioned in the discussion of osteodysplastia. It was concluded that this disorder appears to be one variant of that disease.

Dysosteosclerosis is a term which was introduced by Spranger. Having studied, along with Roy, a patient with this disorder it appears to be a more complicated disorder than its name suggests. Besides the skeletal involvement there may be cutaneous anomalies, which are suggestive lesions of anetodermia and neurologic symptoms characterized by pyramidal signs and psychic regression.

Radiographic Findings

The modeling defect of the diaphyses is accompanied by condensation of epiphyses, of the carpal and

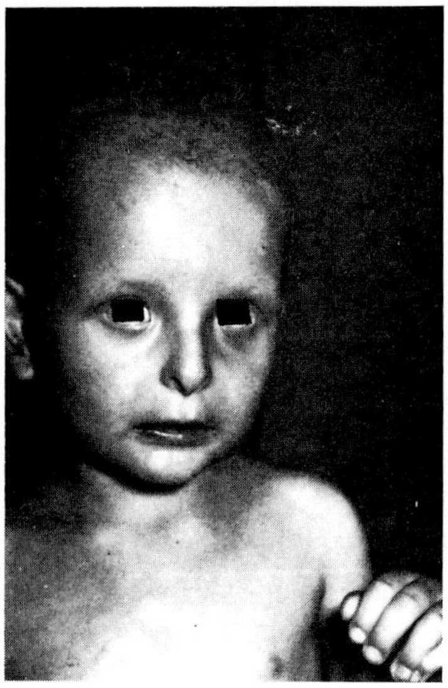

Fig. 3-139. Oculodentoosseous dysplasia. Notice the slender face and microphthalmia. (Courtesy of R. Laplane)

tarsal bones, of the base of the skull, and of vertebrae. The vertebrae are also abnormally formed (Fig. 3-138). Transmission of this disease seems to follow an autosomal recessive mode (Ellis and Field).

The Schwartz-Lelek syndrome is rarely seen and manifests by frontal bossing and genu varum. Radiographic findings include abnormal modeling, metaphyseal lucencies, and a varying degree of craniofacial involvement. Serum alkaline phosphatases are elevated.

Oculo-Dento-Osseous Dysplasia

First described (Meier-Schwickerath et al.) in 1957, this disorder combines anomalies of the facial structures, ocular defects, enamel hypoplasia of the teeth, and syndactyly.

The facial appearance of patients with this syndrome is quite characteristic. The midportion of the face is markedly elongated, the nose is drawn out and prolonged and the hypoplastic nares are oriented in a lateral direction. The chin is small and receding. The smallness of the corneae is frequently associated with microphthalmia. Besides epicanthus there may be other eye disorders (glaucoma, an abnormal iris or persistence of the pupillary membrane). Hair is usually scarce, as are eyebrows and lashes (Fig. 3-139). The enamel hypoplasia results in teeth of a yellowish or brownish color. Occasionally, there is microdontia, precocious eruption, or there are no teeth at all. Syndactyly generally affects the fourth and fifth finger. The latter finger may also be accompanied by camptodactyly or clinodactyly.

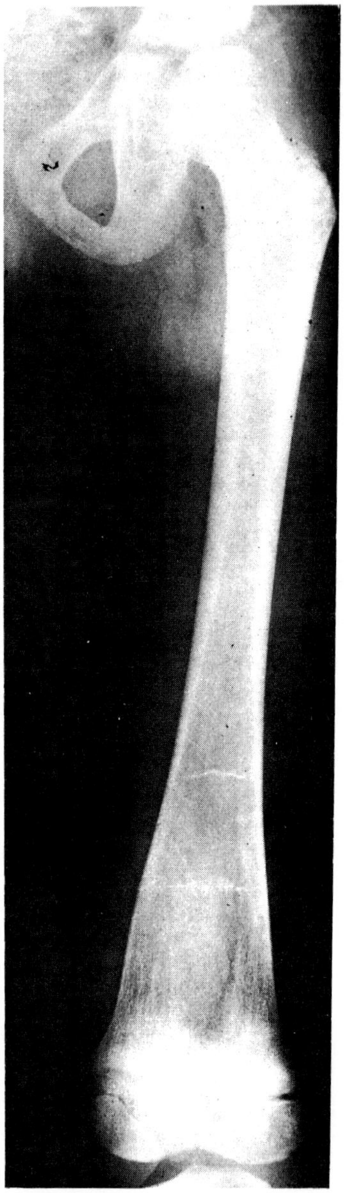

Fig. 3-140. Oculodentooseous dysplasia in an 8-year-old boy. This is a defect of metaphyseal modeling. (Courtesy of R. Laplane)

Radiographic findings include coarse long bones with a modeling defect (Fig. 3-140). Similar changes affect the ribs, the clavicles, and the mandible. The latter has an enlarged horizontal portion and a prominent alveolar ridge. The pelvis is also coarse. In the hand, clinodactyly results from a hypoplastic middle phalanx of the fifth finger. The middle phalanx of toes may be absent. The orbits are smaller than normal and closely set, leading to hypotelorism. Occasionally, thickened cranial vault or facial bones have been noted.

This disorder seems to have an autosomal dominant transmission, but in certain families there may be irregular manifestation of the gene.

REFERENCES

Ostochondrodysplasias: General Works and Articles

BAILEY (J. A.). II. Disproportionate short stature. Diagnosis and management. *Philadelphia, 1973, W. B. Saunders Co., éd.*

BERGSMA (D.) [Ed.]. Birth defects. Atlas and compendium. *Baltimore, 1973, Williams and Wilkins Co., éd.*

BONI (M.), CECILIANI (L.), GHISELLINI (F.) et LENZI (L.). Le condro-osteodisplasie genotipiche. Generalità, Eziopatogenesi, Classificazione, Clinica. *Bologne, 1970, Aulo Gaggi, éd.*

BRAILSFORD (J. F.). Radiology of bones and joints. *Baltimore, 1953, Williams et Wilkins, éd.*

FAIRBANK (H. A. T.). An atlas of general affection of the skeleton. *Edinburgh, 1951, E. et S. Livingstone, éd.*

CAFFEY (J.) et SILVERMAN (F. N.). Pediatric X-ray diagnosis. *5e édit., 1192 p., Chicago, 1967, Year Book med. publ., éd.*

FELSON (B.) [Ed.]. Dwarfs and other little people. *Seminars in Roentgenology, 1973,* **8**, *n° 2. Grune et Stratton, éd.*

HOBAEK (A.). Problems of hereditary chondrodysplasia. *Oslo, 1961, Oslo University Press.*

KAUFMANN (H. J.) [Ed.]. Progress in pediatric radiology. Vol. 4 : Intrinsic diseases of bones. *Basel, 1973, S. Karger, éd.*

KOZLOWSKI (K.) et RUPPRECHT (E.). Klinik und Röntgenbild der Osteochondrodysplasien und Mukopolysaccharidosen. *Berlin, 1972, Akademic-Verlag, éd.*

LAMY (M.) et MAROTEAUX (P.). Les chondrodystrophies génotypiques. *Paris, 1961, Expansion scient. franç., éd.*

MCKUSICK (V. A.). Heritable disorders of connective tissue. *4e édit., Saint Louis, 1972, C. V. Mosby Co., éd.*

Nomenclature internationale des maladies osseuses constitutionnelles. *Ann. Radiol., 1970,* **13**, *455-464.*

POZNANSKI (A. K.). The hand in radiologic diagnosis. *Philadelphia, London, Toronto, 1974, W. B. Saunders Co., éd.*

RUBIN (P.). Dynamic classification of bone dysplasias. *Chicago, 1964, Year Book med. publ., éd.*

SMITH (D. W.). Recognizable patterns of human malformation. Genetic, embryologic, and clinical aspects. *Philadelphia, 1970, W. B. Saunders Co., éd.*

SPRANGER (J. W.), LANGER (L. O., Jr.) et WIEDEMANN (H. R.). Bone dysplasias. An atlas of constitutional disorders of skeletal development. *Stuttgart, 1974, Gustav Fischer Verlag.*

SUGIURA (Y.) et NAKAZAWA (O.). Bone age. Roentgen diagnosis of skeletal development. *Tokyo, 1972, Chugai-Igatu, éd.*

SWISCHUK (L. E.). The beaked, notched, or hooked vertebra. Its significance in infants and young children. *Radiology, 1970,* **95**, *661-664.*

SWOBODA (W. Von). Das Skelet des Kindes. Entwicklung, Fehlbildungen und Erkrankungen. *2e édit., 259 p. Stuttgart, 1969, G. Thieme Verlag, éd.*

VIGLIANI (F.), MARTINELLI (B.) et CAMPAILLA (E.). Le condro-osteodiplasie genotipiche. Evoluzione e prognosi. *Bologne, 1970, Aulo Gaggi éd.*

WIEDEMANN (H. R.). Die grossen Konstitutionskrankheiten des Skeletts. *Stuttgart, 1960, Fischer.*

ABNORMALITIES OF GROWTH

Lethal Chondrodysplasias

CURRAN (J. P.), SIGMON (B. A.) et OPITZ (J. M.). Lethal forms of chondrodysplastic dwarfism. *Pediatrics, 1974,* **53**, *76-85.*

FRACCARO (M.). Contributo allo studio delle malattie del mensenchima osteopoietico, l'Achondrogenesi. *Folia Hered. Path., 1951,* **1**, *190-209.*

GIEDION (A.). Thanatophoric dwarfism. *Helv. paediat. Acta, 1968,* **23**, *175-183.*

GOARD (K. E.) et KOZLOWSKI (K.). Thanatophoric dwarfism II. *Pediat. Radiol., 1973,* **1**, *8-11.*

GOUTIÈRES (F.), AICARDI (J.) et FARKAS-BARGETON (E.). Une malformation cérébrale particulière associée au nanisme thanatophore. *Rev. neurol., 1971,* **125**, *435-440.*

GRAFF (G.), CHEMKE (J.) et LANCET (M.). Familial recurring thanatophoric dwarfism. A case report. *Obstet. Gynec., 1972,* **39**, *515-520.*

HARRIS (R.), PATTON (J. T.) et BARSON (A. J.). Pseudoachondrogenesis with fractures. *Clin. Genet., 1972,* **3**, *435-441.*

HOUSTON (C. S.), AWEN (C. F.) et KENT (H. P.). Fatal neonatal dwarfism. *J. Canad. Ass. Radiol., 1972,* **23**, *45-61.*

LA CHAPELLE (A. DE), MAROTEAUX (P.), HAVU (N.) et GRANROTH (G.). Une rare dysplasie osseuse léthale de transmission récessive autosomique. *Arch. franç. Pédiat., 1972,* **29**, *759-770.*

LANGER (L. O., Jr.), SPRANGER (J. W.), GREINACHER (I.) et HERDMAN (R. C.). Thanatophoric dwarfism. A condition confused with achondroplasia in the neonate, with brief comments on achondrogenesis and homozygous achondroplasia. *Radiology, 1969,* **92**, *285-295.*

LAXOVA (R.), OHARA (P. T.), RIDLER (M. A. C.) et TIMOTHY (J. A. D.). Family with probable achondrogenesis and lipid inclusions in fibroblasts. *Arch. Dis. Childh., 1973,* **48**, *212-216.*

MAJEWSKI (F.), PFEIFFER (R. A.), LENZ (W.), MÜLLER (R.), FEIL (G.) et SEILER (R.). Polysyndaktylie, verkürzte Gliedmassen und Genitalfehlbildungen : Kennzeichen eines selbständigen Syndroms ? *Z. Kinderheilk., 1971,* **111**, *118-138.*

MAROTEAUX (P.), LAMY (M.) et ROBERT (J.-M.). Le nanisme thanatophore. *Presse méd., 1967,* **75**, *2519-2524.*

PARENTI (G. C.). La anosteogenesi : una varieta della osteogenesi imperfetta. *Pathologica, 1936,* **28**, *447-462.*

PARTINGTON (M. W.), GONZALES-CRUSSI (F.), KHAKEE (S. G.) et WOLLIN (D. G.). Cloverleaf skull and thanatophoric dwarfism. Report of four cases, two in the same sibship. *Arch. Dis. Childh., 1971,* **46**, *656-664.*

ROLLAND (J.-C.), BOISRAMÉ (M.), LAUGIER (J.) et DESBUQUOIS (G.). L'achondrogenèse. Aspects cliniques et radiologiques. A propos d'un cas. *Ann. Pédiat., 1973,* **20**, *329-334.*

ROVINSKI (J.), GASGLIA (Mme) et ESKENAZI (R.). Nanisme thanatophore. *Pédiatrie, 1971,* **26**, *75-79.*

SALDINO (R. M.). Lethal short-limbed dwarfism : achondrogenesis and thanatophoric dwarfism. *Amer. J. Roentgenol., 1971,* **112**, *185-197.*

SALDINO (R. M.) et NOONAN (C. D.). Severe thoracic dystrophy with striking micromelia, abnormal osseous development, including the spine, and multiple visceral anomalies. *Amer. J. Roentgenol., 1972,* **114**, *257-263.*

SPRANGER (J.), GRIMM (B.), WELLER (M.), WEISSENBACHER (G.), HERMANN (J.), GILBERT (E.) et KREPLER (R.). Short rib-polydactyly (SRP) syndromes, types Majewski and Saldino-Noonan. *Z. Kinderheilk., 1974,* **116**, *73-94.*

WALKER (M.). A propos d'un cas de forme mineure de l'achondrogenèse. *Thèse Bordeaux, 1974.*

YOUNG (R. S.), POCHACZEVSKY (R.), LEONIDAS (J. C.), WEXLER (I. B.) et RATNER (H.). Thanatophoric dwarfism and cloverleaf skull (« Kleeblattschädel »). *Radiology, 1973,* **106**, *401-405.*

Achondroplasia

ALEXANDER (E., Jr.). Significance of the small lumbar spinal canal : cauda equina compression syndromes dues to spondylosis. Part 5 : Achondroplasia. *J. Neurosurg., 1969,* **31**, *513-519.*

BAILEY (J. A.). II. Orthopaedic aspects of achondroplasia. *J. Bone Jt Surg., 1970,* **52-A**, *1285-1301.*

BARGMAN (G. J.), MACKLER (B.) et SHEPARD (T. H.). Studies of oxidative energy deficiency. I. Achondroplasia in the rabbit. *Arch. Biochem., 1972,* **150**, *137-146.*

BOUVET (J. P.), MAROTEAUX (P.) et FEINGOLD (J.). Etude génétique de l'achondroplasie. *Ann. Génét., 1971,* **14**, *127-131.*

CAFFEY (J.). Achondroplasia of pelvis and lumbosacral spine. *Amer. J. Roentgenol., 1958,* **80**, *449-457.*

CAFFEY (J.). Pediatric X-ray diagnosis. *Chicago, 1967, Year Book med. publ., éd.*

COHEN (M. E.), ROSENTHAL (A. D.) et MATSON (D. D.). Neurological abnormalities in achondroplastic children. *J. Pediat., 1967,* **71**, *367-376.*

DEPAUL. Mémoire sur une maladie spéciale du système osseux développé pendant la vie intra-utérine et qui est généralement décrite sous le nom de rachitisme. *Bull. Acad. Méd. (Paris), 1851,* **16**, *378-379.*

DUVOISIN (R. C.) et YAHR (M. D.). Compressive spinal cord and root syndromes in achondroplastic dwarf. *Neurology, 1962,* **12**, *202-207.*

ELMER (W. A.) et PIERRO (L. J.). The Creeper trait in chickens and growth of tibiotarsi in vitro. *Amer. Zoologist., 1964,* **4**, *381 (abstract).*

ESCAMILLA (R. F.), HUTCHINGS (J. J.), CHOH HAO LI et FORSHAM (P.). Achondroplastic dwarfism. Effects of treatment with human growth hormone. *Calif. Med., 1966,* **105**, *104-110.*

GREBE (H.). Chondrodysplasie. *Roma, 1955, Ed. dell' Istituto G. Mendel, éd.*

HALL (J. G.), DORST (J. P.), TAYBI (H.), SCOTT (C. I.), LANGER (L. O.) et MCKUSICK (V. A.). Two probable cases of homozygotes for the achondroplasia gene. *Birth Defects, Original Articles Series, 1969,* **V** *n° 4, 29-34.*

HAMBURGER (V.). A study of hereditary chondrodystrophia in the chick (« Creeper fowl ») by means of embryonic transplantation. *Proc. Soc. exp. Biol. (N. Y.), 1939,* **41**, *13-15.*

JOHNSON (D. R.) et WISE (J. M.). Cartilage anomaly (can); a new mutant gene in the mouse. *J. Embryol. exp. Morph., 1971,* **25**, *21-31.*

KAUFMANN (E.). Untersuchungen über die sogennante fötale Rachitis (Chondrodystrophia foetalis). *Berlin, 1892, Reiner, éd.*

KIENY (M.) et ABBOTT (U. K.). L'extrait d'embryon diplopode inhibe la croissance des ébauches cartilagineuses normales cultivées in vitro. *C. R. Acad. Sci. (Paris), 1962,* **254**, *1520-1522.*

KONYUKHOV (B. V.) et PASCHIN (Y. V.). Experimental study of the achondroplasia gene effects in the mouse. *Acta Biol. Hung., 1967,* **18**, *285-294.*

KOZLOWSKI (K.) et ZYCHOWICZ (C.). Hypochondroplasie (ein weiterer Beitrag). *Fortschr. Röntgenstr., 1964,* **101**, *531-535.*

LANGER (L. O., Jr.), BAUMANN (P. A.) et GORLIN (R. J.). Achondroplasia. *Amer. J. Roentgenol., 1967,* **100**, *12-26.*

LEFEBVRE (J.), ERRERA (A.) et CHAUREY (M.). Note préliminaire sur la mesure des distances interpédiculaires vertébrales chez l'enfant. *J. Radiol. Electrol., 1958,* **39**, *229-231.*

LERI (A.) et LINOSSIER (Mlle). Hypochondroplasie héréditaire. *Bull. Soc. méd. Hôp. Paris, 1924,* **48**, *1780-1787.*

MACKLER (B.), HAYNES (B.), INAMDAR (A. R.), PEDEGANA (L. R.), HALL (J. G.) et COHEN (M. M., Jr.). Oxidative energy deficiency. II. Human achondroplasia. *Arch. Biochem. Biophys., 1973,* **159**, *885-888.*

MARIE (P.). L'achondroplasie dans l'adolescence et l'âge adulte. *Presse méd., 1900,* **8**, *17-23.*

MAROTEAUX (P.) et LAMY (M.). Achondroplasia in man and animals. *Clin. Orthop., 1964,* **33**, *91-103.*

MÖRCH (E. T.). Chondrodystrophic dwarfs in Denmark. *Opera ex Domo Biol. hered. Hum. Univers. Hafn., 1941,* **3**.

MORGAN (B. C.), AASE (J. M.) et GRAHAM (C. B.). Homozygosity for achondroplasia ? Report of a possible case, with congenital heart disease and severe mental deficit. *Pediatrics, 1970,* **45**, *112-115.*

MURDOCH (J. L.), WALKER (B. A.), HALL (J. G.), ABBEY (H.), SMITH (K. K.) et MCKUSICK (V. A.). Achondroplasia, a genetic and statistical survey. *Ann. hum. Genet., 1970,* **33**, *227-244.*

PARROT (J.). Sur la malformation achondroplasique et le Dieu Ptah. *Bull. S. Anthr., 1878, 3e série,* **1**, *296-308.*

PONSETI (I. V.). Skeletal growth in achondroplasia. *J. Bone Jt Surg., 1970,* **52-A**, *701-716.*

PORAK (C.) et DURANTE (G.). Les micromélies congénitales. Achondroplasie vraie et dystrophie périostale. *Nouv. Iconogr. Salpêt., 1905,* **18**, *481-538.*

RAVENNA (F.). Achondroplasie et chondrohypoplasie. Contribution clinique. *Nouv. Iconogr. Salpêt., 1913,* **26**, *157-184.*

RIMOIN (D. L.), HUGHES (G. N.), KAUFMAN (R. L.), ROSENTHAL (R. E.), MCALISTER (W. H.) et SILBERBERG (R.). Endochondral ossification in achondroplastic dwarfism. *New Engl. J. Med., 1970,* **233**, *728-735.*

RISCHBIETH (H.) et BARRINGTON (A.). Dwarfism. *Treas. hum. Inher., 1912,* **VII-VIII**, *355-573.*

RUDNICK (D.). Differentiation of prospective limb material from Creeper chick embryos in coelomic grafts. *J. exp. Zool., 1945,* **100**, *1-17.*

SCHIEMANN (H.). Ueber Chondrodystrophie (Achondroplasie, Chondrodysplasie). *Wiesbaden, 1967, F. Steiner, éd.*

SEEGMILLER (R.), FRASER (F. C.) et SHELDON (H.). A new chondrodystrophic mutant in mice. Electron microscopy of normal and abnormal chondrogenesis. *J. Cell Biol., 1971,* **48**, *580-593.*

SHEPARD (T. H.), FRY (L. R.) et MOFFETT (B. C., Jr.). Microscopic studies of achondroplastic rabbit cartilage. *Teratology, 1969,* **2**, *13-22.*

SHEPARD (T. H.) et BASS (G. L.). Organ-culture studies of achondroplastic rabbit cartilage : evidence for a metabolic defect in glucose utilization. *J. Embryol. exp. Morph., 1971,* **25**, *347-363.*

SILVERMAN (F. N.). A differential diagnosis of achondroplasia. *Radiol. clin. N. Amer., 1968,* **6**, *225-237.*

WALKER (B. A.), MURDOCH (J. L.), MCKUSICK (V. A.), LANGER (L. O.) et BEALS (R. K.). Hypochondroplasia. *Amer. J. Dis. Child., 1971,* **122**, *95-104.*

WERNER (A.). Compression de la queue de cheval dans l'achondroplasie. A propos de deux observations personnelles. *Praxis, 1964,* **53**, *374-378.*

WOLFF (E.) et KIENY (M.). Recherches sur la nature d'un facteur inhibiteur de la croissance des os longs dans la race du poulet Creeper. *Develop. Biol., 1963,* **7**, *324-341.*

Punctate Epiphyseal Dysplasia

BERGSTRÖM (K.), GUSTAVSON (K.-H.) et JORULF (H.). Chondrodystrophia calcificans congenita (Conradi's disease) in a mother and her child. *Clin. Genet., 1972,* **3**, *158-161.*

COHEN-SOLAL (J.), FAURÉ (Cl.), SARRUT (Mlle S.), LOUBRY (P.), MORENO (J. L.), LEJEUNE (Cl.) et MANDE (R.). Un cas de forme majeure de maladie des épiphyses ponctuées avec étude histologique. *Sem. Hôp. Paris, 1968,* **44**, *2733-2741.*

CONRADI (E.). Vorzeitiges Auftreten von Knochen und eigenartigen Verkalkungskernen bei Chondrodystrophia foetalis hypoplastica. *Z. Kinderheilk., 1914,* **80**, *86-97.*

HÜNERMANN (C.). Chondrodystrophia calcifians congenita als abortive. Form der Chondrodystrophie. *Z. Kinderheilk., 1931,* **51**, *1-19.*

JEUNE (M.), LARBRE (F.), CARRON (R.) et COUETTE (I.). La maladie congénitale des épiphyses pointillées ou calcinose fœtale épiphysaire chondrodystrophiante. *Arch. franç. Pédiat., 1953,* **10**, *914-942.*

MONTLOUIS (H.). Contribution à l'étude de la maladie congénitale des épiphyses pointillées. *Thèse Méd., Toulouse, 1961, n° 32.*

SAUGIER (J.). La maladie congénitale des épiphyses ponctuées (5 observations nouvelles). *Thèse Méd., Paris, 1964.*

SILVERMAN (F. N.). Dysplasies épiphysaires : entité protéiforme. *Ann. Radiol., 1961,* **4**, *833-867.*

SPRANGER (J. W.), OPITZ (J. M.) et BIDDER (U.). Heterogeneity of Chondrodysplasia Punctata. *Hum. Genet., 1971,* **11**, *190-212.*

Diastrophic Dwarfism

KAPLAN (M.), SAUVEGRAIN (J.), HAYEM (F.), DRAPEAU (P.), MAUGEY (F.) et BOULLE (J.). Etude d'un nouveau cas de nanisme diastrophique. *Arch. franç. Pédiat., 1961,* **18**, *981-1001.*

LAMY (M.) et MAROTEAUX (P.). Le nanisme diastrophique. *Presse méd., 1960,* **68**, *1977-1980.*

LANGER (L. O., Jr.). Diastrophic dwarfism in early infancy. *Amer. J. Roentgenol., 1965,* **93**, *398-404.*

PEYTEL (J.). Le nanisme diastrophique. *Lyon, 1966, Simep, éd.*

SEEGMILLER (R.), FRASER (F. C.) et SHELDON (H.). A new chondrodystrophic mutant in mice. Electron microscopy of normal and abnormal chondrogenesis. *J. Cell Biol., 1971,* **48**, *580-593.*

SALLE (B.), PICOT (C.), VAUZELLE (J.-L.), DEFRENNE (P.), MONNET (P.), FRANÇOIS (R.) et ROBERT (J.-M.). Le nanisme diastrophique. A propos de trois observations chez le nouveau-né. *Pédiatrie, 1966,* **21**, *311-327.*

SPRANGER (J.) et GERKEN (H.). Diastrophischer Zwergwuchs. *Z. Kinderheilk., 1967,* **98**, *227-234.*

STANESCU (V.), STANESCU (R.) et MAROTEAUX (P.). Etude histochimique et microchimique du cartilage de croissance tibial dans le nanisme diastrophique et la pycnodysostose. *Ann. Histochim., 1973,* **18**, *177-184.*

WALKER (B. A.), SCOTT (C. I.), HALL (J. G.), MURDOCH (J. L.) et MCKUSICK (V. A.). Diastrophic dwarfism. *Medicine, 1972,* **51**, *41-59.*

Metatropic Dwarfism

CASTEL (Y.), BENARDEAU (M.), DANTOINE (G.), LEROY (J.-P.), BALOUET (G.) et TOUDIC (L.). Nanisme métatropique. *Ann. Pédiat., 1974,* **21**, *101-110.*

COHEN-SOLAL (D. J.). Le nanisme métatropique. *Thèse Méd., Paris, 1972.*

FLEURY (J.), MENIBUS (Cl.-H. de) et HAZARD (E.). Un cas singulier de dystrophie ostéochondrale congénitale (nanisme métatropique de Maroteaux). *Sem. Hôp. Paris, 1966,* **42**, *1661-1664.*

GEFFERTH (K.). Beitrage zur Diagnostik des metatropischen Zwergwuchses. *Z. Kinderheilk., 1968,* **103**, *325-335.*

MARCHESE (G. S.). Una nuova entità morbosa : il nanisme metatropico. *Minerva pediat., 1967,* **19**, *649-653.*

MAROTEAUX (P.), SPRANGER (J.) et WIEDEMANN (H. R.). Der metatropische Zwergwuchs. *Arch. Kinderheilk., 1966,* **173**, *211-226.*

Mesomelic Dwarfism and Other Chondrodysplasias Present at Birth

DÜRR (D. K.). Eine neue Dysostoseform mit Mikromelie bei zwei Geschwistern. *Helv. paediat. Acta, 1968,* **23**, *184-194.*

FREIRE-MAIA (N.) et LENZ (W. D.). Discussion. *Birth Defects Original Article Series, 1969,* **V** *n° 4, 14-16.*

LAMY (M.) et BIENENFELD (C.). La dyschondrostéose. *Analecta Genetica, Roma, 1954,* **1**, *153-164.*

LANGER (L. O.). Mesomelic dwarfism of the hypoplastic ulna fibula mandible type. *Radiology, 1967,* **89**, *654-660.*

MAROTEAUX (P.), ROUX (C.) et FRUCHTER (Z.). Le nanisme micrognathe. *Presse méd., 1970,* **78**, *2371-2374.*

MAROTEAUX (P.), MARTINELLI (B.) et CAMPAILLA (E.). Le nanisme acromésomélique. *Presse méd., 1971,* **79**, *1839-1842.*

NIEVERGELT (K.). Positiver Vaterschaftsnachweis auf Grund erblicher Missbildungen der Extremitäten. *Arch. Klaus-Stift. Vererb.-Forsch., 1944,* **19**, *157-194.*

REINHARDT (K.) et PFEIFFER (R. A.). Ulno-fibulare Dysplasie, eine autosomal dominant vererbte Mikromesomelie ähnlich dem Nievergeltsyndrom. *Fortschr. Röntgenstr., 1967,* **107**, *379-391.*

ROBINOW (M.), SILVERMAN (F. N.) et SMITH (H. D.). A newly recognized dwarfing syndrome. *Amer. J. Dis. Child., 1969,* **117**, *645-651.*

RUPPRECHT (E.), KOZLOWSKI (K.) et HINKEL (G. K.). Sonderform einer epimetaphysären Osteochondrodysplasie. *Helv. paediat. Acta, 1971,* **26**, *311-318.*

VERA-ROMAN (J. M.). Robinow dwarfing syndrome accompanied by penile agenesis and hemivertebrae. *Amer. J. Dis. Child., 1973,* **126**, *206-208.*

WADLINGTON (W. B.), TUCKER (V. L.) et SCHIMKE (R. N.). Mesomelic dwarfism with hemivertebrae and small genitalis (The Robinow Syndrom). *Amer. J. Dis. Child., 1973,* **126**, *202-205.*

WEISSENBACHER (G.) et ZWEYMÜLLER (E.). Gleichzeitiges Vorkommen eines Syndroms von Pierre Robin und einer fetalen Chondrodysplasie. *Mschr. Kinderheilk., 1964,* **112**, *315-317.*

Spondylo-Epiphyseal Dysplasia Congenita and Kniest's Disease

BACH (Ch.), MAROTEAUX (P.), SCHAEFFER (Ph.), BITAN (A.) et CRUMIÈRE (C.). Dysplasie spondylo-épiphysaire congénitale avec anomalies multiples. *Arch. franç. Pédiat., 1967,* **24**, *23-33.*

FARRIAUX (J. P.), DUBOIS (B.) et FONTAINE (G.). La dysplasie spondylo-épiphysaire congénitale. Etude d'une observation. *Pédiatrie, 1971,* **26**, *215-221.*

FRASER (G. R.), FRIEDMANN (A. I.), MAROTEAUX (P.), GLEN-BOTT (A. M.) et MITTWOCH (U.). Dysplasia spondylo-epiphysaria congenita and related generalized skeletal dysplasias among children with severe visual handicaps. *Arch. Dis. Childh., 1969,* **44**, *490-498.*

KOZLOWSKI (K.), FILIPIAK-MIASTROWSKA (I.), NAREBSKA (E.), NOWICKI (S.) et CHYLINSKA (H.). Dysplasia spondylometa-epiphysaria congenita und Dysplasia spondylo-epiphysaria congenita mit Brachymetakarpie und -metatarsie. Ein Beitrag zur Differentialdiagnose der Dysplasia spondylo-epiphysaria congenita. *Fortschr. Röntgenstr., 1971,* **114**, *824-832.*

MARCHAL (C.), DESCHAMPS (J.-P.) et NEIMANN (N.). Dysplasie spondylo-épiphysaire congénitale. *Rev. Pédiat., 1968,* **4**, *23-26.*

MAROTEAUX (P.) et SPRANGER (J.). La maladie de Kniest. *Arch. franç. Pédiat., 1973,* **30**, *735-750.*

MICHAELIS (Von E.), KEMPERDICK (H.) et SPRANGER (J. W.). Dysplasia spondylo-epiphysaria congenita. *Fortschr. Röntgenstr., 1973,* **119**, *429-438.*

SPRANGER (J.) et WIEDEMANN (H.-R.). Dysplasia spondylo-epiphysaria congenita. *Helv. paediat. Act, 1966,* **21**, *598-611.*

SPRANGER (J. W.) et LANGER (L. O., Jr.). Spondylo-epiphyseal dysplasia congenita. *Radiology, 1970,* **94**, *313-322.*

STANESCU (V.) et MAROTEAUX (P.). Anomalie des protéoglycans du cartilage de croissance dans la maladie de Kniest. *C. R. Acad. Sci. Paris, 1974, sous presse.*

Chondro-Ectodermal Dysplasia

BÜTZLER (H.-O.), HENSCHER (L.), MENNICKEN (U.), FRANZ (Chr.) et HILLER (H.-J.). Die Röntgendiagnose der Skelettveränderungen des Ellis-van-Creveld-Syndroms im Wachstumsalter (Literaturanalyse und Bericht über zwei eigene Beobachtungen). *Fortsch. Röntgenestr., 1973,* **118**, *537-552.*

COFFIN (G. S.) et SIRIS (E.). Mental retardation with absent fifth fingernail and terminal phalanx. *Amer. J. Dis. Child, 1970,* **119**, *433-439.*

ELLIS (R. W. B.) et CREVELD (S. van). A syndrome characterized by ectodermal dysplasia, polydactyly, chondrodysplasia and congenital morbus cordis. *Arch. Dis. Childh., 1940,* **15**, *65-84.*

ELLIS (R. W. B.) et ANDREW (J. D.). Chondro-ectodermal dysplasia. *J. Bone Jt Surg., 1962,* **44-B**, *626-636.*

GALLUZZO (A.) et SALVADORI (E.). Un caso di « sindrome di Ellis van Creveld ». Osservato in soggetto adulto (39 anni). *Nunt. radiol. (Roma), 1966, nº 6, 523-540.*

HIROKAWA (K.) et SUZUKI (S.). Ellis-van Creveld syndrome. Report of an autopsy case. *Acta path. jap., 1967,* **17**, *139-143.*

LE MAREC (B.), PASSARGE (E.), DELLENBACH (P.), KERISIT (J.), SIGNARGOUT (J.), FERRAND (B.) et SENECAL (J.). Les formes néo-natales léthales de la dysplasie chondro-ectodermique. A propos de cinq observations. *Ann. Radiol., 1973,* **16**, *19-26.*

McKUSICK (V. A.), EGELAND (J. A.), ELDRIDGE (R.) et KRUSEN (D. E.). Dwarfism in the Amish. I. The Ellis-van Creveld syndrome. *Bull. Johns-Hopk. Hosp., 1964,* **115**, *306-336.*

MONNET (M. P.) et MONNET (Mme F.). Le syndrome d'Ellis-van Creveld. *Rev. lyon. Méd., 1967,* **16**, *47-74.*

MOORE (T. C.). Chondro-ectodermal dysplasia (Ellis-van Creveld syndrome) with bronchial malformation and neonatal tension lobar amphysema. *J. thorac. cardiovasc. Surg. (St. Louis), 1963,* **46**, *1-10.*

MOUCHET (A.) et SEGUIGNOT. Pseudo-achondroplasie. *Bull. Soc. Péd. Paris, 1910,* **12**, *7-16.*

NEIMANN (N.), PIERSON (M.), VIDAILHET (M.), WORMS (Mme A. M.), PLENAT (F.) et FORTIER (G.). Le syndrome d'Ellis-van Creveld et ses rapports avec la dystrophie thoracique asphyxiante. *Pédiatrie, 1973,* **28**, *253-263.*

UEHLINGER (E.). Pathologische Anatomie des Chondroecktodermalen Dysplasie Ellis-van Creveld. *Schweiz. Z. allg. Path., 1967,* **20**, *754-760.*

Asphyxiating Thoracic Dysplasia

BARNES (N. D.), HULL (D.), MILNER (A. D.) et WATERSTON (D. J.). Chest reconstruction in thoracic dystrophy. *Arch. Dis. Childh., 1971,* **46**, *833-837.*

BONNETTE (J.), BRUSSIEUX (J.) et BAUMANN (F.). Dystrophie thoracique asphyxiante familiale. *Sem. Hôp. Paris, 1968,* **44**, *1089-1093.*

BURKLE (F. M.) et BRAVO (A. J.). Asphyxiating thoracic dystrophy. *Clin. Pediat., 1969,* **8**, *165-170.*

COMBE (P.), MICHEL (J.), FAUCHIER (Cl.), RÉGY (J.-M.) et CASENAVE (Cl.). La dystrophie thoracique asphyxiante (Revue générale à propos d'une observation). *Sem. Hôp. Paris, 1969*, **45**, *2211-2223*.

FINEGOLD (M. J.), KATZEW (H.), GENIESER (N. B.) et BECKER (M. H.). Lung structure in thoracic dystrophy. *Amer. J. Dis. Child., 1971*, **122**, *153-159*.

HERDMANN (R. C.) et LANGER. The thoracic asphyxiant dystrophy and renal disease. *Amer. J. Dis. Child., 1968*, **116**, *192-201*.

JEUNE (M.), CARRON (R.), BÉRAUD (C.) et LOAEC (Y.). Polychondystrophie avec blocage thoracique d'évolution fatale. *Pédiatrie, 1954*, **9**, *390-392*.

JEUNE (M.), BÉRAUD (C.) et CARRON (R.). Dystrophie thoracique asphyxiante de caractère familial. *Arch. franç. Pédiat., 1955*, **12**, *886-891*.

LANGER (L. O.). The thoracic pelvic phalangeal dystrophy. *Birth Defects Original Article Series, 1969*, **V** *n° 4, 55-64*.

LECLERC (J.-P.), CANET (J.), LANCRET (P.), CHELLOUL (N.), LE BONT (H.), PESNEL (G.), FABRE (A.) et ALAJOUANINE (P.). Polykystose hépato-pancréato-épididymo-rénale et polydystrophie thoracique néo-natales. Etude anatomo-clinique d'une observation. *Arch. franç. Pédiat., 1971*, **28**, *425-434*.

MAROTEAUX (P.) et SAVART (P.). La dystrophie thoracique asphyxiante. Etude radiologique et rapports avec le syndrome d'Ellis et van Creveld. *Ann. Radiol., 1964*, **7**, *332-338*.

NEIMANN (N.), MANCIAUX (M.), RAUBER (G.), PERNOT (C.) et BRETAGNE-DE KERSAUSON (M. C.). Dystrophie thoracique asphyxiante du nourrisson. *Pédiatrie, 1963*, **18**, *387-397*.

RABUSSON-CORVISARD (Ph.). Association de dystrophie thoracique asphyxiante et de néphropathie chez deux frères. *Thèse Méd., Paris, 1972*.

RAZZI (A.), ROSSO (C.) et DURAND (P.). Contributo anatomopatologico alla distrofia toracica asfissiante del lattante (Malattia di Jeune) e considerazioni sull'utilità terapeutica dell'intervento chirurgico sulle coste. *Minerva pediat., 1965*, **17**, *1823-1827*.

SACREZ (R.), LEVY (J.-M.), HALB (A.), KORN (R.), STOEBNER (Mme), KLEIN (F.) et BEAUVAIS (P.). La dystrophie thoracique asphyxiante. *Pédiatrie, 1966*, **21**, *631-644*.

SHOKEIR (M. H. K.), HOUSTON (C. S.) et AWEN (C. F.). Asphyxiating thoracic chondrodystrophy : association with renal disease and evidence for possible heterozygous expression. *J. med. Genet., 1971*, **8**, *107-112*.

Cleido-Cranial Dysplasia

BACH (Ch.), FAURÉ (C.), SCHAEFER (P.) et JOLLY (J.). La dysostose cléido-crânienne. Etude de six observations. Association à des manifestations neurologiques. *Ann. Pédiat., 1966*, **42**, *67-77*.

COLE (W. R.) et LEVINE (S.). Cleidocranial dysostosis. *Brit. J. Radiol., 1951*, **24**, *549-555*.

CONTE (A.). Considerazioni sulla disostosi cleido-cranica (contributo casistico). *Minerva pediat., 1961*, **13**, *661-667*.

DEBRÉ (R.), LAMY (M.) et SÉE (G.). Etudes et réflexions sur la dysostose cléido-crânienne. *Ann. Méd., 1939*, **46**, *5-25*.

FIORI (M.) et GALLINA (F.). La disostosi da mutazione (disostosi cleido-cranica). *Ortop. Traum. App. mot., 1963*, **31**, *405-425*.

JACKSON (W. P. U.). Osteo-dental dysplasia (cleidocranial dysostosis). The « Arnold Head ». *Acta med. scand., 1951*, **139**, *292-307*.

JOB (J. C.), NAHUM (M.), FAURÉ (C.) et ROSSIER (A.). La dysostose cléido-crânienne. Son polymorphisme. *Arch. franç. Pédiat., 1965*, **21**, *669-686*.

KAUFMANN (H. J.). Röntgenbefunde am kindlichen Becken bei angeborenen Skelettaffektionen und chromosomalen Aberrationen. *Stuttgart, 1964, G. Thieme, éd.*

KEATS (T. E.). Cleidocranial dysostosis : some atypical roentgen manifestations. *Amer. J. Roentgenol., 1967*, **100**, *71-74*.

KITE (J. H.). Congenital pseudarthrosis of the clavicle. *Sth. med. J. (Bgham, Ala.), 1968*, **61**, *703-710*.

KOZLOWSKI (K.), HANICKA (M.) et SYGULSKA-MACHOWA (H.). Dysplasia cleido-facialis. *Z. Kinderheilk., 1970*, **108**, *331-338*.

LASKER (G. W.). The inheritance of cleido-cranial dysostosis. *Hum. Biol., 1946*, **18**, *103-126*.

MARIE (P.) et SAINTON (P.). La dysostose cléido-crânienne héréditaire. *Bull. Soc. méd. Hôp. Paris, 1898*, **15**, *436-442*.

MARTIN (M.). Sur un déplacement naturel de la clavicule. *J. Méd. Chir. Pharmacol., 1765*, **23**, *465-481*.

NOMBALLAIS (G.), WELIN (J.), BUREAU (O.) et GILLOT (F.). A propos d'une observation familiale de dysostose cléido-crânienne. *Rev. Pédiat., 1969*, **2**, *103-115*.

RHINEHART (B. A.). Cleidocranial dysostosis (mutational dysostosis) with a case report. *Radiology, 1936*, **26**, *741-748*.

RUSHTON (M. A.). An anomaly of cementum in cleidocranial dysostosis. *Brit. dent. J., 1956*, **100**, *81-83*.

SCHUCH (P.) et FLEISCHER-PETERS (A.). Zür Klinik der Dysostosis cleidocranialis. *Z. Kinderheilk., 1967*, **98**, *107-132*.

SMITH (N. H. H.). A histologic study of cementum in a case of cleidocranial dysostosis. *Oral Surg., 1968*, **25**, *470-478*.

STOCKS (P.) et BARRINGTON (A.). Hereditary disorders of bone development, cleidocranial dysostosis. *Treasury of human inheritance, 1925*, **III**, *121-139*.

VARESE (L. A.) et LANGE (M. M.). Pseudoartrosi congenita della clavicola. Contributo clinico. *Minerva med. (Turino), 1967*, **19**, *2049-2052*.

WALL (J. J.). Congenital pseudarthrosis of the clavicle. *J. Bone Jt Surg., 1970*, **52-A**, *1003-1009*.

WIEDEMANN (H. R.). Gestörte Ossifikation besonders der bindegewebig präformierten Belegknochen : Die Dysostosis cleidocranialis. *In* H. Opitz et F. Schmid (Ed.), Handbuch der Kinderheilkunde. *Berlin, 1967, Springer-Verlag, éd., p. 129-135*.

WILLICH (E.) et MOSTAFAWY (A.). Die Dysostosis pelvico-cleidocranialis. *Fortschr. Röntgenstr., 1970*, **113**, *49-59*.

ZELLWEGER (H.), THEILER (K.) et LARCHER (F.). Ueber die Dysostosis cleidocranialis. *Helv. paediat. Acta, 1950*, **5**, *264-278*.

Spondylo-Epiphyseo-Metaphyseal Dysplasias: Generalities and Surveys

BAILEY (J. A.). Disproportionate short stature diagnosis and management. *Philadelphia, 1973, W. B. Saunders Co., éd.*

BERNARD (R.) et CAILLOL (P.). Les polyostéochondroses. *Pédiatrie, 1951*, **6**, *269-294*.

CANEPA (G.) et SEGHINI (G.). Osteocondrodistrofia dell' accrescimento. *Arch. Chir. orthop., 1956*, **21**, *26-69*.

CATEL (W.). Differentiale Diagnose von Krankheitssymptomen bei Kindern und Jugendlichen. *3e édit., Stuttgart, 1961, G. Thieme, éd.*

COCCHI (U.). Polytope erbliche enchondrale Dysostosen. *Fortschr. Röntgenstr., 1950,* **72**, *409-435.*

FAIRBANK (H. A. T.). An atlas of general affections of the skeleton. *Edinburgh, 1951, Livingstone, éd.*

HIRSCH (S.). Generalised osteochondrodystrophy. The eccentrochondroplastic form. *J. Bone Jt Surg., 1937,* **19**, *297-313.*

HOBAEK (A.). Problems of hereditary chondrodysplasias. *Oslo, 1961, Oslo University Press, éd.*

LAMY (M.) et MAROTEAUX (P.). Les chondrodystrophies génotypiques. *Paris, 1961, Expansion scient. franç., éd.*

MAROTEAUX (P.), WIEDEMANN (R.), SPRANGER (J.), KOZLOWSKI (K.) et LENZI (L.). Essai de classification des dysplasies spondylo-épiphysaires. *Lyon, 1968, Simep Editions, éd.*

MAROTEAUX (P.). Spondylo-epiphyseal dysplasias and metatropic dwarfism. *Birth Defects Original Articles Series, 1969,* **V** *n° 4, 35-44.*

RUBIN (P.). Dynamic classification of bone dysplasia. *Chicago, 1964, Year Book med. publ., éd.*

Metaphyseal Chondrodysplasias

ALLEMAND (P.). A propos de deux cas d'une forme particulière de dysostose métaphysaire comportant des modifications des phanères et obéissant à un mode de transmission récessif autosomique. *Thèse Méd., Paris, 1966.*

ANDERSON (Ch. M.). Intestinal malabsorption in childhood. *Arch. Dis. Childh., 1966,* **41**, *571-596.*

BURKE (V.), COLEBATCH (J. H.), ANDERSON (C. M.) et SIMONS (M. J.). Association of pancreatic insufficiency and chronic neutropenia in childhood. *Arch. Dis. Child., 1967,* **42**, *147-157.*

COOPER (R. R.), PEDRINI-MILLE (A.) et PONSETI (I. V.). Metaphyseal dysostosis. A rough surfaced endoplasmic reticulum storage defect. *Lab. Invest., 1973,* **28**, *119-125.*

GIEDION (A.), PRADER (A.), HADORN (B.), SHMERLING (D. H.) et AURICCHIO (S.). Metaphysäre Dysostose und angeborene Pankreasinsuffizienz. *Fortschr. Röntgenstr., 1968,* **108**, *51-57.*

GOOR (M.), SAUVAGE (D.), TOURSEL (F.), FARRIAUX (J. P.) et FONTAINE (G.). Contribution à l'étude de la dysostose métaphysaire (présentation d'une observation familiale). *Rev. Pédiat., 1970,* **6**, *531-542.*

GRAM (P. B.), FLEMMING (J. L.), FRAME (B.) et FINE (G.). Metaphysial chondrodysplasia of Jansen. *J. Bone Jt Surg., 1959,* **41-A**, *951-959.*

HAAS (W. H. D. DE), BOER (W. DE) et GRIFFIOEN (F.). Metaphysial dysostosis. A late follow-up of the first reported case. *J. Bone Jt Surg., 1969,* **51-B**, *290-299.*

JANSEN (M.). Ueber atypische Chondrodystrophie (Achondroplasie) and über eine noch nicht beschriebene angeborene Wachstumstörung. *Z. orthop. Chir., 1934,* **61**, *255-286.*

KOZLOWSKI (K.) et SIKORSKA (B.). Dysplasia metaphysaria, typ Vaandrager-Pena. *Z. Kinderheilk., 1970,* **108**, *165-170.*

L'HIRONDEL (J.), CAEN, DARIDON et TILLET. Anémie de Blackfan-Diamond et dysostose métaphysaire récessive autosomique. *Ouest méd., 1967* **20**, *1152-1157.*

MAROTEAUX (P.), SAVART (P.), LEFEBVRE (J.) et ROYER (P.). Les formes partielles de la dysostose métaphysaire. *Presse méd., 1963,* **71**, *1523-1526.*

MCKUSICK (V. A.), ELDRIDGE (R.), HOSTETLER (J. A.), RUANGWIT (U.) et EGELAND (J. A.). Dwarfism in the Amish. II. Cartilage-hair hypoplasia. *Bull. Johns-Hopk. Hosp., 1965,* **116**, *285-326.*

PENA (J.). Disostosis metafisaria. Una revisión. Con aportación de una observación familiar (una forma nueva de la enfermedad). *Radiologia, 1965,* **47**, *3-22.*

RIMOIN (D. L.) et MCALISTER (W.). Metaphyseal dysostosis, conductive hearing loss and mental retardation : a recessivly inherited syndrome. *Birth Defects, Original Article Series,* **VII** *n° 4, 116-122.*

SACREZ (R.), LEVY (J. M.), GODAR (G.) et CASTANIER (J.). Anémie de Blackfan-Diamond associée à des malformations multiples. *Méd. inf., 1965,* **72**, *493-499.*

SCHMID (F.). Beitrag zur Dysostosis enchondralis metaphysaria. *Moschr. Kinderheilk., 1949,* **97**, *393-397.*

SCHMIDT (B. J.), BECAK (W.), BECAK (M. L.), SOIBELMAN (I.), SILVA QUEIROZ (A. da), LORGA (A. P.), SECAF (F.), ANTONIO (C. F.) et ANDRADE CARVALHO (A. de). Metaphyseal dysostosis. *J. Pediat., 1963,* **63**, *106-112.*

SHWACHMAN (H.), DIAMOND (L. K.), OSKI (F. A.) et KHAW (K. T.). The syndrome of pancreatic insufficiency and bone marrow dysfunction. *J. Pediat., 1964,* **65**, *645-663.*

SPAHR (A.) et SPAHR-HARTMANN (I.). Dysostose métaphysaire familiale. Etude de 4 cas dans une fratrie. *Helv. paediat. Acta, 1961,* **16**, *836-849.*

TAYBI (H.), MITCHELL (A. D.) et FRIEDMAN (G. D.). Metaphyseal dysostosis and the associated syndrome of pancreatic insufficiency and blood disorders. *Radiology, 1969,* **93**, *563-571.*

VAANDRAGER (G. J.). Metaphysial dysostosis. *Ned. T. Geneesk., 1960,* **104**, *547-552.*

WEIL (S.). Die metaphysären Dysostosen. *Z. Orthop., 1957,* **89**, *1-16.*

WIEDEMANN (H. R.) et SPRANGER (J.). Chondrodysplasia metaphysaria (Dysostosis metaphysaria) — ein neuer Typ ? *Z. Kinderheilk., 1970,* **108**, *171-186.*

Multiple Epiphyseal Dysplasias

BARRINGTON-WARD (L. E.). Double coxa vara with other deformities occurring in brother and sister. *Lancet, 1912,* **90**, *157-159.*

BOUVET (J. P.), HENRARD (J. CL.), SIAUD (J. R.), PAOLAGGI (J. B.) et AUQUIER (L.). Polyarthropathie dégénérative précoce d'allure inflammatoire. *Rev. Rhum., 1974,* **41**, *123-134.*

BRIEX-CORVOL (M. T.). Poussées douloureuses articulaires cliniquement inflammatoires au cours de la dysplasie polyépiphysaire. *Thèse Méd., Paris, 1969.*

BRILL (W.). Beitrag zur Aetiologie der Perthesshen Erkrankung des Hüftgelenkes und der Köhlerschen Metatarsalerkrankung. *Arch. Orthop. chir., 1926-27,* **24**, *64-83.*

CLÉMENT (R.), GUÉNAUX (G.) et HAGUENAUER (Mlle J.). Dystrophie osseuse épiphysaire chez un enfant de 8 ans. *Bull. Soc. Pédiat., Paris, 1937,* **35**, *547-557.*

FAIRBANK (H. A. T.). Dysplasia epiphysialis multiplex. *Brit. J. Surg., 1947,* **34**, *225-232.*

GORLIN (R. J.), ALPER (R.) et LANGER (L.). Megepiphyseal dwarfism. *J. Pediat., 1973,* **83**, *633-635.*

KAHN (M. F.), CORVOL (M. T.), JURMAND (S. H.), COUTURE (B.), AMOUROUX (J.) et SÈZE (S. DE). Le rhumatisme chondrodysplasique. *Sem. Hôp. Paris, 1970,* **46**, *1938-1953.*

KEHL (X.). Beitrag zur Perthesshen Krankheit. *Bruns Beitr. klin. Chir., 1925,* **138**, *65-66.*

MAROTEAUX (P.), WIEDEMANN (R.), SPRANGER (J.), ZOZLOWSKI (K.) et LENZI (L.). Essai de classification des dysplasies spondylo-épiphysaires. *Lyon, 1968, Simep Editions, éd.*

MONTY (C. P.). Familial Perthes disease resembling multiple epiphysial displasia. *J. Bone Jt Surg., 1962,* **44-B**, *565-568.*

MÜLLER (W.). Die erbliche multiple Störung der epiphysen Verknöcherung als typisches Krankheitsbild. *Fortschr. Röntgenstr., 1939,* **59**, *65-69.*

PFEIFFER (R. A.), JUNEMANN (G.), POLSTER (J.) et BAUER (H.). Epiphyseal dysplasia of the femoral head, severe myopia and perceptive hearing loss in three brothers. *Clin. Genet., 1973,* **4**, *141-144.*

RIBBING (S.). Studien über hereditäre multiple epiphysenstörungen. *Acta radiologica, Suplt.* **34**, *1937.*

SPRANGER (J.). Arthro-ophthalmopathia hereditaria. *Ann. Radiol., 1968,* **11**, *359-364.*

SPRANGER (J.) et WIEDEMANN (H. E.). Dysplasia spondylo-epiphysaria congenita. *Helv. paediat. Acta, 1966,* **21**, *598-611.*

STANESCU (R.). Ultrastructural abnormalities of the chondrocytes in the type of polyepiphyseal dysplasia with a propable autosomal recessive transmission. *Bio. Med. Express, 1974* (sous presse).

STICKLER (G. B.), BELAU (P. G.), FARRELL (F. J.), JONES (J. D.), PUGH (D. G.), STEINBERG (A. G.) et WARD (L. E.). Hereditary progressive arthro-ophthalmopathy. *Mayo Clin. Proc., 1965,* **40**, *433-455.*

STICKLER (G. B.) et PUGH (D. G.). Hereditary progressive arthro-ophthalmopathy. II. Additional observations on vertebral abnormalities, a hearing defect, and a report of a similar case. *Mayo Clin. Proc., 1967,* **42**, *495-500.*

TURPIN (R.) et COSTE (F.). La polyostéochondrite. *Presse méd., 1941,* **49**, *1136-1139.*

WAREMBOURG (H.), RAZEMON (J. P.) et JAILLARD (S.). Sur un cas de dysplasie polyépiphysaire multiple de Fairbank. *Lille méd., 1965,* **10**, *499-504.*

WEINBERG (H.), FRANKLEL (M.), HAKIN (M.) et VAS (E.). Familial epiphysial dysplasia of the lower limbs. *J. Bone Jt Surg., 1960,* **42-B**, *313-332.*

Epiphyseo-Metaphyseal Dysplasias and Complex Dysplasias

COOPER (R. R.), PONSETI (I. V.) et MAYNARD (J. A.). Pseudoachondroplastic dwarfism. A rough-surfaced endoplasmic reticulum storage disorder. *J. Bone Jt Surg., 1973,* **55-A**, *475-484.*

IANNACCONE (G.) et PIERAGOSTINI (P.). La « malattia di Blount » (Tibia vara o osteocondrosi deformante della tibia) : una causa poco nota di genu varum. *Minerva pediat., 1966,* **18**, *178-187.*

LANGENSKIOLD (A.) et RISKA (E. B.). Tibia vara (osteochondrosis deformans tibiae). A survey of seventy one cases. *J. Bone Jt Surg., 1964,* **46-A**, *1405-1420.*

LANGER (L. O.), PETERSEN (D.) et SPRANGER (J.). An unusual bone dysplasia : parastremmatic dwarfism. *Amer. J. Roentgenol., 1970,* **110**, *550-560.*

LÉRI (A.). Dystrophie osseuse généralisée congénitale et héréditaire. La pléonostéose familialc. *Presse méd., 1922,* **30**, *13-16.*

MAROTEAUX (P.) et LAMY (M.). Les formes pseudo-achondroplasiques des dysplasies spondylo-épiphysaires. *Presse méd., 1959,* **67**, *383-386.*

OZONOFF (M. B.) et OGDEN (J. A.). Sjögren-Larsson syndrome with epiphyseal-metaphyseal dysplasia. *Amer. J. Roentgenol., 1973,* **118**, *187-192.*

PAGNIEZ (B.), SAINT-AUBERT (P.), FARRIAUX (J. P.) et FONTAINE (G.). La dysplasie pseudo-achondroplasique. A propos d'une observation. *Ann. Pédiat., 1972,* **19**, *897-903.*

RASK (M. R.). Morquio-Brailsford osteochondrodystrophy and osteogenesis imperfecta : report of patient with both conditions. *J. Bone Jt Surg., 1963,* **45-A**, *561-570.*

SEVASTIKOGLOU (J. A.) et ERIKSSON (I.). Familial infantile osteochondrosis deformans tibiae. Idiopathic tibia vara. A case report. *Acta orthop. scand., 1967,* **38**, *81-87.*

SILFVERSKIOLD (N.). Sur la question de l'achondroplasie atypique et de sa forme périphérique. *Acta radiol. (Stock.), 1926,* **5**, *223-235.*

STANESCU (V.) et MAROTEAUX (P.). Anomalies des protéoglycans du cartilage de croissance de la pseudo-achondroplasie. *C. R. Acad. Sci. Paris, 1973,* **277**, *2585-2588.*

Acrodysplasias

BRAILSFORD (J. F.). The radiology of bones and joint. *1 vol., 4e édit., London, 1948, Churchill, éd.*

FONTAINE (G.), MAROTEAUX (P.), FARRIAUX (J. P.), RICHARD (J.) et ROELENS (B.). Le syndrome tricho-rhino-phalangien. *Arch. franç. Pédiat., 1970,* **27**, *635-647.*

GIEDION (A.). Das tricho-rhino-phalangeale Syndrom. *Helv. paediat. Acta, 1966,* **21**, *475-482.*

GIEDION (A.). Die periphere Dysostose (PD) — ein Sammelbegriff. *Fortschr. Röntgenstr., 1969,* **110**, *507-524.*

GIEDION (A.). Acrodysplasias. Cone-shaped epiphyses peripheral dysostosis, Thiemann's disease and acrodysostosis. *In* Prog. Pediat. Radiol., vol. 4, Intrinsic Diseases of Bones. *Basel, 1973, Karger, éd., p. 325-345.*

GIEDION (A.), BURDEA (M.), FRUCHTER (Z.), MELONI (T.) et TROSC (V.). Autosomal-dominant transmission of the tricho-rhino-phalangeal syndrome. Report of 4 unrelated families, review of 60 cases. *Helv. paediat. Acta, 1973,* **28**, *249-259.*

MAROTEAUX (P.) et MALAMUT (G.). L'acrodysostose. *Presse méd., 1968,* **76**, *2189-2192.*

ROBINOW (M.), PFEIFFER (R. A.), GORLIN (R. J.), MCKUSICK (V. A.), RENUART (A. W.), JOHNSON (G. F.) et SUMMITT (R. L.). Acrodysostosis. *Amer. J. Dis. Child., 1971,* **121**, *195-203.*

SALDINO (R. M.) et MAINZER (F.). Cone-shaped epiphyses (CSE) in siblings with hereditary renal disease and retinitis pigmentosa. *Radiology, 1971,* **98**, *39-45.*

THIEMANN (H.). Juvenile Epiphysenstörungen, idiopatische Erkrankung der Epiphysenknorpel der Fingerphalangen. *Fortschr. Röntgenstr., 1909,* **14** *79-81.*

Platyspondylies

BANNERMAN (R. M.), INGALL (G. B.) et MOHN (J. F.) X-linked spondyloepiphyseal dysplasia tarda : clinical and linkage data. *J. med. Genet., 1971,* **8**, *291-301.*

BARBER (S. H.). An unusual form of familial ostrodystrophy. *Lancet, 1960,* **1**, *1220-1221.*

CLAUSEN (J.), DYGGVE (H. V.) et MELCHIOR (J. C.). Chemical and enzymic studies of a family with skeletal abnormalities associated with mental retardation. *Clin. chim. Acta., 1970,* **29**, *197-207.*

DYGGVE (H. V.), MELCHIOR (J. C.) et CLAUSEN (J.). Morquio-Ullrich's disease. *Arch. Dis. Child., 1962,* **37**, *525-534.*

GRENIER (B.), CASTAING (J.), LAUGIER (J.), MICHEL (J.) et DESBUQUOIS (G.). Deux cas familiaux de dysplasie spondylo-métaphysaire. *Arch. franç. Pédiat., 1969,* **26**, *1015-1026.*

JACOBSEN (A. W.). Hereditary osteochondrodystrophia deformans. *J. amer. med. Ass., 1939,* **113**, *121-124.*

KOZLOWSKI (K.), MAROTEAUX (P.) et SPRANGER (J.). La dysostose spondylo-métaphysaire. *Presse méd., 1967,* **75**, *2769-2774.*

KOZLOWSKI (K.). Platyspondyly in childhood. *Pediat. Radiol., 1974,* **2**, *81-87.*

LE QUESNE (G. W.) et KOZLOWSKI (K.). Spondylometaphyseal dysplasia. *Brit. J. Radiol., 1973,* **46**, *685-691.*

MAROTEAUX (P.), WIEDEMANN (R.), SPRANGER (J.), KOZLOWSKI (K.) et LENZI (L.). La brachyolmie. *In* Essai de classification des dysplasies spondylo-épiphysaires. *Lyon, 1968, Simep Editions, éd., p. 37-40.*

MAROTEAUX (P.), LAMY (M.) et BERNARD (J.). La dysplasie spondylo-épiphysaire tardive. Description clinique et radiologique. *Presse méd., 1957,* **65**, *1205-1208.*

MOURAO (P. A. S.), TOLEDO (S. P. A.), NADER (H. B.) et DIETRICH (C. P.). Excretion of chondroitin sulfate C with low sulfate content by patients with generalized platyspondyly (brachyolmie). *Biochem. Med., 1973,* **7**, *415-423.*

MURDOCH (J. L.) et WALKER (B. A.). A « new » form of spondylometaphyseal dysplasia. *Birth Defects, Original Article Series, 1969,* **V** *n° 4, 368-370.*

SCHMIDT (B. J.), BECAK (W.), BECAK (M. L.), SOIBELMAN (I.), SILVA QUEIROZ (A. da), LORGA (A. P.), SECAF (F.), ANTONIO (C. F.) et ANDRADE CARVALHO (A. de). Metaphyseal dysostosis. Review of literature; study of a case with cytogenetic analysis. *J. Pediat., 1963,* **63**, *106-112.*

SUTCLIFFE (J.). Metaphyseal dysostosis. *Ann. Radiol., 1966,* **9**, *215-223.*

VESTERMARK (S.). Osteochondrodystrophia deformans with mucopolysaccharidosis. *Arch. Dis. Childh., 1965,* **40**, *106-110.*

WIEDEMANN (H. R.) et SPRANGER (J.). Chondrodysplasia metaphysaria (Dysostosis metaphysaria) — ein neuer Typ ? *Z. Kinderheilk., 1970,* **108**, *171-186.*

Dyschondrosteosis

DODINVAL (P.) et COLLARD (M.). Un cas isolé de dyschondrostéose. *Humangenetik, 1965,* **1**, *557-562.*

FELMAN (A. H.) et KIRKPATRICK (J. A.). Dyschondrosteose, Mesomelic Dwarfism of Leri and Weill. *Amer. J. Dis. Child., 1970,* **120**, *329-331.*

LANGER (L. O., Jr.). Dyschondrosteosis, a hereditable bone dysplasia with characteristic roentgenographic features. *Amer. J. Roentgenol., 1965,* **95**, *178-188.*

LERI (A.), LAYANI (F.) et WEILL (J.). La dyschondrostéose, variété nouvelle de nanisme. *Presse méd., 1931,* **39**, *262-264.*

LERI (A.) et WEILL (J.). Une affection congénitale et symétrique du développement osseux : la dyschondrostéose. *Bull. Soc. méd. Hôp. Paris, 1929,* **53**, *1491-1494.*

MOREL PESCAROLO (S.). La dyschondrostéose. Etude de treize observations inédites. *Thèse Méd., Paris, 1964.*

SILVERMAN (F. N.). — Mesomelic dwarfism. *In* Prog. Pediat. Radiol., vol. 4, Intrinsic Diseases of Bones. *Basel, 1973, Karger, éd., p. 546-562.*

OSTEOCHONDRODYSPLASIAS WITH ANARCHIC DEVELOPMENT OF CARTILAGINOUS OR FIBROUS TISSUE

Dysplasia Epiphysealis Hemimelica

BARTA (O.), SCHANZL (A.) et SZEPESI (J.). Dysplasia epiphysialis hemimelica. *Acta orthop. scand., 1973,* **44**, *702-709.*

BIANCHI (M.) et FRASSI (G.). Displasia epifisaria monomelica. *Arch. Ortop., 1963,* **76**, *15-26.*

FAIRBANK (T. J.). Dysplasia epiphysialis hemmimelica. *J. Bone Jt Surg., 1956,* **38-B**, *237-242.*

FÈVRE (M.) et RIGAULT (P.). Fragmentation osseuse hypertrophiante (tarsomégalie, epiphyseal aclasis, dysplasie épiphysaire hémimélique). Le signe de l'hypertrophie épiphysaire tibiale. *Rev. Chir. orthop., 1968,* **54**, *525-534.*

MONTMINY (M.) et GAGNON (P.-A.). Dysplasie épiphysaire hémimélique (tarsomégalie). *Un. méd. Can., 1972,* **101**, *1822-1826.*

MOUCHET (A.) et BELOT (J.). La tarsomégalie. *J. Radiol. Electrol., 1926,* **10**, *289-293.*

THEODOROU (S.) et LANITIS (G.). Dysplasia epiphysialis hemimelica (epiphyseal osteochondromata). Report of two cases and review of the literature. *Helv. paediat. Acta, 1968,* **23**, *195-204.*

Multiple Cartilaginous Exostoses

BETHGE (J. F. J.). Hereditäre, multiple Exostosen und ihre pathogenetische Deutung. *Arch. orthop. Unfall-Chir., 1963,* **54**, *667-696.*

CARDIS (R.). A propos de deux cas d'exostoses cartilagineuses multiples. *Radiol. clin., 1961,* **30**, *209-249.*

CHESTER (D. K.). Multiple cartilaginous exostoses in two generations of dogs. *J. Amer. vet. med. Ass., 1971,* **159**, *895-897.*

FREJKA (B.). Exostoses ostéogéniques multiples. *Rev. Orthop., 1928,* **15**, *225-231.*

HARRIS (H.). A sex-limiting modifying gene in diaphysial aclasis (multiple exostose). *Ann. Eugen. (Camb.), 1948,* **14**, *165-170.*

JAFFE (H. L.). Hereditary multiple exostosis. *Arch. Path. (Chicago), 1943,* **36**, *335-357.*

KEITH (A.). Studies on the anatomical changes which accompany certain growth disorders of the human body. I. The nature of the structural alteration in the disorder known as multiple exostoses. *J. Anat. (Lond.), 1920,* **54**, *101-115.*

KIENBÖCK (R.). Das Ellbogengelenk bei chondraler Dysplasie des Skeletts mit multiplen Exostosen. *Fortschr. Röntgenstr., 1910,* **15**, *104-108.*

LACROIX (P.). Contribution à l'étude de la maladie exostosante. Sur la migration des exostoses au cours de la croissance. *Rev. Orthop., 1950,* **36**, *20-25.*

LANGENSKIÖLD (A.). Normal and pathological bone growth in the light of the development of cartilaginous foci in chondrodysplasia. *Acta chir. scand., 1947,* **95**, *367-385.*

LANGENSKIÖLD (A.). The development of multiple cartilaginous exostoses. *Acta orthop. scand., 1967,* **38**, *259-266.*

LEVEUF (J.). Le problème de la croissance de l'os en longueur, étudié à la lumière de la maladie exostosante. *Rev. Orthop., 1946,* **32**, *5-14.*

MAROTEAUX (P.) et LAMY (M.). La maladie exostosante. *Sem. Hôp. Paris, 1960,* **36**, *172-181.*

MAROTEAUX (P.). La métachondromatose. *Z. Kinderheilk., 1971,* **109**, *246-261.*

MASTRAGOSTINO (S.) et GALLI (G.). Comportamento delle cartilagini di accrescimento nelle esostosi. *Minerva pediat. (Torino), 1957,* **9**, *1559-1561.*

MONTELEONE (M.) et DE ANGELIS RICCIOTTI (F.). Sulle esostosi osteogeniche. Etiopatogenesi. Anatomia patologica. Clinica e terapia. *Ortop. Traum., 1962,* **30**, *117-178.*

MORGAN (J. P.), CARLSON (W. D.) et ADAMS (O. R.). Hereditary multiple exostosis in the horse. *J. amer. vet. med. Ass., 1962,* **140**, *1320-1322.*

MURKEN (J.-D.). Ueber cartilaginäre Exostosen. Zur Klinik, Genetik und Mutationsrate des Krankheitsbildes. *Z. menschl. Vererb. Konstitlehre, 1963,* **36**, *469-505.*

PETIT-DUTAILLIS (D.) et LEREBOULLET (J.). Paraplégie par fibrochondrome des vertèbres dorsales supérieures chez une malade atteinte de maladie ostéogénique. Laminectomie, ablation partielle de la tumeur, amélioration considérable de la paraplégie. *Bull. Soc. Chir., Paris, 1934,* **60**, *691-696.*

POOL (R. R.) et CARRIG (C. B.). Multiple cartilaginous exostoses in a cat. *Vet. Path., 1972,* **9**, *350-359.*

SIGNARGOUT (J.), GUÉGAN (Y.), LE MAREC (B.) et SIMON (J.). Les paraplégies de la maladie des exostoses multiples. A propos de deux observations. *J. Radiol. Electrol., 1973,* **54**, *403-407.*

VINSTEIN (A. L.) et FRANKEN (E. A., Jr.). Hereditary multiple exostoses. Report of a case with spinal cord compression. *Amer. J. Roentgenol., 1971,* **112**, *405-407.*

VIRCHOW (R.). Ueber multiple Exostosen, mit Vorlegung von Präparaten. *Verh. Ges. dtsch. Natur. Aerztz, 64. Versammlung zu Halle, Leipzig, 1892,* **2**, *159-161.*

VITALLI (H. P.). Die Osteochondrome bei Jugendlichen. *Arch. orthop. Unfall-Chir., 1960,* **52**, *270-280.*

Dyschondroplasia and Maffuci's Syndrome

BANNA (M.) et PARWANI (G. S.). Multiple sarcomas in Maffucci's syndrome. *Brit. J. Radiol., 1969,* **42**, *304-307.*

BARBIERI (E.) et CURIONI (G. B.). Degenerazione maligna del morbo di Ollier (Discondroplasia). *Arch. Ortop., 1961,* **74**, *1-12.*

BENTZON (P. G. K.). Roentgenological and experimental studies on the pathogenesis of the dyschondroplasia. *Acta Radiol., 1924,* **3**, *89-111.*

BRADDOCK (G. T.) et HADLOW (V.). Osteosarcoma in enchondromatosis (Ollier's disease). Report of a case. *J. Bone Jt Surg., 1966,* **48-B**, *145-149.*

FONTAN (A.) et BATTIN (J. J.). Chondromatose multiple avec atteinte vertébrale prédominante et nanisme sévère. *J. Méd. Bordeaux, 1965, 2003-2009.*

GRANGES (Y.). A propos d'un cas inédit de syndrome polymalformatif avec gigantisme partiel des extrémités. Etude comparative de 100 cas de syndrome de Maffucci. *Thèse Méd., Lausanne, 1973.*

GRENET (P.), BADOUAL (J.), GALLET (J. P.) et LANGE (C.). Dyschondroplasie et tumeur de l'ovaire. *Ann. Pédiat., 1972,* **19**, *759-764.*

KAST et RECKLINGHAUSEN (Von). Ein Fall von Enchondrom mit ungewöhnlicher Multiplication. *Virchows Arch. path. Anat., 1889,* **118**, *1-18.*

LANGENSKIÖLD (A.) et EDGREN (W.). Imitation of chondrodysplasia by localized roentgen ray injury. An experimental study of bone growth. *Acta chir. scand., 1950,* **99**, *351-373.*

LANGENSKIÖLD (A.). The stages of development of the cartilaginous foci in dyschondroplasia (Ollier's disease). *Acta orthop. scand., 1967,* **38**, *174-180.*

LEWIS (R. J.) et KETCHAM (A. S.). Maffucci's syndrome : functional and neoplastic significance. Case report and review of the literature. *J. Bone Jt Surg., 1973,* **55-A**, *1465-1479.*

MAFFUCCI (A.). Di un caso di encondroma ed angioma multiplo. *Movem. Med. Chir. Napoli, 1881,* **25**, *399-412.*

MAROTEAUX (P.) et LAMY (M.). La dyschondroplasie. Chondromatose multiple du squelette. *Sem. Hôp. Paris, 1960,* **36**, *182-193.*

MURRAY (A. M.) et CRUICKSHANK (B.). Dyschondroplasia. Report of a case. *J. Bone Jt Surg., 1960,* **42-B**, *344-347.*

OLLIER (M.). De la dyschondroplasie. *Bull. Soc. Chir. (Lyon), 1899,* **3**, *22-27.*

Fibrous Dysplasia, Cherubism, and Fibromatosis

ALBRIGHT (F.), BUTLER (A. M.), HAMPTON (A. O.) et SMITH (P. A.). Syndrome characterized by osteotis fibrosa disseminata. *New Engl. J. Med., 1937,* **216**, *727-746.*

BRECK (L. W.). Treatment of fibrous dysplasia of bone by total femoral plating and hip nailing. *Clin. Orthop., 1972, 82-83.*

CAVINA (C.). Cherubismo : rara affezione displatisca familiare delle ossa mascellari. *Minerva stomatol., 1966,* **15**, *830-838.*

CONDON (V. R.) et ALLEN (R. P.). Congenital generalized fibromatosis. Case report, with roentgen manifestations. *Radiology, 1961,* **76**, *444-448.*

DEGOS (R.), CIVATTE (J.), BELAIGH (S.), LARRÈGUE (M.) et BONVALET (D.). Fibromatose juvénile des doigts. *Bull. Soc. franç. Derm. Syph., 1971,* **78**, *6-8.*

DES MARCHAIS (J.), PAQUIN (G.) et GUY (R.). Fibromatose cartilagineuse calcifiante (un cas de fibrome aponévrotique juvénile). *Un. méd. Can., 1972,* **101**, *247-249.*

FOISSIN (B.) et OHANIAN (D.). A propos de deux observations de chérubisme. *Ann. Oto-Laryng. (Paris), 1965,* **82**, *467-472.*

GROSS (C. W.) et MONTGOMERY (W. W.). Fibrous dysplasia and malignant degeneration. *Arch. Otolaryng., 1967,* **85**, *653-657.*

HALL (R.) et WARRICK (C.). Hypersecretion of hypothalamic releasing hormones : a possible explanation of the endocrine manifestations of polyostotic fibrous dysplasia (Albright's syndrome). *Lancet, 1972,* **i**, *1313-1316.*

HARRIS (M.). Cherubism and the osteoclastoma. *Oral Surg., 1968,* **25**, *613-619.*

HUNTER (D.) et TURNBULL (H. M.). Hyperparathyroidism. *Brit. J. Surg., 1931,* **19**, *203-284.*

JAFFE (H. L.). Hyperparathyroidism (Recklinghausen disease of bone). *Arch. Path., 1933,* **16**, *63-112 et 236-258.*

JONES (W. A.). Cystic multilocular disease of the jaws. *Amer. J. Cancer, 1933,* **17**, *946-950.*

JONES (W. A.). Further observations regarding familial multilocular cystic disease of the jaws. *Brit. J. Radiol., 1938,* **25**, *227-241.*

LEEDS (N.) et SEAMAN (W. M. B.). Fibrous dysplasia of the skull and its differential diagnosis. A clinical and roentgenographic study of 46 cases. *Radiology, 1962,* **78**, *570-582.*

LICHTENSTEIN (L.). Polyostotic fibrous dysplasia. *Arch. Surg., 1938,* **36**, *874-898.*

LIÈVRE (J. A.). L'ostéose parathyroïdienne. *Thèse Méd., Paris, 1931, Masson, éd.*

LIÈVRE (J. A.), LIÈVRE (Mme J. A.) et RACT (A.). La dysplasie fibreuse des os. Une série de 34 observations. Nosographie et pathogénie. *Sem. Hôp. Paris, 1966,* **42**, *3252-3263.*

LIÈVRE (J. A.), LEROUX-ROBERT (J.) et LIÈVRE (Mme J. A.). Chérubisme (une observation). *Rev. Rhum., 1972,* **39**, *736-739.*

MANDE (R.), HENNEQUET (A.), LOUBRY (P.), CLOUP (M.) et JULIEN MARIE. Fibromatose congénitale diffuse du nouveau-né à évolution régressive. *Sem. Hôp. Paris, 1965,* **41**, *2584-2593.*

MONTOYA (G.), EVARTS (C. M.) et DOHN (D. F.). Polyostotic fibrous dysplasia and spinal cord compression. Case report. *J. Neurosurg., 1968,* **29**, *102-105.*

RAMON (Y.), BERMAN (W.) et BUBIS (J. J.). Gingival fibromatosis combined with cherubism. *Oral Surg., 1967,* **24**, *435-448.*

RIDDELL (D. M.). Malignant change in fibrous dysplasia. Report of a case. *J. Bone Jt Surg., 1964,* **46-B**, *251-255.*

ROSENCRANTZ (M.). A case of fibrous dysplasia (Jaffe-Lichtenstein) with vertebral fracture and compression of the spinal cord. *Acta orthop. scand., 1965,* **36**, *435-440.*

SACREZ (R.), KLEIN (F.), LÉVY (J. M.), BERLAND (H.), PHILIPPE (E.), KEMPF (Y.), LALHOU et GOLDBACH (R.). Lymphangiectasies osseuses disséminées. *Arch. franç. Pédiat., 1969,* **26**, *537-546.*

SAUVEGRAIN (J.), PARSA (G.), AICARDI (J.) et MANLOT (G.). Lymphangiectasies intra-osseuses et lymphœdème congénital. *Ann. Radiol., 1973* **16**, *1-10.*

STEWART (M. J.), GILMER (W. S.) et EDMONSON (A. S.). Fibrous dysplasia of bone. *J. Bone Jt Surg., 1962,* **44-B**, *302-318.*

STREIT (W.) et KIRSCH (W.). Multiple fibroplastiche Proliferationsherde bei einem Neugeborenen. *Helv. paediat. Acta, 1967,* **19**, *271-276.*

ANOMALIES OF STRUCTURAL DENSITY OF THE DIAPHYSEAL CORTEX OR OF MODELING

Osteogenesis Imperfecta – Juvenile Osteoporosis

AESCHLIMANN (M. I.), GRUNT (J. A.) et CRIGLER (J. F., Jr.). Effects of sodium fluoride on the clinical course and metabolic balance of an infant with osteogenesis imperfecta congenita. *Metabolism, 1966,* **15**, *905-914.*

ALBRIGHT (J. A.) et GRUNT (J. A.). Studies of patients with osteogenesis imperfecta. *J. Bone Jt Surg., 1971,* **53-A**, *1415-1425.*

ALTMANN (F.) et KORNFELD (M.). Osteogenesis imperfecta and otosclerosis : new investigations. *Ann. Otol. (St. Louis), 1967,* **76**, *89-104.*

BANTA (J. V.), SCHREIBER (R. R.) et KULIK (W. J.). Hyperplastic callus formation in osteogenesis imperfecta simulating osteosarcoma. *J. Bone Jt Surg., 1971,* **53-A**, *115-124.*

BIANCHINE (J. W.) et MURDOCH (J. L.). Juvenile osteoporosis (?) in a boy with bilateral enucleation of the eyes for pseudoglioma. *Birth Defects, Original Article Series, 1969,* V *n° 4, 225-226.*

BLECKMANN (H.), KRESSE (H.), WOLLENSAK (J.) et BUDDECKE (E.). Glykosaminoglykan-und Kollagenanalysen bei Osteogenesis imperfecta. *Z. Kinderheilk., 1971,* **110**, *74-84.*

BLÜMCKE (S.) et NIEDORF (H. R.). Histochemical and fine structural studies on the cornea with osteogenesis imperfecta congenita. *Virchows Arch., Abt. B. Zellpath., 1972,* **11**, *124-132.*

BRIARD-GUILLEMOT (M. L.) et FRÉZAL (J.). Communication personnelle.

BROWN (D. M.). Collagen metabolism in fibroblasts from patients with osteogenesis imperfecta. *Abstract. Pediat. res., 1972,* **6**, *394.*

CALKINS (E.), KAHN (D.) et DINER (W. A.). Idiopathic familial osteoporosis in dogs; « osteogenesis imperfecta ». *Ann. N.Y. Acad. Sci., 1956,* **64**, *410-423.*

CASTELLS (S.), INAMDAR (S.), BAKER (R. K.) et WALLACH (S.). Effects of porcine calcitonin in osteogenesis imperfecta tarda. *J. Pediat., 1972,* **80**, *757-762.*

CASTELLS (S.). New approaches to treatment of osteogenesis imperfecta. *Clin. Orthop., 1973,* **93**, *239-249.*

CATTELL (H. S.) et CLAYTON (B.). Failure of anabolic steroids in the therapy of osteogenesis imperfecta. A clinical, metabolic, and biochemical study. *J. Bone Jt Surg., 1968,* **50-A**, *123-141.*

CLOUTIER (M. D.), HAYLES (A. B.), RIGGS (B. L.), JOWSEY (J.) et BICKEL (W. H.). Juvenile osteoporosis : report of a case including a description of some metabolic and microradiographic studies. *Pediatrics, 1967,* **40**, *649-655.*

DEBRÉ (R.), MOZZICONACCI (P.), GRUMBACH (R.) et ATTAL (C.). Dysplasie périostale ou maladie de Porak et Durante. *Sem. Hôp. Paris, 1951,* **31**, *1345-1358.*

DENT (C. E.) et FRIEDMAN (M.). Idiopathic juvenile osteoporosis. *Quart. J. Med., 1965,* **34**, *177-210.*

EASTOE (J. E.), MARTENS (P.) et THOMAS (N. R.). The amino-acid composition of human hard tissue collagens in osteogenesis imperfecta and dentinogenesis imperfecta. *Calcif. Tiss. Res., 1973,* **12**, *91-100.*

ENGFELDT (B.), ENGSTRÖM (A.) et ZETTERSTRÖM (R.). Biophysical studies of the bone tissue in osteogenesis imperfecta. *J. Bone Jt Surg., 1954,* **36-B**, *654-661.*

FALVO (K. A.) et BULLOUGH (P. G.). Osteogenesis imperfecta : a histometric analysis. *J. Bone Jt Surg., 1973,* **55-A**, *275-286.*

FOLLIS (R. H.). Histochemical studies on cartilage and bone. III. Osteogenesis imperfecta. *Bull. Johns-Hopk. Hosp., 1953,* **93**, *386-391.*

FONTAINE (G.), INGELRANS (P.), DUPONT (A.), FARRIAUX (J. P.), DUBOIS (O.), RICHARD (J.), WALBAUM (R.) et LEJEUNE (J.). La fragilité osseuse constitutionnelle. Etude de 23 observations. *Sem. Hôp. Paris, 1968,* **44**, *380-391.*

FRANCIS (M. J. O.), SMITH (R.) et BAUZE (R. J.). Instability of polymeric skin collagen in osteogenesis imperfecta. *Brit. Med. J. 1974,* **1**, *421-423.*

HAEBARA (H.), YAMASAKI (Y.) et KYOGOKU (M.). An autopsy case of osteogenesis imperfecta congenita; histochemical and electron microscopical studies. *Acta path. jap., 1969,* **19**, *377-394.*

HALL (J. G.) et ROHRT (T.). The stapes in osteogenesis imperfecta. *Acta oto-laryng., 1968,* **65**, *345-348.*

HEYS (F. M.), BLATTNER (T. J.) et ROBINSON (H. B. G.). Osteogenesis imperfecta and odontogenesis imperfecta : clinical and genetic aspects in eighteen families. *J. Pediat., 1960,* **56**, *234-245.*

HOLMES (J. R.), BAKER (J. R.) et DAVIES (E. T.). Osteogenesis imperfecta in lambs. *Vet. Rec., 1964,* **76**, *980-984.*

HRENO (A.) et HAUST (D.). Osteogenesis imperfecta congenita. *J. Pediat., 1963,* **62**, *908-914.*

HYAMS (S. W.), KAR (H.) et NEUMANN (E.). Blue sclerae and keratoglobus; ocular signs of a systemic connective tissue disorder. *Brit. J. Ophthal., 1969,* **53**, *53-58.*

JETT (S.), RAMSER (J. R.), FROST (H. M.) et VILLANUEVA (A. R.). Bone turnover and osteogenesis imperfecta. *Arch. Path., 1966,* **81**, *112-116.*

JOWSEY (J.) et JOHNSON (K. A.). Juvenile osteoporosis : bone findings in seven patients. *J. Pediat., 1972,* **81**, *511-517.*

KAPLAN (M.) et BALDINO (C.). Dysplasie périostale paraissant familiale et transmise suivant le mode mendélien récessif. *Arch. franç. Pédiat., 1953,* **10**, *943-950.*

KEATS (T. E.). Diffuse thickening of calvarium in osteogenesis imperfecta. Further observations. *Radiology, 1966,* **86**, *97-99.*

KOSOY (J.) et MADDOX (H. E.). Surgical findings in van der Hoeve's syndrome. *Arch. Otolaryng., 1971,* **93**, *115-122.*

LAPLANE (R.), LASFARGUES (G.) et DEBRAY (P.). Essai de classification génétique des ostéogenèses imparfaites. *Presse méd., 1959,* **67**, *893-895.*

LAURENT (L. E.) et SALENIUS (P.). Hyperplastic callus formation in osteogenesis imperfecta. Report of a case simulating sarcoma. *Acta orthop. scand., 1967,* **38**, *280-290.*

LIÈVRE (J. A.). La fragilité osseuse constitutionnelle (étude de 25 familles comportant 53 malades). *Rev. Rhum., 1959,* **8**, *420-432.*

LINDENFELSER (R.), HASSELKUS (W.), HAUBERT (P.) et KRÖNERT (W.). Zur Osteogenesis imperfecta congenita. Rasterelektronenmikroskopische Untersuchungen. *Virchows Arch., Abt. B. Zellpath., 1972,* **11**, *80-89.*

LOBSTEIN (J. G.). Lehrbuch der pathologischen Anatomie. *Stuttgart, 1835, Wright, éd., bd II, 179.*

MALMQUIST (J.), JAGENBURG (R.) et LINDSTEDT (G.). Familial protein intolerance; possible nature of enzyme defect. *New Engl. J. Med., 1971,* **284**, *997-1002.*

MAROTEAUX (P.) et GILLES (M.). Etude radiologique de l'osteogenesis imperfecta. *Ann. Radiol., 1965,* **8**, *571-583.*

MAROTEAUX (P.) et LAMY (M.). L' « osteogenesis imperfecta » et les difficultés de son diagnostic. *Presse méd., 1965,* **73**, *1535-1540.*

MULDOWNEY (F. P.), O'DONAVAN (D. K.) et GALLAGHER (J. E.). Bone formation in osteogenesis imperfecta; the effect of anabolic steroid therapy. *J. irish med. Ass., 1964,* **54**, *132-135.*

OPHEIM (O.). Loss of hearing following the syndrome of van der Hoeve-de Kleyn. *Acta oto-laryng., 1968,* **65**, *337-344.*

PIEROG (S. H.), FONTANA (V. J.) et FERRARA (A.). Osteogenesis imperfecta. Therapeutic challenge. *N.Y. St. J. Med., 1969,* **69**, *310-313.*

PORAK (C.) et DURANTE (G.). Les micromélies congénitales : achondroplasie vraie et dystrophie périostale. *Nouv. Iconogr. Salpêt., 1905,* **18**, *481-538.*

RAMSER (J. R.), VILLANUEVA (A. R.) et PIROK (D.). Tetracycline-based measurement of bone dynamics in 3 women with osteogenesis imperfecta. *Clin. Orthop., 1966,* **49**, *151-162.*

RANIERI (L.). Aspetti istologici e considerazioni patogenetiche sull'osteogenesi imperfetta. *Atti e memorie della S.O.T.I.M.I., 1963,* **8**, *1-9.*

REICHELT (A.). Operative Behandlungsmöglichkeiten bei der Osteogenesis imperfecta. *Langenbecks Arch. Chir., 1972,* **330**, *238-250.*

RILEY (F. C.), JOWSEY (J.) et BROWN (D. M.). Osteogenesis imperfecta, morphologic and biochemical studies of connective tissue. *Pédiat. Res., 1973,* **9**, *757-768.*

ROBERT (J. M.), GRÉMEAU (J. L.), MOTTER (A.) et GUILHOT (J.). La fragilité osseuse héréditaire. *Lyon méd., 1968,* **99**, *881-982 et 1637-1715.*

RUSSELL (R. G. G.), BISAZ (S.), DONATH (A.), MORGAN (D. B.) et FLEISCH (H.). Inorganic pyrophosphate in plasma in normal persons and in patients with hypophosphatasia, osteogenesis imperfecta and other disorders of bone. *J. clin. Invest., 1971,* **50**, *961-969.*

SCHRÖDER (G.). Osteogenesis imperfecta. *Z. menschl. Vererb. Konstit-Lehre, 1964,* **37**, *632-676.*

SCHWARZ (E.). Hypercallosis in osteogenesis imperfecta. *Amer. J. Roentgenol., 1961,* **85**, *645-648.*

SCOTT (P. P.), MCKUSICK (V. A.) et MCKUSICK (A. B.). The nature of osteogenesis imperfecta in cats. Evidence that the disorder is primarily nutritional, not genetic, and therefore not analogous to the disease in man. *J. Bone Jt Surg., 1963,* **45-A**, *125-134.*

SEEDORFF (K. S.). Osteogenesis imperfecta. A study of clinical features and heredity, based on 55 danish families, comprinsing 180 affected members. *Copenhague, 1949, Universitetsforlaget I Arhus, éd.*

SMARS (G.). Osteogenesis imperfecta in Sweden. Clinical, genetic, epidemiological and socio-medical aspects. *1 vol., Stockholm, 1961, Svenska Borförlaget, éd.*

SOFIELD (H. A.) et MILLAR (E. A.). Fragmentation, realignment, and intramedullary rod fixation of deformities of the long bones in children. *J. Bone Jt Surg., 1959,* **41-A**, *1371-1391.*

SOLOMONS (C. C.) et STYNER (J.). Osteogenesis imperfecta : effect of magnesium administration on pyrophosphate metabolism. *Calcif. Tiss. Res., 1969,* **3**, *318-326.*

SOLOMONS (C. C.) et MILLAR (E. A.). Osteogenesis imperfecta. New perspectives. *Clin. Orthop., 1973,* **96**, *299-303.*

STEIN (R.), LAZAR (M.) et ADAM (A.). Brittle cornea; a familial trait associated with blue sclera. *Amer. J. Ophthal., 1968,* **66**, *67.*

SUMMER (G. K.) et PATTON (W. C.). Intravenous proline tolerance in osteogenesis imperfecta. *Metabolism., 1968,* **17**, *46-53.*

TILEY (F.) et ALBRIGHT (J. A.). Osteogenesis imperfecta : treatment by multiple osteotomy and intramedullary rod insertion. Report of thirteen patients. *J. Bone Jt Surg., 1973,* **55-A**, *701-713.*

VAN DER HEOVE (J.) et KLEIN (A. DE). Blaue Sklera, Knochenbrüchigkeit und Schwerhörigkeit. *V. Graefes. Arch. Ophthal., 1918,* **95**, *81-93.*

VILLANUEVA (A. R.) et FROST (H. M.). Bone formation

in human osteogenesis imperfecta, measured by tetracycline bone labeling. *Acta orthop. scand., 1970,* **41**, *531-538.*

VROLIK (W.). Tabulae ad illustradam embryogenesim hominis in mammallum, tam naturalem quam abnormen. *Amsterdam, 1849, J. Müller, édit.*

WILLIAMS (P. F.), COLE (W. H. J.), BAILEY (R. W.), DUBOW (H. I.), SOLOMONS (C. C.) et MILLAR (E. A.). Current aspects of the surgical treatment of osteogenesis imperfecta. *Clin. Orthop., 1973,* **96**, *288-298.*

Osteopetrosis

ALBERS-SCHÖNBERG (H.). Röntgenbilder einer seltenen Knochenerkrankung. *Münch. med. Wschr., 1904,* **51**, *365-368.*

BARUFFALDI (O.) et LOJODICE (G.). Studio istologico ed istochimico dell'osteopetrosi precoce maligna. *Arch. Putti, Chir. Organi Mov., 1962,* **17**, *20-40.*

BOCQUET (L.), PIUSSANT (C.) et TOUMIEUX (C.). Survie prolongée d'une forme maligne précoce de la maladie d'Albers-Schönberg (documents iconographiques et histologiques). *Bull. Soc. méd. Hôp. Paris, 1966,* **117**, *1227-1233.*

BROWN (D. M.) et DENT (P. B.). Pathogenesis of osteopetrosis : a comparison of human and animal spectra. *Pediat. Res., 1971,* **5**, *181-191.*

DENT (C. E.), SMELLIE (J. M.) et WATSON (L.). Studies in osteopetrosis. *Arch. Dis. Childh., 1965,* **40**, 7-15.

DICK (H. M.) et SIMPSON (W. J.). Dental changes in osteopetrosis. *Oral Surg., 1972,* **34**, *408-416.*

ENELL (H.) et PEHRSON (M.). Studies on osteopetrosis. I. Clinical report of three cases with genetic considerations. *Acta paediat. (Upsala), 1958,* **47**, *279-287.*

ENGFELDT (B.), FAJERS (C. M.), LODIN (H.) et PEHRSON (M.). Studies on osteopetrosis. III. Roentgenological and pathologic-anatomical investigations on some of the bone changes. *Acta paediat. (Upsala), 1960,* **49**, *391-408.*

HOLMES (J. R.). Radiological changes in avian osteopetrosis. *Brit. J. Radiol., 1961,* **34**, *368-377.*

JOHNSTON (C. C., Jr.), LAVY (N.), LORD (T.), VELLIOS (F.), MERRITT (A. D.) et DEISS (W. P., Jr.). Osteopetrosis. A clinical, genetic, metabolic, and morphologic study of the dominantly inherited, benign form. *Medicine, 1968,* **47**, *149-167.*

LICHTENSTEIN (J. R.) et WARSON (R. W.). Syndrome of dental anomalies, curly hair and sclerotic bones. *Birth Defects Original Article Series, 1971,* VII *n° 11, 308-311.*

KLINTWORTH (G. K.). The neurologic manifestations of osteopetrosis (Albers-Schönberg's disease). *Neurology, 1963,* **13**, *512-518.*

MORETTI (S.), CIUCCARELLI (C.), BABINI (L.) et MATTII (M.). Aspetti clinico-radiologici della malattia di Albers-Schönberg. *G. Clin. med., 1965,* **46**, *1010-1028.*

MORRIS (J. W.). Skeletal fluorosis among indians of the american southwest. *Amer. J. Roentgenol., 1965,* **94**, *608-615.*

MORROW (G. III), BARNESS (L. A.), FOST (A.) et RASMUSSEN (H.). Calcium mobilization in osteopetrosis. *Amer. J. Dis. Child., 1967,* **114**, *161-168.*

MURPHY (H. M.). A review of inherited osteopetrosis in the mouse, man and other mammals also considered. *Clin. Orthop., 1969,* **65**, *97-109.*

NEIMANN (N.), PIERSON (M.), MARCHAL (C.) et MICHAUD (C.). Evolution et pronostic de la forme précoce et grave de la maladie d'Albers-Schönberg. *Pédiatrie, 1964,* **19**, *293-307.*

PAUPE (J.), NEZELOFF (Ch.), DENAN (Mme B.) et VIALATTE (J.). L'ostéopétrose avec rachitisme. A propos d'un cas avec étude anatomo-pathologique. *Sem. Hôp. Paris, 1967,* **43**, *2451-2461.*

SEGOND (P. G. L.). Le rétrécissement du canal médullaire des os (à propos d'une observation familiale). *Thèse Méd., Paris, 1972.*

SIMPSON (C. F.) et SANGER (V. L.). A review of avian osteopetrosis : comparisons with other bone diseases. *Clin. Orthop., 1968,* **58**, *271-281.*

SINGH (A.), DASS (R.), HAYREH (S. S.) et JOLLY (S. S.). Skeletal changes in endemic fluorosis. *J. Bone Jt Surg., 1962,* **44-B**, *806-815.*

SJÖLIN (S.). Studies on osteopetrosis. II. Investigations concerning the nature of the anaemia. *Acta paediat. (Upsala), 1959,* **48**, *529-544.*

SRIKANTIA (S. G.) et SIDDIKI (A. H.). Metabolic study in skeletal fluorosis. *Clin. Sci., 1965,* **28**, *477-485.*

TOYAMA (K.), MOUTIER (R.) et LAMENDIN (H.). Résorption osseuse après parabiose chez les rats « op » (ostéopétrose). *C. R. Acad. Sc. Paris, 1974,* **278**, *115-117.*

WALKER (D. G.). Congenital osteopetrosis in mice cured by parabiotic union with normal siblings. *Endocrinology, 1972,* **91**, *916-920.*

WALKER (D. G.). Experimental osteopetrosis. *Clin. Orthop., 1973,* **97**, *158-174.*

ZEITLHOFER (J.) et ZWEYMÜLLER (E.). Die Knochenveränderungen der mit « Rachitis » und Aminoacidurie einhergehenden Osteosklerose Albers-Schönberg. *Z. Kinderheilk., 1963,* **88**, *475-489.*

Pycnodysostosis

ALMEIDA (L. M. de). Contribution à l'étude génétique de la pycnodysostose. *Ann. Génét., 1972,* **15**, *99-101.*

BAKER (R. K.), WALLACH (S.) et TASHJIAN (A. H.). Plasma calcitonin in pycnodysostosis : intermittently high basal levels and exaggerated responses to calcium and glucagon infusion. *J. clin. Endocrin., 1973,* **37**, *46-55.*

BALTHAZAR (E.), SMITH (E. H.) et MOSKOWITZ (H.). Pycnodysostosis : an unusual case. *Brit. J. Radiol., 1972,* **45**, *304-307.*

COLLADO-OTERO (F.). Una forma más de distrofia ósea. *Acta pediát. esp., 1956,* **14**, *1-27.*

DUSENBERRY (J. F., Jr.) et KANE (J. J.). Pycnodynostosis. Report of three new cases. *Amer. J. Roentgenol,. 1967,* **99**, *717-723.*

ELMORE (S. M.), NANCE (W. E.), MCGEE (B. J.), ENGEL DE MONTMOLLIN (M.) et ENGEL (E.). Pycnodysostosis, with a familial chromosome anomaly. *Amer. J. Med., 1966,* **40**, *273-282.*

JANECKA (J.) et BRUNA (J.). Pycnodysostosis im Röntgenbild. *Fortschr. Röntgenstr., 1973,* **118**, *n° 3, 298-305.*

MAROTEAUX (P.) et LAMY (M.). La pycnodysostose. *Presse méd., 1962,* **70**, *999-1002.*

MAROTEAUX (P.) et LAMY (M.). The malady of Toulouse-Lautrec. *J. amer. med. Ass., 1965,* **191**, *715-717.*

SARNSETHSIRI (P.), HITT (O. K.), EYRING (E. J.) et FROST (H. M.). Tetracycline-based study of bone dynamics in pycnodysostosis. *Clin. Orthop., 1971,* **74**, *301-312.*

SEDANO (H. D.), GORLIN (R. L.) et ANDERSON (V. E.). Pycnodysostosis. Clinical and genetic considerations *Amer. J. Dis. Child., 1968,* **116**, *70-77.*

STANESCU (V.), MAXIMILAN (C.), POENARU (S.), FLOREA (I.), STANESCU (R.), IONESCO (V.) et IOANITIU (D.). Syndrome héréditaire dominant réunissant une dysostose cranio-faciale particulière, une insuffisance de croissance d'aspect chondrodystrophique et un épaississement massif de la corticale des os longs. *Rev. franç. Endocr. clin., 1963,* **4**, *219-231.*

STANESCU (V.), STANESCU (R.) et MAROTEAUX (P.). Etude histochimique et microchimique du cartilage de croissance tibial dans le nanisme diastrophique et la pycnodysostose. *Ann. Histochim., 1973,* **18**, *179-186.*

WEISMANN-NETTER (R.) et LORCH (P.). Nanisme familial avec densification généralisée du squelette et dysgénésies polytopiques. *Sem. Hôp. Paris, 1956,* **32**, *2713-2719.*

Melorheostosis

ABRAHAMSON (M. N.). Disseminated asymptomatic osteosclerosis with features resembling melorheostosis, osteopoikilosis, and osteopathia striata. Case report. *J. Bone Jt Surg., 1968,* **50-A**, *991-996.*

CAMPBELL (C. J.), PAPADEMETRIOU (T.) et BONFIGLIO (M.). Melorheostosis. A report of the clinical, roentgenographic, and pathological findings in fourteen cases. *J. Bone Jt Surg., 1968,* **50-A**, *1281-1304.*

DUME (Th.), SCHULTE-BRINKMANN (W.) et STURM (A., Jr.). Osteopoikilie mit Hyperostose. *Dtsch. med. Wschr., 1971,* **96**, *422-428.*

LERI (A.) et LIÈVRE (J. A.). La mélorhéostose, l'hyperostose d'un membre « en coulée ». *Presse méd., 1928,* **36**, *801-805.*

LERI (A.), LOISELEUR et LIÈVRE (J. A.). Une nouvelle observation de mélorhéostose. Etude clinique, anatomique et expérimenale. *Bull. Soc. méd. Hôp. Paris, 1930,* **54**, *1210-1217.*

MAROTEAUX (P.) et LAMY (M.). La mélorhéostose chez l'enfant. *Sem. Hôp. Paris, 1961,* **37**, *3470-3475.*

MAROTEAUX (P.) et LAMY (M.). Mélorhéostose, ostéopœcilie et sclérodermie en bandes. *Sem. Hôp. Paris, 1961,* **37**, *3476-3480.*

MORRIS (J. M.), SAMILSON (R. L.) et CORLEY (C. L.). Melorheostosis. Review of the literature and report of an interesting case with a nineteen-year follow-up. *J. Bone Jt Surg., 1963,* **45-A**, *1191-1206.*

MÜLLER-ALBERTI (W.). Ein Beitrag zum Krankheitsbilde der Melorheostose. *Z. Orthop., 1941,* **72**, *194-211.*

PUTTI (V.). L'osteosi eburneizzante monomelica (una nuova sindrome osteopatica). *Chir. Organi Mov., 1927,* **11**, *335-361.*

WAGERS (L. T.), YOUNG (A. W.) et RYAN (S. F.). Linear melorheostotic scleroderma. *Brit. J. Derm., 1972,* **86**, *297-301.*

WALLENSTEIN (S.). Melorheostosis Leri. *Acta chir. scand., 1952* **102**, *463-474.*

Osteopoecily

ALBERS-SCHÖNBERG (H.). Eine seltene, bisher nicht bekante Strukturannomalie des skelettes. *Fortschr. Röntgenstr., 1915,* **23**, *174-178.*

BLOOR (D. U.). Case of osteopathia striata. *J. Bone Jt Surg., 1954,* **36-B**, *261-265.*

CLAUS (H. G.). Gibt es eine streifige Form des Osteopoikilie ? *Fortschr. Röntgenstr., 1964,* **101**, *522-530.*

CULVER (G. J.) et THUMASATHIT (C.). Osseous changes of osteopathia striata and Pyle's disease occurring in a patient with an 11 year follow-up. A case report. *Amer. J. Roentgenol., 1972,* **116**, *640-643.*

GEHWEILER (J. A.), BLAND (W. R.), CARDEN (T. S., Jr.) et DAFFNER (R. H.). Osteopathia striata, Voorhoeve's disease. Review of the roentgen manifestations. *Amer. J. Roentgenol., 1973,* **118**, *450-455.*

GINSBURG (L. D.), SEDANO (H. O.) et GORLIN (R. J.). Focal dermal hypoplasia syndrome. *Amer. J. Roentgenol., 1970,* **110**, *561-571.*

GOLTZ (R. W.), HENDERSON (R. R.), HITCH (J. M.) et OTT (J. E.). Focal dermal hypoplasia syndrome. A review of the literature and report of two cases. *Arch. Derm. Syph. (Chicago), 1970,* **101**, *1-11.*

GOLTZ (R. W.), PETERSON (N. C.), GORLIN (R. J.) et RAVITS (H. G.). Focal dermal hypoplasia. *Arch. Derm. Syph. (Chicago), 1962,* **86**, *708-717.*

GONZALEZ (A. R.), LLEDIAS (J. A. C.) et LÔPEZ (A. C.). Osteopoiquilia hereditaria asociada a otras malformaciones. *Rev. clin. esp., 1962,* **85**, *203-206.*

HURT (R. L.). Osteopathia striata-Voorhoeve's disease : report of case presenting features of osteopathia striata and osteopetrosis. *J. Bone Jt Surg., 1953,* **35-B**, *80-96.*

LARRÈGUE (M.), MAROTEAUX (P.), MICHEL (Y.) et FAURÉ (C.). L'ostéopathie striée, symptôme radiologique de l'hypoplasie dermique en aires. *Ann. Radiol., 1972,* **15**, *287-295.*

LEDOUX-LEBARD (R.), CHABANEIX et DESSANE. L'ostéopœcilie, forme nouvelle d'ostéite généralisée. *J. Radiol. Electrol., 1916,* **2**, *133-134.*

MELNICK (J. C.). Osteopathia condensans disseminata (osteopoikilosis). Study of a family of 4 generations. *Amer. J. Roentgenol., 1959,* **82**, *229-238.*

RAVAULT (P. P.), LEJEUNE (E.), MAÎTREPIERRE (J.), BOUVIER (M.), VAUZELLE (J. L.) et BANSSILLON (V.). A propos de trois nouvelles observations d'ostéopœcilie ponctuée. *Rev. Rhum., 1965,* **32**, *335-341.*

SCHIMPF (A.), ROTH (W.) et KOPPER (J.). Dermatofibrosis lenticularis disseminata mit Osteopoikilie. Buschke-Ollendorf Syndrom. *Dermatologica, 1970,* **141**, *409-420.*

SCHORR (W. F.), OPITZ (J. M.) et REYES (C. N.). The connective tissue nevus-osteopoikilosis syndrome. *Arch. Derm., (Chicago), 1972,* **106**, *208-214.*

VOORHOEVE (N.). L'image radiologique non encore décrite d'une anomalie du squelette. *Acta radiol., 1924,* **3**, *407-427.*

Diaphyseal Dysplasia – Cranio-Diaphyseal Dysplasia

BATTAGLIA (L.) et VENTURI (R.). La poliosteopatia addensante simmetrica ereditaria (malattia di Camurati-Engelmann). Studio clinico ed anatomo-patologico. *Chir. Organi Mov., 1960,* **49**, *179-196.*

BENABDERRAHMANE (M.), SIEGENTHALER (P.), UHLMANN (C.) et WETTSTEIN (P.). Le syndrome de Camurati-Engelmann. A propos d'un cas et revue de la littérature. *Schweiz. med. Wschr., 1969,* **99**, *1204-1212.*

BRAHAM (R. L.). Multiple congenital abnormalities with diaphyseal dysplasia (Camurati-Engelmann's syndrome). *Oral. Surg., 1969,* **27**, *20-26.*

CAMURATI (M.). Di un raro caso di osteite simmetrica ereditaria degli arti inferiori. *Chir. Organi Mov., 1922,* **6**, *622-665.*

CLAWSON (D. K.) et LOOP (J. W.). Progressive diaphyseal dysplasia (Engelmann's disease). *J. Bone Jt Surg., 1964,* **46-A**, *143-150.*

COCKAYNE (E. A.). Case for diagnosis. *Proc. roy. Soc. Med., 1920,* **13**, *132-136.*

ENGELMANN (G.). Ein Fall von Osteopathia hyperostotica (Sclerosis) multiplex infantilis. *Fortschr. Röntgenstr., 1929,* **39**, *1101-1106.*

FOSMOE (R. J.), HOLM (R. S.) et HILDRETH (R. C.). Van Buchem's disease (Hyperostosis corticalis generalisata familiaris). A case report. *Radiology, 1968,* **90**, *771-774.*

HUNDLEY (J. D.) et WILSON (F. C.). Progressive diaphyseal dysplasia. Review of the literature and report of seven cases in one family. *J. Bone Jt Surg., 1973,* **55-A**, *461-474.*

JOSEPH (R.), LEFÈBVRE (J.), GUY (E.) et JOB (J. C.). Dysplasie cranio-diaphysaire progressive. Ses relations avec la dysplasie diaphysaire progressive de Camurati-Engelmann. *Ann. Radiol. (Sem. Hôp. Paris), 1958,* **1**, *1-14.*

LENNON (E. A.), SCHECHTER (M. M.) et HORNABROOK (R. W.). Engelmann's disease. Report of a case with a review of the literature. *J. Bone Jt Surg., 1961,* **43-B**, *273-284.*

MACPHERSON (R. J.). Craniophyseal dysplasia, a disease or group of diseases. *J. Canad. Ass. Radiol., 1974,* **25**, *22-32.*

MOTTRAM (M. E.) et HILL (H. A.). Diaphyseal dysplasia. Report of a case. *Amer. J. Roentgenol., 1965,* **95**, *162-167.*

RUELLE (M.) et DUBOIS (J. L.). A propos de deux cas familiaux de sclérose diaphysaire multiple (syndrome de Camurati-Engelmann). *Rev. Rhum., 1964,* **7**, *345-348.*

SPARKES (R. S.) et GRAHAM (C. B.). Camurati-Engelmann disease. Genetics and clinical manifestations with a review of literature. *J. Med. Genet., 1972,* **9**, *73-85.*

TRUNK (G.), NEWMAN (A.) et DAVIS (Th. E.). Progressive and hereditary diaphyseal dysplasia. *Arch. intern. Med., 1969,* **123**, *417-422.*

Osteoectasia With Hyperphosphatasemia. Osteodysplastia. Fronto-Metaphyseal Dysplasia

BAKWIN (H.), GOLDEN (A.) et FOX (S.). Familial osteoectasia with macrocranium. *Amer. J. Roentgenol., 1964,* **91**, *609-617.*

CAFFEY (J.). Familial hyperphosphatasemia with ateliosis and hypermetabolism of growing membranous bone; review of the clinical, radiographic and chemical features. *Prog. Pediat. Radiol., 1973,* **4**, *438-468.*

DANKS (D. M.), MAYNE (V.), HALL (R. K.) et MCKINNON (M. C.). Frontometaphyseal dysplasia. A progressive disease of bone and connective tissue. *Amer. J. Dis. Child., 1972,* **123**, *254-258.*

FANCONI (G. von), MOREIRA (G.), UEHLINGER (E.) et GIEDION (A.). Osteochalasia desmalis familiaris. Hyperostosis corticalis deformans juvenilis, chronic idiopathic hyperphosphatasia, osteoectasia and macrocranium. *Helv. paediat. Acta, 1964,* **19**, *279-295.*

GORLIN (R. J.) et COHEN (M. M., Jr.). Frontometaphyseal dysplasis. *Amer. J. Dis. Child., 1969,* **118**, *487-494.*

HOLT (J. F.), THOMPSON (G. R.) et ARENBERG (I. K.). Frontometaphyseal dysplasia. *Radiol. clin. (Nth Amer.), 1972,* **10**, *225-243.*

MAROTEAUX (P.), CHOURAKI (L.) et COSTE (F.). L'ostéodysplastie (syndrome de Melnick et de Needles). *Presse méd., 1968,* **76**, *715-718.*

MARSHALL (W. C.). A chronic progressive osteopathy with hyperphosphatasia. *Proc. roy. Soc. Med., 1962,* **55**, *238-239.*

MELNICK (J. C.) et NEEDLES (C. F.). An undiagnosed bone dysplasia; a 2 family study of 4 generations and 3 generations. *Amer. J. Roentgenol., 1966,* **97**, *39-48.*

SCHEEPER (J. H.). A patient with skeletal abnormalities due to dysplasia and hypoplasia of the muscular system. *Radiol. clin. biol., 1967,* **37**, *339-348.*

SWOBODA (W.). Hyperostosis corticalis deformans juvenilis : ungewöhnliche generalisierte Osteopathie bei zwei Geschwister. *Helvet. paediat. Acta, 1958,* **13**, *185-188.*

THOMPSON (R., Jr.), GAULL (G. E.), HORWITZ (S. J.) et SCHENK (R. K.). Hereditary hyperphosphatasia. Studies of three siblings. *Amer. J. Med., 1969,* **47**, *209-219.*

Endosteal Hyperostosis. Narrowing of the Medullary Canal

CAFFEY (J.). Congenital stenosis of medullary spaces in tubular bones and calvaria in two proportionate dwarfs, mother and son ; coupled with transitory hypocalcemic tetany. *Amer. J. Roentgenol., 1967,* **100**, *1-14.*

HANSEN (H. G.). Sklerosteose. *In* vol. 6, Handbuch der Kinderheilkunde. *Berlin, Gottingen, Heidelberg, New York, H. Opitz and F. Schmid, ed., 1967, p. 351-355.*

KENNY (F. M.) et LINARELLI (L.). Dwarfism and cortical thickening of tubular bones. Transient hypocalcemia in a mother and son. *Amer. J. Dis. Child., 1966,* **111**, *201-207.*

MAROTEAUX (P.), FONTAINE (G.), SCHARFMAN (W.) et FARRIAUX (J. P.). L'hyperostose corticale généralisée à transmission dominante (type worth). *Arch. franç. Pédiat., 1971,* **28**, *685-698.*

RUSSELL (W. J.), BIZZOZERO (O. J., Jr.) et OMORI (Y.). Idiopathic osteosclerosis. A report of 6 related cases. *Radiology, 1968,* **90**, *70-76.*

SEGOND (P. G. L.). Le rétrécissement du canal médullaire des os. *Thèse Méd., Paris, 1972.*

TRUSWELL (A. S.). Osteopetrosis with syndactyly. A morphologic variant of Albers-Schönberg's disease. *J. Bone Jt Surg., 1958,* **40-B**, *208-218.*

VAN BUCHEM (F. S. P.), HADDERS (H. N.), HANSEN (J. P.) et WOLDRING (M. G.). Hyperostosis corticalis generalisata. Report of seven cases. *Amer. J. Med., 1962,* **33**, *387-397.*

VAN BUCHEM (F. S. P.). The pathogenesis of hyperostosis corticalis generalisata and calcitonin. *Proc. kon. nederl. Akad. Wet., 1970,* **73**, *243-253.*

VAN BUCHEM (F. S. P.). Hyperostosis corticalis generalisata. Eight new cases. *Acta med. scand., 1971,* **189**, *257-267.*

WITKOP (C. J.). Congenital anomalies of the face and associated structures. *Springfield, 1961, C. C. Thomas, éd., Pruzansky, 202.*

WORTH (H. M.) et WOLLIN (D. G.). Hyperostosis corticalis generalisata congenita. *J. canad. Ass. Radiol., 1966,* **17**, *67-74.*

Anomalies of Metaphyseal Modeling

BAKWIN (H.) et KRIDA (A.). Familial metaphyseal dysplasia. *Amer. J. Dis. Child., 1937,* **53**, *1521-1527.*

CARLSON (D. H.) et HARRIS (G. B. C.). Craniometaphyseal dysplasia. *Radiol., 1972,* **103**, *n° 1, 147-151.*

COHN (M.). Konstitutionelle Hyperspongioserung des Skelets mit partiellem Riesenwuchs. *Fortschr. Röntgenstr., 1933,* **47**, *293-298.*

ELLIS (R. W. B.). Osteopetrosis. *Proc. roy. Soc. Med., 1933-1934,* **27**, *1563-1571.*

FIELD (C. E.). Albers-Schönberg disease. An atypical case. *Proc. roy. Soc. Med., 1938,* **32**, *320-324.*

GORLIN (R. J.), SPRANGER (J.) et KOSZALKA (M.). Genetic craniotubular bone dysplasias and hyperostoses. A critical analysis, *Birth Defects, Original Articles Series, 1969,* V *n° 4, 79-95.*

GUIBAUD (P.), HERMIER (M.), AJACQUES (J. C.), BŒUF (J. P.) et LARBRE (F.). La dysplasie cranio-métaphysaire. *Pediatrie, 1973,* **28**, *149-161.*

HOLT (J. F.). The evolution of cranio-metaphyseal dysplasia. *Ann. Radiol., 1966,* **9**, *209-214.*

JACKSON (W. P. U.), ALBRIGHT (F.), DREWRY (G.), HANELIN (J.) et RUBIN (M. I.). Familial metaphyseal dysplasia and cranio-metaphyseal dysplasia; their reation to leontiasis ossea and osteopetrosis; disorders of « bone remodeling ». *Arch. intern. Med., 1954,* **94**, *871-885.*

LELEK (I.). Camurati-Englmann'sche Erkrankung. *Fortschr. Röntgenstr., 1961,* **94**, *702-712.*

LIÈVRE (J. A.) et FISCHGOLD (H.). Leontiasis ossea chez l'enfant (ostéopétrose partielle probable). *Presse méd., 1956,* **64**, *763-765.*

MEYER-SCHWICKERATH (G.), GRUTERICH (E.) et WEYERS (H.). Mikrophthalmussyndrome. *Klin. Mbl. Augenheilk., 1957,* **131**, *18-30.*

MALPUECH (G.), RAYNAUD (E. J.), MERLE (J.) et ESPINASSE (G.). La dysplasie cranio-métaphysaire. Etude clinique et génétique d'une observation. *Arch. franç. Pédiat., 1974,* **31**, *71-76.*

MILLARD (D. R., Jr.), MAISELS (D. O.), BATSTONE (J. H. F.) et YATES (B. W.). Craniofacial surgery in craniometaphyseal dysplasia. *Amer. J. Surg., 1967,* **113**, *615-621.*

MILLER (A. L.), LEHMAN (R. H.) et GERETTI (R.). Unusual audiological findings in cranial metaphyseal dysplasia. *Arch. Otolaryng. (Chicago), 1969,* **89**, *83-86.*

PEASE (C. N.) et NEWTON (G. G.). Metaphyseal dysplasia due to lead poisoning in children. *Radiology, 1962,* **79**, *233-240.*

PYLE (E. C.). A case of unusual bone development. *J. Bone Jt Surg., 1931,* **13**, *874-876.*

ROSS (M. W.) et ALTMAN (D. H.). Familial metaphyseal dysplasia. Review of the clinical and radiologic feature of Pyle's disease. *Clin. Pediat., 1967,* **6**, *143-149.*

ROY (C.), MAROTEAUX (P.), KREMP (L.), COURTECUISSE (V.) et ALAGILLE (D.). Un nouveau syndrome osseux avec anomalies cutanées et troubles neurologiques. *Arch. franç. Pédiat., 1968,* **25**, *893-905.*

RUBIN (P.). Dynamic classification of bone dysplasias. *Chicago, 1964, Year Book Med. publ., éd.*

SCHENK (R.), MERZ (W. A.), MÜLHBAVER (R.), RUSSELL (R. G. G.) et FLEISCH (H.). Effect of ethane 1-hydroxy-1, 1-diphosphanate (EHDP) and dichloromethylene diphosphonate on the calcification and resorbtion of cartilage and bone in the tibia epiphysis and metaphysis of rat. *Calcif. Tiss. Res., 1973,* **11**, *196-214.*

SCHWARZ (E.). Craniometaphyseal dysplasia. *Amer. J. Roentgenol., 1960,* **84**, *461-466.*

SPRANGER (J.), PAULSEN (K.) et LEHMANN (W.). Die kraniometaphysäre Dysplasie (Pyle). *Z. Kinderheilk., 1965,* **93**, *64-79.*

SPRANGER (J.), ALBRECHT (Ch.), ROHWEDDER (H. J.) et WIEDEMANN (H. R.). Die Dysosteosklerose, eine Sonderform der generalisierten Osteosklerose. *Fortschr. Röntgenstr., 1968,* **109**, *504-512.*

TAYSI (K.), SAY (B.), FIRAT (T.) et GURSU (G.). Case report, Oculodentodigital dysplasia syndrome. *Acta paediat. scand., 1971,* **60**, *235-238.*

WALKER (N.). Pyle's disease or cranio-metaphyseal dysplasia. *Ann. Radiol., 1966,* **9**, *197-207.*

4 The Dysostoses

This term implies the presence of a single skeletal malformation, occurring either completely isolated or, in association with other similar involvement.

Dysostoses can be located in either the skull, the face, the spine, the limbs, or in their most distal segment. We will, therefore, separately investigate these five areas.

CRANIAL DYSOSTOSES

We refer here to the different types of craniosynostosis which result from premature closure of sutures and lead to various developmental problems depending on their location. We will not, however, discuss microcephaly, localized or generalized defects of cranial vault development accompanied by neurologic lesions, or skeletal manifestations that are secondary or contingent (see p. 310). Basilar impression will be discussed along with anomalies of the cervicooccipital region (see p. 160).

Following the approach taken by Laitinen and other authors, we have distinguished two groups of craniosynostoses which are dependent on whether there is early closure of a single suture or another associated malformation.

ISOLATED CRANIOSYNOSTOSES

There are several varieties of isolated craniosynostoses. They include scaphocephaly which results from premature closure of the sagittal suture and which has a high incidence; brachycephaly which results from closure of the coronal suture and is rarely seen; oxycephaly, which is seen with the same incidence as scaphocephaly and results from sagittal suture closure as well as coronal and in an unusual case, of the lambdoid suture; trigonocephaly which is due to early closure of the metopic suture, and finally, plagiocephaly which is the result of the early closure of a single suture.

There is also an unusual type of craniosynostosis which affects the lambdoid suture and leads to a flattened occipital region and an anterior prominence of the forehead.

Clinical Findings

The presence of a craniosynostosis can be noted at various ages and under various circumstances. In some patients we know at birth that the skull has an unusual configuration, in other cases it will manifest later. Abnormal vision or severe headaches may sometimes be the initial signs. Finally, the pediatrician may notice the condition at a routine checkup.

In order to understand the morphologic alterations, we must recall that growth of the cranial vault occurs perpendicularly to the sutures. This fact implies that a longitudinal craniosynostosis will prevent further lateral growth, while early closure of the coronal sutures will lead to a stop in anteroposterior growth. In the first situation we have a scaphocephaly characterized by excessive length, frontal bossing, and a reduced lateral diameter. The second situation results in brachycephaly characterized by a short widened skull and often, exophthalmus.

The mixed craniosynostoses simultaneously involve the sagittal and coronal sutures, and occasionally the lambdoid suture which resutls in an appearance of oxycephaly or turricephaly. The forehead is unusually high and flat and there may be mild exophthalmus (Fig. 4-1). Under these circumstances there is an unusual variety of different forms according to timing and the sequence of suture closure.

In trigonocephaly we note a reduced width of the forehead, and a median ridge which gives the skull a triangular shape. The eyes may be somewhat close together and the face appears narrow.

In plagiocephaly we see a unilateral deformity which is dependent on the location of the involvement. Coronal cranial synostosis results in a flattened forehead on the involved side and of the frontal rim. The eyebrow is high in position and the ipsilateral eye protrudes slightly. A number of ophthalmologic problems may be associated with plagiocephaly. These include exophthalmus, and frequent strabism which is occasionally related to eyeball protrusion. Most frequently,

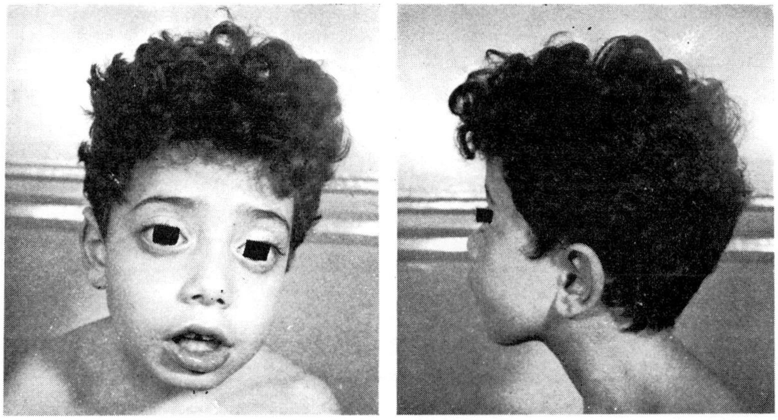

Fig. 4-1. Turricephalic deformity of the skull. The forehead is unusually high and flat.

however, there does not seem to be any direct connection of this finding with the craniostenosis. Loss of visual acuity, sometimes leading to blindness, results from optic atrophy. This complication may be due to various mechanisms. Intracranial hypertension, acute angulation of the optic nerve resulting from a deformity of the anterior or middle fossa, or compression or abnormal vascularization resulting from the mentioned mechanisms are some of the causative factors. We should be aware that the incidence of ocular complications varies considerably from one type of involvement to the other. It is quite exceptional in craniosynostosis of the sagittal suture and may be seen if the coronal suture is involved, whether isolated or in combination with others. In the latter situation there will be a higher incidence of complications.

Mental retardation should not be considered to be caused by or secondary due to a deformity of the skull. However, its incidence is particularly high in such patients. Electroencephalography and gasencephalography are normally in isolated craniosynostosis. Study of the eye ground, however, may show signs of capillary stasis as well as atrophy of the optic disk.

Radiographic Findings

Radiographic studies should help in defining the exact localization of a synostosis as well as in determining its extent. A suture's entire length can be affected, resulting in a complete loss of its linear or interdigitated appearance (Fig. 4-2). In other cases, we only note a suture in the act of closing with dense borders. Some types are rapidly progressive and follow-up studies will reveal the fast advance of closure.

No further review of the different modifications of the skull's form is necessary (Fig. 4-3). It should be added, however, that the basal angle is particularly flat in longitudinal synostosis but remains normal if the coronal sutures are involved. Contrary to this is the opening of the orbital angle which is formed by the roof of the orbit and the clivus and assumes a vertical position with the roof of the orbit. Digital impressions may be very marked corresponding to the effect of cerebral convolution pressure upon the internal table. Careful examination of the optic canals is always recommended, as they may be abnormal in shape. In isolated craniostenosis they are, however, rarely narrow.

Pathogenesis and Genetic Data

Even though synostosis can result from an abnormal metabolic process, as vitamin D resistant rickets or hypophosphatasia, the vast majority of the cases occur isolated and remain unexplained. There are, however, a number of pedigrees on record supporting the thought that they might be of genetic origin. The exact mode of transmission is not yet clear. The incidence appears to be higher in boys. Several pedigrees suggest a dominant transmission, while others are suggestive of a recessive disorder. The present conclusion is that there are probably several genes involved.

As to the pathogenesis of the malformation itself, we know very little. Certain studies, particularly those done by Moss or Müke suggest that premature synostosis is only a symptom. In some patients Moss has shown that there is a correlation between early closure of the metopic suture and abnormal development in the base of the skull for those who suffer from cleft palate. Müke insists on the coexistence of intracranial hypertension with changes of the volume of the skull

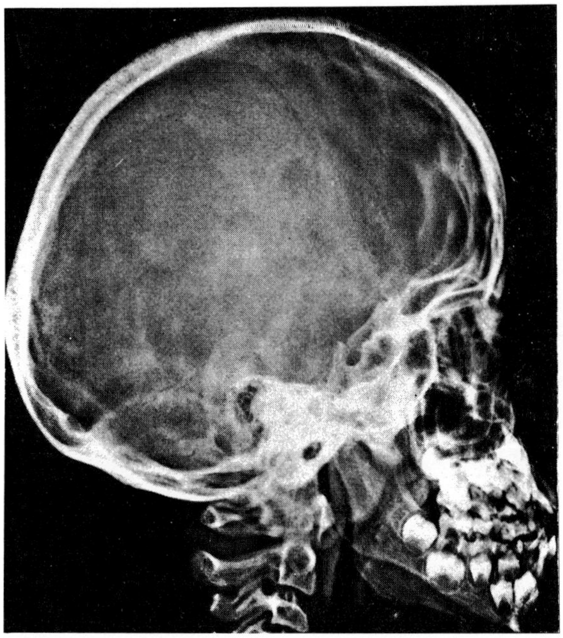

Fig. 4-2. Secondary brachycephaly resulting from premature closure of the coronal sutures in a 7-year-old girl.

and brain. Histologic studies in carniosynostoses demonstrate that the dura mater is abnormally dense and fibrotic. It remains a well documented fact that craniosynostosis can be a secondary manifestation of metabolic disturbances such as hypophosphatasia (see p. 218). Treatment will be discussed at the end of this chapter.

CRANIOSYNOSTOSES ASSOCIATED WITH OTHER MALFORMATIONS

The three diseases which will be mentioned here are craniofacial dysostosis, acrocephalosyndactyly, and clover leaf skull.

Craniofacial Dysostosis (Crouzon's Disease)

Clearly defined by Crouzon in 1912, this disorder is characterized by craniostenosis and hypoplasia of the facial structures.

Clinical Studies

In spite of the fact that the craniofacial alterations are present at birth, this disease can occasionally be overlooked. Then complications such as a visual disturbance, may lead the patient to seek help. Unfortunately, it is sometimes too late.

The most characteristic clinical finding of the skull is a marked protrusion of the anterior fontanelle which is similar to a "clown's hat." A lateral crista can extend into the region of the coronal sutures or a midline crista may descend towards the nasal root (Fig. 4-4). In other cases there can be an increased AP diameter with marked frontal bossing. Finally, craniosynostosis can present in the same fashion as oxycephaly. Involvement of the facial structures is always prominent. The midface and orbits are sunken, the bridge of the nose is flat and wide, and there is marked exophthalmus. Maxillary hypoplasia leads to a very prominently appearing mandible. The palate is very high with a narrow roof. Malaligned teeth are frequently seen and at times one can note supernumerary or anomalous teeth.

Ocular complications are frequently present. Errors in refraction, strabism, and nystagmus may be noted. Hypoacusis, as well as complete deafness and anosmia have been described in Crouzon's disease. Some authors emphasize respiratory difficulties which are secondary to the facial anomalies (Lemariey). Mental retardation is seen less frequently, and to a lesser extent than in acrocephalosyndactyly. However, the incidence of cranial nerve compression and of intracranial hypertension are arguments for cautious prognosis. This leads to the recommendation of repeated careful follow-up studies in these patients.

Radiographic Findings

Skull films confirm the coronal and sagittal craniosynostosis along with the prominent bulge in the area of the anterior fontanelle in the brachycephalic patient. There are usually markedly increased digital impressions. The thickness of the cranial vault is uneven and in several areas it is rather thin, for instance, in the region of the frontal bossing. The base of the skull is shortened and has a tendency to become vertical. The planum ethmoidale is oblique inferiorly and posteriorly, and the sella turcica is pushed down and forward. The cerebellar fossa is abnormally deep. The maxilla is markedly hypoplastic and recessed. The maxillary sinuses are small and their floor is high in location just as the fossa nasalis (Fig. 4-5).

Genetic Data

Crouzon's disease is unquestionably transmitted as a dominant disorder, an observation already made by Crouzon. However, we must insist on the various degrees of manifestation in this disease. One family

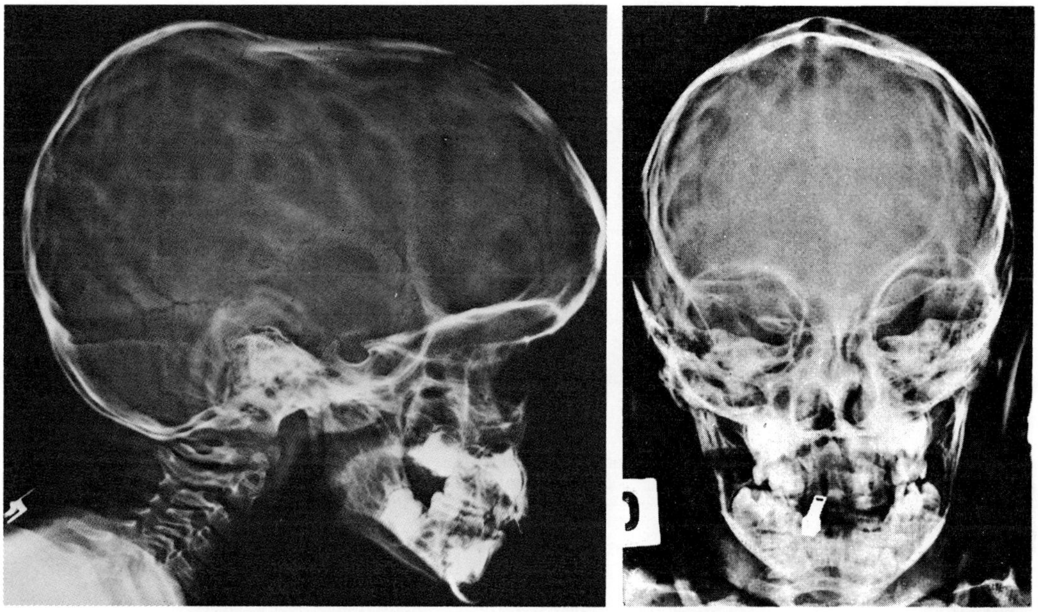

Fig. 4-3. Scaphocephaly in a 4-year-old girl. There is complete disappearance of the sagittal suture on the AP film.

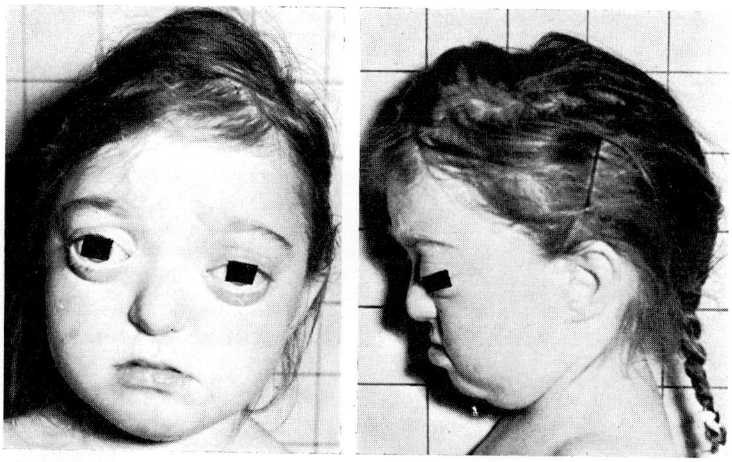

Fig. 4-4. Craniofacial dysostosis with a deformity of the upper portion of the skull which looks like a "clown's cap." There is exophthalmus and insufficient development of the facial structures and marked protrusion of the mandible.

may have persons with deformities of the skull, sometimes to a very marked degree. while others only have signs of partial craniosynostosis and very mild facial involvement. It may be rather difficult to recognize the minor forms or "formes frustes" and to distinguish them from craniosynostosis.

On the other hand, there are several observations on record which suggest the possibility of recessive transmission. Therefore, genetic heterogeneity can not be ruled out.

We would also like to add that some observations of coexisting syndactyly are on record. This fact has led

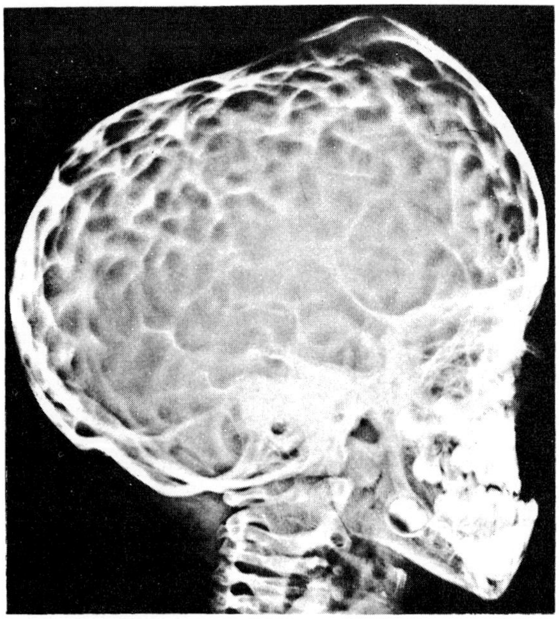

Fig. 4-5. Craniofacial dysostosis in a 3-year-old girl. Besides the prominent frontal bulge, there is excessive formation of digital impressions and hypoplasia of the facial bones.

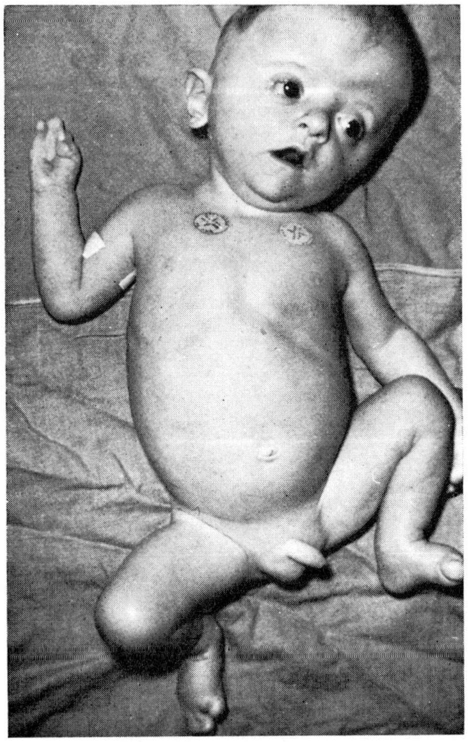

Fig. 4-6. Acrocephalosyndactyly. An association of cranial and distal skeletal malformation.

to a classification by McKusick which is based on the Vogt type of acrocephalysyndactyly. This condition has been cited as an argument in confirming the identity of two different diseases (Cruvellier). We do not feel that this can be maintained.

The pathophysiology of this disorder is unknown.

Acrocephalosyndactyly

Described originally by Apert this disorder associates anomalies of the skull with syndactyly of the fingers and toes.

For this discussion we would like to focus on the most typical variant of this syndrome, which is also the one most frequently seen. Still, it should be emphasized that there are other similar disorders with the association of syndactyly and acrocephaly.

Clinical Findings

Acrocephalosyndactyly is discovered at birth because of the severe changes which are fully evident. The excessive height of the skull is striking, and involves, in particular, the forehead which is flat or slightly protruding in appearance (Fig. 4-6). The occipital region is almost parallel with the neck. The root of the nose is flat. The nose itself often looks like the beak of an eagle or parrot. Hypertelorism and exophthalmus are generally seen and the palpable fissures have a slightly oblique course inferiorly and laterally. The mouth is kept open. A divided palate is often present, and sometimes there is a deep medial groove or a particularly high vault.

The abnormal hands and feet vary considerably from one patient to another. All fingers and toes may be fused. The hand is reduced to one or two vertical grooves which suggest the form of fingers. More frequently, however, fusion involves only the second to the fifth finger and a malformed, but preserved, thumb is present (Fig. 4-6). Finally, one may encounter a patient with only a mild degree of syndactyly between the two middle or the two lateral fingers. The fingernails are also malformed. Sometimes they may be combined in one single mass, but most frequently there are individual nails present, at least in a rudimentary form. The same can be said for the toenails.

A severe degree of mental retardation is frequently associated with these anomalies and aggravates the prognosis of acrocephalosyndactyly. Gasencephalography often leads to the detection of agenesis in the corpus callosum.

Ocular complications are the same as those described in the preceding chapters.

Radiographic Findings

Reduction in AP diameter of the skull along with its abnormal height are striking. Upon viewing some of the radiographs one is tempted to think that they are the result of technical errors and that they should be looked at in a tilted position because the craniocaudal diameter of the skull is clearly larger than its length (Fig. 4-7). Digital impressions are recognized early. The thickness of the vault is usually uneven and the frontal region is particularly thin. The base of the skull is markedly oblique and the angle formed by the clivus and the groove of the orbit tends to reach 180°. The former seems almost to be a prolongation of the orbital roof.

On hand films the metacarpals are usually all present, however, their arrangement is not always regular, since some frequently have an oblique axis. The ground phalanges of the second to fifth finger are individually formed, but a distal synostosis between two of them, for instance the third and the fourth finger may be noted. The phalanges of the thumb are usually fused and are grossly triangular or quadrangular in appearance. The middle and distal phalanges of the other fingers are difficult to identify. No finger has more than one of these elements and there may be different types of local fusion. Thus, an arch may be formed from the second to the fifth finger (Fig. 4-8).

In the foot the phalanx of the first toe is often fused with the second resulting in an irregular mass which is combined with a disorganized arrangement of the other toes. This is also seen in the hand.

Clinical Types and Genetic Data

Acrocephalosyndactyly is most frequently present in an isolated patient. Coronal synostosis is present from birth and the sagittal suture may follow soon after. Dominant mutation seems likely. As in achondroplasia there is a significantly elevated paternal age.

Other Types

Acrocephalosyndactyly is not the only syndrome which combines acrocephaly and syndactyly. A large number of publications have appeared on similar associations, but relate to a number of different facts and findings. Besides the classical form of Apert, McKusick distinguishes four other types.

Among those that we would like to single out is the Chotzen type, which is transmitted as a dominant disorder. It refers to acrocephaly with brachycephaly and is combined with an unusual facial appearance, a deviation of the nasal septum, hypertelorism, ptosis, small malformed ears, and prognatism. The partial syndactyly involves the second and third finger and the corresponding toes (Fig. 4-9). Affected males have cryptorchidism.

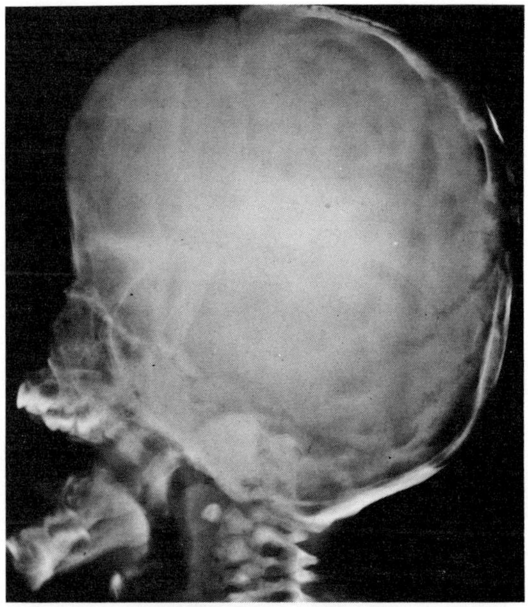

Fig. 4-7. Acrocephalosyndactyly in an 18-month-old boy. The forehead is unusually high and straight.

The type described by Pfeiffer is also transmitted as a dominant. The trapezoid appearance of the ground phalanx of the thumb, along with the varus deviation of the big toe with its almost triangular first phalanx in the presence of a hypertrophic first metatarsal are the most characteristic signs.

A number of authors have described other findings which await confirmation. This is in reference to the observations made by Wardenburg, and Hermann and Opitz of mandibular hypoplasia, brachydactyly, absent nails, congenital cardiac and genital malformations, retarded growth, and mental development. We would also like to note Summit's observation of a probably recessive form which is combined with obesity. All these conditions have only a moderate degree of acrocephaly. Another type which is distinctly different from the preceeding one has been described by Carpenter under the name of acrocephalopolysyndactyly (Fig. 4-10). In such patients one will note polydactyly associated with syndactyly. Clinically there may also be a coxa vara, a slight degree of obesity, as well as insufficient genital development.

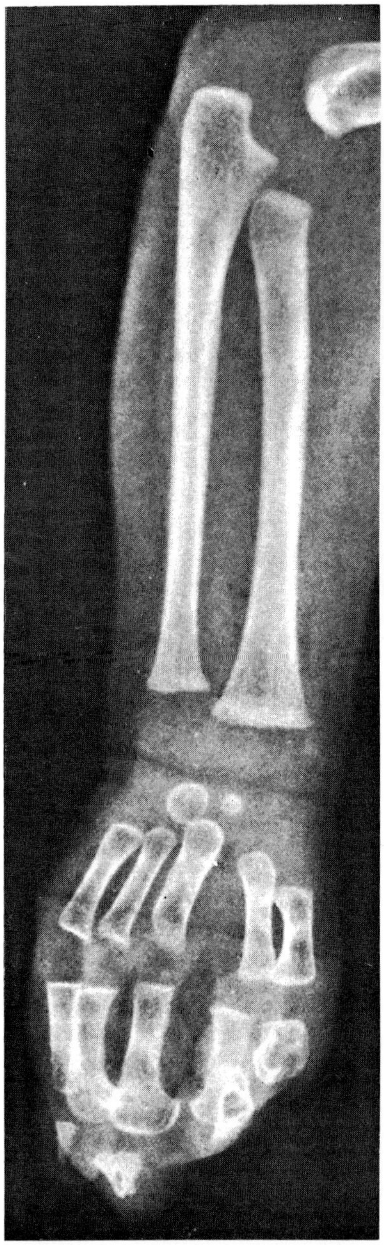

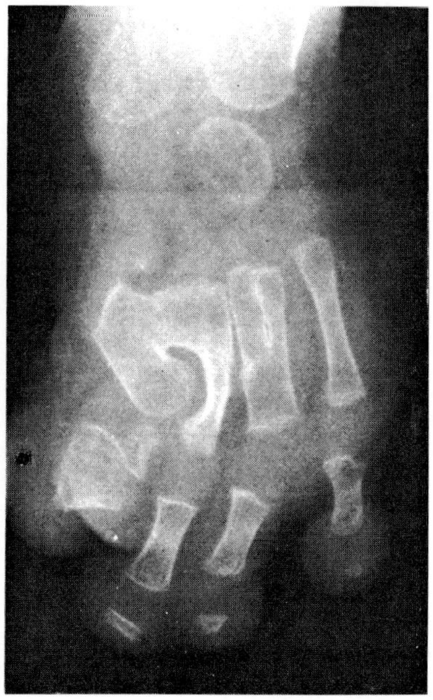

Fig. 4-8. Acrocephalosyndactyly in an 18-month-old boy.

A further condition, Noack's syndrome, is occasionally related to the group of acrocephalopolysyndactylies. Under this term the dominant transmission of a simple duplication of the terminal phalanx of the big toe has been described. The autonomy of such a syndrome seems difficult to ascertain.

We would also like to recall that Apert has already proposed that a disorder combining acrocephaly with anomalies of the forearms and elbows be designated as "acrocephalosynanky."

Clover Leaf Skull

Recognized as a special entity by Holtermüller and Wiedemann, this is a monstrosity of the skull with a trilobed appearance. The clover leaf appearance may be visualized in the AP view and is the result of the premature closing of the coronal, lambdoid, and squamosal sutures. The volume of the skull is markedly increased with a large bulge at the frontal and temporal regions (Fig. 4-11). Exophthalmus is combined with maxillary hypoplasia, macrostomy, macroglossy, dental anomalies, and prognatism. A growth deficit is noted in the majority of patients observed.

It is likely that this combination of malformations does not correspond to a single entity. A number of patients show the combination with the radiographic appearance of thanatophoric dwarfism (see p. 33). This combination is fatal, whereas other patients (Feingold, Neumarker) have shown entirely different skeletal findings, some with ankylosis of the elbow (Comings, Angle et al.), a clubbed foot, and lack of phalanges (Schuch et al.). Whatever the actual situation, this is a serious disorder and is mostly fatal. However, we must be aware that occasionally a patient does survive with all the stigmata of severe mental retardation and other malformations.

The etiology is still under discussion and may not be connected with just one single mode. In addition to genetic factors (see p. 34) radiation during pregnancy has been incriminated (Schuch).

There are further dysostoses of the skull. Some of these, such as bathrocephaly, must be considered normal variants (see p. 23), while others like cranium bifidium or lacunar skull will be discussed with the neurologic anomalies (see p. 310).

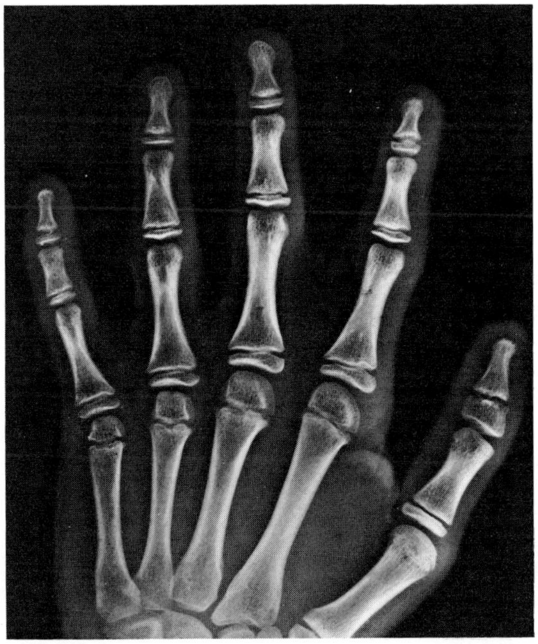

Fig. 4-9. Chotzen syndrome in an 14-year-old boy. Syndactyly mainly involves the 2nd and 3rd fingers. Compare with Fig. 4-8. (Courtesy of P. Mabille)

Treatment

The treatment of craniosynostoses presents a complex problem about which there is considerable disagreement. Premature craniosynostoses as well as those which rapidly develop must be operated upon early. Intervention consists of the creation of a new suture line either by the removal of the closed suture or a parallel excision of bone. If there has already been a major deformity, remodeling must be attempted by resecting flaps and their subsequent rotation or inversion (Rougerie et al.). There are advocates of total craniectomy, a procedure that should be performed prior to the age of two.

Where craniosynostosis is discovered late, we would feel that it is not necessary to treat every patient. A careful follow-up with attention to the eyegrounds is recommended. Surgical correction only seems sensible, for very strong esthetic reasons or when there are early signs of papillary stasis. Certain craniosynostoses, for example, scapocephaly rarely lead to early cerebral complications. If there is an associated mental retardation one can obviously not expect to improve this through surgical intervention.

In craniofacial dysostoses treatment for the craniosynostosis is combined with that for facial deformity. Complex techniques have been recently standardized and have been successfully used. Thus, it is now posible to elevate entire structures of the upper and midface bringing them into a more normal position (Tessier).

In the approach to acrocephalosyndactyly several authors insist on the association of hydrocephalus which they treat by shunting (Hogan and Bauman).

FACIAL DYSOSTOSES

Facial dysplasias are noted in a number of disorders studied in this book, particularly in several types of dwarfism, where they form an important symptomatic element. We will not return to them here nor to isolated anomalies of the facial or mandibular bones. The most frequent lesion is a cleft palate, often associated with other malformations and syndromes which are too numerous to list (Gorlin et al.). We have indicated this in our presentation of diastrophic dwarfism.

We would like to recall here that a cleft palate is very often accompanied by pathology of the hands and the feet. This is the case, for instance, in the popliteal-pterygium syndrome, to hypoplasias or agenesis of fingers, syndactyly, malformation of the foot, either in varus or in valgus, shortening of the tibia, and genital anomalies, in particular, cryptorchidism. We would also like to refer to the dominant type of lip fistula and cleft lip or palate syndrome (Gorlin and Pidborg) seen in combination with clubbed foot or syndactyly. In the ectromelia and ichtyotis syndrome ectodermal dys-

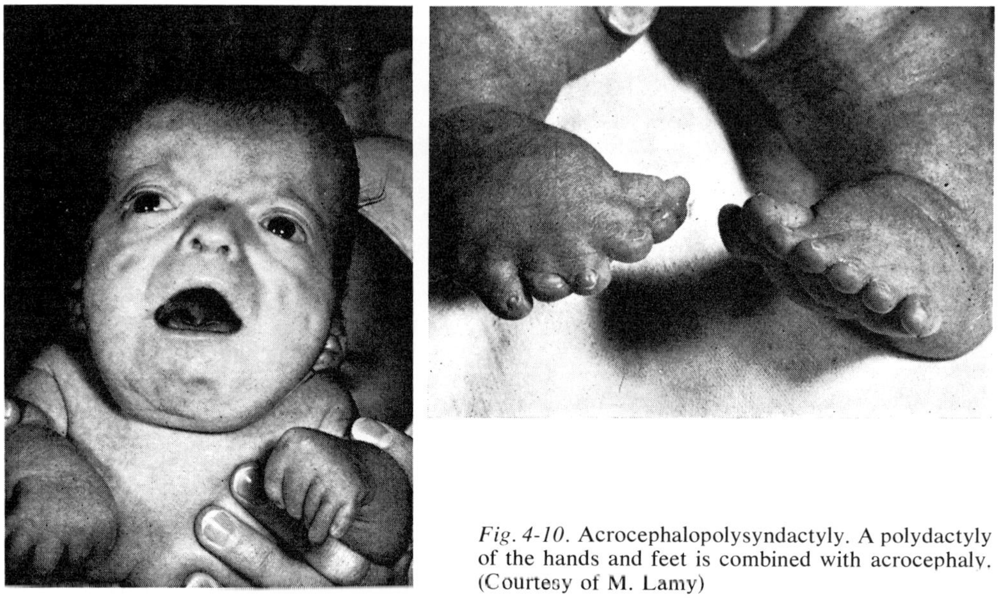

Fig. 4-10. Acrocephalopolysyndactyly. A polydactyly of the hands and feet is combined with acrocephaly. (Courtesy of M. Lamy)

plasia—ectrodactyly and cleft palate—also a harelip may occur together as described by Rüdiger and Freire-Maïa. There can be a combination of absent fingers or a split hand with ectodermal anomalies such as hypotrychosis and dental anomalies. Dominant transmission has been reported in several families (Brill et al., Robinson et al.). In other cases besides the cleft palate we note polydactyly. This is a frequent finding in glossopalatine ankylosis and in anomalies of the hand and feet. In such a case there is a small tongue fixed to the roof of the mouth at the upper alveolar border, a reduced number of teeth, and an absence of incisors. This is in addition to various anomalies of the extremities which include syndactyly, hypoplastic fingers, clinodactyly, and the absence of tarsal bones.

We will not emphasize any further these different syndromes, but will discuss four different dysostoses which electively affect the face. These are mandibulofacial dysostosis, mandibular hypoplasia (Pierre Robin syndrome), the oculo-mandibulo-facial syndrome of Hallerman-Streiff-François and the Basal-Cell Carcinoma Syndrome.

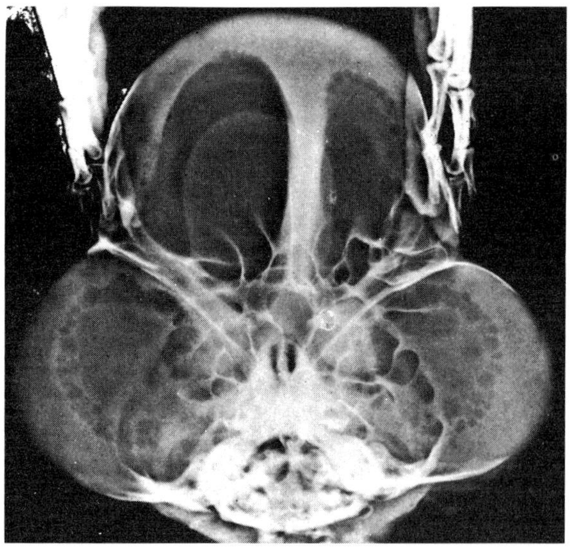

Fig. 4-11. Clover leaf skull. (Courtesy of H. R. Wiedemann)

Mandibulofacial Dystostosis

Although well defined by Francheschetti and Zwahlen, but sometimes referred to as the Treacher-Collins syndrome, this disorder is recognized at birth because of its abnormal facial appearance. Marked hypoplasia of the maxillary malar processes is combined with an antimongoloid slant of the palpebral fissures and coloboma in the outer portion of the lower lid. The external ear is usually small and malformed with atresia of the external canal and preauricular appendices. The mouth is too big and blind fistulae are often located between the lateral angle of the mouth and ears. There is frequently also a cleft palate. The mandible is hypoplastic with malaligned teeth (Fig. 4-12). Abnormal

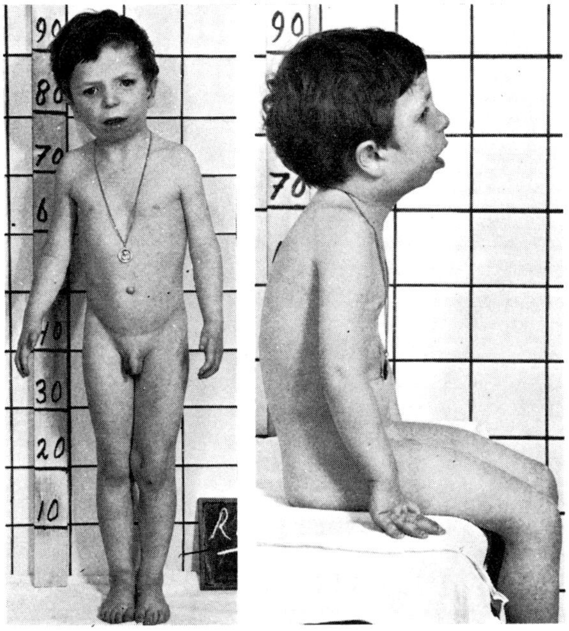

Fig. 4-12. Mandibulofacial dysostosis. There is also hypoplasia of the thumb.

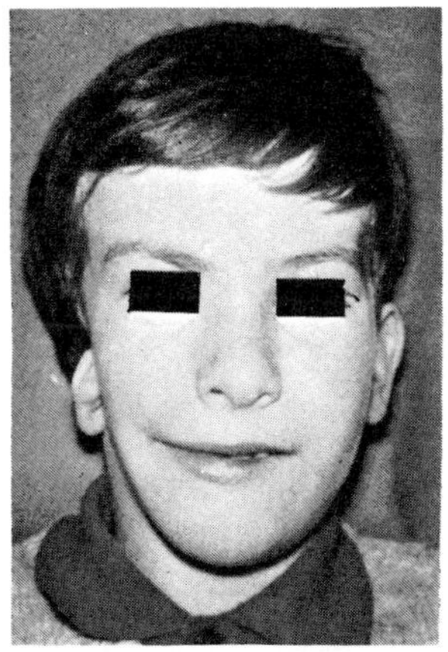

Fig. 4-13. Goldenhar's syndrome. This boy suffers from unilateral involvement of the right side. (Courtesy of A. Mugnier)

findings involving the hands, such as deformed fingers, syndactyly, aplasia or hypoplasia of the thumb are not uncommon. Sometimes there is even a more serious involvement of the arms – radioulnar synostosis, radial aplasia, and even phocomelia. Prognosis is guarded since these patients encounter not only esthetic problems, but also deafness due to abnormal transmission or hypoacusis. In addition, 15 to 20 per cent of all patients affected have mental retardation.

On lateral skull films the anterior portion of the base of the skull is short, the mandible is hypoplastic, and the maxillary sinus is insufficiently developed both in the growing child and in the adult. On AP views the orbits are low in relation to the ethemoids. The zygomatic apophysis of the temporal bone is hypoplastic and on special views it is possible to also recognize the hypoplastic malar process and the orbital apophyses of the maxilla (Water's view).

Transmission of this disorder is dominant but genetic manifestation varies. An abnormally developed first and second branchial arch appears to be the cause. The mechanism of these events is unknown. Therapy attempts to correct the facial anomalies through transplants of skin and cartilage (Longacre), and the correction of the abnormal ear. The coloboma will be excised and autoplastic correction can usually close the defect. Surgical elongation of the superior branch of the mandible must be accompanied by concentrated orthodontic efforts to counteract the maligned teeth. Tympanoplasty can help to inprove deafness, even though its results are somewhat questionable.

Besides mandibulofacial dysostosis there are several other closely related syndromes. We will only mention the oculoauriculovertebral syndrome of Goldenhar, the oculovertebral syndrome of Weyers and Thier, and the otomandibular dysostosis of François and Haustrate.

The oculoauriculovertebral syndrome reveals ocular anomalies, most frequently subconjunctival lipodermoids and epibulbar dermoids as well as unilateral, coloboma, and ptosis. Preauricular appendices usually close to the tragus can be accompanied by a blind fistula and anomalies of the outer ear resulting in deafness. This ear involvement is unilateral. We emphasize the high incidence of facial asymmetry with macrostomia along with anomalies of dental articulation (Fig. 4-13). Radiographic study will confirm the facial structure and temporal bone defects (Malar hypoplasia, asymmetry of the petrous portion of the temporal bone, and atresia of the external or internal auditory canal, Bowen et al.). In addition there will be vertebral anomalies electively affecting the cervical spine and the first thoracic vertebrae in the form of fusion, hemivertebrae, and supernumerary vertebrae.

This syndrome most frequently occurs isolated. It is, however, possible that a genetic factor is involved and an observation of concordant monozygotic twins (Terhaar) appears to support this.

The oculovertebral syndrome of Weyers and Thier combines microphthalmia or anophthalmia, vertebral or rib malformations with unilateral mandibulofacial dy-

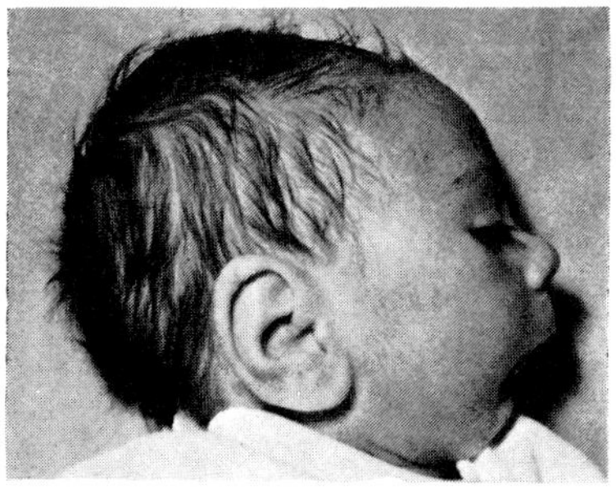

Fig. 4-14. Pierre Robin syndrome. Mandibular hypoplasia. (Courtesy of A. Mugnier)

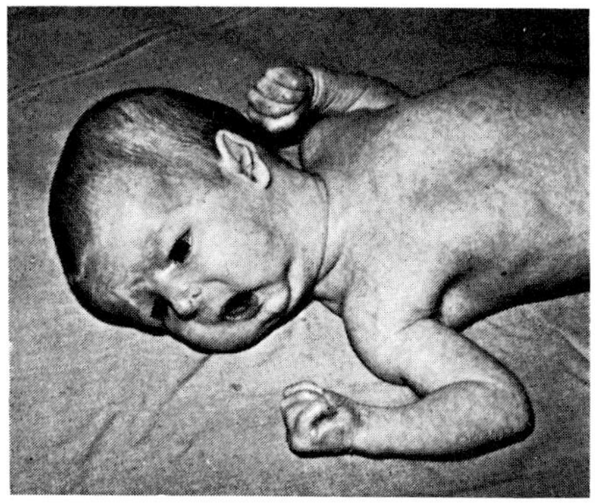

Fig. 4-15. Oculomandibulofacial syndrome. (Courtesy of Menget)

sostosis. The vertebral involvement is localized mainly in the lumbar area in the form of block formation or wedged vertebral bodies.

Otomandibular dysostosis of François and Haustrate combines agenesis of the mandible, which is occasionally unilateral, anomalies of the temporomandibular joint and dental malalignment, with an atresia of the external auditory canal and a malformed ear.

One should not confuse mandibulofacial dysostosis with its closely related form of maxillonasal dysostosis (Binder's syndrome). This name can lead to confusion, but patients have a typical appearance with a hypoplastic, almost vertically positioned nose and a small maxilla (Delaire et al.). Micronasal dysplasia is a distinct entity with the midportion of the face narrowed resulting in a small pucked up nose.

Mandibular Hypoplasia (Pierre Robin Syndrome)

This syndrome is the combination of mandibular hypoplasia, glossoptosis and cleft palate. It is frequently associated with further visceral, ocular, and bony malformation (Fig. 4-14). Most frequently involved are the hands and feet—syndactyly, shortened fingers or metacarpals—but occasionally long bones may be involved (Assemany et al., Walden et al.). The Pierre Robin syndrome has also been noted in combination with arthrogryposis, diastrophic dwarfism, and, in particular, with micrognathic dwarfism (see p. 66).

The combination of these malformations may result in critical clinical conditions with a high mortality. Glossoptosis may lead to aspiration and a severe respiratory disturbance requiring emergency measures. Alimentation by gastric tubing in the prone position may be required. The difficulties have a tendency to decrease as the patient becomes older. Prognosis will depend largely on the degree of mental retardation or on other malformations. Familial observations (Bixler and Christian) support genetic factors as the origin of this syndrome. A similar condition could be produced experimentally by injecting purine desoxyguanosine (Cocke), into the embryo.

There are a number of further developmental anomalies of the mandible, but their discussion goes beyond the scope of this book and would be of special interest mainly to stomatologists. We would just like to mention the recessive observation by Buchignani which combines thinning and the absence of a mandibular angle with other skeletal anomalies, such as scoliosis, thin ribs, and cortical widening of long bones. In acrofacial dysostosis there is a median mandibular fissure (see p. 175).

Elsahy and Waters have described a dominant disorder under the term branchio-sceleto-genital syndrome. These patients, in addition to mandibular hypoplasia and malaligned teeth, have other craniofacial malformations which include brachycephaly, hypertelorism, ptosis, strabism, maxillary and mandibular cysts as well as an occasional cleft palate or bifid uvula, mental retardation, hypospadias, and occasionally spinal or thoracic anomalies.

The Oculo-Mandibulo-Facial Syndrome (Hallermann-Streiff-François Syndrome)

Already noted by Aubry in 1893 the definition of this syndrome is the result of the contributions by the authors, whose name it now carries. The essential features are craniofacial dysplasia, along with ocular and dental anomalies. Frequently associated abnormalities of skin, and hair, and dwarfism are recognized.

The craniofacial disproportion is characterized by marked frontal bossing, a small face, minimal development of the nose similar to a parrot's beak, and retro-

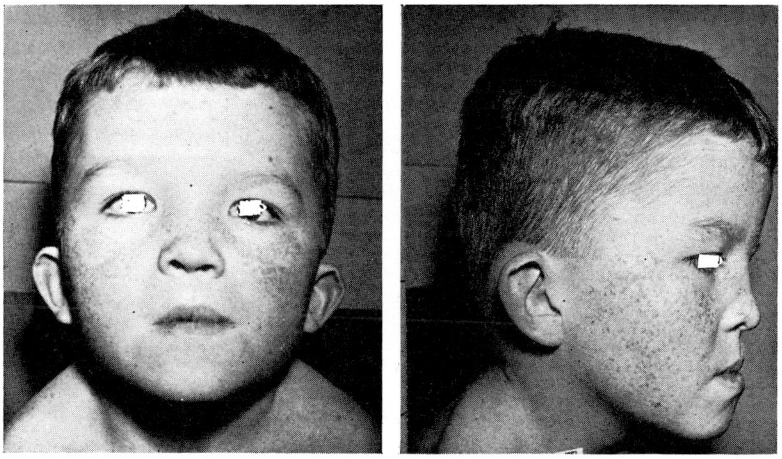

Fig. 4-16. Basal cell Nevus syndrome with its characteristic facial appearance and prominent cheeks. (Courtesy of O. Schweisguth)

gnathism (Fig. 4-15). Cataracts and microphthalmia are always present. Further anomalies of the eyes including strabism, nystagmus, blue sclerae, and a number of eye ground changes may be noted. The teeth are poorly aligned, are abnormally formed, and frequently show early signs of caries. Their eruption is irregular and individual teeth are totally absent. Frequently there is atrophy of the skin and hypotrichosis. Dwarfism has been noted in about half of all patients affected.

Radiographic study reveals a thin cranial vault, sometimes poorly mineralized, with delayed closure of the anterior fontanelle. The shape of the skull varies, but is most frequently brachycephalic. Frontal and parietal bossing is commonly present. The facial structures, especially the orbits, are relatively small. The mandible is hypoplastic with shortened upper rami and anterior displacement of the temporomandibular joints. The condyle may be poorly formed, and the long bones and ribs are thin. There is sometimes development of a scoliosis.

The genetic transmission of this syndrome is not yet well established. There are indications that we may be possibly dealing with a dominant disorder, most frequently resulting from a mutation, as there has been an observation of a father and son (Guyard et al.).

The syndrome described by Cohen seems to be closely related. It is the combination of similar ocular and facial anomalies with obesity, hypotonia, mental retardation, and abnormalities of hands and feet. The hands, especially their distal portions, are narrow with thin fingers. One such family with affected brothers and sisters suggests a recessive mode of transmission, but it is still too early to separate this syndrome from that described by Hallermann-Streiff and François.

Basal-Cell Carcinoma Syndrome

This unusual dominant disorder is characterized by the presence of basal-cell carcinomas with early manifestation during childhood and an abnormal craniofacial morphology. Occasionally there may be further skeletal malformations.

Clinical appearance, besides cutaneous involvement, reveals frontal and temporal bossing and excessive development of the supraorbital structures. The bridge of the nose is wide and there may be hypertelorism. Mandibular prognatism is frequently noted and may be combined with mandibular cysts. These lesions may be noted prior to the appearance of the cutaneous manifestations. Such cysts may become unusually large and can affect the patient's appearance considerably (Fig. 4-16). Kyphoscoliosis is not unusual. The thorax is narrow, and is sometimes deformed as a pigeon chest.

Radiographic study confirms the widened skull, and the clear lytic zones within the horizontal ending branches of the mandible. Several types of vertebral anomalies—vertebral fusion, spina bifida oculta—may accompany kyphoscoliosis. We often note anomalies of ribs, such as bifid ribs, synostosis or absence of ribs (Fig. 4-17). Shortening of the fourth and fifth metacarpals has been seen in some cases. Due to the malignant characteristics of the skin lesions this is a very serious disorder.

A number of other facial anomalies with varying degrees of skeletal involvement could have been discussed in this chapter. A large group is well described elsewhere with the teratologic disorders (Duhamel). Greig's hypertelorism in itself does not seem to be a distinct disease entity. The most clearly defined form

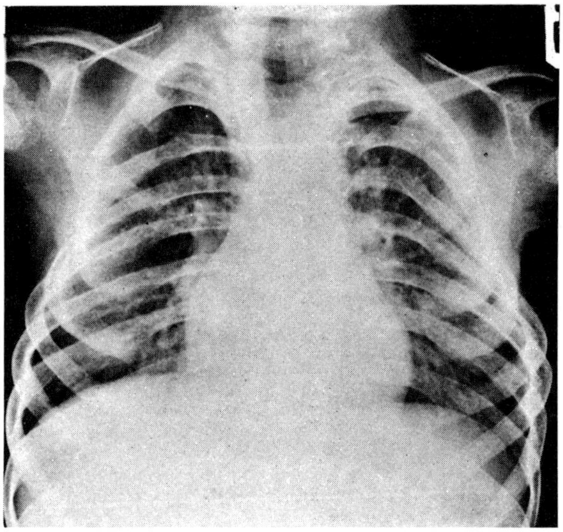

Fig. 4-17. Basal cell Nevus syndrome in an 8-year-old boy. Note the short 2nd, 3rd and, 4th ribs with the narrowed upper segments of the thorax. (Courtesy of O. Schweisguth)

is that described by Sedano as frontonasal dysplasia. This is a combination of hypertelorism, a widened nasal base, and an indication of a minimal median cleft of the tip of the nose and occasionally of the upper lip. There is great variability in the expression of this malformation, since it sometimes is just barely noticeable, while in others there is indeed marked separation of the wings of the nose. Twinning seems to occur with an unusually high incidence in such families (Cohen et al.).

DYSOSTOSES WITH ELECTIVE TRUNK INVOLVEMENT

In this chapter we will successively discuss spinal dysostoses and anomalies of the shoulder and pelvic girdles.

SPINAL DYSOSTOSES

A large number of anomalies of vertebral development can be seen and we will not attempt to offer an exhaustive discussion. Schematically such anomalies may involve the vertebral bodies and the posterior arches. The first group is composed of sagittal fissures, lateral or posterior hemivertebra, aplasia of the vertebral body, or congenital vertebral block formation by fusion of two or several bodies. Involvement of the posterior arch can be limited to the pedicles, the lateral or median portion, or to the spinous processes resulting in a defect within the different segments mentioned. There may be a wider defect with partial or total aplasia of the posterior arch or a synostosis. Anomalies of the vertebral apophyses can also be seen.

The incidence of these anomalies differs markedly and their clinical significance varies greatly with their exact location. Sometimes there are multiple defects. They may be adjacent and can result in serious disorders. Occasionally, they are part of a larger complex of defects. For example, there have been a number of patients with hemivertebra formation and supernumerary ribs in combination with incontinentia pigmenti and shortened extremities, syndactyly, or a dislocated hip. A separate description is in order for lesions of the suboccipital region, the lumbosacral area, and the spondylocostal dysostoses.

Abnormal Segmentation

Such defects can involve all vertebral bodies, but most frequently are noted in the cervical spinal area. This may simply be the result of the fact that such lesions are most readily noted. Generally, this type of anomaly is referred to as the Klippel-Feil syndrome, in spite of the fact that we are not necessarily dealing with a well defined syndrome, but rather with a spectrum of clinical and radiographic malformations.

In its most severe form patients present with an unusually short neck, a low hairline and a marked limitation in head movements. Difficulty with thoracic mobility may also be noted (Fig. 4-18). A high positioned scapula is not unusual as is the presence of a pterygium colli.

Other patients may only reveal the presence of torticollis or a cervical or thoracic scoliosis. A stiff neck along with mild local discomfort may be the only manifestations of this malformation.

Utilizing radiographic criteria Feil distinguished three different types of anomalies. These are complete fusion of the cervical spine which may extend down to the first thoracic vertebra, synostosis of two vertebrae involving one or two interspaces, and finally, the combination of one of these with involvement of the thoracic or lumbar spine.

The most readily described alterations are in the second group and refer, for example, to the fusion of two neighboring vertebral bodies, C2-C3 or C5-C6. It is, however, not at all unusual to note further malformations, such as hemivertebra. In the majority of patients we are dealing with complex malformations which may involve partial fusion of the body or arches,

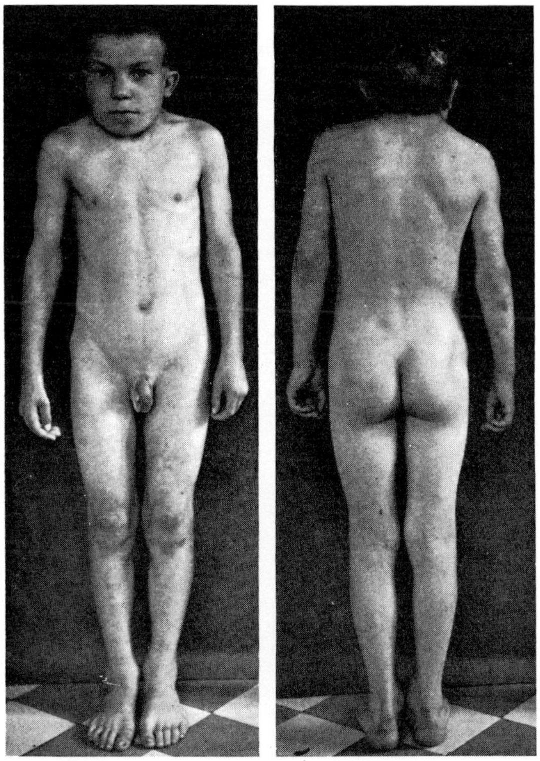

Fig. 4-18. Klippel-Feil syndrome. (Taken from Pédiatrie, CMC, Flammarion)

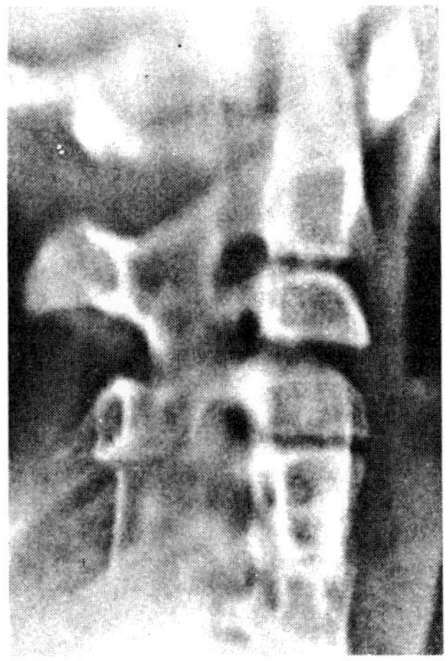

Fig. 4-19. Klippel-Feil syndrome in a 7-year-old boy. Note the posterior fusion of the 2nd and 3rd cervical vertebrae and the block formation of the last 3 cervical bodies.

lack of vertebrae, asymmetry of a number of vertebral bodies, or hemivertebrae which may result in a seriously disturbed posture (Fig. 4-19). A similarly complex situation must be expected in involvement of the thoracic or lumbar spine. In these patients we are also faced with anomalies of the ribs, which may be absent, fused, or bifid.

All these facts suggest that this group of anomalies is heterogeneous, which is supported by genetic data. In the chapter on chromosomal aberrations we will see that translocation of one chromosome in the 13-15 group may be responsible for these types of malformation. In other patients, however, the disorder is definitely genetic. It has been shown (Gunderson et al.) that C2-C3 fusion may be transmitted as a dominant trait, whereas C5-C6 fusion occurred as an autosomal recessive disorder in the families that were studied. They noted in two families the presence of a dominant gene that caused fusion at different levels. Finally, it should not be overlooked that many isolated cases which are indicators of these malformations are acquired, and not genetically determined.

In the presence of a spinal lesion the prognosis is always in keeping with the nature and extent of the lesion. In the second group, according to Feil, there are usually late complications resulting from the development of a secondary arthrosis or from trauma. This does not hold true for the other groups, because an association with several malformations may be incompatible with survival and because the neurologic disturbances are not unusual. These patients will suffer mainly from sensory, sympathetic, or vasomotor troubles, sometimes even from quadriplegia, and sometimes in combination with cerebellar or cranial nerve involvement. Most frequently these neurologic disorders can not be explained on the basis of bony compression alone. A coexisting neurologic anomaly is possible.

There is a particular association between spinal lesions and deafness, mentioned in 1936 by Jalladeau. In these cases deafness seems to be the result of an underlying complex of anomalies of the internal ear, as has been demonstrated by the tomographic studies of Palant and Carter. Wilderwanck has described a complex of malformations under the term of cervico-oculo-acoustic syndrome. These consist of anomalies of the vertebral column similar to those described for the Klippel-Feil syndrome. The deafness is secondary to anomalies of the internal ear and includes abducens paralysis, sometimes with retraction of the bulbus of one or both eyes. Facial palsy may also be noted. The combination of a Klippel-Feil syndrome with pterygium colli, ptosis, and a high arched cleft palate together with camptodactyly, has been described as Nilson's syndrome (Moldenhauer).

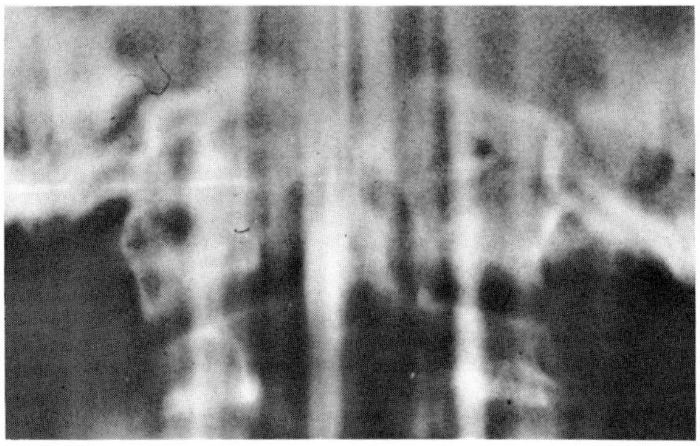

Fig. 4-20. Occipitoatlantoid block in a 10-year-old boy. AP tomograms reveal that there is no longer a visible line between the occiput and the atlas and that the lateral borders are in direct continuity. (Courtesy of J. Sauvegrain)

Anomalies of the Cervico-occipital Region

These anomalies fall into three groups, as suggested by Sauvegrain and Mareschal: vertebral block formation, malformations of the basi-occipital, and anomalies of the odontoid.

Vertebral Blocks

We can distinguish several types.

The occipito-atlantoid block results from the fusion of the atlas with the occipital. This fusion may be incomplete, sometimes involving only the posterior arch. In a number of patients the fusion also involves the anterior arch or the lateral mass (Fig. 4-20). Unilateral block formation is quite frequently seen. Such patients may come to our attention clinically because of torticollis. This condition is best visualized on AP tomograms. The severity of this malformation usually results from hypoplasia of the atlas. Hypoplasia of the atlas causes a repositioning of the dens at the level of the foramen magnum. Neurologic symptoms stem from this malposition.

In occipital-transverse blocks there is fusion between the apophysis of the atlas, an extra apophysis, and the analogous formation at the base of the skull. The result is solid bridging. Sometimes a synchrondrosis may persist. This anomaly may be unilateral or bilateral and can be associated with an assimilation of the atlas.

Block formation between the second and third cervical vertebrae has a high incidence, whereas fusion between the atlas and the epistropheus is rare.

Malformations of the Basioccipital Bone

Aplasia of the basioccipital results in an anterior displacement of the foramen magnum. There is a high position of its posterior border, while the posterior fossa is located at a considerably lower level than normal. The occipital condyles face anteriorly and the petrous bones are high in location. Sometimes this aplasia is limited to a simple anomaly of the basilar pyramid, which is much smaller than usual. The demonstration of such a basilar impression, if only mildly present, requires careful radiographic study. On the lateral view, it is best to use either the line of Chamberlain which connects the posterior end of the bony palate to the posterior border of the foramen magnum, or the line of MacGregor, where the latter landmark is replaced by the most inclined point of the occipital squama. Normally there is projection of the apophysis of the dens below or just at this line. In order to be certain that there is indeed basilar impression, the apophysis must be 7 to 9 mm too high (Fig. 4-21).

On AP films the best help can be gained from the digastric line of Fischgold and Metzger which connects the two mastoid notches (digastric fossae) where the medial surface of the mastoid meets with the base of the skull (Fig. 4-21). In normal individuals the dens will always remain below this line. In basilar impression it will reach or even situate itself above this line. The upper border of petrous bone is oblique, inferiorly and medially.

Basilar impression is often associated with other anomalies. Its incidence is high in a number of constitutional skeletal disorders, especially in osteogenesis imperfecta, and occasionally in cleidocranial dysplasia (see pp. 62, 105). Resulting neurologic symptoms are not always parallel to the radiologic severity, and, conversely, a mild degree of basilar impression can be accompanied by severe nervous malformations.

Sometimes only a rudimentary occipital vertebra, reduced to a small portion of the posterior arch may be present or an anterior intermediary structure. A third condyle, which articulates with the anterior arch of the atlas, has also been described. Finally, cervical spondylolisthesis can occur at the level of the second and third cervical vertebrae.

A careful follow-up of these patients is mandatory. One should not actively treat them if there are no clinical manifestations. Unlike the case of adults, it is quite unusual to encounter neurologic complications during childhood. Guidance for their future professional career is important for these children and they should avoid all hard forms of labor. If there is a beginning dislocation, an orthopedic support must be worn. If neurologic symptoms are impending, surgical intervention is advised. One should never overlook the possibility of neighboring malformations in vertebral anomalies. Where a mechanical support of the spine is needed, the patient may also require a support of the base of the skull.

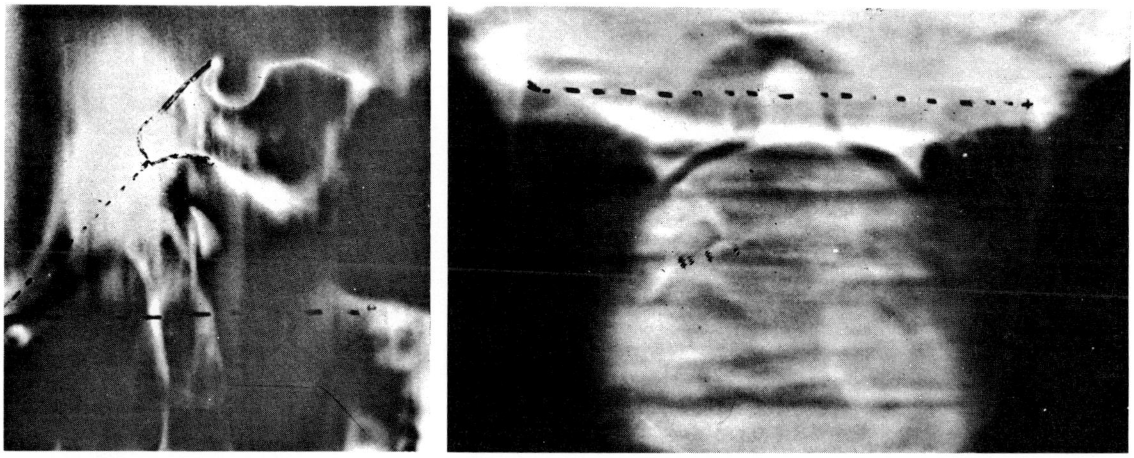

Fig. 4-21. Basilar impression in a 12-year-old girl. Both AP and lateral tomograms. The line of Chamberlain and the foramen magnum have been marked (*left*) and also the digastric line (*right*). (Courtesy of J. Sauvegrain)

Anomalies of the Dens

Quite frequently there is a small os odontoid or a small extra center of ossification at the tip of the dens. During infancy there is normally an ossification center which appears from two to four years of age and fuses towards the twelfth year. Sometimes this supernumerary ossicle seems to be part of the dens, but sometimes it may appear as separate and slightly displaced laterally on an AP film. If there has been trauma (Fig. 4-22), there may be some difficulty in properly distinguishing this finding from a fracture.

In some chondrodysplasias there may be hypoplasia or morphologic anomalies of the apophysis of the dens, as in Morquio's disease, and in metatropic dwarfism. The potential seriousness of these malformations, especially in a defect of closure, is due to the danger of atlanto-axial dislocation with the secondary problem of compression of the cervical portion of the spinal cord.

Anomalies of the Lumbosacral Region

Sacralization of the fifth lumbar vertebra is much less serious than anomalies of the first cervical vertebra, since there is usually a normally sized L5 (Fig. 4-23) and local pain only in adults. Such transitional anomalies result from arthrosis. However, abnormal posture, especially scoliosis, is not unusual in such individuals. We cannot discuss all the possible anatomic variants of this region.

Spondylolisthesis, however, deserves careful attention, since it is not uncommon during childhood. This anomaly, most frequently involving L5, results from a congenital defect of the posterior arch in the region of the isthmus.

Clinically, such patients have lumbar pain of varying intensity, sometimes radiating to the legs. There may be contracture of the lumbosacral musculature and painful flexion. It is, however, not unusual to recognize this finding during a radiographic study for unrelated problems.

One of the key findings is the anterior sliding of the lower-most lumbar vertebra with a disruption of the curve formed by the posterior borders of the lumbar and sacral vertebral bodies (Fig. 4-24). The anomaly of the isthmus can frequently be shown only in oblique views, in which it is always located at the inferior border of the superior articular apophyseal facette. Once this anomaly has been recognized, regular radiographic follow-up is advised, since anterior sliding of L5 may precipitate or aggravate neurologic problems because of nerve root compression or stretching. In cases that worsen seriously, surgical fixation by posterior spine fusion is necessary. Usually an individual with agenesis of a large number of vertebral segments does not survive. Patients with lumbo-sacral agenesis usually do.

In the most frequently seen type of such a disorder, there is a lack of development of the gluteal muscles. Because of this, Foix and Hillemand call such individuals "patients without buttocks." The most severely involved individuals, those with total lumbar agenesis, have skin bands, especially in the popliteal region, together with abduction and flexion of the legs. This gives the newborn the aspect of a "Buddha." There is lumbar kyphosis with a protrusion of the lowermost vertebral body present. Neurologic symptoms are variable depending on the degree of involvement. The

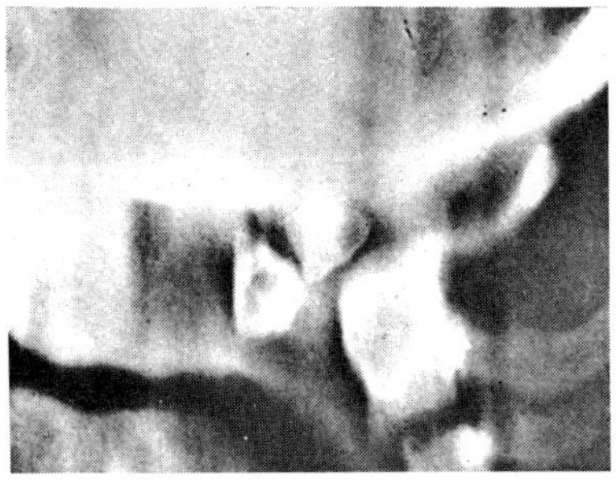

Fig. 4-22. Tomographic appearance of the dens in a 4-year-old boy. (Courtesy of J. Sauvegrain)

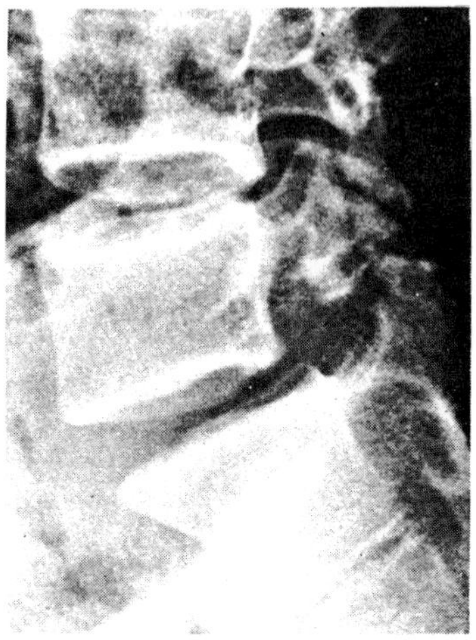

Fig. 4-24. Spondylolisthesis in a 15-year-old boy. There is marked malalignment between the lower and posterior corner of L5 and the upper posterior corner of S1.

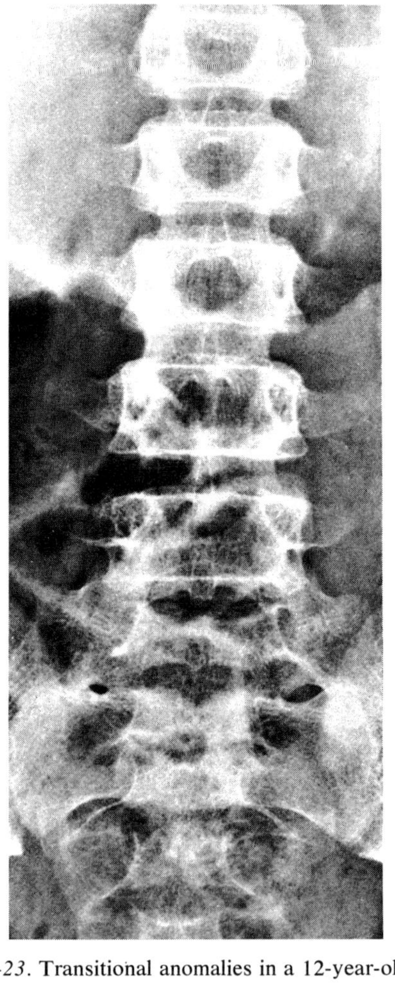

Fig. 4-23. Transitional anomalies in a 12-year-old boy.

spectrum may extend from total paraplegia with anesthesia of the legs in high agenesis at L1 to simple saddle anesthesia with amyotrophia, where the aplasia of the sacrum is limited to the region below S2. Abnormal urinary control is often a problem, but the involvement of the rectal sphincter may improve with age. Radiographically, there may be a more or less extensive involvement. Sometimes one or two abnormal sacral elements persist, but agenesis of the rest of the sacrum and of the coccyx may be complete, and even abnormal development above may be recognized—sacralisation of L5, vertebral fusion, spina bifida. In other patients there is complete aplasia of the lumbosacral spine, sometimes even involving the last thoracic vertebrae, but agenesis may be less extensive or unilateral. In such a situation this may result in asymmetrical and/or abnormal development of the pelvis. Occasionally, there may only be involvement of the coccyx, which complicates the problem of early diagnosis. Lumbosacral agenesis is seen only in isolated cases, and genetic factors seem to play only a minor role in its occurrance. A number of authors have noted the relatively high incidence of such lesions in infants of diabetic mothers (Lenz and Kucera).

Spondylocostal Dysostoses

These dysostoses combine abnormal spinal segmentation and malformations of ribs. Clinically, such patients have an unusually short trunk and neck. Only rarely is this condition painful during infancy. Radio-

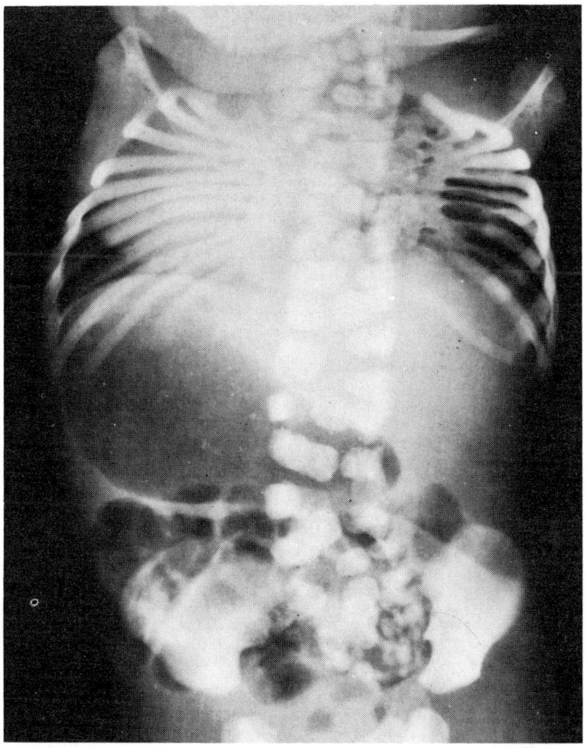

Fig. 4-25. Spondylocostal dysostosis. (Courtesy of L. Guéraud)

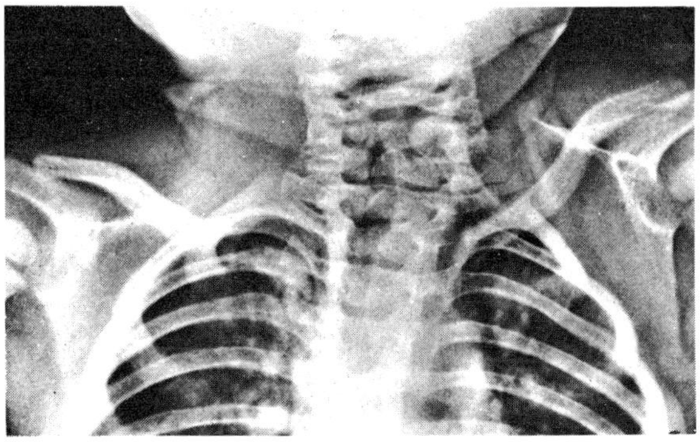

Fig. 4-26. Sprengel's deformity of the left scapula in a 1-year-old boy. There are also a number of anomalies of the cervical vertebrae.

graphically, the vertebral anomalies are comparable to those described in the preceding chapter: vertebral block formation, hemivertebra, and clefts. There is a reduced number of ribs, and they are hypoplastic or fused. Sometimes there is a mild degree of widening of the iliac wings. In this group we can distinguish two different types of lesions. The first, isolated by Rimoin, is characterized by much less severe clinical and radiographic anomalies and a dominant genetic transmission. The second, described by Moseley and by Pochaczevsky, et al., is transmitted as an autosomal recessive disorder. Shortening of the trunk is very marked, and there is anterior sternal protrusion. Numerous hemivertebrae are present, and the vertebrocostal articulations are positioned close to one another resulting in the fanning out of all the ribs like the wings of a butterfly (Fig. 4-25). Many of these patients die early in life from respiratory infection. Spondylocostal dysostosis is associated with mesomelic dwarfism and can be transmitted as a dominant disorder (see p. 51). There are a number of isolated dysostoses of the thorax. They are still undefined and may be confused with the asphyxiating thoracic dysplasia of Jeune. Rabushka has described a dominant type, clinically evident by a bell-shaped or very narrow thorax. Respiratory infection occurs frequently, but does not seem to seriously endanger survival. In the baby, radiographs will reveal thin, short, and horizontally placed ribs. This slender appearance is quite different from that seen in Jeune's disease. Eventually the ribs will become oblique, and the thorax assumes a triangular aspect. The rest of the skeleton is normal.

ANOMALIES OF THE BONES OF THE SHOULDER AND PELVIC GIRDLES

Morphologic anomalies of the clavicle do not receive much attention outside of what has already been described in cleidocranial dysplasia (see p. 62). The most important anomaly of the scapula is Sprengel's deformity, scapula alata (Fig. 4-26). The unilateral disorder most frequently results from a lack of normal anatomic descent of the scapula, which can be rather large, and slightly reduced in its height, and which can have an inner hook-like angle. Sometimes there is a bony connection with ribs or vertebral apophyses. The congenital elevation of the scapula is very frequently combined with malformations of the spine and ribs (see p. 158). Even though this lesion occurs most frequently in an isolated fashion, in some families there is well documented dominant transmission (Wilson et al.).

Among pelvic anomalies, those of the acetabulum have particular importance because of the inherent risk of dislocation or subluxation of the femoral head. Sacral agenesis can result in narrowing and abnormal form of the pelvis. Agenesis or hypoplasia of the iliac wings is rare. It can occasionally be associated with hypoplasia of the scapulae and of the clavicles (Ko-

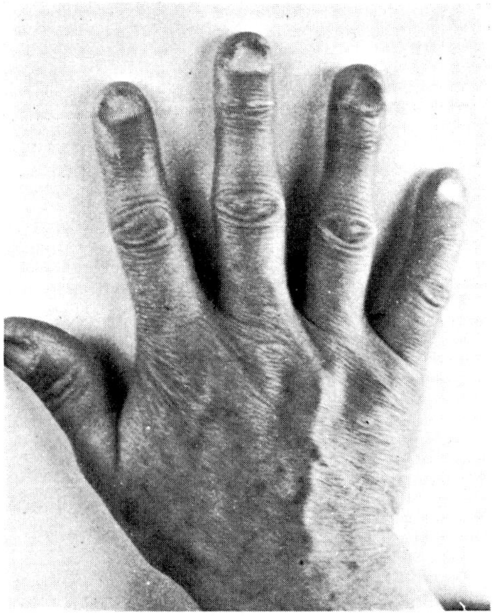

Fig. 4-27. Onychoosteodysostosis. Notice the irregular clubbed appearance of the nails.

senow et al.). We shall focus on osteoonychodysostosis, a disorder with a most unusual manifestation, that of iliac horns.

Osteoonychodysostosis

This syndrome associates abnormal fingernails with a number of skeletal changes involving especially the patella, elbow, and pelvis. These characteristics have only been slowly recognized since the iliac horns, representing one of its most characteristic features, were only discovered by Kieser in 1939. These were already present, but had not been appreciated on the original radiographs shown in Turner's publication. In spite of its name, osteoonychodysplasia, this disorder should be grouped with the dysostoses. Other terms occasionally used are the "nail patella syndrome" or, in French, "onycharthrose."

Clinical Findings

The disorder is recognized at different ages, most frequently because of symptoms resulting from the patellar involvement. Such symptoms are late learning of, or difficult walking, instability of the knee joints resulting in frequent falls in younger children, sometimes with local pain after long walks, and sometimes genu valgum (Alain and Rigault). Rarely there are complaints related to a hypoplastic elbow or the anomalies of the nails. The growth of these patients is normal, but careful palpation and inspection will reveal the presence of small and laterally displaced patellae. Sometimes they are even absent, and the normal patellar contour is replaced by a local depression. There is, however, no significant articular limitation. The mobility of the patella itself can be excessive, especially towards the medial side. Studies of the arms may show limitation of pronation and supination and also of extension of the forearm. The nails are small and concave, or bulging, striated, and rough. They sometimes appear greyish or discolored and are fragile and brittle (Fig. 4-27). Muscular anomalies, usually atrophy or pterygia, have been occasionally noted. It is entirely possible that the muscular atrophy at least in part is secondary to the bony defect. Sometimes there is clubfoot. Lester has reported on the presence of heterochromia of the iris. The total prognosis of such patients would be quite good, if there were not some patients who eventually develop serious nephropathy. This occurs not infrequently, and often during infancy is evidenced by an isolated albuminuria and slow progression.

Radiographic Findings

The most easily recognizable symptoms are those of the knees, elbows, and the pelvis. It should, however, be noted that in about one-half of the cases not all of these changes are present. Most frequently the patellae are small, often bipartite, and laterally dislocated. In very young infants it may be difficult to properly identify, and one should insist on lateral films. There may be absence of the local thickening of the tendon in the area of the patella, which normally results from its local cartilaginous presence (Fauré). There is frequently hypertrophy of the medial condyle, whereas the lateral condyle is rather hypoplastic. The intercondylar fossa is usually shallow. Some alterations of the proximal extremity of the tibia have also been described, such as protrusion of the anterior tuberosity and an abnormal slump of the medial plateau (Fig. 4-28). On films of the elbow there is frequently hypoplasia of the radial head, with posterior, and sometimes also lateral, subluxation. This dislocation is favored by a hypoplastic humeral condyle (Fig. 4-29). The radial neck is often narrow, deviating somewhat laterally and posteriorly. On AP views there is a wide space between radius and ulna. The iliac horns are the third major radiographic sign. They occur somewhat less frequently than the previously described changes. However, if present, this finding will reliably establish the diagnosis of osteoonychodysostosis. They are located at the external surface of the iliac bone, slightly

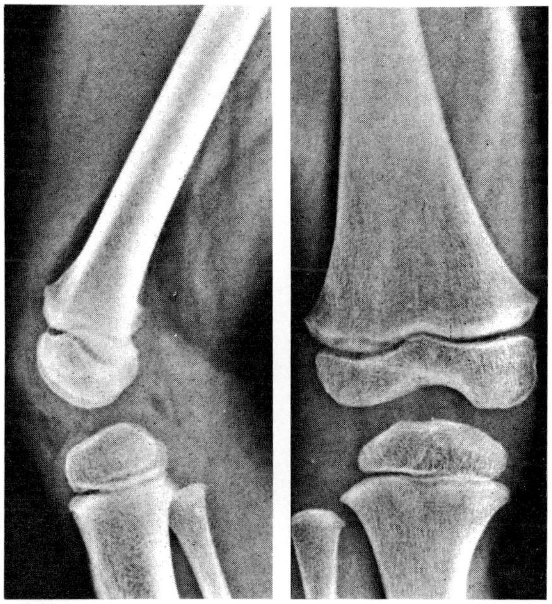

Fig. 4-28. Onychoosteodysostosis in a 5-year-old girl. Note that the patella is absent. (Courtesy of P. Royer)

outside of the sacroiliac line, and are visible from the first days of life. They are spurs, grossly pyramidal in shape, with an oblique lateral and posterior orientation. Most frequently, they occur bilaterally, but they are sometimes asymmetrical (Fig. 4-30). Emphasis should also be placed on the characteristically abnormal form of the iliac wings. There is a very prominent appearance of the anterior superior iliac spine and an almost vertical crista in its anterior portion. The anterior border of the iliac wing is concave and may form a notch. Coxa valga can be present. Slight malformations of the shoulder have been reported, such as hypoplasia of the scapula, excessive projection of the acromion, or the lateral end of the clavicle, and small lateral exostoses of the humerus. These findings, possibly in combination with others only rarely noted—the small size of some of the carpal bones, lack of a pair of ribs, large parietal foramina—are evidence of the fact that the skeleton is indeed more or less involved in osteoonychodysostosis.

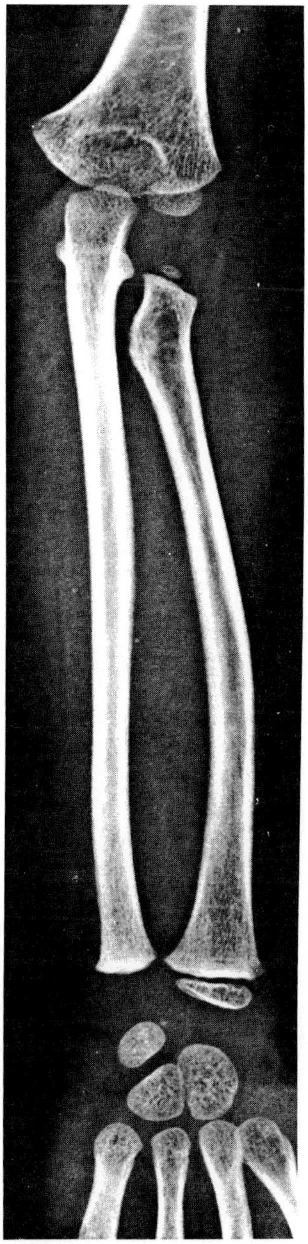

Fig. 4-29. Onychoosteodysostosis in a 5-year-old girl. Note the abnormal shape of the proximal radial end. (Courtesy of P. Royer)

Genetic Data and Pathology

Autosomal dominant transmission has been established, and there is a connection between the responsible gene and that for the blood groups A, B, and O. Pathologic and ultrastructural studies have been directed mainly towards the involvement of the kidneys. Most authors insist on the finding of a thickened glomerular basement membrane (Morita). Sometimes there are collagen fibers within the mesangium and may also be found in the thickened portion of the basement membrane and transparent islands by electron microscopy (Bennett et al.).

The pathophysiology of this disease is entirely un-

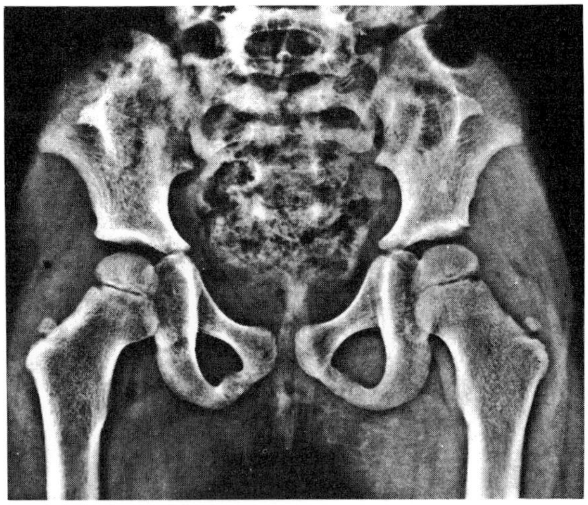

Fig. 4-30. Osteoonychodysostosis in a 5-year-old girl. Notice the bilateral iliac horns. (Courtesy of P. Royer)

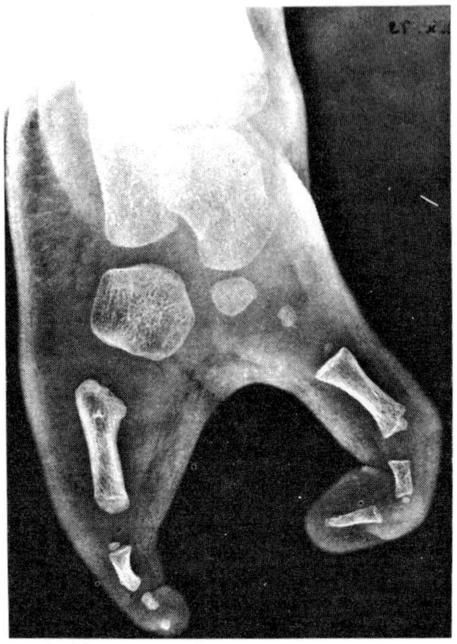

Fig. 4-31. Foot deformity of the "lobster claw" type in a young adult. (Courtesy of M. Lamy)

known. A close relationship between the accumulation of abnormal fibers in the kidneys and the skeletal malformations is hard to establish. Therapy must limit itself to the surgical correction of the anomalies, especially in the case of the dislocation of the patella, and the resulting instability of the knee.

DYSOSTOSES WHICH ELECTIVELY INVOLVE THE LIMBS

First, we shall look into the different types of aplasias or agenesis and congenital bowing of bones. A discussion of some segmental anomalies follows.

AGENESIS OF BONES—PHOCOMELIAS

There are numerous types of phocomelias resulting from a lack of formation of bones of limbs. First, we will attempt to clarify their classification. This will be followed by an analysis of etiologic possibilities.

Classification

We shall adopt here, with some modifications, the classification of Frantz and O'Rahilly, distinguishing between terminal aplasias, phocomelias, and lateral hemiaplasias.

The terminal aplasias refer to the absence of the most distal portions of a limb. Depending on the extent, we can distinguish amelia or total absence of a limb, total hemi-melia in a patient with total lack of the forearm and of the hand, or the inferior portion of the leg, and partial hemi-melia, where there is still persistence of a portion of the forearm or the lower half of the leg. Acheria and apodia are characterized by the total absence of the hands or of the feet. And finally adactylia or aphalangia—absence of fingers or phalanges, may be partial or total.

Phocomelias are characterized by aplasia of the mid or proximal segment of a limb, while the hand or foot are preserved. It is possible to distinguish between complete phocomelias, a situation where hands and feet are directly attached to the body, proximal phocomelias, which focus mainly on the length of the arms, and distal phocomelias, with aplasia of the forearm or the middle third of the legs.

The term lateral hemi-aplasias refers to the absence of one of the bones of the forearm or the lower leg. It is our impression that special attention should be given to this malformation because of its relative frequency.

The bony agenesias of the hand are particularly complex. Occasionally, all fingers are involved or total agenesis; more often there is absence of the last phalanx or "transverse agenesis." In other instances there is a somewhat more metameric distribution: radial, absence of the thumb or the first, second, and third fingers; ulnar, absence of the ringfinger or fingers four and five. Such agenesias may be accompanied in the former type by a lack of formation of the radius and in the latter, of the ulna. Aplasia of the median territory may result in a cleft hand, also called lobster claw deformity (Fig. 4-31). Often it is difficult in the presence of a hand showing only two or three fingers to be certain how to identify those elements. In such a situation it may be helpful to carefully analyze the bones of the carpus: the absence of the cuneiform, the pisiform, and of the lateral portion of the hamatum will orient towards agenesis of the fifth finger, for instance, whereas an absence of the capitatum would rather point to agenesis of the midfinger (Bouvet). The lack of formation of the pelvic girdle is a rare malformation, most frequently associated with total agenesis of all structures below. Besides total or partial aplasia of the bone, it is possible to recognize simple hypoplasia. Femoral hypoplasia is seen most frequently, and is often accompanied by coxa vara (see p. 171).

Any attempt at classifying a single case is artificial, since in a given individual there may be several anomalies. It would be very difficult to group them in a rigid system. For instance, a patient may suffer from bilateral absence of the femur combined with hypoplasia of the lower segment, clubfoot, and a total absence of the forearm as in the case of Ring.

Etiology

Familial study confirms the complexity of this group of afflictions. Terminal aplasias most frequently seem to occur isolated, whereas acheria, partial or complete adactylia of the hands or of the feet, and complete aphalangia may sometimes be transmitted as recessive disorders (Freire Maia, Toledo).

It appears important to differentiate the so-called lobster claw deformity of the hand or of the foot. The midportion of the hand is split, the middle fingers are absent, and hypoplasia of the third metacarpal bones is present. In the most severe forms the hands and feet appear like two plates of a claw. Each plate is formed by the fusion of the lateral fingers, conserving, on the whole, their skeletal structure (Fig. 4-31). In other patients there is only an absence of the middle finger. Sometimes there is a reduction of the claw to a single plate, and this is called ectrodactyly. This type of malformation can be seen in isolated cases, but in certain families it is transmitted as a dominant. Vogel distinguishes two types. In the first type there is a major involvement of the feet—the hand may also be involved, but never by itself. This type is always transmitted as a dominant lesion. The second type has a more variable appearance. A single hand may be affected, feet are not always involved, and their aspect is not always that of a typical split hand or foot. The responsible gene seems to have irregular manifestation, and generations may be skipped.

Amputation of the extremities can be part of more complex syndromes. In the Hanhart syndrome, where four different types have already been separated, a birdheaded face is combined with micrognathia, dental anomalies, and amputations of extremities (Garner and Bixler). Absence of the tongue, and other oral anomalies, can be associated with agenesis of extremities of varying severity. There may be total absence of the forearm and of the hand or only that of a single finger. This is the case in the aglossia-adactylia syndrome (Fig. 4-32).

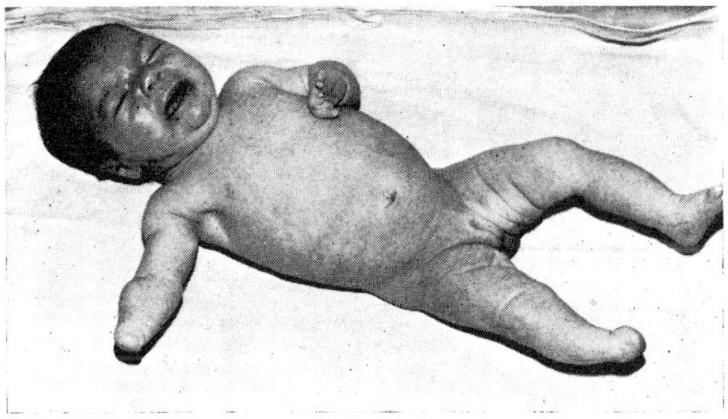

Fig. 4-32. Aglossiaadactylia syndrome. (Courtesy of C. Piussan)

Phocomelias usually occur in single individuals. Renewed interest in these phocomelias has unhappily been precipitated by the prescription of the drug thalidomide during pregnancy. Yet recessive transmission of certain types of phocomelia has also been signaled in the syndrome described by Hermann and others. Hall and Greenberg have proposed to designate this as "the syndrome of hypomelia, hypotrichosis and facial hemangioma." Developmental defects of the bones of the forearm and of the leg are associated with hypotrichosis, and a median hemangioma of the face with local dysmorphism—minimal wings of the nose and micrognatia. The incidence of hemiaplasias of only one arm or one leg is quite irregular. Involvement of fibula and radius occurs most frequently. Usually these are isolated cases occurring in a family, but there have been some observations of dominant or recessive transmission. When discussing the hematologic disorders, we shall see that partial radial aplasia can be accompanied by an aplastic anemia or thrombocytopenia. Sometimes there is an association with a ventricular septal defect—ventriculo-radial dysplasia, or with craniosynostosis (Greitzer et al.). Tibial aplasia can be accompanied by the absence of the thumb and polydactyly and may be transmitted as a dominant (syndrome of Werner; see p. 178). Fibular aplasia can also be transmitted but as a recessive lesion. We have followed this in a particular form of dominant mesomelic dwarfism.

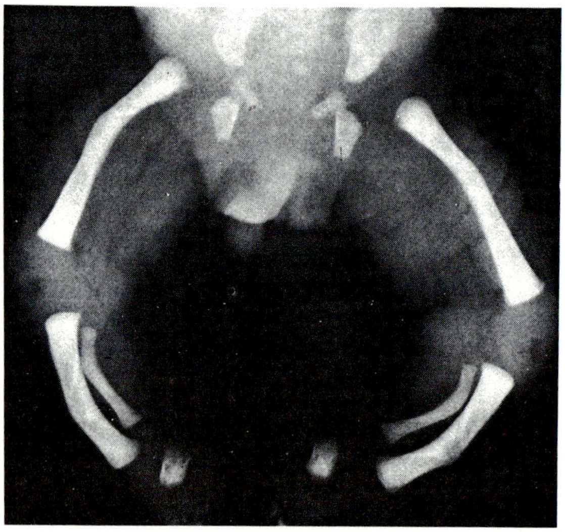

Fig. 4-33. Campomelic syndrome with bowing of the femur and tibia. Note the marked dislocation of the fermoral heads and hypoplasia of the equally bowed fibula.

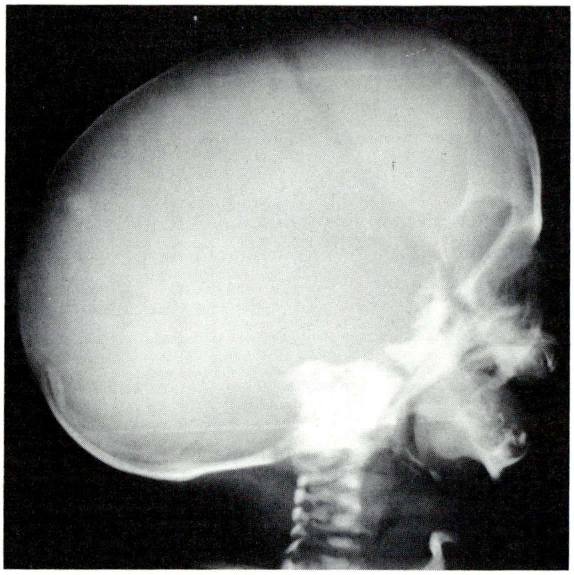

Fig. 4-34. Campomelic syndrome with all the facial structures severely underdeveloped.

No further discussion of severe morphologic disorders of the limbs is attempted. The therapeutic approach is extensively discussed in the orthopedic literature.

CONGENITAL BOWING OF LONG BONES

Congenital bowing of the long bones can be more or less generalized, or limited to a single bone, usually the tibia. First, we shall discuss the campomelic syndrome, so far the most well defined entity in this group. Isolated bowing of the tibia will be dealt with subsequently.

The Campomelic Syndrome

This disorder is recognized from birth because of shortening and bowing of the lower extremities. Height is around 45 cm. The thighs are held in abduction, and the tibias are angulated posteriorly. The face may be flattened, the chin small, and a cleft palate may be noted. Frequently there is rapid deterioration and death of the patient. This may result from respiratory complications resulting from the very narrow thorax or from laryngotracheal anomalies.

Radiographically, there is marked bowing of the femora and tibias, with an anterior and lateral convexity. The involvement of the femur is slightly above the midportion of the bone, whereas in the tibia the lower third is affected. The fibula is hypoplastic, and the pelvis is markedly narrow resulting from agenesis of the sacral wings and the narrowing of the iliac wings. Dislocated hips are the rule (Fig. 4-33). Occasionally there may be bowing of the humerus, but except for the hypoplasia of the scapula, the upper extremities will be almost normal. The ribs are thin and markedly oblique, and the chest has a tapering appearance. The vertebral bodies may be slightly wedged. The skull may be larger than normal in its transverse diameter, and the facial structures are markedly hypoplastic, as is the mandible (Fig. 4-34).

We have observed two sisters (Baggio), and familial transmission has been reported in Thormon et al., involving two brothers and their half-sister. It is thus likely that transmission is genetically determined. There are other observations of multiple bowing of long bones that have not yet been properly classified, seemingly of a different origin and having a much better prognosis (Caffey, Stüve and Wiedemann). Purely mechanical theories offered in an attempt to explain congenital bowing of long bones are not adequate to explain the variety of symptoms seen in the campomelic syndrome. Thus its pathogenesis is totally unknown. Study of growth cartilage reveals markedly disorganized cells at the base of the columnar zone (Stanescu).

The campomelic syndrome should not be confused with the embryopathy due to aminopterine or methotrexate taken during pregnancy. In such babies there

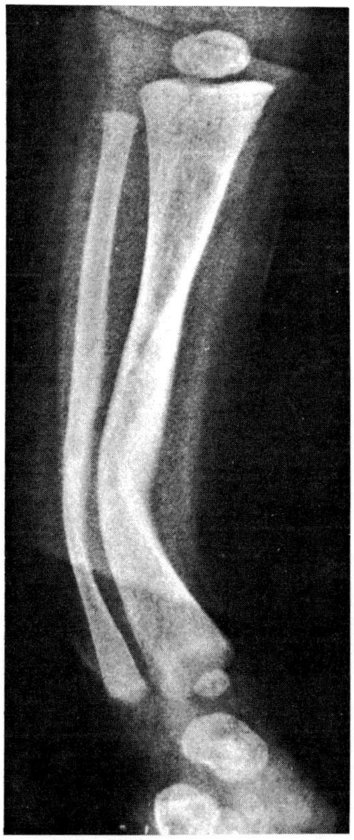

Fig. 4-35. Congenital bowing of the tibia and fibula in a patient with von Recklinghausen's disease. The structure of the tibia is markedly abnormal. (Courtesy of J. Lefevbre)

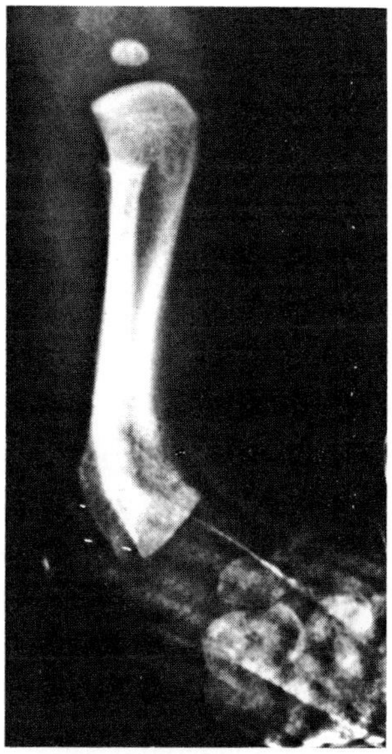

Fig. 4-36. Congenital posterior bowing of the tibia and fibula with anterior concavity.

may be micrognathia, cleft palate, clubfoot, and even a dislocated hip. Still, there should not be any bowing of the long bones of the legs. On the other hand, there may be acrocephaly and absence or anomalies of fingers or toes (Milunski).

ISOLATED BOWING OF THE TIBIA

As proposed by Heyman and Herndon, three large groups of congenital bowing can be distinguished, each with an entirely different prognosis.

The first type one which accompanies congenital aplasia of the fibula, was mentioned above.

The second type is bowing of the lower third of the tibia, most frequently with an anterior convexity. Sometimes the radiograph will show a clear pseudocystic defect in the neighborhood of its bend. This type of bowing frequently later results in pseudarthrosis. This appears towards two to four years, and may be provoked by orthopedic therapeutic efforts. There are some infants who already at birth have a congenital pseudarthrosis of the tibia. Radiographically this appears as two individual fragments with somewhat irregular and thin adjacent segments (Fig. 4-35). The prognosis in this type of bowing must be extremely cautious. Surgery of such pseudarthrosis is often very difficult and problematic (Judet et al.). In a number of such patients this is a local manifestation of neurofibromatosis or osseous fibromas. The presence of cartilaginous inclusions have also been recorded.

A third type of tibial bowing is also located at the lower third of the bone, but its convexity has a posterior tip (Fig. 4-36). This form of tibial bowing, unlike the preceding type, has a very good prognosis. Its course is spontaneously regressive, and if required, surgical correction can be considered without reservation.

SEGMENTAL ANOMALIES OF LIMBS

We shall limit our attention to the main types of segmental anomalies of the limbs, and to their related syndromes.

The most frequently seen anomalies affecting the arms are those of the forearms. There is an isolated type of symmetrical shortening of the humeri, and this dominant affection was occasionally considered to be a localized form of achondroplasia.

Congenital dysostoses of the elbow are not rare. This was emphasized in the discussion of onychodysostosis. Beals has also described a dominant affection under the name auriculo-osteodysplasia. It is manifested clinically by small size, anomalies of the elbow—hypoplasia of humeral condyle with or without dislocation of the radial head, and anomalies of the external ear—a long earlobe with a small posterior lobulus. Dislocated hips may be also present.

Several authors have mentioned the presence of partial hypoplasia of both bones of the forearm, in association with corneal opacities and sometimes mandibular anomalies. This appears to be a dominant disorder in the family studied by Pillay—ophtalmo-mandibulo-melico-dysplasia, whereas in the case of Mietens and Weber, brothers and sisters were affected and suffered from mental retardation and several neurologic anomalies. This is also true of the observations of rather complex anomalies by Klemm—absent radius and malformed extremities.

The most frequently noted local disorders are Madelung's deformity and radioulnar synostosis. The former was discussed at length in the chapter on dyschondrosteosis. The isolated occurrence of this deformity is due only to the minor manifestation of the gene for this disease. The transmission is dominant, and females are affected at a higher rate.

Radio-ulnar synostosis manifests itself by a limitation of movements of the forearm. Usually bilateral, it will result in a fixation of the hand in pronation and in a more or less complete lack of ability to pronate and supinate. Radiographically, the synostosis is located most frequently at the most proximal end of both bones, and it is accompanied by bowing of the radius and deformity of the radial head (see Fig. 8-3, p. 286). Synostoses in the middle or distal region are seen only exceptionally.

Radio-ulnar synostosis can be seen in certain chromosomal aberrations (see p. 286), but it can also be transmitted as a dominant lesion. Still, the expression of the gene is variable, and some individuals in affected families will only have a deformity of the proximal ends of radius and ulna.

Other types of synostoses of rare occurrence have been described (Feldmüller). If these afflictions of the radius and humerus are associated with further synostoses of the carpal and tarsal bones and combined with symphalangism, we are dealing with the syndrome of multiple synostoses (see p. 174).

In the lower extremities, femoral involvement occurs most frequently. Hypoplasia of the femur may occasionally be accompanied by coxa vara, but these two anomalies may occur separately. Congenital pseudarthrosis refers to agenesis and dislocation of the upper portion of the femur, which remains connected to the femoral head, still located in the acetabulum. Localized hypoplasia of the distal portion is unusual. These different types of femoral anomalies do not appear to occur as a familial trait. They may however be bilateral in location (Bailey and Beighton).

Tibiofibular synostosis is rarely seen (Grobelski). Sirenomelia resulting from the fusion of both legs is a lethal disorder and a teratologic curiosity.

The patella can be involved in different ways. There may be complete duplication or just two separate centers of ossification. We have already discussed the patellar involvement as a key symptom in osteoonychodysostosis (see p. 164).

In the cerebro-hepato-renal syndrome of Zellweger (Bowen et al.), the most characteristic involvement is that of the patella (Poznanski et al.). We find multiple calcifications associated with a malformed foot—clubfoot or metatarsus adductus—and combined with camptodactyly and forced flexion of joints. Affected babies show hypotonia, mongoloid facies, ocular anomalies—cataract, glaucoma and corneal opacities, and genital anomalies—clitoris hypertrophy.. Besides the frequently present cerebral anomalies, pathologic study will show renal cysts and hepatic alterations resulting in hepatomegaly. These patients die during infancy. The disorder is probably transmitted as an autosomal recessive.

DYSOSTOSES WITH ELECTIVE INVOLVEMENT OF THE HANDS AND OF THE FEET

The complexity of the disorders in this group requires a subdivision. After a discussion of the anomalies of the carpal and tarsal bones, we shall present a more or less generalized discussion of abnormal metacarpal and phalangeal development and of the isolated malformations of the thumb.

ANOMALIES OF THE CARPAL AND TARSAL BONES

There are numerous anatomic variants of the carpal bones. The most frequently seen are the duplication of the scaphoid, supernumerary bones, and possibly fusions of the semilunar and cuneiforme. There may also be lack of a scaphoid. Most of these, such as the fusion of the hamatum and capitatum as mentioned in the discussion of the Ellis van Creveld syndrome, are never diagnosed or noted at the time of a radiographic study.

It is more important to be familiar with the variants of the tarsal bones, because they may actually be responsible for local disorders. Problems of clubfeet shall not be discussed here, since this is not a primary anomaly of the skeleton, but it can be a component of certain disorders, especially diastrophic dwarfism (see p. 45), and trisomies 13 and 18 (see p. 303). Equinovarus is also one of the characteristic findings in the rare syndrome of Freeman-Sheldon (see p. 269).

Fusion of tarsal bones, which may be a dominant anomaly, is not recognized at birth, but only towards 14 or 15 years, because of a painful flat foot. Calcaneoscaphoid synostosis, which is most frequently seen, usually occurs bilaterally. Synostoses between astragalus and scaphoid or calcaneus occur considerably more rarely as just calcaneo-cuboid synostosis. Treatment will consist of a medio-tarsal and sub-talar double arthrodesis.

In some exceptional patients there may be association between a more or less complete carpal and tarsal fusion transmitted as a dominant lesion. Such is the case as one of the key findings in the syndrome of multiple synostoses (see p. 174). This can also be the case in acropectoro-vertebral dysplasia (type F; Grosse et al.) and transmitted as a dominant. This is also associated with complex anomalies of the fingers and toes—a broad thumb with a rudimentary duplication or a lack of fingers. A protruding sternum, a funnel chest, spina bifida oculta of L5 or S1 are further findings of this syndrome. In the dominant syndrome (Forney et al.), there is, in addition to the bony anomalies, congenital heart disease and deafness.

Another anomaly of the tarsal bones is duplication of cuneiforme or supernumerary bones. Among the latter the most frequently encountered is the os tibiale externum located above and medially to the tuberosity of the scaphoid. Occasionally local pain may be present during adolescence (Fig. 4-37).

In the dominant digitocalcaneal dysmophism described by Sallis and Beighton vertical angulation of the calcaneus is associated with a flexion deviation of the fingers.

METACARPO OR METATARSOPHALANGEAL ANOMALIES

We shall focus mainly on the brachydactylies, symphalangism, polydactyly, syndactyly, camptodactyly, and finally, the orodigitofacial syndrome, in which the anomalies of the fingers are one of the main symptoms. Some of these anomalies are seen relatively frequently in the general population, and it is important to be aware that many anomalies of fingers are present in a large segment of patients with malformation syndromes or mental retardation. We shall refer to some selected examples, but cannot attempt to give a general survey.

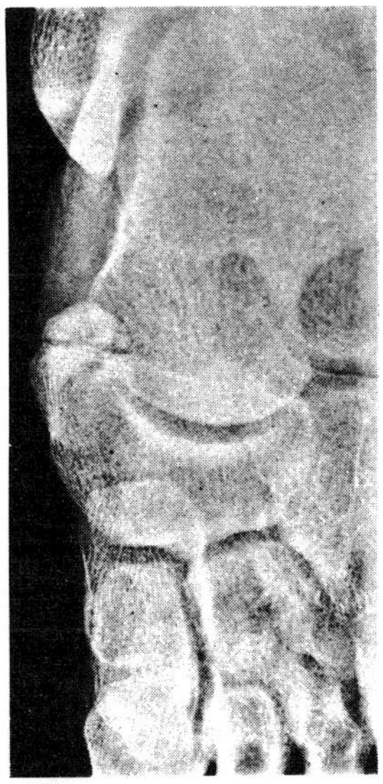

Fig. 4-37. Os tibial externum. (Courtesy of J. Lefevbre)

The Brachydactylies

Shortening of bony elements of the hand is often seen in a number of chondrodysplasias as discussed earlier. In some of these, such a finding is a key to diagnosing an underlying lesion, such as multiple epiphyseal dysplasia of the Léri-Silverköld type, for instance. We limit here the term brachydactyly to those patients who do not show the metaphyseal or epiphyseal changes typical for a constitutional skeletal disorder. Admittedly there is an arbitrary element in this type of distinction, since certain patients with brachydactyly also do have reduced height. This latter seems to be an expression of a more generalized skeletal involvement rather than one simply occurring with a shortening of the hands. It is important to carefully distinguish true brachydactylies and brachymetapodies, where shortening electively involves the metacarpals as well as brachydactyly of the thumb as shall be seen later. The real forms of brachydactyly, as has been proposed by Bell, can be further divided into three sub-groups. Brachydactylies of type A have elective involvement of the middle phalanx which is transmitted as a dominant. The proximal phalanx of the thumb and the toe may also be involved. Affected individuals usually are of small size—brachydactyly of the Farabee-type (Fig. 4-38, *Top, left*). The most common form of brachydactyly involves electively

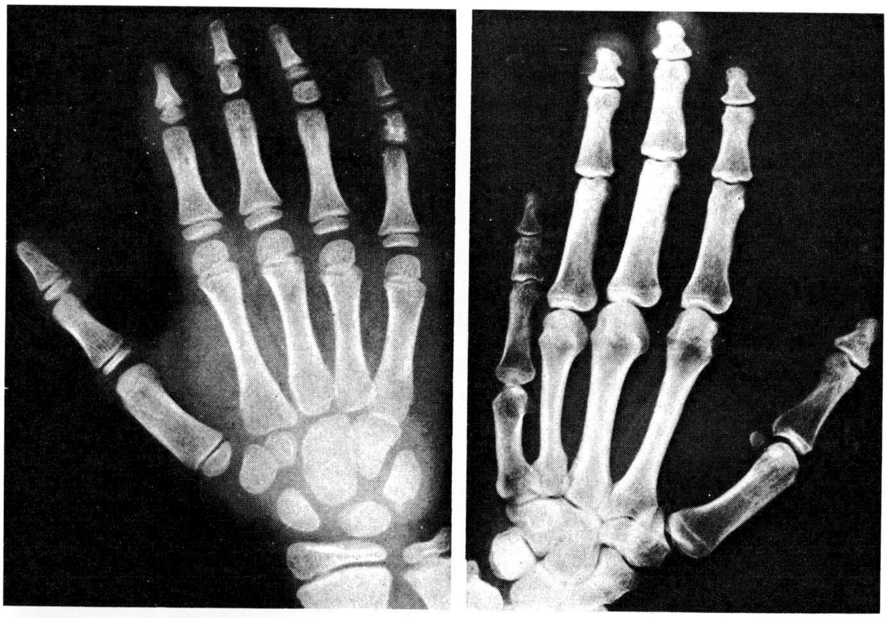

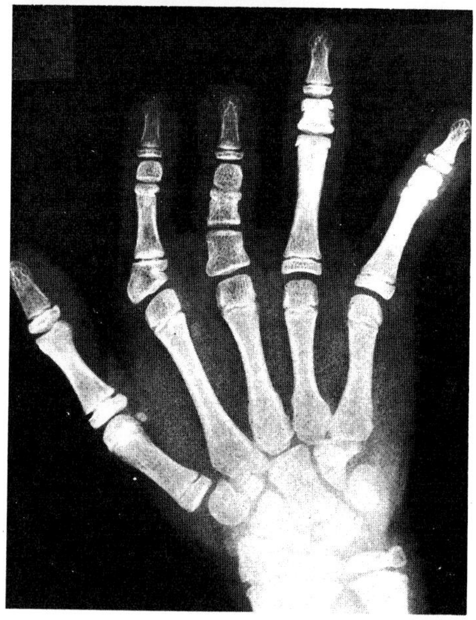

Fig. 4-38. Different types of brachydactyly with varying involvement of the middle phalanges (*top, left*), the distal phalanges (*top, right*), or of a more complex type (*bottom*). (Courtesy of R. Walbaum)

the fifth finger and leads to its bowing because of a trapezoid deformity of the phalanx, clinodactyly. This anomaly is commonplace and inherited as a regularly dominant trait. Isolated brachydactyly of the middle phalanx of the index finger, however, is very unusual.

In brachydactyly type B there is associated involvement of the very short or absent terminal phalanx with that of the middle phalanx (Fig. 4-38, *Top, right*). Occasionally there is mild syndactyly. In Sorsby's syndrome coloboma of the macula is combined with this type of brachydactyly and has a dominant transmission.

Brachydactyly of type C is more complex. Besides shortening of the middle phalanx of the second, third, and fifth fingers, and occasionally of their terminal phalanx, there may be supernumerary phalanges present as well as symphalangism. The metacarpals are also involved. Transmission is also dominant. A closely related type of brachydactyly is that of Vidal (Fig. 4-38, *Bottom*).

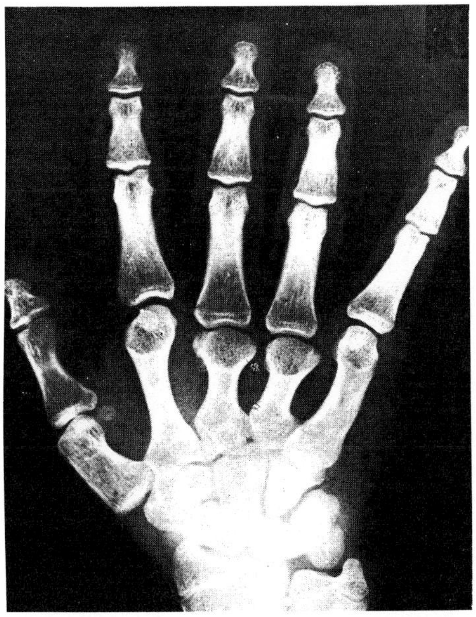

Fig. 4-39. Brachymetacarpalia. (Courtesy of R. Walbaum)

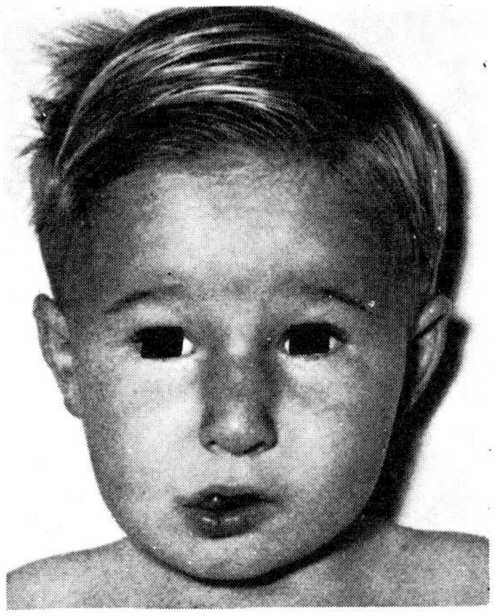

Fig. 4-40. Syndrome of multiple synostoses with facial disproportion.

Brachymetapody may be responsible not only for the shortening of metacarpals but also for their square and massive appearance. Most frequently this is accompanied by shortening of the phalanges, which have a similar square aspect (Fig. 4-39). The individuals involved usually are short, and it would appear that this dominant disorder actually results from diffusely disturbed enchondral growth, which may lead to its being listed as a dysostosis in the future. There are however other types of brachymetapodies. The syndrome described by Ruvalcaba and collaborators showed marked shortening of the metatarsals and of the distal phalanges. The study was of two brothers with mental retardation and facial dysproportion. Elective shortening of the fourth and fifth metacarpals is also one of the characteristic findings in certain syndromes such as Turner's syndrome, which will be discussed under the chromosomal aberrations or pseudo-hypoparathyroidism.

Brachydactyly can also be accompanied by syndactyly, and in particular by an absence of fingers. In the patients observed by Keutel, brachydactyly of the distal phalanges was associated with multiple stenoses of pulmonary arteries, inner ear deafness, and calcification of cartilage in the ear, nose, and trachea. Transmission in these cases was most likely by an autosomal recessive mode.

A special place must also be reserved for the syndrome of aplasia of the pectoralis muscle and dysdactyly of Poland. This disorder is characterized by unilateral symbrachydactyly associated with aplasia of the pectoralis major muscle of the same side. Most frequently there is smallness of the fingers with syndactyly of the first phalanx. In some patients there has also been a partial or total lack of middle fingers leading to a split hand. The humerus of the involved side may be slightly shortened. There also may be a mild deformity of the nose characterized by a poorly developed cartilaginous portion (Poland). Finally, there may be absence of the mammary gland of the involved side. This may only be noted at puberty. This syndrome occurs most frequently in individual patients, but there have been some familial observations—involvement of one parent or a cousin—which may suggest a genetic factor. The occurrence of acute leukemia has been reported several times in this syndrome (Walters et al.).

Anomalies of a somewhat similar type as in the syndrome of Poland have also been noted in the Moebius syndrome, where patients are affected by facial diplegia and paralysis of the oculomotor muscles, the muscles of the tongue, and those of mastication. Aplasia of the pectoralis, costal or vertebral malformations, and occasionally clubfoot may also be present.

Symphalangism

Symphalangism is characterized by a lack of interphalangeal articular differentiation. We can distinguish two types of symphalangism depending on whether the proximal or distal phalangeal joints are involved. Distal symphalangism is seen only rarely. There are

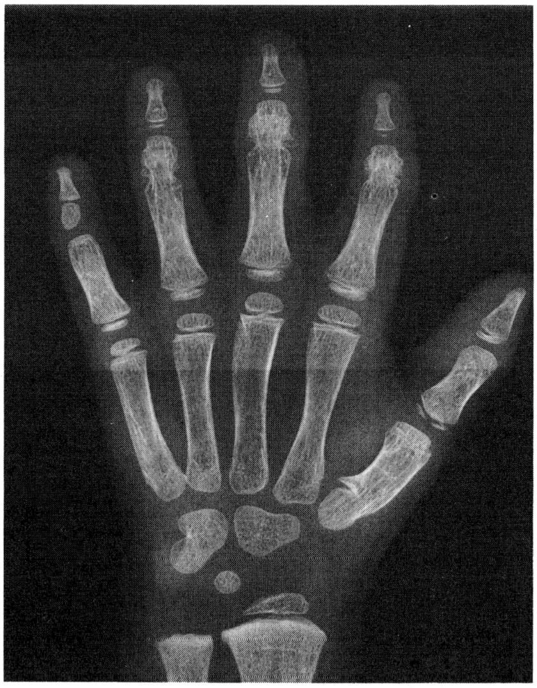

Fig. 4-41. Syndrome of multiple synostoses in a 3-year-old boy. There is fusion between the 2nd and 3rd phalanges which is not yet fully completed, and between the carpal elements.

hardly more than five observations recorded in the literature. Occasionally only a single finger (Schwartz) is affected. There is a higher incidence of the proximal type, and it appears to be part of a more generalized disorder, the syndrome of multiple synostoses.

The Syndrome of Multiple Synostoses

This disorder is usually recognized at birth, because of rigidity of the fingers or elbows.

The facial appearance is somewhat unusual. Those affected have a pointed nose and a wide nasal bridge (Fig. 4-40). Study of the hand will reveal marked interphalangeal rigidity of the second to the fifth finger, combined with absence of the corresponding skinfolds. Occasionally there may be partial or total amputation of the terminal phalanx of one or several fingers. Limitation of mobility of the wrist may be noted. The feet may be similarly involved. Sometimes there is underdevelopment of the toenails. Limitation of movements of the foot and of the tibiotalar joint may be present, but these findings are quite variable. There may also be involvement of the elbow, but this finding may be totally lacking. There are, however, patients whose elbows are completely blocked bilaterally. Another infrequent finding is deafness. Its onset is hardly ever noted before adolescence. It is a result of disturbed transmission. Beyond the deafness itself, the prognosis depends simply on the functional involvement. Growth is not affected.

Radiographic Findings

The phalangeal synostoses are not always identical and occur at different ages. In very early infancy there is a persisting narrow line between the first and second phalanges. The appearance of the second phalanx is quite variable. In some patients it may be almost normal, in others markedly shortened and hypoplastic. The terminal phalanx also has a variable appearance. It may be totally amputated at its most distal extremity or completely absent. The second and third metacarpals frequently are abnormally formed distally, and have a coarse aspect. Fusion of the carpal bones occurs in a completely irregular way. Most frequently they combine in two or three blocks. One block may combine the capitatum and hamatum with the scaphoid, and another the semilunar, trapezium, and trapezoid. Or the trapezium may combine with the first metacarpal bones (Fig. 4-41).

In the feet we also note great variability: symphalangism, sometimes amputation of toes, and massive or partial fusions of tarsal bones, especially between the cuboid and metatarsals. Involvement of the elbow is not invariably found either. Radiohumeral synostosis is characteristically present, since this by itself is an unusual malformation. Some cases, however, do not show complete fusion, but rather a marked deformity of the ends of the bones at the elbow. Some patients have an entirely normal elbow..

Genetic Data

The transmission of this disorder is dominant, but there can be a variable manifestation of the genes within a given family.

Polydactyly

Polydactyly is characterized by the presence of extra fingers. Most frequently, these are somewhat malformed.

There are a number of different types of polydactyly which cannot easily be classified. Usually we distinguish polydactyly by duplication of the thumb—preaxial polydactyly, or by duplication of the little finger—

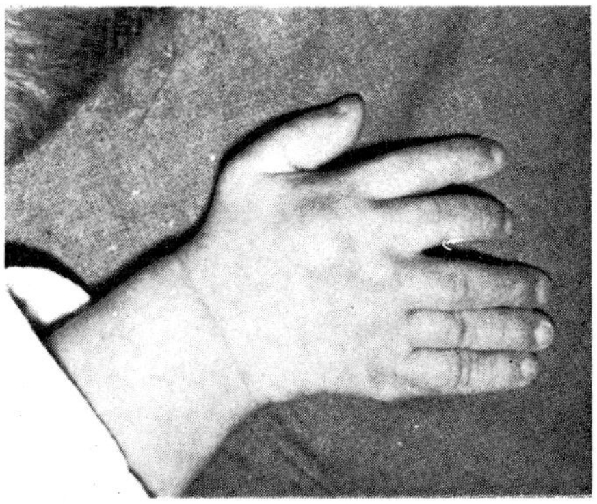

Fig. 4-42. Polydactyly.

postaxial polydactyly, and finally by duplication of the middle finger, which occurs somewhat more rarely. The duplication can manifest at the level of a joint. This results in a complete duplication distal to this point or by a duplication within one of the metacarpal or the phalangeal bones. An occasional patient has triplication of the thumb or of the fifth finger.

Another unusual type of polydactyly includes the duplication of the ulna and of the fingers two to five in the absence of the radius. This anomaly has been designated by Duhamel as schizomelia. It may also affect the lower extremity, where there may be a total absence of the fibula in the presence of two tibias. In such patients there will be either total lack of or marked hypoplasia of the thumb. Pfeiffer has described an analogous condition occurring as a dominant familial lesion with duplication of the fibula in the absence of a tibia.

In the most frequently seen type of polydactyly there is also malformation of the extra fingers. Sometimes there is simply a small appendage without skeletal elements, in others there may be reduction to just one or two phalangeal elements. More rarely the finger will be virtually normal (Fig. 4-42). Syndactyly is frequently also present, and occasionally the duplication manifests itself as a markedly wide first or fifth finger, and sometimes just by a broad appearance of the second phalanx of the thumb, if this is the only involved region. Duplication of the thumb may be accompanied by triphalangism.

The radiographic appearance is correspondingly variable. Duplication may similarly affect the metacarpal or phalangeal bones, but there may simply be bifidity of a metacarpal bone, isolated duplication of the phalanges or of the terminal phalanx only. This is most frequently the case at the distal end of the thumb. There is enormous variability in the appearance of the extra bony elements. As a rule, these extra bones are unusually slender or otherwise abnormally shaped.

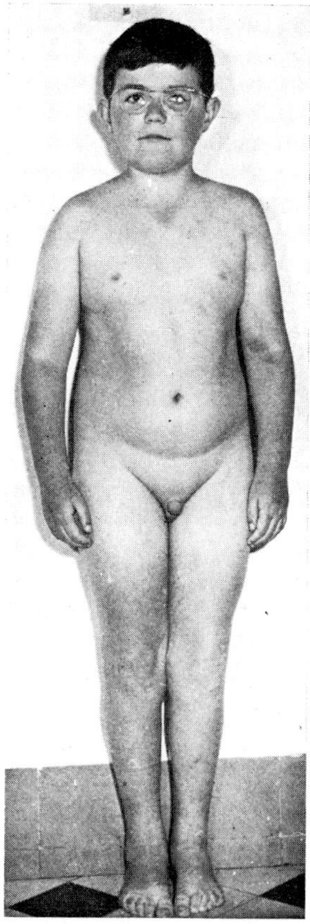

Fig. 4-43. Laurence-Moon-Biedl syndrome. (Taken from: Pédiatrie, CMC, Flammarion)

Polydactyly is frequently a dominant trait, but with variable expressivity. It may be one of the key elements of a syndrome, as it is in the Ellis-van-Creveld syndrome (see p. 58), the syndrome of Werner (see p. 178) or the Laurence-Moon-Bardet-Biedl syndrome. The associated anomalies are retinitis pigmentosa, obesity, hypogonadism, and mental retardation. This disorder is inherited as an autosomal recessive (Fig. 4-43). In the acrofacial dystososis of Weyers there is a combination of postaxial hexadactyly of the hands and feet with a midline fissure at the mandibular symphysis and other anomalies of the median incisors. The transmission is autosomal dominant.

In the Ullrich-Feichtiger syndrome, typus Rostockiensis or dyscraniopygophalangy, hexadactyly of the hands and feet is combined with facial dysmorphism, including micrognathia, anomaly of the external ear—and cryptorchidism (Weber, Plöchl).

Therapy of polydactyly is the surgical removal of the extra elements. This operation should be accomplished at about the midpoint of the first year.

Syndactyly

Syndactyly is characterized by the firm connection of two or several fingers. Several dominant types have been described. The most frequent one is a complete or partial syndactyly of the second and third fingers, which may be associated with the same phenomenon involving the second and third toes. Sometimes radiography will show fusion of the terminal phalanges. Isolated partial syndactyly of the second and third toes is quite frequently seen in the general population. Syndactyly of the fourth and fifth fingers is more rarely noted. The fifth finger is short with hypoplasia of its middle phalanx. Involvement is usually symmetrical, but the foot may not be involved (Johnston and Kirby). In rare instances there may be an associated fusion of the fourth and fifth metacarpals. All fingers may be fused, and such a condition may be combined with other skeletal anomalies (Cenani et al.).

Syndactyly may accompany polydactyly, and most frequently affects the third and fourth finger, or sometimes all of them (Haas). In some families we note the association of such an anomaly with cranio facial dysmorphism. This includes the fronto-digital syndrome of Marshall and Smith, involving a prominent forehead, and the familial observations by Hootnick and Holmes manifesting with hypertelorism.

Amongst the different types of syndactyly it would seem that acrosyndactyly (Walsh) should be considered separately. Here the fusion involves the distal portion of the finger with a free interval in its proximal portion. This malformation is associated with amputations of the fingers and congenital ridges. In more than one third of the patients there is involvement of the toes, and almost the same incidence of clubfoot. This anomaly does not seem to be familial.

Syndactyly may be part of a more complex entity, such as the following syndromes: acrocephalosyndactyly (see p. 148), autosomal recessive syndactyly, which is a cryptophthalmus syndrome involving the absence of the eyelids and genital or facial malformations, cleft palate or hairlip (Sugar) or the focal dermal hypoplasia syndrome. In the latter there is elective involvement of the second and third finger, or occasionally absence of a finger or polydactyly (see p. 120). Syndactyly may also be associated with an autosomal recessive or sex linked type of mental retardation (Scott et al.), or with a chromosomal aberration such as trisomy 21.

Therapy is limited to surgical intervention in an attempt to separate the involved fingers completely. This should be done at about 18 months or slightly earlier, particularly where the syndactyly is between two fingers with a markedly different rate of growth, such as thumb and index finger or the ring and little fingers, especially when one of these begins to be in a constantly flexed position. The operation is frequently much more complex than it would seem from looking at the hand.

Camptodactyly

This anomaly involves primarily soft tissue structures and has only a secondary effect on the underlying skeleton. Clinically there is a fixed flexion deformity of the proximal interphalangeal joint. This may result in some functional disturbance, when several fingers are similarly affected. Radiographic study of the involved finger in the lateral view may only show a slight curving of the tip of the first phalanx with a slightly anterior orientation of its articular surface. The normal articular concavity of the second phalanx is sometimes slightly displaced posteriorly and there may be a mild degree of subluxation. The fifth finger is very frequently involved, and occasionally several other fingers. Confusion must be avoided between camptodactyly and clinodactyly of the fifth finger. In the latter there is shortening and abnormal shape of the middle phalanx resulting in an incurved, but not a flexed, finger. Congenital polydactyly can be transmitted as an autosomal dominant disorder. It is part of many syndromes, such as the Freeman-Sheldon syndrome, oculodentodigital dysplasia, focal dermal hypoplasia, the orodigitofacial syndrome and the syndrome of Moldenhauer. Numerous other familial and dominant observations are on record combining captodactyly or other forms of fixed flexion deformity of the fingers with a number of different malformations including cleft palate, clubfoot (Gordon, et al.), deafness (Stewart and Bergström), and facial dysmorphism (Emery and Nelson).

Therapy is largely limited to an attempt at mobilizing the camptodactyly. This can be by extension of the finger, and, in the most severe cases, by surgical intervention. The results of such measures, however, are not convincing.

Other digital anomalies, including megalodactyly, where one or several fingers are excessively large, could also be discussed here. This hypertrophy may simultaneously involve bone and soft tissues. Some observers emphasize that the nerves are particularly thick in these lesions. The etiology is totally unknown. Delta-shaped middle phalanges, another rare anomaly, is recognized by a triangular aspect of the middle phalanges, with a proximal epiphysis outlining the distal border, and its retracted shape.

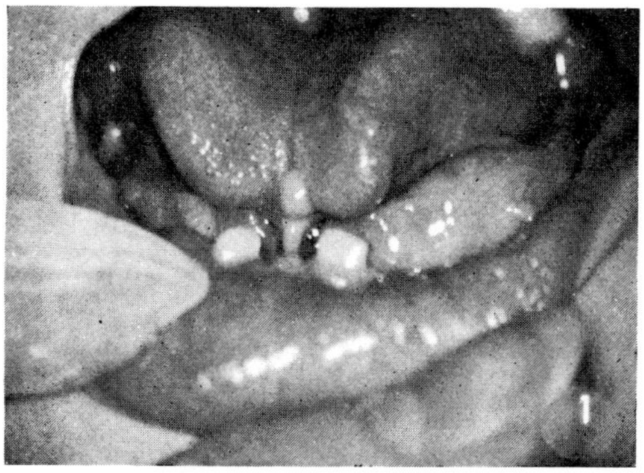

Fig. 4-44. Orodigitofacial syndrome. (Courtesy of A. Mugnier)

The Oro-Digito-Facial Syndrome

Described by Papillon, Léage and Psaume, this is the association of malformations of the hands and feet with those of the face and mouth. There may be incomplete syndactyly, clinodactyly, or brachydactyly. Involvement of the toes is somewhat less frequently seen, and is less dramatic. Polydactyly is unusual. The facial appearance includes slight frontal bossing, hypertelorism with epicanthus, a tiny and narrow nose results from hypoplasia of the alar cartilage, a mild midline defect of the upper lip, and dry and sparse hair. The tongue is large and lobulated, and has a very short frenulum. The palate is high, and sometimes there is a cleft of the soft palate. In addition there may be multiple gingival bands and dental anomalies – extra teeth, lack of teeth, particularly the lateral incisors, and enamel hypoplasia (Fig. 4-44). Half of the patients also suffer from mental retardation. Radiographically, the most typical finding is the shortening and square shape of the bony structures of the hands and feet, combined with irregular radiolucency and the presence of irregularly shaped islands of abnormally radiolucent tissue within central microgeodes (Fig. 4-45). This finding however is only recognized in about one-fourth of all patients. On lateral skull films there is an increase of the basal angle and an oblique anterior fossa. This results from the elevation of the cribriform plate and the small wings. The ascending branch of the mandible is often hypoplastic. This disorder is almost exclusively seen in females and therefore in all likelihood is fatal in males. It is possible, but not yet conclusively proven, that the gene responsible for its transmission might be located on the X-chromosome.

Therapy mainly concentrates on the surgical correction of the cleft palate and attention to the dental malalignment.

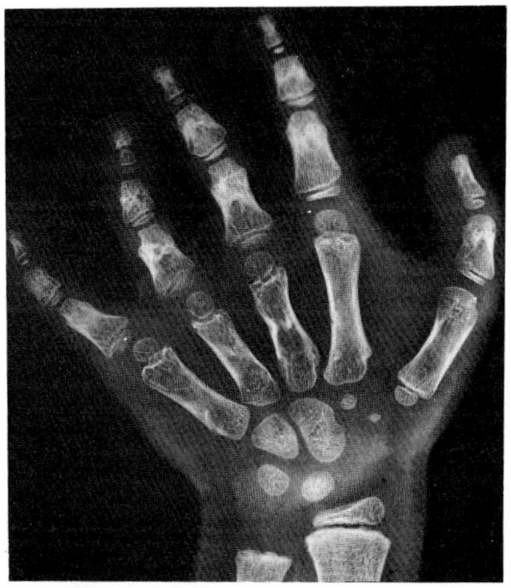

Fig. 4-45. Orodigitofacial syndrome. Note the presence of many small geodes within the phalanges. (Courtesy of M. L. Briard)

A similar condition is the syndrome of Mohr, with recessive transmission. The oral anomalies are however less dramatic, and a cleft palate is only rarely present. This syndrome is characterized by a partial duplication or enlargement of the big toe and sometimes by hexadactyly of the hand. This is only rarely noted in the orodigitofacial syndrome. The hair is normal, but deafness occurs frequently. The intellectual development is normal.

Radiographically, we have not yet seen microgeodes involving the phalanges in the Mohr syndrome. There is, however, a very broad, sometimes almost doubled, appearance of the phalanges of the big toe, and of the first metatarsal (Fig. 4-46). Further anomalies of the foot are occasionally present, such as a large cuboid and an extra cuneiforme. Widening of the metaphyses of the long bones has been reported (Rimoin).

Anomalies of the Thumb

The thumb is frequently the site of local malformations. An elective development of the thumb and of the big toe may be one of the elements of a dominant syndrome described (Stern et al.) as the hand-foot-uterus syndrome. In this condition there is an abnormal origin of the thumb and insufficient rotation. There may also be clinodactyly of the fifth finger and shortening of the large toe. Radiographically, there is shortening of the first metacarpal and first metatarsal bone, and also of the middle phalanx of the big toe. The end

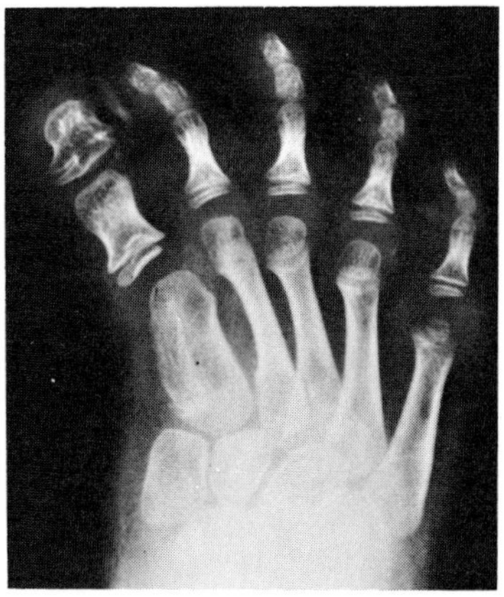

Fig. 4-46. Mohr's syndrome in an 8-year-old boy. There is abnormal development of the 1st metatarsal and of the bones of the big toes. (Courtesy of J. C. Dayras)

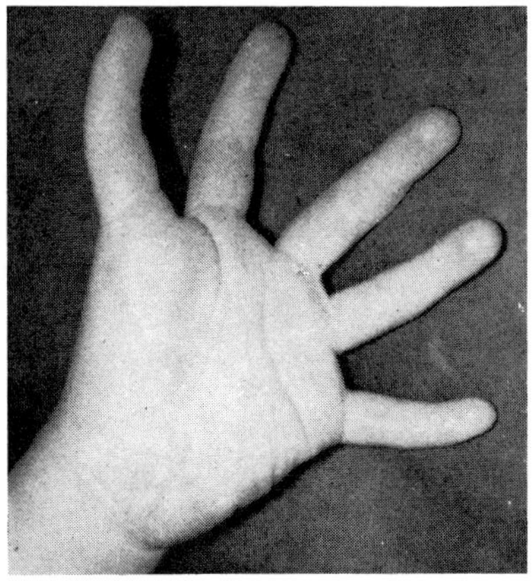

Fig. 4-47. Triphalangeal thumb in a patient with the Holt-Oram syndrome. (Courtesy of I. Emerit)

phalanx of the thumb and of the big toe is pointed. In addition, there is occasionally abnormal fusion of elements of the carpals and of the tarso-metatarsal region. Uterine anomalies can include a duplication with a bifid uterus, a total separation of double uterus, and a septate vagina.

Total absence of the thumb combined with polydactyly of the toes is one of the characteristic findings of the syndrome of Werner. Well studied by Pashayan and others, this syndrome combines in its complete form polydactyly of the foot, and occasionally of the hand, with a lack of the thumb. Tri-phalangeal fingers are arranged in the same plane, and there is aplasia or hypoplasia of the tibia. This disorder seems to be transmitted by a dominant gene with variable expressivity.

We shall now turn to a discussion of, and emphasis on, specific malformations of the thumb, triphalangism, and the syndrome of Holt-Oram.

Triphalangism of the Thumb

Schematically we can distinguish two different types. In one there is an almost normal morphology of this thumb since opposition is maintained. In the other, however, there is almost no morphological difference from the other four fingers (Fig. 4-47).

Radiographically, the first type is characterized by the presence of an extra wedge-shaped bony element of usually small size. This results in a medial or lateral deviation of the last phalanx. In the second type there may also be some degree of malformation of the intermediary bony phalangeal element, but this may be much more developed and practically comparable to that of the four other fingers.

According to Swanson and Brown both types can be transmitted as dominant lesions. The former, however, is not frequently seen in isolated patients, as is the latter, and it may more often by unilateral. Triphalangism of the thumbs is not always an isolated finding. It can be associated with aplastic anemia of a type close to the Blackfan-Diamond syndrome (Murphy and Lubin). Other sometimes familial observations of triphalangism of the thumb are on record in combination with dysplastic toenails and deafness (Quazi et al., Walbaum et al.).

The Holt-Oram Syndrome

This syndrome was isolated in 1960, and many familial observations have already been carefully studied. It is the association of an atrial septal defect of the ostium secundum and a disturbed heartrate with anomalies of the thumb. The first finger distally orients itself parallel to the other fingers, and often, but not always, has a third bony element (Fig. 4-48). In some patients there may be absence of the thumb, and occasionally there is a malformed thumb on one side and no thumb on the other. The first metacarpal may be of abnormal size, larger or smaller than average. Shortening of the middle phalanx of the fifth finger and clinodactyly are frequently present. Anomalies of carpal bones can be quite variable. The most frequently noted anomaly refers to the scaphoid, and sometimes an extra bony element may be present (Poznanski). Slight irregularity of the metaphysis of radius and ulna have been reported, together with an unusually long styloid process of the ulna.

The elbow sometimes shows an abnormal epicondylar prominence. Also there may be anomalies of the

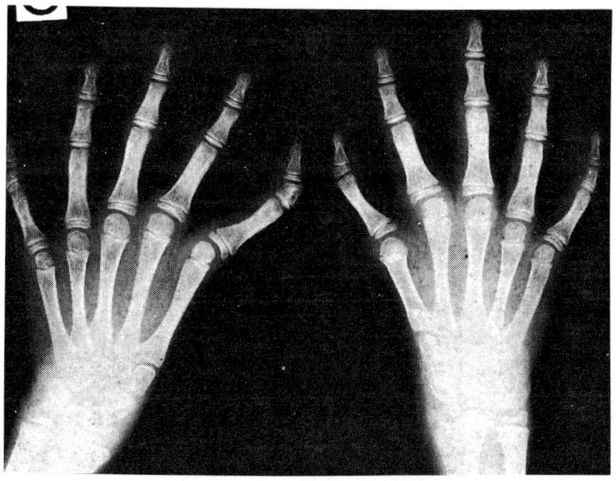

Fig: 4-48. Anomalies of the hand in a patient with the Holt-Oram syndrome. (Courtesy of I. Emerit)

shoulder: a small scapula, a short clavicle widened at its lateral end, and deformity of the humeral head. The sternum is also frequently involved. It may be short and protruding or almost at right angles to its normal position. A funnel chest has been reported. Somewhat more severe anomalies, such as total absence of the radius and hemivertebra have been described (Piussan et al.).

The Holt-Oram syndrome is transmitted as an autosomal dominant disorder, but there is variability of the manifestations of the gene, particularly with respect to the anomaly of the thumb.

Under the title cardiofacioskeletal syndrome, Blank has described a syndrome which combines the Holt-Oram syndrome with facial anomalies close to those of the Goldenhar syndrome.

THE ACRO-OSTEOLYSES

Osteolysis, or the progressive disappearance of one or several skeletal elements, is a very complex phenomenon. Schematically we can distinguish between two separate groups of disorders: massive osteolysis and acro-osteolysis. The different types of massive osteolysis, well described by Gorham, are characterized by a more or less rapid destruction of one or several elements of the skeleton. The onset always is referable to a single bone. Its etiology is still poorly understood, but there are post-traumatic cases. Such osteolytic processes can be characterized by local proliferation of a capillary tissue, almost similar to a hemangioma. We shall therefore study this problem, in the chapter on vascular tumors (see p. 392).

The acro-osteolyses result in the progressive disappearance of bone of the hands and of the feet. In the adult they are most frequently secondary to other disorders, such as syringomyelia, tabes, and rheumatoid arthritis. This is not the case in the pediatric age group. Acrodystrophic neuropathy, or Thévenard's syndrome, may have its onset during adolescence. Findings are a combination of peripheral sensory impairment, trophic changes, and ulcers, primarily of the soles of the feet. This condition will be discussed with the neurologic disorders (see p. 319).

We thus limit our discussion here mainly to idiopathic acro-osteolysis in its two main types. In one the onset involves the distal phalanges, whereas in the other onset electively involves the carpal and tarsal bones. In both types there is a marked variability in the age of onset.

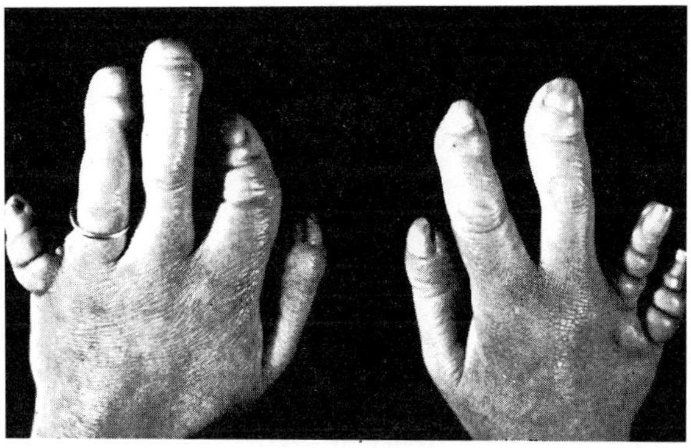

Fig. 4-49. Acroosteolysis with an "opera glass" deformity of several fingers.

ACRO-OSTEOLYSIS WITH DISTAL ONSET

The distal phalanges of the affected fingers are square in appearance while the toes and the nails become elliptic. The progressive shortening of the fingers is similar to a "lorgnette (opera glasses)" as described by Léri. Later there may also be deformity of the hand and of the wrist (Fig. 4-49). Usually there is no uniformity of the destruction present, since the fingers are affected to a markedly differing degree. As a rule, there is parallel development of changes of the feet. The evolution of the lesions is quite variable. In some instances they seem to progress in a regular and steady fashion and thus lead to considerable destruction, whereas, in other instances, there may be a trend towards stabilization.

Radiographically, the first changes are seen in the distal phalanges of fingers and toes. These may completely disappear. Sometimes there may still be some visible calcified or bony fragments within the zone of

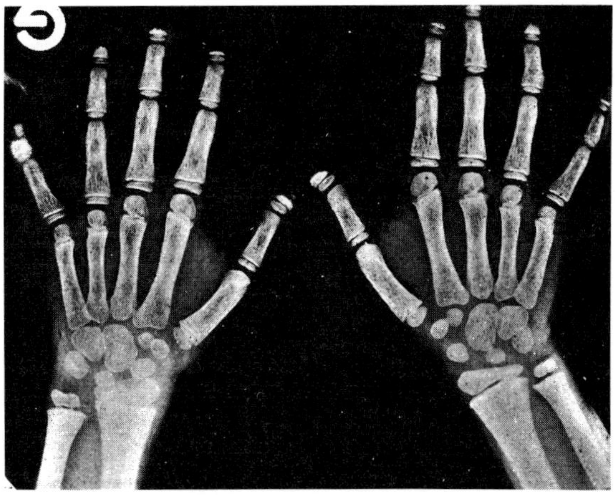

Fig. 4-50. Acroosteolysis with onset in the most distal segment in a 6-year-old boy. The ends of the distal phalanges and of the middle phalanges of the 5th finger have disappeared.

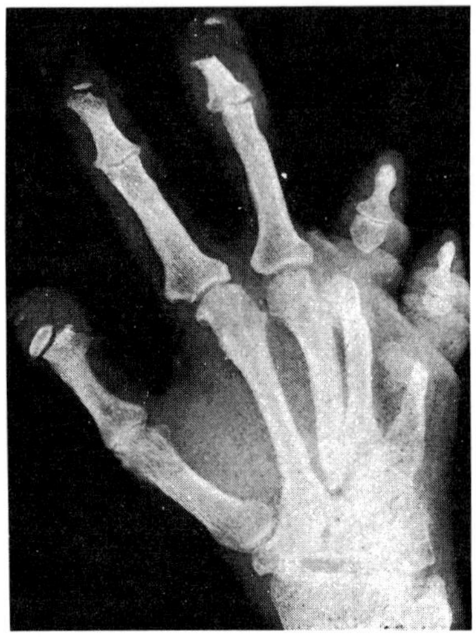

Fig. 4-51. Acroosteolysis with peripheral onset. Mother of the patient seen in Fig. 4-50. This comparison offers an idea of the progressive character of this disorder.

destruction (Fig. 4-50). Eventually other skeletal elements are affected. The distal ends of the phalanges or of the metacarpals are eroded from the sides, become narrow, and eventually disappear. The diaphysis assumes the characteristic appearance of a "sucked sugar cone." The carpal or tarsal areas may be involved with dramatic local changes, including loss of size, and finally, the reduction of the carpal elements to a small unidentifiable bony mass (Fig. 4-51). The same sequence of events takes place with the feet. In one patient other osteolyses have been noted involving the mandible and the clavicles (Harnasch). The disorder is heterogeneous, as suggested by genetic data. In some families a dominant transmission was noted (Lamy), whereas in others there was autosomal recessive transmission (Joseph et al.). Hajdu and Cheney have described a special dominant type which seems to begin with its manifestation in adolescence and is accompanied by an abnormal laxity and fractures and deformity of the skull in combination with early shedding of teeth. Radiographically, there is osteoporosis involving long bones as well as the spine. The vertebral bodies take the shape of a biconcave lens. Sometimes there is also abnormal metaphyseal modelling. The occipital region of the skull is elongated like a bun, sutures are widened, and many wormian bones are noted along with signs of basilar impression. The mandible is small, sometimes with a total lack of the lamina dura. These findings are reminiscent of osteogenesis imperfecta, but there are only a few fractures seen in such patients. Herrman has proposed for this type the name arthrodentoosteodysplasia, and Young, mandibulo-acraldysplasia.

Other patients suffer from plantar ulcerations, which would seem to suggest a possible relationship with those of Thévenard (Giaccai). Similar osteolytic findings can be seen during the course of progeria and in congenital insensitivity to pain (see Fig. 10-20 p. 319). In pycnodystosostosis we also note the disappearance of the distal end of the phalanges, however this is not a progressive lesion.

TYPE WITH CARPO-TARSAL ONSET

Affected patients usually will first complain of walking difficulties or a swelling of the wrists. Local inspection shows shortening of the wrists. The carpal region is swollen, and movements at the wrist, particularly flexion, are markedly limited. Some patients show local hyperlaxity. Later there is shortening of the forearms. The development of the lesions involving the feet is equally progressive. Initially there is a flat or often cavus appearance. Walking becomes more and more difficult.

Several authors have also emphasized the high incidence of renal disease in this type, since chronic nephritis may lead to death in such patients during early adult life. The progression of the bony lesions, however, seems to slow down, with stabilization in adolescence.

Radiographically, the earliest lytic changes involve the carpal and tarsal bones. Often bone age is ad-

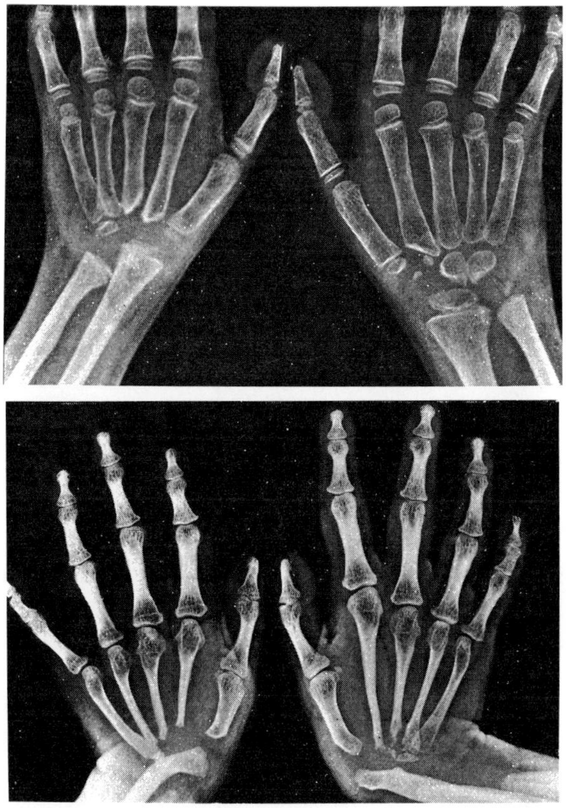

Fig. 4-52. Osteolysis beginning in the carpal region. These films were taken 12 years apart and show the progression of osteolysis. (Courtesy of J. Marie)

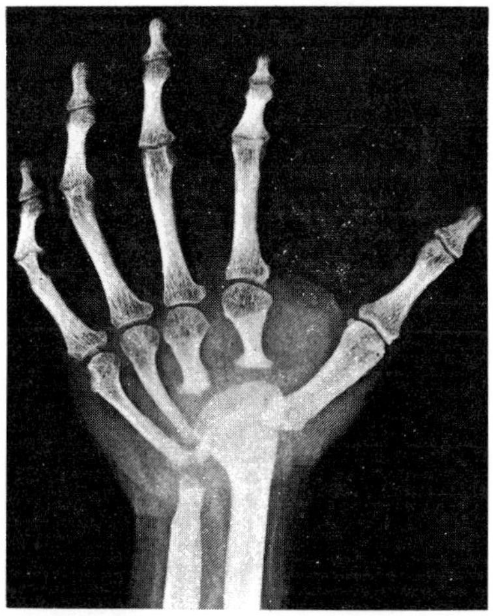

Fig. 4-53. Dermochondrocorneal dystrophy of François. (Courtesy of H. R. Wiedemenn)

vanced at the beginning of these manifestations (Fig. 4-52). This finding is especially well seen in patients with unilateral predominance. The bony elements of the carpus may later disappear almost completely, and the lytic process will then involve the bones of the forearm and the metacarpals. In the foot there is never complete disappearance of the tarsal bones. Lysis will be particularly dramatic in the medio-tarsal region, involving the scaphoid and the cuneiforme cunoid.

This type is transmitted as a dominant disorder, and it appears that the expressivity of the gene can be quite variable. Certain patients may only suffer from nephropathy, and others, only from osteolysis.

Another autosomal recessive type (Torg et al.) leads to a fusiform appearance of the fingers, pescavus and limitation of movements of several joints—knee, elbow, and hips—combined with subcutaneous nodules. Radiographically, osteoporosis is associated with osteolysis, not only of the carpal and tarsal bones, but also of the interphalangeal joints, and, though this has not been clearly described by these authors, most probably of other bony extremities.

Another disorder with marked osteolytic involvement has been described by François as dermochondrocorneal dystrophy (Fig. 4-53). Skeletal lesions are combined with corneal opacities and xanthomathous nodules of the skin in many regions such as the extensor surface of the joints of the fingers, the toes, the elbow, the external ear, and the nose. Sometimes there is an even wider involvement of the skeleton and of the joints of the extremities. In patients with this very unusual syndrome early hypercholestorolemia, albuminuria, and electroencephalographic anomalies have also been noted. Transmission probably follows an autosomal recessive mode. Somewhat similar osteolytic findings can be seen in patients with the Winchester syndrome (see p. 244).

The pathophysiology of all these types of acro-osteolysis is unknown. It is very likely that there is no uniform mechanism responsible for all of them. In certain patients local hypervascularisation of the lytic zone has been documented, and it is possible that vascular pathology may play a role. But it is equally likely that neural factors also play a role, as is suggested by observations with associated trophic disturbances.

Whatever the actual cause, these osteolyses are severe, because of their progressive character, and because of the possibility of a concomitant renal disorder, which may complicate matters in a patient suffering from acro-osteolysis with the onset by carpotarsal involvement.

REFERENCES

Isolated Craniostenoses. Clover Leaf Skull

ANDERSON (F. M.) et GEIGER (L.). Craniosynostosis. A survey of 204 cases. *J. Neurosurg., 1965,* **22**, *229-240.*

ANDERSON (H.) et PARANHOS GOMES (S.). Craniosynostosis. Review of the literature and indications for surgery. *Acta paediat. scand., 1968,* **57**, *47-54.*

ANGLE (C. R.), MCINTIRE (M. S.) et MOORE (R. C.). Cloverleaf skull : Kleeblattschädel-deformity syndrome. *Amer. J. Dis. Child., 1967,* **114**, *198-202.*

BENNETT (K. A.). Craniostenosis : a review of the etiology and a report of new cases. *Amer. J. phys. Anthrop., 1967,* **27**, *1-10.*

COMINGS (D. E.). The Kleeblattschädel syndrome — a grotesque form of hydrocephalus. *J. Pediat., 1965,* **67**, *126-129.*

FEINGLOD (M.), O'CONNOR (J. F.), BERKMAN (M.) et DARLING (D. B.). Kleeblattschädel syndrome. *Amer. J. Dis. Child., 1969,* **118**, *589-594.*

FREEMAN (J. M.) et BORKOWF (S.). Craniostenosis. Review of the literature and report of thirty-four cases. *Pediatrics, 1962,* **30**, *57-70.*

GAUDIER (B.), LAINE (E.), FONTAINE (G.), CASTIER (C.) et FARRIAUX (J.-P.). Les craniosynostoses (étude de vingt observations). *Arch. franç. Pédiat., 1967,* **24**, *775-792.*

HOLTERMÜLLER (K.) et WIEDEMANN (H.-R.). Kleeblattschädel-Syndrom. *Med. Mschr., 1960,* **14**, *439-446.*

LAITINEN (L.). Craniosynostosis. *Ann. Paediat. Fenn., 1956, supplém. 6.*

MOSS (M. L.). The pathogenesis of premature cranial synostosis in man. *Acta anat. (Basel), 1959,* **37**, *351-370.*

MÜKE (R.). Neue Gesichtspunkte zur Pathogenese und Therapie der Kraniosynostose. *Acta neurochir. (Wien), 1972,* **26**, *191-250.*

NEUMÄRKER (K.-J.) et NEUMÄRKER (M.). Klinischer und neuroradiologischer Beitrag zum Kleeblattschädelsyndrom. *Z. Kinderheilk., 1972,* **113**, *151-160.*

PEMBERTON (J. W.) et FREEMAN (J. M.). Craniosynostosis. A review of experience with forty patients with particular reference to ocular aspects and comments on operative indications. *Amer. J. Ophthal., 1962,* **54**, *641-650.*

SCHUCH (A.) et PESCH (H.-J.). Beitrag zum Kleeblattschädel-Syndrom. *Z. Kinderheilk., 1971,* **109**, *187-198.*

Craniofacial Dysostosis. Acrocephalosyndactyly

ALFIERI (A.), ALU (C.) et CECCARINI (M.). Dysostose cranio-faciale héréditaire (contribution à l'étude des rapports entre la maladie d'Apert et la maladie de Crouzon). *J. Génét. hum., 1967-1968,* **16**, *1-14.*

APERT (E.). De l'acrocéphalosyndactylie. *Bull. Soc. méd. Hôp. Paris, 1906,* **23**, *1310-1330,*

APERT (E.). Association de l'acrocéphalie avec des malformations symétriques des coudes (acrocéphalosynankie). *Bull. Soc. méd. Hôp. Paris, 1926,* **50**, *1432-1434.*

BARTSOCAS (C. S.), WEBER (A. L.) et CRAWFORD (J. D.). Acrocephalosyndactyly type III : Chotzen's syndrome. *J. Pediat., 1970,* **77**, *267-272.*

BLANK (C. E.). Apert's syndrome (a type of acrocephalosyndactyly), observations on a british series of thirty-nine cases. *Ann. hum. Genet., 1960,* **24**, *151-164.*

BONAMOUR (G.) et BONNET (M.). Les manifestations ophtalmologiques des dystrophies cranio-faciales. *J. Méd., Lyon, 1962,* **43**, *1839-1854.*

CARPENTER (G.). Case of acrocephaly with other congenital malformations. *Proc. roy. Soc. Med., 1909,* **2**, *45-53.*

CHOTZEN (F.). Eine eigenartige familiäre Entwicklungsstörung. *Mschr. Kinderheilk., 1932,* **55**, *97-122.*

CLERC (P.) et DEUMIER (R.). La surdité dans les dysplasies osseuses et les dysmorphies cranio-faciales. *Ann. Oto-Laryng. (Paris), 1958,* **75**, *852-874.*

CRUVEILLER (J.). Maladie d'Apert Crouzon. *Thèse Méd., Paris, n° 767, 1964.*

DUNN (F. H.). Non familial and non hereditary craniofacial dysostosis : a variant of Crouzon's disease. *Amer. J. Roentgenol., 1960,* **84**, *472-478.*

DUNN (F. H.). Apert's acrocephalosyndactylism. *Radiology, 1962,* **78**, *738-743.*

GNAMEY (D.) et FARRIAUX (J. P.). Syndrome dominant associant polysyndactylie, pouces en spatule, anomalies faciales et retard mental (une forme particulière de l'acrocéphalo-polysyndactylie de type Noack). *J. Génét. hum., 1971,* **19**, *299-316.*

HERRMANN (J.) et OPITZ (J. M.). An unusual form of acrocephalosyndactyly. *Birth Defects, Original Article Series, 1969, V n° 3, 39-42.*

HOGAN (G. R.) et BAUMAN (M. L.). Hydrocephalus in Apert's syndrome. *J. Pediat., 1971,* **79**, *782-787.*

JUBERG (R. C.) et CHAMBERS (S. R.). Case report. An autosomal recessive form of craniofacial dysostosis (the Crouzon's syndrome). *J. med. Genet, 1973,* **10**, *89-94.*

KALOUSTIAN (V. M. Der), SINNO (A. A.) et NASSAR (S. I.). Acrocephalopolysyndactyly, type II (Carpenter's syndrome). *Amer. J. Dis. Child., 1972,* **124**, *716-718.*

LEHRER (H. Z.) et FAMILIANT (J. W.). A concordant craniofacial dysostosis with enlarged parietal foramina in twins. *Radiology, 1969,* **92**, *127-130.*

LEMARIEY (A.), PAQUELIN (F.) et THOMAS (R.). La dysostose cranio-faciale de Crouzon. *Ann. Oto-Laryng. (Paris), 1962,* **79**, *773-788.*

NOACK (M.). Ein Beitrag zum Krankheitbild der Akrozephalosyndactylie (Apert). *Arch. Kinderheilk., 1959,* **160**, *168-171.*

PFEIFFER (R. A.). Dominant erbliche Akrocephalosyndaktylie. *Z. Kinderheilk., 1964,* **90**, *301-320.*

ROUGERIE (J.), DEROME (P.) et ANQUEZ (L.). Craniosténoses et dysmorphies cranio-faciales. Principes d'une nouvelle technique de traitement et ses résultats. *Neurochirurgie, 1972,* **18**, *429-440.*

SALDINO (R. M.), STEINBACH (H. L.) et EPSTEIN (C. J.). Familial acrocephalosyndactyly (Pfeiffer's syndrome). *Amer. J. Roentgenol., 1972,* **116**, *609-622.*

SCHÖNENBERG (H.). Akrocephalosyndaktylie (Apert-Syndrom). *Mschr. Kinderheilk., 1972,* **120**, *12-16.*

SUMMITT (R. L.). Recessive acrocephalosyndactyly with normal intelligence. *Birth Defects, Original Article Series, 1969, V n° 3, 35-58.*

TEMTAMY (S. A.). Carpenter's syndrome : acrocephalosyndactyly. An autosomal recessive syndrome. *J. Pediat., 1966,* **69**, *111-120.*

TEMTAMY (S.) et MCKUSICK (V. A.). Synopsis of hand malformations with particular emphasis on genetic factors. *Birth Defects, Original Article Series, 1969, V n° 3, 125-184.*

TESSIER (P.). Traitement des dysmorphies faciales propres aux dysostoses cranio-faciales (DCF) (maladies de Crouzon et d'Apert). Ostéotomie totale du massif facial. Déplacement sagittal du massif facial. *Neurochirurgie, 1971,* **17**, *295-322.*

TRIDON (P.) et THIRIET (M.). Malformations associées de la tête et des extrémités. *Paris, 1966, Masson et Cie, éd.*

VOGT (A.). Dyskephalie (Dysostosis craniofacialis, maladie de Crouzon, 1912) und eine neuartige Kombination dieser Krankheit mit Syndactylie der 4 Extremitäten (Dyskephalodactylie). *Klin. Mbl. Augenheilk., 1933,* **90**, *441-454.*

WAARDENBURG (P. J.). Eine merkwurdige Kombination von angeborenen Missbildungen doppelseitiger Hydrophtalmus verbunden mit Akrokephalosyndactylie, Herzfehler, Pseudohermaphroditismus und anderen Abweichungen. *Klin. Mbl. Augenheilk., 1934,* **92**, *29-44.*

Facial Dysostoses. Mandibulofacial Dysostoses

BARTSOCAS (C. S.) et PAPAS (C. V.). Popliteal pterygium syndrome : evidence for a severe autosomal recessive form. *J. med. Genet., 1972,* **9**, *222-226.*

BIMLER (H. P.). Ueber die microrhine Dysplasie. *Fortschr. Kieferorthop., 1965,* **26**, *417-434.*

BINDER (K. H.). Dysostosis maxillo-nasalis, ein arhinencephaler Miszbildungskomplex. *Dtsch. zahnärztl. Z., 1962,* **6**, *438-444.*

BOWEN (D. I.), COLLUM (L. M. T.) et REES (D. O.). Clinical aspects of oculo-auriculo-vertebral dysplasia. *Brit. J. Ophthal., 1971,* **55**, *145-154.*

BRILL (C. B.), HSU (L. Y. F.) et HIRSCHHORN (K.). The syndrome of ectrodactyly, ectodermal dysplasia and cleft lip and palate : report a family demonstrating a dominant inheritance pattern. *Clin. Genet., 1972,* **3**, *295-302.*

BROCHER (J. E. W.) et KLEIN (D.). Die Dysostosis mandibulofacialis im Röntgenbild. *Fortschr. Röntgenstr., 1960,* **93**, *67-79.*

BUDDEN (S. S.) et ROBINSON (G. C.). Oculoauricular vertebral dysplasia. Its association with sensorineural deafness and other abnormalities. *Amer. J. Dis. Child., 1973,* **125**, *431-433.*

BÜNNIGE (M.). Angeborene Zungen-Munddach-Verwachsung. *Ann. paediat. (Basel), 1960,* **195**, *173-180.*

CHRISTIAENS (L.), WALBAUM (R.), FARRIAUX (J. P.) et FONTAINE (G.). A propos de deux cas de dysplasie oculo-auriculo-vertébrale. *Pédiatrie, 1966,* **21**, *935-942.*

COLLINS (E. T.). Cases with symmetrical congenital notches in the outer part of each lower lid and defective development of the malar bones. *Trans. ophthal. Soc. U.K. 1933,* **20**, *190-192.*

DELAIRE (J.), BILLET (J.), LE DIASCORN (H.) et COUTURIER (J. C.). Le syndrome de Binder (quatre observations). *Rev. Stomatol. (Paris), 1970,* **71**, *257-269.*

FRANCESCHETTI (A.) et KLEIN (D.). The mandibulofacial dysostosis. A new hereditary syndrome. *Acta ophthal., 1949,* **27**, *144-224.*

FRANÇOIS (J.) et HAUSTRATE (L.). Anomalies colobomateuses du lobe oculaire et syndrome du premier arc. *Ann. Oculist. (Paris), 1954,* **187**, *340-368.*

FREIRE-MAIA (N.). A newly recognized genetic syndrome of tetramelic deficiencies, ectodermal dysplasia, deformed ears and other abnormalities. *Amer. J. hum. Genet., 1970,* **22**, *370-377.*

GOLDENHAR (M.). Associations malformatives de l'œil et de l'oreille, en particulier le syndrome dermoïde épibulbaire, appendices auriculaires, « fistula auris congenita » et ses relations avec la dysostose mandibulo-faciale. *J. Génét. hum., 1952,* **1**, *243-282.*

GORLIN (R. J.), JUE (K. L.), JACOBSEN (U.) et GOLDSCHMIDT (E.). Oculo-auriculovertebral dysplasia. *J. Pediat., 1963,* **63**, *991-999.*

GORLIN (R. J.) et PINDBORG (J. J.). Syndromes of the head and neck. *New York, 1964, McGraw-Hill Book Co., éd.*

GORLIN (R. J.), SEDANO (H. O.) et CERVENKA (J.). Popliteal pterygium syndrome. A syndrome comprising cleft lip-palate, popliteal and intercrural ptetygia, digital and genital anomalies. *Pediatrics, 1968,* **41**, *503-509.*

GORLIN (R. J.), ČERVENKA (J.) et PRUZANSKY (S.). Facial clefting and its syndromes. *Birth Defects, Original Article Series, 1971,* VII *n° 11, 3-49.*

HECHT (F.) et JARVINEN (J. M.). Heritable dysmorphic syndrome with normal intelligence. *J. Pediat., 1967,* **70**, *927-935.*

IDE (C. H.), JARUDI (N.), BINGHAM (H.) et WOLLSCHLAEGER (P. B.). Oculo-auriculo-vertebral (Goldenhar's syndrome). *Brit. J. Ophthal., 1972,* **56**, *911-913.*

KIND (H. P.). Popliteales Pterygiumsyndrom. *Helv. paediat. Acta, 1970,* **25**, *508-516.*

KLEIN (D.). Un curieux syndrome héréditaire : chéilo-palatoschizis avec fistules de la lèvre inférieure associé à une syndactylie, une onychodysplasie particulière, un ptérygion poplité unilatéral et des pieds varus équins. *J. Génét. hum., 1962,* **11**, *65-71.*

LONGAGRE (J. J.). The surgical management of mandibulo-facial dysostosis. *J. Génét. hum., 1964,* **13**, *351-384.*

MONNET (P.), BOULEZ (N.), NEUMANN (E.), MAYNARD (Y.) et HUMBERT (G.). Deux cas de dysostose mandibulo-faciale ou syndrome de Franceschetti. *Pédiatrie, 1960,* **15**, *537-544.*

PIERSON (M.), TRIDON (P.) et THIRIET (M.). A propos d'un complexe malformatif associant gueule de loup, rideau fibreux intermaxillaire, brides poplitées et syndactylies. *Rev. Pédiat., 1966,* **2**, *177-180.*

POMERLEAU (D.) et AMYOT (M.). Le syndrome oculo-auriculo-vertébral. *Un. méd. Can., 1972,* **101**, *462-465.*

ROBINSON (G. C.), WILDERVANCK (L. S.) et CHIANG (T. P.). Ectrodactyly, ectodermal dysplasia, and cleft lip-palate syndrome. Its association with conductive hearing loss. *J. Pediat., 1973,* **82**, 107-109.

ROVIN (S.), DACHI (S. F.), BORENSTEIN (D. B.) et COTTER (W. B.). Mandibulofacial dysostosis, a familial study of five generations. *J. Pediat., 1964,* **65**, *215-221.*

RÜDIGER (R.), HAASE (W.) et PASSARGE (E.). Association of ectrodactyly, ectodermal dysplasia, and cleft lip-palate. *Amer. J. Dis. Child., 1970,* **120**, *160-163.*

SAUVEGRAIN (J.) et NAHUM (H.). Hypertélorisme essentiel. *J. Radiol. Electrol., 1962,* **43**, *528-531.*

SUGAR (H. S.). The oculoauriculovertebral dysplasia syndrome of Goldenhar. *Amer. J. Ophthal., 1966,* **62**, *678-682.*

TERHAAR (B.). Oculo-auriculo-vertebral dysplasia (Goldenhar's syndrome) concordant in identical twins. *Acta Genet. med. (Roma), 1972,* **21**, *116-124.*

TRELAT (U.). Sur un vice de conformation très rare de la lèvre inférieure. *J. Méd. Chir. prat., 1869,* **40**, *442-445.*

WEYERS (H.) et THIER (C. J.). Malformations mandibulo-faciales et délimitation d'un syndrome oculo-cérébral. *J. Génét. hum., 1958,* **7**, *143-173.*

Pierre Robin Syndrome. Hypertelorism

ASSEMANY (S. R.), KAJII (T.) et GARDNER (L. I.). Syndrome of phocomelia with mandibular hypoplasia. *Helv. paediat. Acta, 1971,* **26**, *403-409.*

BIXLER (D.) et CHRISTIAN (J. C.). Pierre Robin syndrome occurring in two related sibships. *Birth Defects, Original Article Series, 1971,* VII *n° 11, 67-71.*

BORSELLI (L.). Lineamenti clinici, biometrici, radiologici e neurologici dell'ipertelorismo. *Minerva pediat., 1964,* **16**, *905-918.*

BUCHIGNANI (J. S.), COOK (A. J.) et ANDERSON (L. G.). Roentgenographic findings in familial osteodysplasia. *Amer. J. Roentgenol., 1972,* **116**, *602-608.*

CENTA (A.) et RASORE-QUARTINO (A.). La sindrome di Pierre Robin. Studio di sette casi. *Minerva pediat., 1967,* **19**, *2042-2048.*

COCKE (W., Jr.). Experimental production of micrognathia and glossoptosis associated with cleft palate (Pierre Robin syndrome). *Plast. reconstr. Surg., 1966,* **38**, *395-403.*

COCOZZA (G.) et FEROLA (R.). Considerazioni sulla sindrome ipertelorica di Greig nei suoi rapporti con altre cranio-sinostosipatologiche. *Pediatria (Napoli), 1958,* **66**, *592-613.*

COHEN (M. M., Jr.), SEDANO (H. O.), GORLIN (R. J.) et JIRASEK (J. E.). Frontonasal dysplasia (median cleft face syndrome) : comments on etiology and pathogenesis. *Birth Defects, Original Article Series, 1971,* VII *n° 11, 117-119.*

DUHAMEL (B.), HAEGEL (P.) et PAGES (R.). Morphogenèse pathologique. « Des monstruosités aux malformations ». *Paris, 1966, Masson, éd.*

ELSAHY (N. I.) et WATERS (W. R.). The branchio-skeleto-genital syndrome. A new hereditary syndrome. *Plast. reconstr. Surg., 1971,* **48**, *542-550.*

FANDRE (M.), COFFIN (R.), PENNAFORTE (F.) et PUIG (M.-Th.). Le syndrome de Pierre Robin. *Ann. Méd. Reims, 1967,* **4**, *93-98.*

GROS (Ch.), SACREZ (R.), LEVY (J. M.), WALTER (J. P.) et FRANCFORT (F. F.). Hypertélorisme avec malformations cranio-faciales encéphaliques et vertébrales multiples. *J. Radiol. Electrol., 1963,* **44**, *635-638.*

GROUCHY (J. DE), SALMON (Ch.), SALMON (D.) et MAROTEAUX (P.). Délétion du bras court d'un chromosome 13-15, hypertélorisme et phénotype haptoglobine HpO dans une même famille. *Ann. Génét., 1966,* **9**, *80-85.*

JERESATY (R. M.), HUSZAR (R. J.) et BASU (S.). Pierre Robin syndrome. Cause of respiratory obstruction, cor pulmonale and pulmonary edema. *Amer. J. Dis. Child., 1969,* **117**, *710-716.*

PENA (J.), MORENO DE ORBE (M.), BURGUERA (B.), SUAREZ NUNEZ (J. M. D.), TABOADA (R.) et DOMINGUEZ (J.). Cinco observaciones de Sindrome de Pierre Robin. Con una nota sobre la evolucion longitudinal. *Rev. esp. Pediat., 1965,* **21**, *703-726.*

PENDL (G.) et ZIMPRICH (H.). Ein Beitrag zum Syndrom des Hypertelorismus Greig. *Helv. paediat. Acta, 1971,* **26**, *319-325.*

SACREZ (R.), FRANCFORT (J.-J.), GIGONNET (J.-M.), BEAUVAIS (P.) et BOLL (G.). A propos de la débilité intellectuelle et d'anomalies associées à la triade symptomatique du syndrome de Pierre Robin. *Sem. Hôp. Paris, 1967,* **43**, *28-33.*

SEDANO (H. O.), COHEN (M. M., Jr.), JIRASEK (J. E.) et GORLIN (R. J.). Frontonasal dysplasia. *J. Pediat., 1970,* **76**, *906-913.*

WALDEN (R. H.), LOGOSSO (R. D.) et BRENNAN (L.). Pierre Robin syndrome in association with combined congenital lengthening and shortening of the long bones. *Plast. reconstr. Surg., 1971,* **48**, *80-82.*

Oculo-Mandibulo-Facial Syndrome. Basal Cell Carcinoma Syndrome

AUBRY (M.). Variété singulière d'alopécie congénitale; alopécie suturale. *Ann. Derm. Syph. (Paris), 1893,* **4**, *899-900.*

COHEN (M. M., Jr.), HALL (B. D.), SMITH (D. W.), GRAHAM (C. B.) et LAMPERT (K. J.). A new syndrome with hypotonia, obesity, mental deficiency and facial, oral, ocular, and limb anomalies. *J. Pediat., 1973,* **83**, *280-283.*

FERRIER (P. E.) et HINRICHS (W. L.). Basal-cell carcinoma syndrome. *Amer. J. Dis. Child., 1967,* **113**, *538-545.*

FRANÇOIS (J.). A new syndrome. Dyscephalia with bird face and dental anomalies, nanism, hypotrichosis, cutaneous atrophy, microphthalmia, and congenital cataract. *Arch. Ophthal., 1958,* **60**, *842-862.*

GUYARD (M.), PERDRIEL (G.) et CERUTI (F.). Sur deux cas de syndrome dyscéphalique à tête d'oiseau. *Bull. Soc. franç. Ophtal., 1962,* **62**, *443-447.*

HALLERMANN (W.). Vogelgesicht und Cataracta congenita. *Klin. Mbl. Augenheilk., 1948,* **113**, *315-318.*

KURLANDER (G. J.), LAVY (N. W.) et CAMPBELL (J. A.). Roentgen differentiation of the oculodentodigital syndrome and the Hallermann-Streiff syndrome in infancy. *Radiology, 1966,* **86**, *77-86.*

LAMY (M.), JAMMET (M.-L.), MAROTEAUX (P.) et AJJAN (N.). La dyscéphalie (syndrome de Hallermann-Streiff-François). *Arch. franç. Pédiat., 1965,* **22**, *929-938.*

MEERKOTTER (V. A.) et SHEAR (M.). Multiple primordial cysts associated with bifid rib and ocular defects. *Oral Surg., 1964,* **18**, *498-503.*

SCHWEISGUTH (O.), GÉRARD-MARCHANT (R.) et LEMERLE (J.). Nævomatose basocellulaire, association à un rhabdomyosarcome congénital. *Arch. franç. Pédiat., 1968,* **25**, *1083-1093.*

STREIFF (E. B.). Dysmorphie mandibulo-faciale (tête d'oiseau) et altérations oculaires. *Ophtalmologica (Basel), 1950,* **120**, *79.*

Spinal and Costal Dysostoses

AMUSO (S. J.) et MANKIN (H. J.). Hereditary spondylolisthesis and spina bifida. Report of a family in which the lesion is transmitted as an autosomal dominant through three generations. *J. Bone Jt Surg., 1967,* **49-A**, *507-513.*

ASSEMANY (S. R.), MUZZO (S.) et GARDNER (L. I.). Syndrome of phocomelic diabetic embryopathy (Caudal dysplasia). *Amer. J. Dis. Child., 1972,* **123**, *489-491.*

BANTA (J. V.) et NICHOLS (O.). Sacral agenesis. *J. Bone Jt Surg., 1969,* **51-A**, *693-703.*

CARNEY (R. G.) et CARNEY (R. G., Jr.). Incontinentia pigmenti. *Arch. Derm., 1970,* **102**, *157-162.*

CASTROVIEJO (I. P.), RODRIGUEZ-COSTA (T.) et CASTILLO (F.). Spondylothoracic dysplasia in three sisters. *Develop. Med. Child Neurol., 1973,* **15**, *348-354.*

CHAPTAL (J.), JEAN (R.), BONNET (H.), DOSSA (D.) et FONVILLE (Cl.). Agénésie du sacrum : quatre observations. *Pédiatrie, 1965,* **20**, *793-804.*

DAVID-SAAL (C.). Les agénésies lombo-sacrées. *Thèse Méd., Paris, 1971.*

FOIX (C.) et HILLEMAND (P.). Dystrophie cruro-vésicofessière par agénésie sacro-coccygienne. *Rev. neurol., 1924,* **40**, *450-468.*

Godlewski (S.) et Dry (J.). Les anomalies congénitales de la charnière cervico-occipitale. *Paris, 1964, Expansion scient. franç., éd.*

Graf (K.). Angeborene Taubstummheit und okzipitozervikale Skelettmissbildung (Wildervanck-Syndrom). *Pract. oto-rhino-laryng. (Basel), 1968,* **30**, *82-89.*

Gunderson (C. H.), Greenspan (R. H.), Glaser (G. H.) et Lubs (H. A.). The Klippel-Feil syndrome : genetic and clinical reevaluation of cervical fusion. *Medicine (Baltimore), 1967,* **46**, *491-512.*

Jalladeau (J.). Malformations congénitales associées au syndrome de Klippel-Feil. *Thèse Med., Paris, 1936*

Klippel (M.) et Feil (A.). Un cas d'absence des vertèbres cervicales avec cage thoracique remontant jusqu'à la base du crâne. *Nouv. Iconogr. Salpêt., 1912,* **25**, *223-250.*

Klippel (M.) et Feil (A.). Anomalie de la colonne vertébrale par absence des vertèbres cervicales, cage thoracique remontant jusqu'à la base du crâne. *Bull. Soc. anat. Paris, 1912,* **87**, *185-188.*

Lamy (M.), Garcin (R.), Duperrat (B.), Aussannaire (M.), Jammet (M.-L.) et Touraine (R.-L.). L'incontinentia pigmenti (maladie de Bloch-Sulzberger). *Arch. franç. Pédiat., 1958,* **15**, *577-585.*

Lenz (W.) et Kucera (J.). L'étiologie de la régression caudale (agénésie du sacrum). *Méd. Hyg. (Genève), 1967,* **25**, *241-243.*

Lourie (H.). Sacral agenesis. Case report. *J. Neurosurg., 1973,* **38**, *92-95.*

Moldenhauer (E.). Zur Klinik des Nielson-Syndroms. *Derm. Wschr., 1964,* **150**, *594-601.*

Morrison (S. G.), Perry (L. W.) et Scott (L. P. III). Congenital Brevicollis (Klippel-Feil syndrome) and cardiovascular anomalies. *Amer. J. Dis. Child., 1968,* **115**, *614-620.*

Moseley (J. E.) et Bonforte (R. J.). Spondylothoracic dysplasia. A syndrome of congenital anomalies. *Amer. J. Roentgenol., 1969,* **106**, *166-169.*

Palant (D. I.) et Carter (B. L.). Klippel-Feil syndrome and deafness. *Amer. J. Dis. Child., 1972,* **123**, *218-221.*

Pfeiffer (R. A.). Zur Frage der Vererbung der Incontinentia pigmenti Bloch-Siemens. *Z. menschl. Vererb. Konstit. Lehre, 1960,* **35**, *469-493.*

Pizon (P.). Les anomalies vertébrales lombo-sacrées d'origine ostéogénétique. *J. Radiol. Electrol., 1962,* **43**, *32-44.*

Pochaczevsky (R.), Ratner (H.), Perles (D.), Kassner (G.) et Naysan (P.). Spondylothoracic dysplasia. *Radiology, 1971,* **98**, *53-58.*

Rabushka (S. E.), Love (L.) et Kadison (H. I.). Isolated thoracic dysostosis. *Radiology, 1973,* **106**, *161-165.*

Rimoin (D. L.), Fletcher (B. D.) et McKusick (V. A.). Spondylocostal dysplasia. A dominantly inherited form of short-trunked dwarfism. *Amer. J. Med., 1968,* **45**, *948-953.*

Sauvegrain (J.) et Mareschal (J.-L.). Malformations de la charnière cranio-cervicale chez l'enfant. A propos de 35 observations. *Ann. Radiol., 1972,* **15**, *263-277.*

Simonin (J. L.). Le spondylolisthésis lombaire. Indications respectives du traitement médical et chirurgical. *Gaz. méd. Fr., 1969,* **76**, *5011-5021.*

Singh (S. P.), Rock (E. H.) et Shulman (A.). Klippel-Feil syndrome with unexplained apparent conductive hearing loss. A case report. *Laryngoscope, 1969,* **79**, *113-117.*

Thalhammer (O.), Lachmann (D.) et Scheibenreiter (S.). « Caudale Regression » beim Kind einer 18 jährigen Frau mit Prädiabetes. *Z. Kinderheilk., 1968,* **102**, *346-355.*

Weber (V.), Schneider (H. J.) et Haberlandt (W.). Pathogenetische und genetische Fragen beim Klippel-Feil Syndrom, vergleichende Betrachtungen bei zwei Vettern. *Fortsch. Röntgenstr., 1973,* **119**, *209-215.*

Wildervanck (L. S.). Een geval van aandoening van Klippel-Feil, gecombineerd met abducensparalyse, retractio bulbi en doofstomheid. *Ned. T. Geneesk., 1952,* **96**, *2752-2755.*

Zünkeler (K. G.). Ueber die Variationen der Wirbelsäule. Vergleichende Betrachtung bei Mensch und Tier. *Z. menschl. Vererb. Konstitlehre, 1963,* **36**, *431-468.*

Anomalies of the Bones of the Shoulder and the Pelvis

Alain (J. L.) et Rigault (P.). Onycho-arthro-dysplasie héréditaire. *Rev. Chir. orthop., 1972,* **58**, *623-628.*

Bennett (W. M.), Musgrave (J. E.), Campbell (R. A.), Elliot (D.), Cox (R.), Brooks (R. E.), Lovrien (E. W.), Beals (R. K.) et Porter (G. A.). The nephropathy of the nail-patella syndrome. *Amer. J. Med., 1973,* **54**, *304-319.*

Cowell (H. R.). Hereditary onycho-osteodysplasia. Report of a kindred with dysplasia of the fifth finger. *Clin. orthop. rel. Res., 1971,* **76**, *43-53.*

Darlington (D.) et Hawkins (C. F.). Nail-patella syndrome with iliac horns and hereditary nephropathy. Necropsy report and anatomical dissection. *J. Bone Jt Surg., 1967,* **49-B**, *164-174.*

Deragna (S.) et Cocciante (G.). Sprengel's congenital deformity. A clinical contribution. *Panminerva med., 1967,* **9**, *108-111.*

Duncan (J. G.) et Souter (W. A.). Hereditary onycho-osteodysplasia. The nail-patella syndrome. *J. Bone Jt Surg., 1963,* **45-B**, *242-258.*

Fauré (C.) et Petrel (Ph.). L'ostéo-onycho-dysplasie héréditaire. *Ann. Radiol., 1968,* **11**, *376-388.*

Fong (E. E.). « Iliac-horns » (symetrical bilateral central posterior iliac processes) case report. *Radiology, 1946,* **47**, *517-518.*

Hakosalo (J.), Similä (S.), Vesa (L.) et Järvi (J.). Renal abnormalities in hereditary onycho-osteodysplasia. *Ann. Paediat. Fenn., 1968,* **14**, *55-60.*

Kieser (W.). Die sog. Flughaut beim Menschen. *Z. menschl. Vererb. Konstit. Lehre, 1939,* **23**, *594-619.*

Kosenow (W.), Niederle (J.) et Sinios (A.). Becken-Schulter-Dysplasie. *Fortschr. Röntgenstr., 1970,* **113**, *39-48.*

Lester (A. M.). Familial dyschondroplasia associated with anonychia and other diformities. *Lancet, 1936,* **ii**, *1519-1521.*

Mande (R.), Loubry (P.) et Roustan (R.). L'onycho-ostéo-dysplasie héréditaire. *Sem. Hôp. Paris, 1967,* **43**, *34-41.*

Morita (T.), Laughlin (L. O.), Kawano (K.), Kimmelstiel (P.), Suzuki (Y.) et Churg (J.). Nail-patella syndrome. Light and electron microscopic studies of the kidney. *Arch. intern. Med., 1973,* **131**, *271-277.*

Silverman (M. E.), Goodman (R. M.) et Cuppage (F. E.). The nail-patella syndrome. Clinical findings and ultrastructural observations in the kidney. *Arch. intern. Med., 1967,* **120**, *68-74.*

TURNER (J. W.). A hereditary arthro-dysplasia associated with hereditary dystrophy of the nails. *J. amer. med. Ass., 1933,* **100**, *882-884.*

WILSON (M. G.), MIKITY (V. G.) et SHINNO (N. W.). Dominant inheritance of Sprengel's deformity. *J. Pediat., 1971,* **79**, *818-821.*

Dysostoses Electively Involving the Extremities

BAGGIO (P.). Communication personnelle.

BAILEY (J. A. II) et BEIGHTON (P.). Bilateral femoral dysgenesis. *Clin. Pediat., 1970,* **9**, *668-674.*

BAIN (A. D.) et BARRETT (H. S.). Congenital bowing of the long bones : report of a case. *Arch. Dis. Childh., 1959,* **34**, *516-524.*

BEALS (R. K.). Auriculo-osteodysplasia. A syndrome of multiple osseous dysplasia, ear anomaly, and short stature. *J. Bone Jt Surg., 1967,* **49-A**, *1541-1550.*

BIRCH-JENSEN (A.). Congenital deformities of the upper extremities. *In* Opera ex Domo Biologiae hereditariae humanae Universitatis hafniensis, vol. 19. Copenhague, *1949, Ejnar Munksgaard, éd.*

BOUVET (J. P.). Communication personnelle.

BOWEN (P.), LEE (C. S. N.), ZELLWEGER (H.) et LINDENBERG (R.). Familial syndrome of multiple congenital defects. *Bull. Johns-Hopk. Hosp., 1964,* **114**, *402-414.*

CAFFEY (J.). Prenatal bowing and thickening of tubular bones, with multiple cutaneous dimples in arms and legs. *Amer. J. Dis. Child., 1947,* **74**, *543-562.*

DANLOS, APERT et FLANDIN. Micromélie congénitale. *Nouv. Iconogr. Salpêt., 1909,* **22**, *682-688.*

DAUM (R.), HEISS (W.) et WENZ (W.). Die menschliche « Sirene ». Ein Beitrag aus klinisch-röntgenologischer Sicht. *Z. Kinderheilk., 1969,* **105**, *296-302.*

DRESHER (C. S.) et MACDONELL (J. A.). Total amelia. *J. Bone Jt Surg., 1965,* **47-A**, *511-516.*

DUHAIME (M.), SIMONEAU (R.), DAZIONO (L.), FAVREAU (J. C.), GAUTHIER (B.) et LABELLE (P.). Les pseudarthroses congénitales du tibia (quinze observations). *Un. méd. Can., 1972,* **101**, *1832-1837.*

FELDMÜLLER (M.). Ein Beitrag zur kongenitalen Aplasie des Humeroradialgelenkes (HRS). *Fortschr. Röntgenstr., 1972,* **117**, *69-71.*

FELMAN (A. H.) et KIRKPATRICK (J. A., Jr.). Madelung's deformity : observations in 17 patients. *Radiology, 1969,* **93**, *1037-1042.*

FOCK (G.) et SULAMAA (M.). Congenital short femur. *Acta orthop. scand., 1965,* **36**, *294-300.*

FRANTZ (C. H.) et O'RAHILLY (R.). Congenital skeletal limb deficiencies. *J. Bone Jt Surg., 1961,* **43-A**, *1202-1224.*

FREIRE-MAIA (N.). The handless and footless families of Brazil. *Lancet, 1970,* **i**, *519-520.*

FUHRMANN (W.), STEFFENS (CH.) et ROMPE (G.). Dominant erbliche doppelseitige Dysplasie und Synostose des Ellenbogengelenks mit symmetrischer Brachymesophalangie und Brachymetakarpie sowie Synostosen im Finger-, Hand-und Fusswurzelbereich. *Humangenetik, 1966,* **3**, *64-75.*

GARNER (L. G.) et BIXLER (D.). Micrognathia, an associated defect of Hanhart's syndrome, types II and III. *Oral Surg., 1969,* **27**, *601-606.*

GREITZER (L. J.), JOWES (K. L.), SCHNALL (B. S.) et SMITH (D. W.). Craniosynostosis radial aplasie syndrome. *J. Pédiat., 1974,* **84**, *723-724.*

GRISLAIN (J.), MAINARD (R.), BERRANGER (P. de), BRELET (G.), CADUDAL (J. L.) et BILLET (J.). Aglossie-adactylie et syndrome d'Hanhart. A propos de deux observations. *Pédiatrie, 1971,* **26**, *353-364.*

GROBELSKI (M.). Die angeborene tibiofibulare Synostose am distalen Ende des Unterschenkels. *Arch. orthop. Unfall-Chir., 1965,* **57**, *190-193.*

HALL (C. B.), BROOKS (M. B.) et DENNIS (J. F.). Congenital skeletal deficiencies of the extremities. *J. amer. med. Ass., 1962,* **181**, *590-599.*

HALL (B. D.) et GREENBERG (M. H.). Hypomelia-hypotrichosis-facial hemangioma syndrome (pseudothalidomide, SC-syndrome, SC-phocomelia syndrome). *Amer. J. Dis. Child., 1972,* **123**, *602-604.*

HANHART (E.). Ueber die Kombination von Peromeli mit Mikrognathie, ein neues Syndrom beim Menschen, entsprechend der « Akroteriasis congenita » von Wriedt und Mohr beim Rinde. *Arch. Klaus-Stift. Vererbforsch., 1950,* **25**, *531-544.*

HARRIS (L. C.) et OSBORNE (W. P.). Congenital absence or hypoplasia of the radius with ventricular septal defect : ventriculoradial dysplasia. *J. Pediat., 1966,* **68**, *265-272.*

HERRMANN (J.), FEINGOLD (M.), TUFFLI (G. A.) et coll. A familial dysmorphogenetic syndrome of limb deformities, characteristic facial appearance and associated anomalies : the « pseudothalidomide » or « SC-syndrome ». *Birth Defects, Original Article Series, 1969,* V *n° 3, 81-89.*

HEYMAN (C. H.) et HERNDON (C. M.). Congenital posterior angulation of tibia. *J. Bone Jt Surg., 1949,* **31-A**, *571-580.*

HOHMANN (G.). Beitrag zur radio-ulnaren Synostose. *Arch. orthop. Unfall-Chir., 1962,* **54**, *523-525.*

HOLENSTEIN (P.). Die kongenitale Fibulaaplasie : ihre Differentialdiagnose und Behandlung. *Helv. paediat. Acta, 1965,* **20**, *118-127.*

JUDET (J.), RIGAULT (R.) et ROY (C. R.). Traitement des pseudarthroses congénitales de la jambe par décortication, fixateur externe et greffe secondaire de renforcement. *Rev. Chir. orthop., 1968,* **54**, *503-510.*

KELLN (E. E.), BENNETT (C. G.) et KLINBERG (W. G.). Aglossia-adactylia syndrome. *Amer. J. Dis. Child., 1968,* **116**, *549-552.*

KEUTEL (J.), KINDERMANN (I.) et MÖCKEL (H.). Eine wahrscheinlich autosomal recessiv vererbte Skeletmissbildung mit Humeroradialsynostose. *Humangenetik, 1970,* **9**, *43-53.*

KLEMM (E.). Minderwuchs infolge multipler enchondraler Dysostose bei zwei Geschwistern mit Hornhauttrübungen und Sturge-Weber syndrom. *Mschr. Kinderheilk., 1960,* **108**, *356-361.*

KOIVIKKO (A.). Ventriculoradial dysplasia in a mongoloid infant. *Ann. clin. Res., 1970,* **2**, *79-81.*

LAMY (M.) et BIENENFELD (C.). La dyschondrostéose. *Analecta Genet., 1954,* **1**, *153-164.*

LEE (F. A.), ISAACS (H., Jr.) et STRAUSS (J.). The « Campomelic » syndrome. Short life-span dwarfism with respiratory distress, hypotonia, peculiar facies, and multiple skeletal and cartilaginous deformities. *Amer. J. Dis. Child., 1972,* **124**, *485-496.*

MADELUNG (O. W.). Die spontane Subluxation der Hand nach Vorne. *Verh. dtsch. Ges. Chir., 1878,* **7**, *259-276.*

MAROTEAUX (P.), SPRANGER (J.), OPITZ (J. M.), KUCERA (J.), LOWRY (R. B.), SCHIMKE (R. N.) et KAGAN (S. M.). Le syndrome campomélique. *Presse méd., 1971,* **79**, *1157-1162.*

MASSERMAN (R. L.), PETERSON (H. A.) et BIANCO (A. J.). Congenital pendarthrosis of the tibia. *Clinic. Orthop., 1974,* **99**, *140-145.*

MIETENS (C.) et WEBER (H.). A syndrome characterized by corneal opacity nystagmus, flexion contracture of the elbows, growth failure and mental retardation. *J. Pediat., 1966,* **69**, *624-629.*

MILUNSKI (A.), GRAEF (J. W.) et GAINOR (M. F.). Metothrexate-induced congenital malformation. *J. Pédiat., 1968,* **72**, *790-795.*

NEVIN (N. C.), DODGE (J. A.) et KERNOHAN (D. C.). Aglossia-adactylia syndrome. *Oral Surg., 1970,* **29**, *443-446.*

PFEIFFER (R. A.). Morphologie der Thalidomid-Embryopathie. *VIIIe Congrès de l'Union thérapeutique internationale, Bruxelles, 1963, 51-69.*

PILLAY (V. K.). Ophthalmo-mandibulo-melic dysplasia. An hereditary syndrome. *J. Bone Jt Surg., 1964,* **46-A**, *858-862.*

POZNANSKI (A. K.), NOSANCHUK (J. S.), BAUBLIS (J.) et HOLT (J. F.). The cerebro-hepato-renal syndrome (CHRS) (Zellweger's syndrome). *Amer. J. Roentgenol., 1970,* **109**, *313-322.*

THORMON (T. F.), DE FRAITES (E. B.) et ANDERSON (B. S. et E. E.). Familial camptomelic dwarfism. *J. Pediat., 1973,* **83**, *841-843.*

RING (P. A.). Congenital abnormalities of the femur. *Arch. Dis. Childh., 1961* **36**, *410-417.*

SCHMICKEL (R. D.), HEIDELBERGER (K. P.) et POZNANSKI (A. K.). The campomelique syndrome. *J. Pediat., 1973,* **82**, *299-302.*

STANESCU (V.), communication personnelle.

STANNUS (H. S.) et WILSON (S. A. K.). La micromélie humérale bilatérale congénitale et ses relations avec l'achondroplasie. *Nouv. Iconogr. Salpêt., 1911,* **24**, *463-471.*

STÜVE (A.) et WIEDMANN (H.-R.). Angeborene Verbiegungen langer Röhrenknochen, eine Geschwisterbeobachtung. *Z. Kinderheilk., 1971,* **111**, *184-192.*

TOLEDO (S. P. A.), SALDANHA (P. H.), BORELLI (A.) et CINTRA (A. B. U.). Further data on acheiropody. *J. Génét. hum., 1972,* **20**, *253-258.*

VANNI (E.). La sinostosi radio-ulnare congenita. *Minerva med., 1962,* **53**, *3519-3523.*

VOGEL (F.). Verzögerte Mutation beim Menschen ? *Ann. hum. Genet., 1957,* **22**, *132-137.*

Anomalies of Carpus, Tarsus, the Metacarpals, and the Fingers

ANDREASEN (E.). Calcaneo-navicular coalition. Late results of resection. *Acta orthop. scand., 1968,* **39**, *424-432.*

ANTONUTTI (A.) et STRUKELJ (L.). Sulla sindrome dell'os tibiale externum. *Friuli med.,* **19**, *3-14.*

BALCI (S.), SAY (B.) et ERDAL (R.). Laurence-Moon-Biedl syndrome in presumably identical twins. *Humangenetik, 1971,* **13**, *328-332.*

BELL (J.). On brachydactyly and symphalangism. *Treas. hum. Inherit., 1951,* **5**, *1-31.*

BENE (M.), RADU (H.), KOCSIS (M.) et RADU (A.). Le syndrome de Laurence-Moon-Bardet-Biedl. *Ann. pédiat., 1969,* **16**, *57-61.*

BURAGGI (G. L.) et PEDOJA (G.). La brachimetapodia. Contributo allo studio delle malformazioni dei metacarpei e dei metatarsei. *Radiol. med. (Torino), 1961,* **47**, *814-830.*

CENANI (A.) et LENZ (W.). Totale Syndactylie und totale radioulnare Synostose bei zwei Brüdern. Ein Beitrag zur Genetik der Syndaktylien. *Z. Kinderheilk., 1967,* **101**, *181-190.*

CHRISTIAENS (L.), DEMINATTI (M.), WALBAUM (R.) et DEBEUGNY (P.). A propos d'une famille atteinte de brachydactylie héréditaire type Vidal. *Lille méd., 1965,* **10**, *686-691.*

CLAISSE (R. H.). Une forme spéciale de symphalangisme : la biphalangie généralisée par synostose interphalangienne proximale avec brachymétapodie des premiers rayons. *Rev. Rhum., 1965,* **32**, *118-125.*

CURRARINO (G.) et WALDMAN (I.). Camptodactyly. *Amer. J. Roentgenol., 1964,* **92**, *1312-1321.*

DALLOZ (J. C.) et NOCTON (F.). Le syndrome de Moebius. A propos de deux observations nouvelles. *Arch. franç. Pédiat., 1964,* **21**, *1025-1047.*

DANIEL (G. H.). Case of hereditary anarthrosis of index finger with associated abnormalities in proportion fingers. *Ann. Eugen., 1936,* **7**, *281-297.*

DREWES (J.) et GÜNTHER (D.). Angeborene Fusswurzelsynostosen. *Radiologe (Berl.), 1966,* **6**, *225-231.*

DUBOIS (H. J.). Nievergelt-Pearlman syndrome. Synostosis in feet and hands with dysplasia of elbows. Report of a case. *J. Bone Jt Surg.,* **52-B**, *325-329.*

DUBOST (E.), PICARD (J. M.), ECARLAT (B.) et HERNANDEZ (C.). Trois formes d'anomalies congénitales des membres. *J. Radiol. Electrol., 1960,* **41**, *579-583.*

DUHAMEL (B.), HAEGEL (P.) et PAGES (R.). Morphogenèse pathologique. « Des monstruosités aux malformations ». *Paris, 1966, Masson, éd.*

EMERY (A. E. H.) et NELSON (M. M.). Case report. A familial syndrome of short stature, deformities of the hands and feet and an unusual facies. *J. med. Genet., 1970,* **7**, *379-382.*

FORNEY (W. R.), ROBINSON (S. J.) et PASCOE (D. J.). Congenital hear disease, deafness and skeletal malformations : a new syndrome ? *J. Pediat., 1966,* **68**, *14-26.*

GLICENSTEIN (J.), PENNECOT (G. F.) et DUHAMEL (B.). Le syndrome de Poland. 17 nouvelles observations. *Ann. chir. Plast., 1974,* **19**, *47-54.*

GNAMEY (D.), WALBAUM (R.), SAINT-AUBERT (P.) et FONTAINE (G.). Brachydactylie héréditaire de type C. Etude clinique et génétique de trois familles. *Ann. Pédiat., 1971,* **18**, *438-449.*

GORDON (H.), DAVIES (D.) et BERMAN (M.). Camptodactyly, cleft palate, and club foot : a syndrome showing the autosomal-dominant pattern of inheritance. *J. med. Genet., 1969,* **6**, *266-274.*

GROSSE (F. R.), HERRMANN (J.) et OPITZ (J. M.). The F-form of acro-pectoro-vertebral dysplasia : the F-syndrome. *Birth Defects, Original Article Series, 1969, V n° 3, 48-63.*

HAAS (S. L.). Bilateral complete syndactylism of all fingers. *Amer. J. Surg., 1940,* **50**, *363-366.*

HARLE (T. S.) et STEVENSON (J. R.). Hereditary symphalangism associated with carpal and tarsal fusions. *Radiology, 1967,* **89**, *91-94.*

HAWS (D. V.) et MCKUSICK (V. A.). Farabee's brachydactylous kindred revisited. *Bull. Johns-Hopk. Hosp., 1963,* **113**, *20-30.*

HOEFNAGEL (D.) et GERALD (P. S.). Hereditary brachydactyly. *Ann. hum. Genet., 1966,* **29**, *377-382.*

HOOTNICK (D.) et HOLMES (L. B.). Familial polysyndactyly and craniofacial anomalies. *Clin. Genet., 1972,* **3**, *128-134.*

JACQUEMAIN (B.). Die angeborene Windmühlenflügelstellung als erbliche Kombinationsmissbildung. *Z. Orthop., 1966,* **102**, *146-154.*

JOHNSTON (O.) et KIRBY (V. V.). Syndactyly of the ring and little finger. *Ann. J. hum. Genet., 1955,* **7**, *80-82.*

JONES (G. B.). Delta phalanx. *J. Bone Jt Surg., 1964,* **46-B**, *226-228.*

KITE (J. H.). Congenital syndactylism of fingers. *Sth. med. J. (Bgham, Ala.), 1958,* **51**, *160-164.*

Le Marec (B.). La polydactylie. Maladie ou symptôme. *Thèse Méd., Rennes, 1969.*

Mace (J. W.), Kaplan (J. M.) et Schanberger (J. E.). Poland's syndrome : report of seven cases and review of the literature. *Clin. Pediat., 1972,* **11**, *98-102.*

Maroteaux (P.), Bouvet (J. P.) et Briard (M.-L.). La maladie des synostoses multiples. *Nouv. Presse méd., 1972,* **1**, *3041-3044.*

Marshall (R. E.) et Smith (D. W.). Frontodigital syndrome : a dominantly inherited disorder with normal intelligence. *J. Pediat., 1970,* **77**, *129-133.*

O'Rahilly (R.). A survey of carpal and tarsal anomalies. *J. Bone Jt Surg., 1953,* **35-A**, *626-642.*

Otto (F. M. G.). Die « cranio-carpo-tarsal Dystrophie » (Freeman und Sheldon). Ein kasuistischer Beitrag. *Z. Kinderheilk., 1953,* **73**, *240-250.*

Pearl (L.), Chow (J. F.) et Friedman (E.). Poland's syndrome. *Radiology, 1971,* **101**, *619-623.*

Pearlman (H. S.), Edkin (R. E.) et Warren (R. F.). Familial tarsal and carpal synostosis with radial-head subluxation (Nievergelt's syndrome). *J. Bone Jt Surg., 1964,* **46-A**, *585-592.*

Pfeiffer (R. A.) et Roeskau (M.). Agenesie der Tibia, Fibulaverdoppelung und spiegelbildliche Polvdaktylie (Diplopodie) bei Mutter und Kind. *Z. Kinderheilk., 1971,* **111**, *38-50.*

Plöchl (E.). Zum Ullrich-Feichtinger-Syndrom (Dyskraniopygophalangie). *Pädiat. Pädol., 1969,* **5**, *276-280.*

Poland (A.). Deficiency of pectoralis muscle. *Guy's Hosp. Rep., 1841,* **6**, *191-193.*

Poznanski (A. K.), Pratt (G. B.), Manson (G.) et Weiss (L.). Clinodactyly, camptodactyly, Kirner's deformity, and other crooked fingers. *Radiology, 1969,* **93**, *573-582.*

Poznanski (A. K.). Foot manifestations of the congenital malformation syndromes. *Seminars Roentgenol., 1970,* **5**, *354-366.*

Robinson (G. C.), Wood (B. J.), Miller (J. R.) et Baillie (J.). Hereditary brachydactyly and hip disease. *J. Pediat., 1968,* **72**, *539-543.*

Ruvalcaba (R. H. A.), Reichert (A.) et Smith (D. W.). A new familial syndrome with osseous dysplasia and mental deficiency. *J. Pediat., 1971,* **79**, *450-455.*

Sallis (J. G.) et Beighton (P.). Dominantly inherited digito-talar dysmorphism. *J. Bone Jt Surg., 1972,* **54-B**, *509-515.*

Schreiber (A.). Symmetrische Fuss- and Handwurzelsynostosen in 4 Generationen. *Z. Orthop., 1968,* **104**, *197-202.*

Schwarz (E.) et Rivellini (G.). Symphalangism. *Amer. J. Roentgenol., 1963,* **89**, *1256-1259.*

Scott (C. R.), Bryant (J. I.) et Graham (C. B.). A new craniodigital syndrome with mental retardation. *J. Pediat., 1971,* **78**, *658-663.*

Seringe (Ph.), Allaneau (Cl.), Fores (Cl.) et Guimbaud (P.). Le syndrome de Bardet-Biedl et ses troubles endocriniens. *Ann. Endocrin. (Paris), 1969,* **30**, *641-657.*

Smith (R. J.) et Kaplan (E. B.). Camptodactyly and similar atraumatic flexion deformities of the proximal interphalangeal joints of the fingers. *J. Bone Jt Surg., 1968,* **50-A**, *1187-1204.*

Sorsby (A.). Congenital coloboma of the macula, together with an account of the familial occurrence of bilateral macular coloboma in association with atypical dystrophy of hands and feet. *Brit. J. Ophthal., 1935,* **19**, *65-90.*

Staheli (L. T.), Clawson (D. K.) et Capps (J. H.). Bilateral curving of the terminal phalanges of the little fingers. Report of two cases. *J. Bone Jt Surg., 1966,* **48-A**, *1171-1176.*

Steinberg (A. G.) et Reynolds (E. L.). Further data on symphalangism. *J. Hered., 1948,* **39**, *23-27.*

Stewart (J. M.) et Bergstrom (L.). Familial hand abnormality and sensorineural deafness : a new syndrome. *J. Pediat., 1971,* **78**, *102-110.*

Strasburger (A. K.), Hawkins (M. R.), Eldridge (R.), Hargrave (R. L.) et McKusick (V. A.). Symphalangism : genetic and clinical aspects. *Bull. Johns-Hopk. Hosp., 1965,* **117**, *108-127.*

Sugar (H. S.). The cryptophthalmos-syndactyly syndrome. *Amer. J. Ophthal., 1968,* **66**, *897-899.*

Temtamy (S.) et McKusick (V. A.). Synopsis of hand malformation with particular emphasis on genetic factors. *Birth Defects, Original Article Series, 1969,* V, *125-184.*

Thorne (F. L.), Posch (J. L.) et Mladick (R. A.). Megalodactyly. *Plast. reconstr. Surg., 1968,* **41**, *232-239.*

Tünte (W.) et Kersting (D.). Spiegelbildliche Verdoppelung von Ulna und ulnaren Handanteil bei fehlendem Radius (« mirror-hand »). *Z. Orthop., 1967,* **103**, *490-498.*

Walsh (R. J.). Acrosyndactyly. A study of twenty-seven patients. *Clin. orthop., 1970,* **71**, *99-111.*

Walters (T. R.), Reddy (B. N.), Bailon (A.) et Vitale (L. F.). Poland's syndrome associated with leukemia. *J. Pediat., 1973,* **82**, *889.*

Weber (J. W.) et Schwarz (H.). Der Typus Rostockiensis Ullrich-Feichtiger. Dyskranio-pygo-phalangie. *Helv. Paediat. Acta, 1960,* **15**, *163-170.*

Weyers (H.). Hexadactylie, Unterkieferspalt und Oligodontie, ein neuer Symptomenkomplex. Dysostosis acro-facialis. *Ann. paediat. (Basel), 1953,* **181**, *45-60.*

Wildervanck (L. S.), Goedhard (G.) et Meijer (S.). Proximal symphalangism of fingers associated with fusion of os naviculare and talus and occurrence of two accessory bones in the feet (os paranaviculare and os tibiale externum) in an European-Indonesian-Chinese family. *Acta genet. (Basel), 1967,* **17**, *166-177.*

Wilkinson (R. H.). Tarsal coalition. *Postgrad. Med., 1970,* **47**, *69-71.*

Oro-Facio-Digital Syndrome. Anomalies of the Thumb. Holt-Oram Syndrome

Blank (E.). A cardio-facial-skeletal syndrome. *Amer. J. Roentgenol., 1972,* **116**, *634-639.*

Cotta (H.) et Jäger (M.). Die familiäre Triphalangie des Daumens und ihre operative Behandlung. *Arch. orthop. Unfall-Chir., 1965,* **58**, *282-290.*

Emerit (I.), Grouchy (J. de), Vernant (P.), Corone (P.) et Gennes (J.-L. de). Communication interauriculaire. Troubles du rythme et malformation des membres supérieurs. Un nouveau syndrome malformatif. *Sem. Hôp. Paris, 1964,* **40**, *2560-2566.*

Emerit (I.), Grouchy (J. de), Laval-Jeantet (M.), Corone (P.) et Vernant (P.). Malformations complexes des membres supérieurs associées à une cardiopathie congénitale. *Acta genet. med. (Roma), 1962,* **14**, *132-163.*

Fuhrmann (W.), Stahl (A.) et Schroeder (T. M.). Das oro-facio-digitale Syndrom. Zugleich eine Diskussion der Erbgänge mit geschlechts-begrenztem Letaleffekt. *Hum. Genet., 1966,* **2**, *133-164.*

FUHRMANN (W.) et STAHL (A.). Zur Differentialdiagnose von Papillon-Léage-Psaume-Syndrom und Mohr-Syndrom. *Hum. Genet., 1970,* **9**, *54-63.*

HOLT (M.) et ORAM (S.). Familial heart disease with skeletal malformations. *Brit. Heart. J., 1960,* **22**, *236-242.*

JOHNSON (C. F.). Abnormal thumbs and physical diagnosis. Anomalies of the thumbs as signs of congenital disorders in organ systems. *Clin. Pediat. (Phila.), 1970,* **9**, *131-143.*

KAUFMAN (R. L.), RIMOIN (D. L.), MCALISTER (W. H.) et HARTMANN (A. F.). Variable expression of the Holt-Oram syndrom. *Amer. J. Dis. Child., 1974,* **127**, *21-25.*

MAJEWSKI (F.), LENZ (W.), PFEIFFER (R. A.) et TÜNTE (W.). Das oro-facio-digitale Syndrom. Symptome und Prognose. *Z. Kinderheilk., 1972,* **112**, *89-112.*

MOHR (O. L.). A hereditary sublethal syndrome in man. *Arh. Norske Videnskad (Oslo), 1941,* **14**, *1-18.*

MURPHY (S.) et LUBIN (B.). Triphalangeal thumbs and congenital erythroid hypoplasia : report of a case with unusual features. *J. Pediat., 1972,* **81**, *987-989.*

PASHAYAN (H.), FRASER (F. C.), MCINTYRE (J. M.) et DUNBAR (J. S.). Bilateral aplasia of the tibia, polydactyly and absent thumb in father and daughter. *J. Bone Jt Surg., 1971,* **53-B**, *495-499.*

PAPILLON-LEAGE et PSAUME (J.). Une malformation héréditaire de la muqueuse buccale. Brides et freins anormaux. *Rev. stomat., 1954,* **55**, *209-227.*

PAPILLON-LEAGE et PSAUME (J.). Une nouvelle malformation héréditaire. Dysmorphie des freins buccaux. Huit observations. *Actualités odonto-stomat., 1954,* **25**, *7-26.*

PFEIFFER (R. A.), MAJEWSKI (F.) et MANNKOPF (H.). Das Syndrom von Mohr und Claussen. *Klin. Pädiat., 1972,* **184**, *224-229.*

PIUSSAN (C.), RISBOURG (B.), BENS (J. L.), CRUNELLE (R.) et BOULANGER (J. C.). Syndrome de Holt-Oram et dysplasies thoraco-digitales. *Rev. Pédiat., 1973,* **9**, *27-35.*

POZNANSKI (A. K.), GALL (J. C., Jr.) et STERN (A. M.). Skeletal manifestations of the Holt-Oram syndrome. *Radiology, 1970,* **94**, *45-53.*

QAZI (Q. H.) et SMITHWICK (E. M.). Triphalangy of thumbs and great toes. *Amer. J. Dis. Child., 1970,* **120**, *255-257.*

RIMOIN (D. L.) et EDGERTON (M. T.). Genetic and clinical heterogeneity in the oral-facial-digital syndromes. *J. Pediat., 1967,* **71**, *94-102.*

SCHWARZ (E.) et FISH (A.). Roentgenographic features of a new congenital dysplasia. *Amer. J. Roentgenol., 1960,* **84**, *511-517.*

STERN (A. M.), GALL (J. C., Jr.), PERRY (B. L.), STIMSON (C. W.), WEITKAMP (L. R.) et POZNANSKI (A. K.). The hand-foot-uterus syndrome. A new hereditary disorder characterized by hand foot dysplasia, dermatoglyphic abnormalities, and partial duplication of the female genital tract. *J. Pediat., 1970,* **77**, *109-116.*

SWANSON (A. B.) et BROWN (K. S.). Hereditary triphalangeal thumb. *J. Hered., 1962,* **53**, *258-265.*

VAILLAUD (J. C.), MARTIN (J.), SZEPETOWSKY (G.) et ROBERT (J. M.). Le syndrome oro-facio-digital. Etude clinique et génétique à propos de 10 cas observés dans une même famille. *Rev. Pédiat., 1968,* **4**, *383-392.*

WALBAUM (R.), FONTAINE (G.), LIENHARDT (J.) et PIQUET (J. J.). Surdité familiale avec ostéo-onychodysplasie. *J. Génét. hum., 1970,* **18**, *101-108.*

WERNER (P.). Ueber einen seltenen Fall von Zwergwuchs. *Arch. Gynäk., 1915,* **104**, *278-300.*

Acro-Osteolyses

BÉBE (M.). Ostéopathies et néphropathies : étude de leur rapport à propos de deux cas d'acro-ostéolyse associée à une insuffisance rénale. *Thèse Méd., Paris, 1962.*

BÉBE (M.). Acro-ostéolyse essentielle, anomalies squelettiques congénitales et néphrite chronique avec défaillance rénale. Maladie de Julien Marie et M. Derot. *Ann. Pédiat., 1974,* **50**, *532-552.*

BERTHOUX (F.), ROBERT (J.-M.), ZECH (P.), FRIES (D.) et TRAEGER (J.). Acro-ostéolyse essentielle à début carpien et tarsien avec néphropathie. *Arch. franç. Pédiat., 1971,* **28**, *615-630.*

CHENEY (W. D.). Acro-osteolysis. *Amer. J. Roentgenol., 1965,* **94**, *595-607.*

FRANÇOIS (J.). Dystrophie dermo-chondro-cornéenne familiale. *Ann. Oculist., 1949,* **182**, *409-442.*

GIACCAI (L.). Familial and sporadic neurogenic acro-osteolysis. *Acta radiol. (Stockh.), 1952,* **38**, *17-29.*

GORHAM (L.-W.). Disappearing bones. *J. Bone Jt Surg., 1955,* **37-A**, *985-1004.*

HAJDU (N.) et KAUNTZE (R.). Cranioskeletal dysplasia. *Brit. J. Radiol., 1948,* **21**, *42-48.*

HARNASCH (H.). Die Akroosteolyse, ein neues Krankheitbild. *Fortschr. Rontgenstr., 1950,* **72**, *352-359.*

HERRAULT (A.), COHEN-SOLAL (J.), DUHAMEL (A.) et GOUYON (F. de). Acro-ostéolyses idiopathiques de l'enfant. A propos d'une observation. *Ann. Pédiat., 1965,* **41**, *714-721.*

HERRMANN (J.). Arthro-dento-osteodysplasia (Hajdu-Cheney syndrome). Review of a genetic « acro-osteolysis » syndrome. *Z. Kinderheilk., 1973,* **114**, *93-110.*

JOSEPH (R.), NEZELOF (Ch.), GUÉRAUD (L.) et JOB (J. C.). Acro-ostéolyse idiopathique familiale. Renseignements fournis par la biopsie. *Ann. Pédiat., 1959,* **35**, *82-89.*

KLAUS (E.), ROĆEK (V.) et BURDA (M.). Ein Fall von idiopathischer Acroosteolyse. *Radiologe (Berl.), 1969,* **9**, *167-170.*

KOHLER (E.), BABBITT (D.), HUIZENGA (B.) et GOOD (T. A.). Hereditary osteolysis. A clinical, radiological and chemical study. *Radiology, 1973,* **108**, *99-105.*

KOZLOWSKI (K.), HANICKA (M.) et GARAPICH (M.). Neurogene ulcerierende Akropathie (Akroosteolyse-Syndrom). *Mschr. Kinderheilk., 1971,* **119**, *169-175.*

LAMY (M.) et MAROTEAUX (P.). Acro-ostéolyse dominante. *Arch. franç. Pédiat., 1961,* **18**, *693-702.*

LAMY (M.), FREZAL (J.) et LAUT (J.). Un syndrome acropathique héréditaire. *Presse méd., 1963,* **71**, *1837-1840.*

MCPHERSON (R. I.), WALKER (R. D.) et KOWALL (M. H.). Essential osteolysis with nephropathy. *J. canad. Ass. Radiol., 1973,* **24**, *98-103.*

MARIE (J.), SALET (J.), LEVÈQUE (B.) et SAUVEGRAIN (J.). Syndrome ostéodystrophique de nature congénitale probable réalisant l'association d'une ostéolyse essentielle progressive des os des extrémités des membres et d'anomalies malformatives vertébrales et costales. *Presse méd., 1956,* **64**, *2173-2176.*

PAPAVASILIOU (C. G.), GARGANO (F. P.) et WALLS (W. L.). Idiopathic nonfamilial acro-osteolysis associated with other bone abnormalities. *Amer. J. Roentgenol., 1960,* **83**, *687-691.*

REMKY (H. von) et ENGELBRECHT (G.). Dystrophia dermo-chondro-cornealis (François). *Klin. Mbl. Augenheilk., 1967,* **151**, *319-331.*

THIEFFRY (S.) et SORREL-DÉJERINE (J.). Forme spéciale d'ostéolyse héréditaire et familiale à stabilisation spontanée, survenant dans l'enfance. *Presse méd., 1958,* **66**, *1858-1861.*

TORG (J. S.), DIGEORGE (A. M.), KIRKPATRICK (J. A., Jr.) et TRUJILLO (M. M.). Hereditary multicentric osteolysis with recessive transmission : a new syndrome. *J. Pediat., 1969,* **75**, *243-252*

TORG (J. S.) et STEEL (H. H.). Sequential roentgenographic changes occurring in massive osteolysis. *J. Bone Jt Surg., 1969,* **51-A**, *1649-1655.*

WIEDEMANN (H. R.). Zur François'schen Krankheit. Dystrophia dermo-chondro-cornealis familiaris. *Arztl. Woch., 1958,* **13**, *905-909.*

YOUNG (L. W.), RADEBAUGH (J. F.), RUBIN (P.), SENSENBRENNER (J. A.) et FIORELLI (G.). New syndrome manifested by mandibular hypoplasia, acroosteolysis, stiff joints and cutaneous atrophy (mandibulo-acral dysplasia) in two unrelated boys. *Birth Defects, Original article, series VII, 1971,* n° 11, *291-297.*

Part Three:

Metabolic Skeletal Disorders

This part of our discussion deals with the disorders of metabolism of phosphorus and calcium, and those of the metabolism of glucides and lipids.

Renal tubular disorders which also possibly affect the skeleton will be discussed, together with the inheritable anomalies of the metabolism of phosphorus and calcium. Homocystinuria, aspartylglycosaminuria, phenylketonuria, and Wilson's disease will be treated with neurologic disorders in the third part of this book.

5 Disorders of the Metabolism of Phosphorus and Calcium

A few general comments on metabolism and its regulation will be followed by the successive study of avitaminoses and hypervitaminoses, endocrine disorders, genetic metabolic diseases, and renal and intestinal osteopathies.

Sometimes we will step slightly beyond the limits implied by the title, since a number of deficiencies or endocrine disorders with skeletal manifestations stem from causes outside those limits.

GENERAL COMMENTS ON THE METABOLISM AND CONTROL OF CALCIUM

We are attempting to cover essential information needed to understand the classification and mechanism of skeletal anomalies seen with disorders which affect calcium metabolism.

CALCIUM METABOLISM

In the chapter on the anatomy and physiology of bone it was stated that bone is formed from calcium phosphate. Since this is the most prevalent electrolyte in the body, forming 1.6 per cent of the total body weight, it assumes great significance.

From birth to adulthood there is a rapid increase in the calcium content in the body. The full term newborn baby has a calcium reserve of about 30 g, as compared to 1,100 g in an adult. Furthermore, there is a marked decrease in the calcium content towards the end of gestation. At 7 months of gestation the fetus contains only 8 g of calcium, thus, during the ninth month this value practically doubles.

To a large degree, this calcium is fixed in the skeleton – 98 to 99 per cent – in the form of calcium phosphate or carbonate. Within the plasma calcium circulates in its free ionized form – 50 per cent, and is partly bound to acid radicals, such as citric acid, and partly bound in its ultrafiltrable form – 5 per cent, or in combination with proteins. The total calcemia is close to 100 mg/1 or five milliequivalents.

Besides its physiologic role within the body in ossification, calcium is a significant factor in the permeability of cellular membranes, in the activation of a number of enzymatic systems, and in decreasing neuromuscular excitability.

Calcium intake occurs exclusively through the oral ingestion, milk and its derivatives together with certain vegetables and dried fruits being the main source. Alimentary calcium is absorbed from the intestine by active and passive mechanisms. Several factors influence this absorption, especially parathyroid hormones and vitamin D, which influences active resorption. On the other hand, fatty acids, phytic acids, thyroid hormones or cortisol have an inhibiting effect on calcium resorption.

In the normal person calcium absorption depends on the amount of calcium ingested and on the need of the organism. Adaptation to a low calcium intake seems to be inadequate in certain persons as has been shown by Malm. This may influence certain types of osteoporosis, at least in the adult. Too large an amount of calcium may inhibit the absorption of phosphates. This may happen when the Ca/P ratio, normally around 0.8, increases beyond 3, but it has not been reliably proven.

Several studies have demonstrated the presence of a transport protein for calcium (Wasserman). Synthesis of this protein is inhibited by a lack of vitamin D and by renal insufficiency. This synthesis, however, occurs at a higher rate if there is a lack of calcium, and is stimulated by vitamin D.

Calcium is eliminated in the stool and urine. The loss by sweat is negligible in the milder climates, but in infants it must be seriously considered in climates where considerable postprandial sweat loss may occur. The eliminated calcium in the stools can be either that which is secreted and not absorbed with the digestive juices, or nonabsorbed alimentary calcium. The former is referred to as endogenous calcium and its amount is close to 40-60 mg/day during infancy and 150 mg/day during adolescence. The percent of the ingested calcium not present in the stools is referred to as the utilization coefficient of calcium. This value depends on the patient's age and type of nutrition. It is very high in breast-fed babies, where it may be above 70 per cent. If, however, cow's milk is fed, this value is around 35 to 45 per cent. In periods of accelerated growth there is a high value, especially during prepuberty, during which time it is above 30 per cent and may go as high as 50 per cent. Except for these periods, the factor remains between 25 and 30 per cent. It is important to be familiar with these variations in order to correctly interpret the digestive utilization coefficient.

Calciuria consists of filtrated calcium which is not reabsorbed. Renal tubular secretion is still under discussion. Physiologic calciuria during childhood is expressed in mg/kg/24 h. This value depends to some degree on intake, but it is further under the influence of a number of factors, such as parathormone, growth hormone, vitamin D, sodium chloride content, acid-overload, protide concentration, and water diuresis. On the average it is either at or slightly below 3 mg/kg/24 h. Calciuria higher than 6 mg is considered the upper limit of normal. There are nocturnal and seasonal variations of the degree of calciuria. The latter seems to be in direct relation to sunlight exposure.

FACTORS AFFECTING CALCIUM REGULATION

Normally there is a regulating mechanism maintaining calcemia within narrow limits. This stability is indispensable for growth and normal skeletal mineralization, and for normal muscular contractility. There are numerous factors which affect this regulating mechanism. Experimentally, a calcium free diet has lead initially to disturbed growth, retarded skeletal maturation, and osteoporosis. This is not seen in humans even under conditions of extreme poverty, in which large parts of the population subsist on 200 mg per day. This amount seems to be sufficient to prevent a marked deficit in calcium. Still, we will see that this mechanism is at least in part responsible for a particular type of osteopathy occurring in premature babies. Low intake levels can exacerbate certain abnormal conditions, such as disturbed intestinal absorption or idiopathic hypercalciuria.

Normally the essential regulatory role belongs to the skeleton itself. Because of the enormous surface it presents for exchange, it is the site of the many different regulatory factors which have their effect on calcemia.

Abnormal renal function can have an effect on calcium metabolism by causing an electrolyte imbalance. Disturbed intestinal absorption also adversely affects the calcium metabolism.

There are two key factors responsible for the regulation of calcemia. We will first discuss vitamin D and endocrine factors, and specifically, among the latter, the effects of parathormone and thyrocalcitonin. We will point out that in the light of the most recent discoveries vitamin D has an action that is very close to that of a hormone.

Vitamin D

The importance of vitamin D in calcium regulation has been known for years, but it was not until very recently that its proper metabolic role was clearly defined. De Luca and Kodicek have clarified a number of important points by demonstrating that vitamin D is transformed within the body into a number of metabolites, the most active being 1-25-di-hydroxycholecalciferol. The substance is formed within the kidney, and presently is considered to be the hormonal form of vitamin D. 25-hydroxycholecalciferol, the circulating form of vitamin D, and the precursor of the active dihydroxylate metabolite, is formed in the liver.

The synthesis of 1-25-di-hydroxycholecalciferol is relative to the serum calcium concentration. The synthesis occurs at a quicker rate when the value is low, and may completely stop when calcemia is markedly high. We can thus conclude that in the regulation of calcemia, the kidney, as well as the parathyroids, plays the role of an endocrine organ.

Vitamin D accumulates within the body, especially within the intestinal mucosa, the kidneys, adipose tissue, and the circulating blood. It is transported by α_2-globuline. After it has been transported into a cell it is transformed into two active metabolites. These will eventually reach the location of their specific effect, the bone and the intestinal mucosa. Excretion occurs mainly by the biliary tract and through the intestine. In the urine we find only small amounts as glycoconjugates or in the form of other water soluble complexes.

Vitamin D acts mainly on the intestinal calcium resorption and on the skeleton. The exact nature of these influences are still not fully understood. Absorption of calcium, under the influence of vitamin D, takes place over the entire extent of the small intestine. Calciuria and tubular phosphate reabsorption are increased by physiologic amounts of vitamin D. Vitamin D has a liberating effect on calcium in the skeleton and in high doses can be responsible for hypercalcemia. While treating rickets hypocalcemia can be temporarily seen after therapy with vitamin D. This results from an avidity for, and insufficient availability of calcium.

The normal infant needs about 400 to 800 U/day of vitamin D. Vitamin D must be added to the regular food. This supplementation should be maintained up to the age of five. The synthesis by the skin of vitamin D under the effect of the sun's rays varies according to local climate, atmospheric pollution, and the degree of skin pigmentation. Lack of vitamin D is responsible for rickets. Still, its excessive intake can be equally dangerous to the child. If doses higher than 5000 U/day are ingested continuously over a long period of time—some years—the result may be hypercalciuria, hypercalcemia, and arterial or renal calcifications.

Hormonal Factors

Parathormone

Parathormone plays an important role by its elective effects on the bones and kidneys. It liberates calcium and phosphorus from bone. The exact mechanism of this action is still under discussion. Parathormone seems to increase the solubility of calcium. It increases hydrogen ions by a liberation of citrate—the citric acid theory of Newmann, and the lactate theory of Vaes. Furthermore, it stimulates the formation of osteoclasts, which can remodel bone, and it appears to have a direct effect on osteocytes and their environment (Talmage). Finally, it can alter matrix. Calcium bound to collagen would thus be able to penetrate into the extracellular space (Belanger). This latter function is the result of the activity of acid hydrolases with its cellular excretion induced by parathormone (Vaes).

At the cellular level, the first effect of parathormone is to increase the permeability of its membranes to calcium. There follows an increase of the intra-cellular calcium content, and its subsequent departure from the cell. There is also an effect of increasing cyclic AMP.

Parathormone creates this effect by *increasing phosphate diuresis* and by *decreasing renal tubular reabsorption.* In physiologic amounts it will bring about an increased renal tubular reabsorption of calcium. If given in large amounts, there will be increased calciuria, usually secondary to hypercalcemia. The effects of this complex action are an elevation of serum calcium and the lowering of serum phosphorus. Parathyroid secretion is stimulated by a drop of the plasma concentration of ionized calcium.

Calcitonin

Calcitonin is secreted by the parafollicular cells of the thyroid, which are rich in mitochondria, the C cells discovered by Copp and others in 1962.

This hormone, similar to parathormone, has a direct but opposite effect on bone. It reduces osteolysis, and this results in a decrease of calcemia and of phosphoremia. It increases phosphaturia, but its action is independent of vitamin D. Young individuals, and those with a very active skeletal metabolism, seem to be particularly sensitive to the action of calcitonin.

Other hormones do have some influence on calcium metabolism, but this action is weaker than that of parathormone or calcitonin. Cortisone inhibits osteogenesis and diminishes intestinal calcium resorption. Thyroid hormone also reduces the latter and increases the exchange within the skeleton. Somatotropic hormone increases intestinal resorption and calciuria and reduces tubular reabsorption of phosphates. The sexual hormones have an anabolic effect on the skeleton.

CLASSIFICATION OF SKELETAL DISEASES SECONDARY TO AN ABNORMAL METABOLISM OF PHOSPHORUS AND CALCIUM

We have divided this chapter into four sections. The first part will be a discussion of Avitaminoses and Hypervitaminoses, in so far as they have skeletal effects, and osteopathy of premature babies. Endocrine disorders and their effect on the skeleton and the metabolism of phosphorus and calcium are grouped in part two. In the third part we lump together genetic disorders of calcium metabolism, especially the vitamin D resistant types of rickets, idiopathic hypercalciuria, hypophosphatasia and idiopathic hypercalcemia. Renal osteopathies and abnormal intestinal resorption are covered in the fourth part, with special focus on their skeletal manifestations.

AVITAMINOSES AND HYPERVITAMINOSES

DEFICIENCY RICKETS

Methods of preventing rickets are well known and easily accomplished, but this is still a relatively frequent disorder. We shall not attempt to offer a complete description of the pathophysiology and of the clinical details, however, some of the key elements shall be recalled. Emphasis is placed on certain radiographic findings of a potentially misleading character which could cause errors in diagnosis during the phase of growth.

Clinical Findings

Rickets is seen mainly in babies between 6 and 18 months old. The onset may be much earlier, and there may also be patients with a much later onset, especially in the presence of a chronic skin lesion. There is a high incidence of rickets in babies with marked skin pigmentation, especially in those from economically deprived living conditions.

The infant suffering from rickets is most frequently brought to our attention because of bowing of the lower extremities or a disturbed gait. Sometimes hospitalization is precipitated by a fracture, a tetanic episode or an upper respiratory infection. Careful, systematic investigation often leads to a much earlier recognition of this disease.

In its mildest form clinical investigation will simply reveal metaphyseal widening, which can be palpated at the distal end of radius and fibula. A costal rosary results from a similar widening of the chondrocostal junction. This finding should never be confused with the normal local step effect as is felt when one palpates from the sternum towards the lateral portion of the ribs. Its recognition requires careful palpation moving laterally towards the medial portion, in other words from the rib onto the sternum. The finding of craniotabes or pingpong ball phenomenon, when palpating the region of the occipital squama does not have a particularly significant value before the fifth month of life.

Often there are other more dramatic findings accompanying the metaphyseal flaring, especially bowing of the lower extremities, electively involving the distal third of the tibia with a medial concavity. This is not a constant finding, and an anterior concavity or genu valgum may also be noted. The thorax is frequently flat with a decreased AP diameter and a depression in the region below the breasts. A functional deficit or crepitation may be the result of a fracture.

Many other symptoms are considered to be characteristic for rickets, but their diagnostic value appears to be open to question considering the wide individual variability in such areas as the widening of sutures or late dental eruption. Usually mention is also given to hypotonia, hyperchromic anemia and a somewhat poor general condition of such babies. These symptoms often point to a variety of deficiencies, and are the result of the poor living conditions so frequently associated with rickets. Tetany resulting from serious respiratory disturbance occasionally leads to the recognition of rickets.

If there is no treatment, there is further increase of the deformities and also a marked growth deficit, which is not well understood. If vitamin D is given, there will be progressive disappearance of the skeletal changes. Sometimes however late sequelae may be noted radiographically.

Radiographic Findings

During the course of rickets, there are abnormal findings affecting the metaphyses, epiphyses and the diaphyses.

The earliest alterations are those of the metaphyses. In mild involvement the only visible findings may be irregularities of the metaphyseal border, which may appear comblike or fringed. Its form may be concave and widened, and its lateral contours spread out. The space between the metaphyseal line of ossification and the corresponding epiphysis is wider than normal (Fig. 5-1). The epiphyseal ossification center appears late, has an abnormal transparence and its structure is lacy. Sometimes the contours are also soft and irregular.

The aspect of the diaphyseal cortex is variable. In the majority of cases there is loss of cortical thickness. This is usually noted in hypocalcemic patients. Looser-Milkman's lines, and sometimes real fractures, are seen only in severe cases. In about one-third of the patients, there is a thick appearance of the cortex with a corticodiaphyseal ratio above 50 per cent. The borders are ill-defined, which results in difficulties with measuring. There are patients in whom sub-periosteal resorption is clearly visible, quite similar to that seen in hyperparathyroidism. This resorption occurs almost exclusively at the level of the femoral neck and the phalanges.

Diaphyses are frequently bowed, a finding varying somewhat with the age at the onset of rickets (Royer). In very early onset, while the baby is mostly in a horizontal position, it is sometimes possible to note bowing of the clavicles. The upper extremities become deformed when the baby is somewhat older and begins to move around on all fours. Tibial bowing with anterior convexity also seems to appear prior to assuming the upright position. Lateral bowing is the hallmark of the baby already assuming the upright position. If bowing is already old, there is usually marked cortical thickening of the concavity of the affected long bones, which in no way should detract from the actual diagnosis.

An increased radiolucency of other skeletal parts such as the pelvis and spine, together with abnormal,

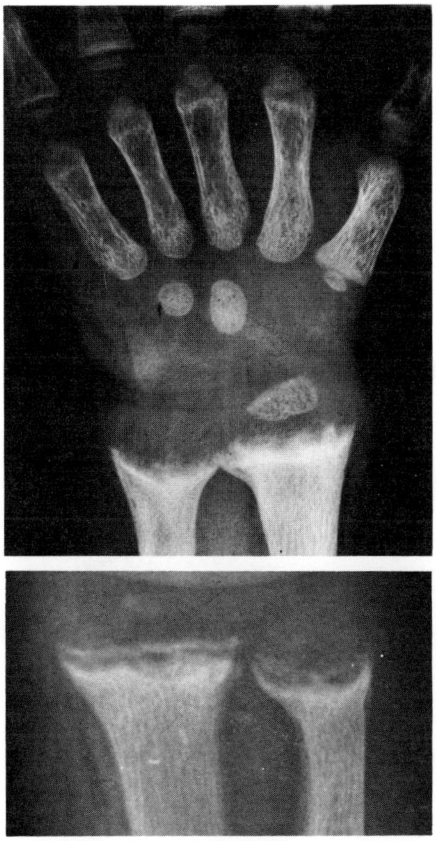

Fig. 5.1. Two different patients 7 and 9 months old with (*top*) acute stage and (*bottom*) healing stage of rickets.

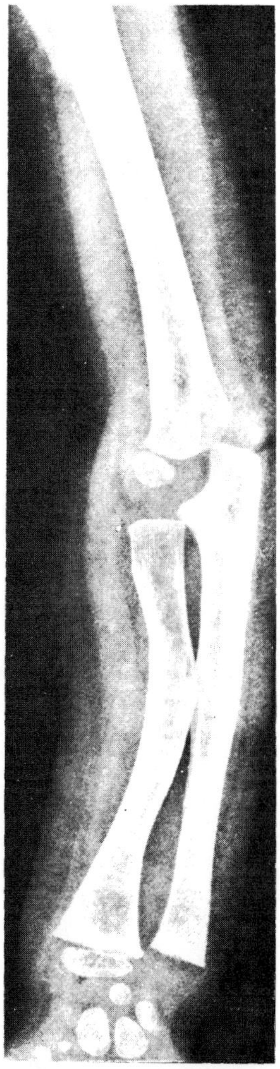

Fig. 5-2. A 23-month-old infant during the healing phase of deficiency rickets. Note the dense lines at the metaphyseal ends of the forearm, the modeling defect, and the double outline of the cortex. (Courtesy of J. Lefebvre)

thin and lacy trabeculation may be noticeable in severe cases. The ill-defined aspect of the ribs and the flaring at the costal ends can be very striking. Chest radiographs will reveal mildly opacified lungfields, sometimes with prominent hilar or peri-hilar regions contrasting with the increased radiolucency of the skeleton. In severe cases a reticulo-nodular pattern will be noted, and sometimes localized atelactasis combined with localized emphysema of one of the apical lungfields.

Besides delayed ossification at the sutures and a possible persistence of the fontanelle, it should be remembered that these patients have a certain risk of developing craniosynostosis and thickening of the skull. Craniosynostosis occurs only exceptionally in deficiency rickets, in spite of the figure of 10 per cent given by some authors. We consider this figure to be too high. Thickening of the skull affects by preference the frontal and occipital bone and will only be seen during the second year of life or later. It may persist for a long time.

During spontaneous healing or under treatment, there is progressive disappearance of these lesions and the distance between the epiphyses and the metaphyses will again become normal. Quite frequently we can note the appearance of a dense band at the metaphyseal border (Fig. 5-2). Immediately adjacent to this there is often a clear zone, which will calcify later, but this lucency may persist for a considerable time. The metaphyseal ends may for a while appear as if they contain noncalcified tissue. The

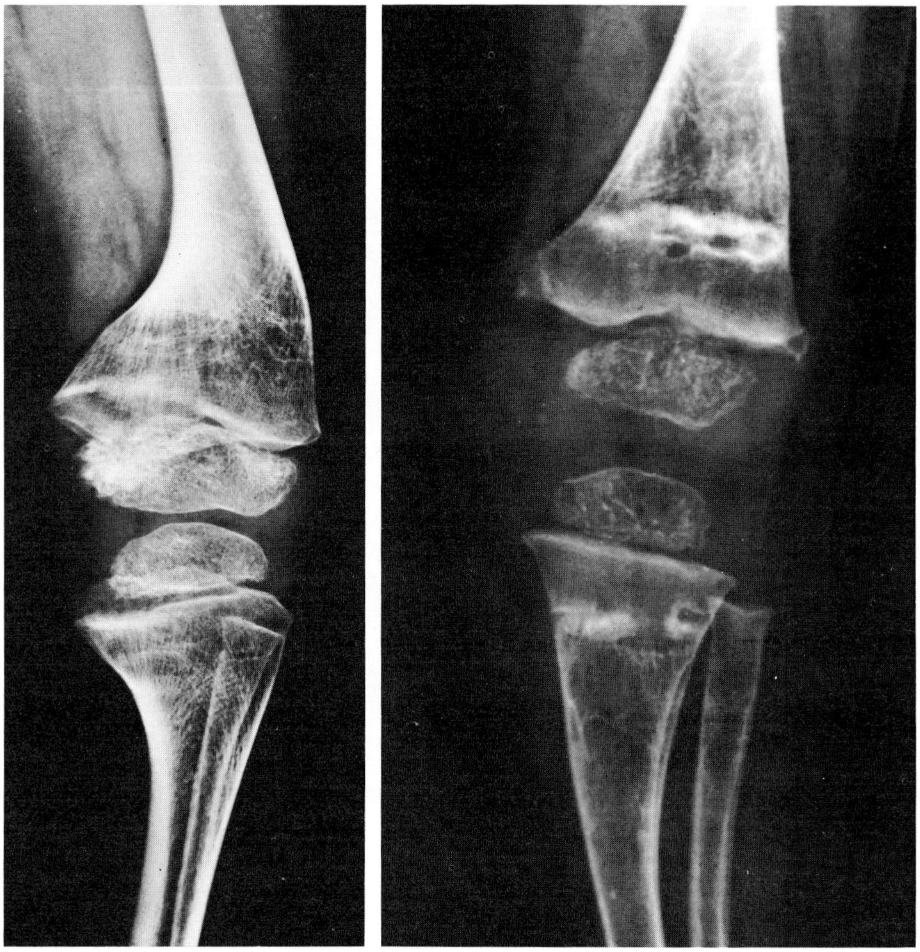

Fig. 5-3. Late radiographic findings after rickets. (*Left*) 3-year-old girl with a modeling defect of the metaphyses. (*Right*) 2-year-old boy with persisting chondroid inclusion. (Courtesy of J. Guivarch)

epiphyses may be encircled by a thin line resulting in a double contour. The diaphyseal area, particularly in severe involvement, will show appositional growth around the old diaphysis, which seems to give it a second outer bony contour.

The spine during this stage frequently shows a double contour of the vertebrae similar to what is seen in the epiphyses, but it persists much longer. Occasionally this finding can be helpful in a retrospective diagnosis. The calcification of rib lesions may result in a continuous opaque band, a symptom that should not be confused with pleural thickening.

Later, rickets may result in marked skeletal sequelae, often not recognized as relating to the basic disease. We have already referred to the zone of increased radiolucency immediately above the growth zone, the vertebrae with double contour and craniosynostosis. Other symptoms include affected metaphyseal modeling, inclusion of chondroid tissue islands, bowing and disturbed growth. These changes are seen in a case of severe rickets which has gone without treatment for a prolonged time.

The metaphyseal modeling defect is recognized by widening of the metaphyses at their diaphyseal end. These alterations are somewhat reminiscent of Pyle's disease, but there is no concomitant widening of the diaphyseal cortices. Careful analysis of the metaphysis often reveals the presence of a more lucent region corresponding to growth during the active phase of rickets. This region is separated from the metaphyseal border by a zone of normal density, laid down during healing (Fig. 5-3, *Left*).

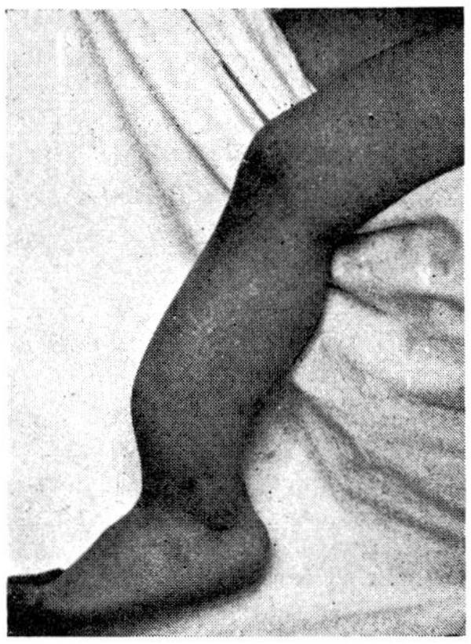

Fig. 5-4. Healed rickets. Marked bowing with anterior convexity of tibia. (Courtesy of J. Guivarch)

Inclusions of chondroid tissue first localized in the immediate neighborhood of the line of ossification sometimes persist after healing and migrate towards the diaphysis just as do chondromas, to which they have a similarity (Fig. 5-3, *Right*). The bowing of long bones, tends to spontaneously heal, but may persist over a prolonged period of time. Occasionally corrective surgery is necessary.

Rickets of excessively long duration may result in serious growth retardation and sometimes in scoliosis, appearing at first sight almost like chondrodysplasia. There are individual cases of a particularly severe degree, where the growth spurt after healing does not occur normally or only to an insufficient degree.

A possible example of such effects may be toxopachyosteosis, described by Weissmann-Netter. It manifests itself as a growth deficit combined with anterior convexity of the tibiae. It is our opinion that most of the cases published under this heading should be classified as rickets (Fig. 5-4). Study of the cases in the literature has led to the recognition of minor anomalies, such as a mild degree of coxa vara, bowing of the diaphyses and pelvic deformity indicative of previous osteomalacia. On the other hand there are unquestionable cases of rickets, which have been found with documented persistence of similar findings after healing (Epitalbra-Schnebelen) (Fig. 5-5).

Biologic Findings

During the course of rickets there are constant anomalies of the metabolism of phosphorus and calcium. The great majority of patients have low values for serum phosphorus, but calcium may be normally present or only slightly low. It is unusual to have normal phosphorus value in the presence of low calcium

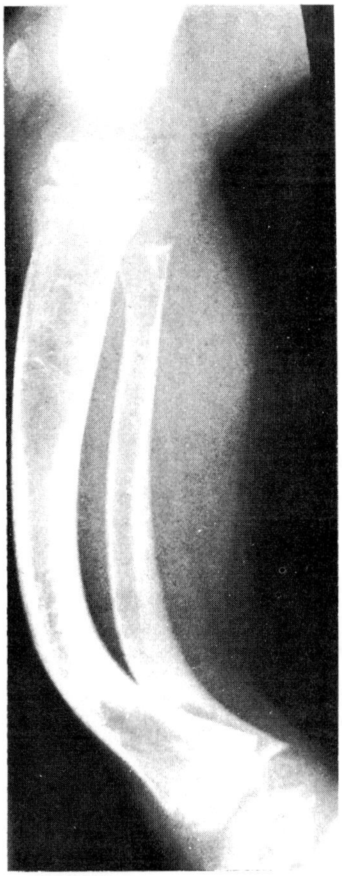

Fig. 5-5. A late sequelae of rickets which are identical to the bowing and deformity described under the name toxopachyosteosis. (Weissmann-Netter syndrome) in a 6-year-old boy. (Courtesy of J. Guivarch)

in the serum. The alcaline phosphatases of the serum are constantly elevated as are the values for fecal calcium and phosphorus. Calciuria may be normal, but in the majority of cases is markedly low.

The parathyroids, in a large number of patients, will attempt to compensate the calcium loss resulting from the lack of vitamin D, and from the disturbed intestinal calcium resorption. Interference by parathormone explains the many patients with normo-calcemia, and lowered phosphoremia. It can reduce tubular reabsorption of phosphorus. Lowering of calcemia would result in those cases in which the parathyroids cannot bring about normalization of serum calcium.

There is a high incidence of hyperchloremic acidosis. If this is present investigations for tubular function should *not* be performed. Such studies are sometimes initiated erroneously by physicians not familiar with this problem. Usually there is also hyperaminoaciduria and hypochromic anemia.

During treatment, vitamin D leads to an increase of phosphoremia, which will go well beyond the normal, possibly as high as 80 mg/l. In the most severe cases there are variable biochemical alterations. Without additional calcium intake, an increase of phosphoremia can be accompanied by a drop of serum calcium with the inherent risk of a serious tetanic seizure. If calcium is supplemented phosphoremia and calcemia will return to normal values without first reaching excessively high values for the former. Fecal phosphorus and calcium will be lowered while calciuria and phosphaturia, initially low, will slowly increase. Within one or two weeks there is normalization of these parameters, but the values for alkaline phosphatases remain high for a prolonged period of time.

Pathology and Pathogenesis

The characteristic histologic alteration of rickets is the persistence of noncalcified osteoid bony tissue. Normally, when newly formed bone is laid down, as soon as vessels invade from the growth cartilage, there is immediate calcification. This does not occur in rickets.

Calcification beginning along the columnar cartilage is effective, the invasion by blood vessels is disorderly and the zone of provisional calcification is not resorbed. The cartilaginous cells continue to proliferate, and this zone becomes much larger than normal. There is no cartilaginous hypertrophy, but only a defect in its normal maturation. There are also anomalies of structure of collagen with the presence of afibrillar material in the neighborhood of these cells, occurring secondarily to a defect of maturation.

During treatment the first noticeable response is the deposition of calcium salts immediately around the growth cartilage. Avitaminosis D negatively affects metabolism of calcium, and only secondarily of phosphorus. Disturbed intestinal resorption is the primary defect leading to this deficit. We have referred to the fact that vitamin D also has a direct action on calcification. Secondarily, lack of calcium results in parathyroid hyperactivity, and subsequent increased phosphorus elimination. This effect is sometimes insufficient to relieve calcemia.

Hyperaminoaciduria of rickets is still poorly understood, but it is corrected rapidly by vitamin D. It does not appear to be related to a constitutional anomaly which would predispose one to rickets, as has been proposed by some authors. Fraser has shown that there is a positive correlation between hyperaminoaciduria and hyperparathyroidism, which might possibly have an effect on tubular reabsorption of amino acids.

Treatment and Prevention

Therapy of rickets requires a total dose of 200,000 U of vitamin D. This may be given in a single dose or daily doses of 2000 to 4000 U during 6 to 12 weeks. Calcium supplementation is indispensable for patients suffering from or threatened by tetany, and for severely affected patients with considerable loss of skeletal calcium. This will limit hypocalcemia and it will also result in rapid remineralization. The usually prescribed dosage is 0.5 to 1 g/day.

To prevent rickets a daily dose of 400 U vitamin D is necessary, which should be routinely given for the 18 initial months of life and later during the winter. This preventive approach is even more necessary when children live in generally poor conditions, lack exposure to sunshine and have highly pigmented skin. In a mild climate such babies are especially prone to develop rickets. Under these circumstances, it is advisable to give 2000 U/day to prevent the disease.

It should be remembered that in the bigger child rickets may still develop because of disturbed intestinal resorption—steatorrhea, or as a result of chronic skin disorders, such as eczema. Prolonged treatment with anticonvulsant or neuroleptic drugs can lead to rickets. It is proper to increase the dosage of vitamin D in infants so treated. These drugs seem to have an activating effect on the hepatic hydrolases and to accelerate transformation of vitamin D into its more polar and biologically inactive derivatives. 25-hydroxycalciferol appears to be highly effective in the treatment of this type of rickets, since it is quite possible that this derivative escapes inactivation better than vitamin D (Royer and Arsane).

OSTEOPATHY OF PREMATURITY

Very premature babies can develop a peculiar bony disorder, which has been widely recognized following the description by Friis-Hansen and by Rossier. In its most severe form this disorder is a combination of skeletal lesions, a hepatic icterus and a subacute pulmonary process.

Clinical Findings

This disorder is recognized most frequently because of the appearance of icterus and more rarely of a lung pathology between 6 weeks and 3 months of age. Clinically, the skeletal lesions are hardly noted. There may be a rosary of the thorax and slight metaphyseal flaring. Occasionally, however, there is a functional lesion accompanied by local swelling of soft tissues. Such findings may lead one to suspect a spontaneous fracture. The icterus is usually of moderate degree, the urine may be dark, and the stools occasionally colorless. Frequently there is hepatomegaly. Pulmonary involvement may be clinically noted because of dyspnea, accompanied by cough and cyanosis. Usually there is fever and some general weakness. Auscultation often is normal. Occasionally there are fine rales in both lungfields. Other infections, mainly staphylococcal can be seen.

Usually these patients will improve, but rarely death can result from pulmonary complication. The skeletal lesions will heal, usually without sequelae. There are, however, several cases on record with local changes of the femoral head and residual coxa valga.

Radiographic Findings

Skeletal studies show excesive radiolucency of bones, especially the diaphyses of the long bones. The cortical areas are thin and often have a double contour. Spontaneous fractures occur in about half of the cases. The metaphyses are cupped, with uneven and fringed borders as in rickets. The ossification centers are delayed in appearance and irregular in structure (Fig. 5-6).

The involvement of the ribs is particularly striking. Besides the unusual transparency there are frequent fractures of ribs, usually at the transition from the posterior to the middle third. The respiratory problems and pulmonary complications most likely are to a large extent caused by these fractures. There are marked similarities with the rachitic lung changes, in that diffuse inhomogenous pulmonary opacities give them an ill-defined aspect.

Under therapy rapid disappearance of these findings is the rule. Repair may be exuberant, as has been pointed out by Boissière, et al. There may be hypertrophic callus formation or thick diaphyseal periosteal bone deposits. Abnormal findings involving the femoral head and neck sometimes persist after healing. Follow-up chest films may reveal the presence of segmental opacification or bullae.

Biochemical Data and Pathogenesis

Serum calcium is most often low and sometimes excessively so. This explains the high incidence of tetany. Alkaline phosphatase is usually elevated. Serum phosphorus however is normal.

In the presence of icterus the values for prothrombine and proconvertine are usually low. Other liver function tests may occasionally be abnormal.

These premature infants frequently suffer from marked anemia.

Two disorders seem to precipitate the symptoms: severe hypocalcemia of prematurity, and disturbed tubular phosphorus reabsorption. Supplementation of calcium, vitamin D and protides has resulted in the complete disappearance of this disorder in those centers where such policies have been put into effect. The pulmonary pathology is secondary to rib pathology. The icterus is not a constant feature and does not play the central role originally attributed to it.

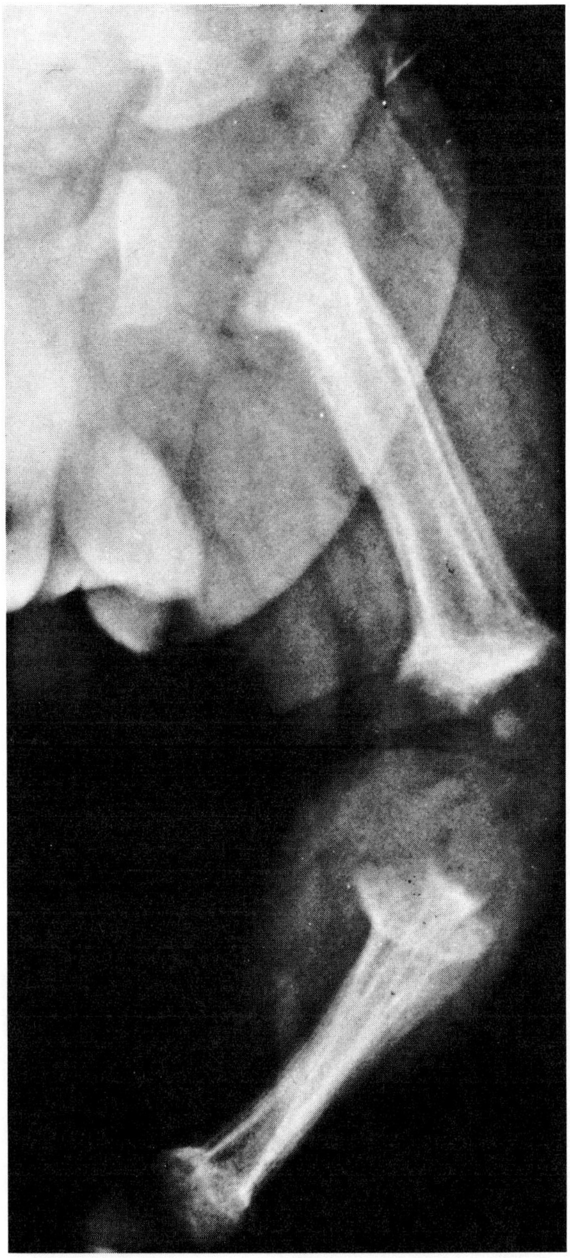

Fig. 5-6. Generalized osteopathy in prematurity. (Courtesy of H. Boissière)

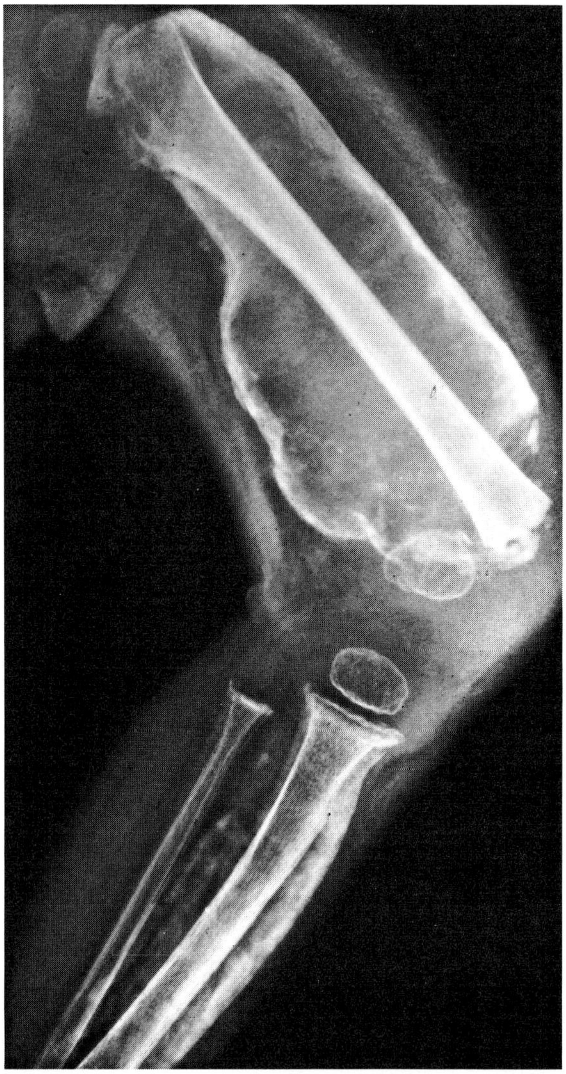

Fig. 5-7. Scurvy in a 1-year-old boy. There are enormous hematomas, and widened metaphyses with a hyperlucent submetaphyseal line. (Courtesy of P. Royer)

Treatment

Therapy for the icterus or the pulmonary involvement are not discussed here. Therapy must complement the efforts directed against the skeletal lesions: the administration of vitamin D and calcium. Vitamin D should be given in the dosage of 3000 to 6000 U/day and calcium at least 50 mg/kg/day. Disturbed intestinal resorption secondary to icterus may occasionally justify parenteral administration.

Prophylaxis consists in the administration of high doses of vitamin D in all small prematures by supplementation of 2000 U/day in combination with 50 mg/kg/day of supplemental calcium. If there is icterus present these dosages should be doubled or tripled.

SCURVY

Rickets unhappily is still a lesion seen with some regularity, scurvy has almost completely disappeared. Therefore such a diagnosis should be advanced with great care and only after having eliminated all the other much more frequently seen conditions, especially "the battered child" syndrome (see p. 345). Scurvy occurs in young infants. Discovery results from local changes. Uusually there is fever, local pain and limitation of movements of one extremity, leading to the radiographic recognition of the underlying changes.

Hemorrhagic manifestations are responsible for the clinical symptoms. There may be some petechiae, located by preference on the face. Gingival hemorrhages frequently accompany erupted teeth, but subperiosteal hemorrhages are characteristic. Severe local pain and limitation of motion is noted, and occasionally a pseudo-paralysis (Hutinel). Local swelling of the soft tissues can be prominent. Palpation reveals an underlying bony lesion. Rosary formation from subperiosteal hemorrhage at the chondroosteal junctures may be noted. Fever is usually present during the development of this disorder. This may result from superinfection, or simply from the resorption of hematomas. Frequently we note hypochromic anemia, hypophosphoremia and hypoproteinemia.

Radiographically, scurvy is recognized by diffuse osteoporosis, fractures and subperiosteal hematomas. Increased radiolucency of the skeleton is a generalized phenomenon involving the diaphyses and epiphyses. The cortex of the long bones is very narrow. Trabeculation is poorly developed. Immediately next to the metaphyseal border a dense band is separated from the rest of the diaphysis by a markedly radiolucent zone, where the bone has completely lost its structure. This dense line is unusually long and the metaphysis shows acute widening at its site (Fig. 5-7). The epiphyses show a clear central zone, a lacy periphery, and a somewhat dense border at the articular surface. This finding is especially clearcut in the knee.

Pathologic fractures are frequently seen. They are located mostly in the metaphyseal region, just below the line of ossification. Sometimes they simply result in a rupture of the cortex.

Initially the hematoma will show up as an irregular density in the soft tissues adjacent to the affected bone. Secondary calcification will form a complete cylinder surrounding the diaphysis. Its borders are irregular, lacy, but always clearcut. Under the influence of vitamin C there is progressive resorption of the hematoma. The metaphyseal modeling deficit can persist for a considerable length of time.

After healing a circular density around the epiphyseal centers can persist, as occasionally does the abnormal increased central radiolucency. The dense metaphyseal band will migrate towards the diaphysis while the cortex may assume a double contour similar to that seen in rickets.

Histologic study of the growth cartilage reveals a disturbed growth zone, with swelling, or a complete cessation of enchondral ossification.

The diagnosis is confirmed when the vitamin C-level of leukocytes is close to zero. Therapy consists of high doses of ascorbic acid, 100 to 200 mg/day. If there is also an intestinal disturbance vitamin C should be given parenterally. Therapy should be continued for at least 3 months.

HYPERVITAMINOSIS A

We shall not deal here with acute vitamin A intoxication, but rather with the effect of a prolonged intake of high amounts. This is a rare disorder, but a number of cases have been reported from different parts of the world.

Hypervitaminosis A is most frequently recognized because of unusual irritability combined with a loss of appetite, pain in extremities, disturbed gait, weakness of the lower extremities, and sometimes fractures. In an unusual situation there may be growth arrest. Palpation of the extremities is painful. Craniotabes is occasionally noted together with a dry skin with excoriations and sometimes loss of hair. Some patients can no longer walk. Radiologic study shows mild bowing of the diaphyses, and mainly a thickening of the cortex of long bones combined with abnormal modeling of the metaphyses immediately next to the growth cartilage, which itself may be reduced in height. This cartilage may show abnormal density and slight irregularity at the metaphyseal border. In extreme cases there may be premature closure of cartilaginous zones.

Intoxication of only short duration and with a relatively low dosage has also been described in babies. This led to a lack of bony density and cupping and irregularity of the metaphyseal ends of long bones (Persson et al.).

It is difficult to specify the exact level of vitamin A that may lead to such a disorder, since it appears that there is an individual sensitivity. The clinical symptoms will disappear after the vitamin A intake has been terminated, but the growth disturbance may be definitive, if there has been closure of growth zones. A possible similar role of carotene is still under discussion. Some authors have suggested that the small size of certain population groups may actually be the result of an excessive intake of carotenoids.

HYPERVITAMINOSIS D

The danger of an excessive intake of vitamin D is now recognized worldwide. Because of this there are now only very sparse incidences of this hypervitaminosis.

Most frequently intoxication of vitamin D is recognized because of loss of appetite, nausea or vomiting, and because of a most prominent excessive thirst and polyuria. Sometimes acute accidents secondary to dehydration with hyperchloremia may be seen. The symptom is a convulsive crisis, a collapse or a coma, simulating tuberculous meningitis.

The distribution of the local lesions is quite different from that of infantile cortical hyperostosis (see p. 343) with which it could be confused. In the former there is no involvement of the mandible, one of the key symptoms of the latter.

The prognosis depends on the degree of nephrocalcinosis present. If severe, irreversible renal damage may result. In infants there has been death from dehydration or cerebral hemorrhage. The bony lesions however will completely disappear.

Radiographically there is a lack of density of the skeleton with small zones of condensation immediately next to the growth zones. Sometimes this condensation is quite prominent, forming dense bands similar to those seen in heavy metal poisoning. In some exceptional cases generalized osteosclerosis has been present (De Wind). Finally, fine calcium deposits may be noted within articular structures. The calcifications known to occur within the walls of vessels or within the kidney are not seen radiologically.

Biochemical study reveals an increase of plasma calcium in all its fractions. Phosphorus is usually normal, and a decrease of plasma magnesium has been reported, also alcalosis, most likely as the result of vomiting. Calciuria is high. Often there is an increase of plasma-urea and a disturbed concentration of urine, which may simulate renal failure.

Histologic study shows that the bony trabeculae are surrounded by wide osteoid seams reminiscent of rickets, but there is normal calcification. Studies in the rat have resulted in the recognition of increased bony resorption with accelerated calcium metabolism. This

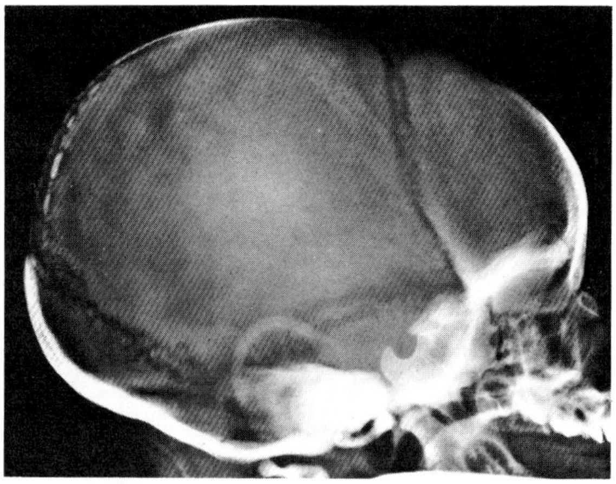

Fig. 5-8. Myxedema in a 5-month-old baby. The base of the skull has a somewhat dense appearance, but there is insufficient mineralization in the neighborhood of the sutures. Note the numerous wormian bones.

may result from the excessive formation of ostoid tissue.

Severe cases with coma or dehydration should be treated with calcitonin, which will quickly bring down the calcemia. It should be given in combination with a general regimen low in calcium and therapy with cortisone. Obviously an immediate termination of any vitamin D intake is mandatory.

SKELETAL LESIONS RESULTING FROM ENDOCRINE DISTURBANCES

Two endocrine glands play a primary role in the development of the skeleton: the thyroid and the parathyroids. These will be first considered. Subsequent discussion of other endocrine disorders will be offered, within the framework of their main skeletal manifestations.

HYPOTHYROIDISM

Disturbed skeletal growth and dwarfing are the most significant results of hypothyroidism.

The bony changes are a complex association of delayed growth and maturation, epiphyseal dysgenesis with metaphyseal changes and an unusually dense bony structure. The relative importance of any one of these changes depends on the age of the patient and the exact type of the disorder.

In athyreosis at birth there is only a mild lack of growth. The main symptoms are the infiltration of the skin, the abnormal facial appearance and the general condition and behavior of the baby.

Radiologically the most prominent findings are a marked delay in bone age and especially epiphyseal dysgenesis, which sometimes allows one to recognize the onset of the disorder prenatally. The distal femoral epiphyses and those of the proximal tibia are not visible, while the astragalus, the calcaneus and the cuboid have an irregular or fragmented structure. Ossification of the skull is deficient and the base of the skull may be unusually dense (Fig. 5-8). Changes of the vertebral bodies will not be seen before 3 to 6 months. In the newborn period one has to be careful in the presence of an unusually dense appearance of all the long bones, since normally the cortex may be quite thick at this age.

In the bigger child the symptoms consist of a combination of retarded skeletal maturation and epiphyseal dysgenesis. The latter is the most characteristic finding, but we should also insist on the finding of an unusually dense skeleton. Delayed maturation does not only involve the epiphyses, the carpal and tarsal bones, but also the vertebrae and the craniofacial structures. This is usually a generalized and symmetrical effect, and the ratio of the bone age to height age is usually below 1. This finding is not seen in other conditions.

Once the ossification centers have appeared radiologically, they have a spongy character, they are frequently fragmented or have several isolated centers of ossification. This finding is most striking in the region of the femoral head, but can be seen elsewhere. Depending on the location, it may be a good indicator of the onset of hypothyroidism (Fig. 5-9). Thus involvement of the femoral head, the first cuneiforme and of the first carpal centers of ossification result from an onset of the disease before 1 year. Metacarpal or metatarsal pseudo-epiphyses are seen with an unusually high incidence. Epiphyseal dysgenesis can be rather prominent in patients with mild clinical signs of hypothyroidism. The clinical differentiation of such patients from those with multiple epiphyseal dysplasia may be difficult. The degree of disturbed growth and maturation, the thickness of the cortex and the elective involvement of the femoral head, where multiple centers are quite typically seen in hypothyroidism will be supporting arguments. If this differentiation appears impossible, one should determine the level of plasma iodine and obtain a thyroid scintigram.

Besides the epiphyseal involvement Royer has emphasized metaphyseal alterations of the femoral neck, which are often quite clearcut. This region may be somewhat short, wide and irregularly lacy in outline.

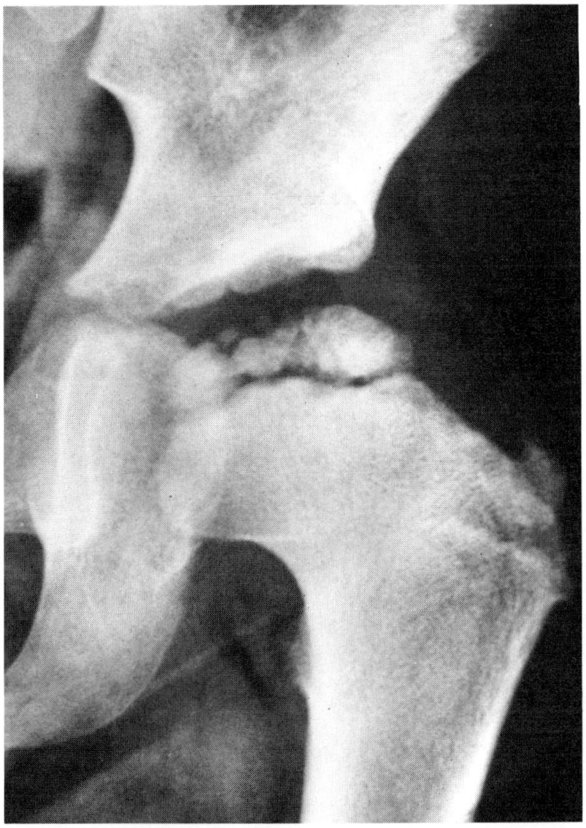

Fig. 5-9. Hypothyroidism in an 8-year-old girl. There is severe dysgenesis of the upper femoral epiphysis with fragmentation and an abnormal shape and outline.

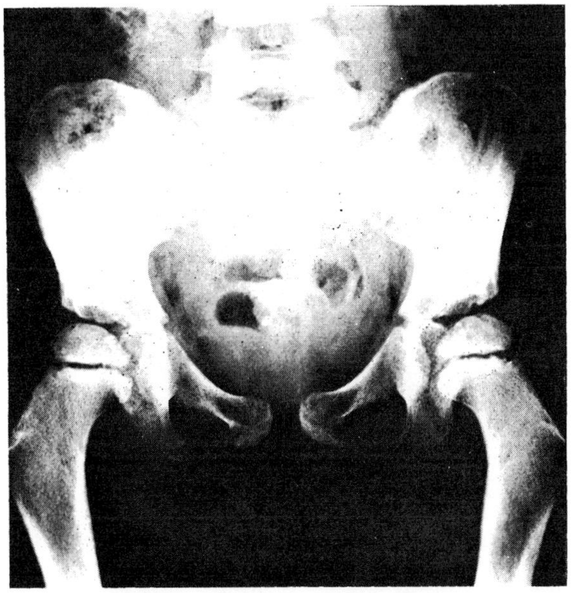

Fig. 5-10. Ectopic thyroid in a 7-year-old boy. The most striking finding is that of a slight irregularity in the proximal femoral metaphysis.

This finding can also be noted at the distal end of radius, ulna and tibia. It may be accompanied by the disappearance of the perichondral ring and by lateral widening of the metaphyseal border, forming a small spur. In some exceptional patients there may be an isolated finding of such metaphyseal changes. This seems to be the case particularly in patients with an ectopic location of the thyroid. The epiphyses develop somewhat late, but without recognizable morphologic alteration (Fig. 5-10). The diagnosis may be relatively difficult in such patients and will have to lean heavily on the discovery and evaluation of a severely retarded bone age.

Late vertebral maturation is another important sign of hypothyroidism. The findings are reduced height of the vertebral body and an abnormal persistence of the ovoid form and of the arterial vascular groove (channel of Hahn). One of the key findings is the wedged appearance of one lumbar vertebra, usually the second, combined with an anterior spur. This anomaly results in a lumbar kyphosis, and should not lead to a confusion with some types of spondylo-epiphyseal dysplasia or one of the mucopolysaccharidoses. Lack of an anterior tongue-formation projecting to other vertebrae will help in differentiating these, and especially to eliminate the possible diagnosis of Morquio's disease (Fig. 5-11). The delayed maturation of the craniofacial structures may be recognized by the following findings: widening of sutures and an abnormally long persistence of fontanelles. The synchondroses of the base close after considerable delay and the pneumatisation of the sinus is equally slow. There is an increased basal angle. All these findings are noted in patients with hypothyroidism of long standing. This somewhat diminishes their diagnostic value. The dental development is relatively less delayed. The sella remains within the plane of the cranial base and often appears somewhat ballooned with a wide superior opening. This finding is most marked in patients diagnosed and treated *late* for hypothyroidism. It can also be noted under therapy.

Condensation of the skeleton electively involves the long bones and the skull. The cortex is abnormally thick, and the metaphyses may get very close together or even completely obliterate the medullary canal (Fig. 5-12). A dense transverse band at the level of the growth cartilage is quite often present and a dense ring around the epiphyses is sometimes noted. Mégevand, Mathieu and Royer emphasize the presence of a local-

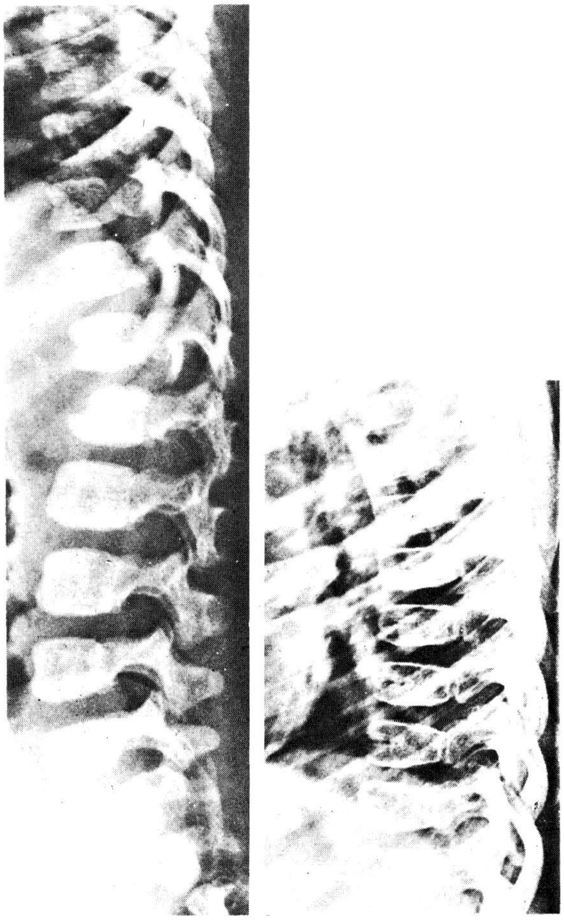

Fig. 5-11. Hypothyroidism. (*Left*) A 2-year-old infant with wedging of the spine. (Courtesy of A. Rossier) (*Right*) 7-year-old boy with an ectopic thyroid.

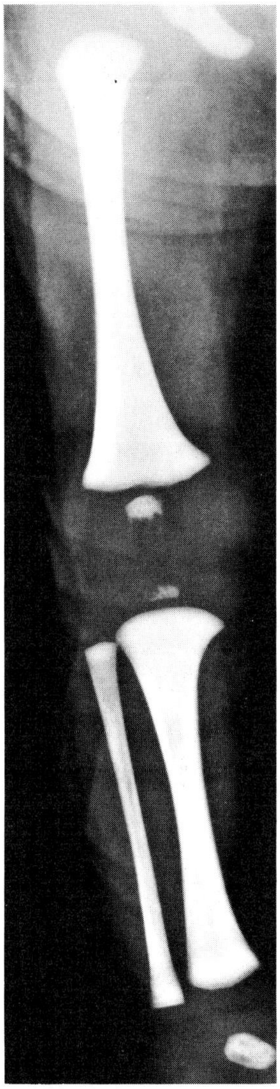

Fig. 5-12. Infant with hypothyroidism. Note the unusual dense appearance of the skeleton. (Courtesy of C. Fauré).

ized periosteal reaction. Thickening of the cranial structures involves the vault and the base together with the facial bones, especially the orbital borders. This thickening contrasts with the widening of the sutures, which helps to differentiate this disorder from other lesions in which unusually dense bones are found, especially idiopathic hypercalcemia.

In an exceptional patient especially in early infancy, the skeleton may be even denser, leading to confusion with osteopetrosis (Albers-Schönberg). Extra-skeletal calcification has been reported, especially in nephrocalcinosis, which results from prolonged disease.

Under therapy maturation of the skeleton will resume after 2 to 4 months, depending on the dosage of thyroid extract given and the age of the patient. Catch-up growth of the bone age is significantly more rapid before 1 year of age, as is growth in length. During therapy careful follow-up of the development of the bone age and the growth of the patient is important, since too rapid an acceleration of the former carries the danger of premature closure of the growth centers.

Epiphyseal dysgenesis will disappear, but persists as long as the bone age has not caught up with the chronological age. Prior to this stage, even new centers of ossification, appearing under therapy, are fragmented. The vertebral alterations will also be corrected, just as will the abnormal density of the skeleton. This may take several months. At the beginning of therapy, and with patients who have minimal thyroid activity, there may be a pseudo-scurvy appearance of the metaphyses, with a dense metaphyseal zone adjacent to a clear area, and with double ringed epiphyseal centers (Lelong).

A special point should be mentioned in reference to the lack of rickets in patients with hypothyroidism and an occasional occurrence during growth under hormone therapy.

Biochemical study sometimes shows hypercalcemia, but this is not a constant finding. The test of provoked hypercalcemia in some cases will show marked hypercalcemia and a delayed return to normal values (Royer et al.). Thus there seems to be a defect of the homeostasis of serum calcium with a resulting incapability of the organism to counterbalance disturbed calcium values. Sometimes there is marked calciuria, especially during therapy. This explains the high incidence of nephrocalcinosis during hypothyroidism. Pathophysiologic studies have shown that thyroxine has a simultaneous effect on the metabolism of phosphorus and calcium, and consequently on the skeleton. It results in an increase of the accumulation of calcium, osteolysis and osteoclastic resorption, together with reduced intestinal calcium resorption. In hypothyroidism, studies of ^{45}Ca show a reduced uptake and osteolysis (Job et al.). This delay of osteolysis is very marked and in all likelihood offers an explanation for the increased skeletal density. The intestinal resorption coefficient for calcium may be elevated and thyroid therapy will diminish this. Thyroxine has an elective effect on ossification of membranous bone and on skeletal maturation, but also on the development of growth cartilage. It is needed for the proliferation and hypertrophy of chondrocytes and also for the invasion of cartilage by vessels. The lack of thryoid hormone results in a defective development and late maturation of the columnar cartilage within the epiphyses. Vascular penetration does not occur within the center of the future epiphysis, rather, it occurs at several points, resulting in the presence of several ossification centers.

From these observations we conclude that, if calcitonin plays a role, in bringing about the symptoms of hypothyroidism, thyroxine is also important. This substance largely corrects the abnormalities noted during calcium perfusion. Delayed bony metabolism and increased intestinal resorption are obvious results of its lack. Vitamin D does not seem to play a major role here, but its somewhat parallel action may add its effect to that of hypothyroidism.

HYPERTHYROIDISM

Bony changes of hyperthyroidism are seen in an occasional adolescent, but mainly in adults, especially women after menopause. Prominent findings are osteoporosis with thin cortices and a rarefaction of the bony trabeculae, sometimes accompanied by geodes. This osteoporosis is most prominent within the spine and pelvis. This results in a high incidence of fractures and skeletal pain, especially within the spine. Advanced bone age and growth are prominent during childhood. Excessive height is present in roughly one half of all patients, especially in younger children during the early phase of the disease. This finding does not seem to be a direct expression of the degree of hyperthyroidism. There is wide variability of abnormally advanced bone age. Sometimes there is uneven involvement of some epiphyses, which will make interpretation of the bone age quite difficult, sometimes with a disparity of several years.

Usually the values for calcium and phosphorus are normal. Still, hypercalcemia has been noted, as has been an elevation of the level of phosphorus together with an increased renal tubular resorption of phosphorus. There may be markedly increased elimination of stool calcium. Experimentally there is diminished intestinal resorption of calcium (Noble).

In hyperthyroidism there seems to be an excessive mobilization of calcium from the skeleton. This has been documented by histologic study and occasionally by radiology. Hypercalcemia has been detected clinically, sometimes together with hypercalciuria, as has been proven by strontium studies (Eisenberg).

HYPOPARATHYROIDISM

Skeletal changes are not in the foreground of the symptoms of chronic hypoparathyroidism during infancy. Most frequently as a result of abnormal metabolism of phosphorus and calcium there is tetany, laryngeal spasm, convulsions, headaches, abdominal pain, fatigue or psychic depression. Sometimes there are abnormal skin findings: cutaneous moniliasis, eczema, loss of teeth, alopecia, and cataract.

Radiologically, bones can be entirely normal, but in some newborns or babies cortical hyperostosis can be noted. This may affect the femurs, tibias, fibulas and the humeri, and often results in a double contour (Fig. 5-13).

An unusually dense appearance of the skeleton is quite regularly noted in the older child. Long bones have a thick cortex with dense metaphyseal bands alternating with clear zones. Vertebral bodies and the pelvis can also be unusually dense (Fig. 5-14). Reduced trabeculation may sometimes give the bones a somewhat striated aspect. The inner table of the skull may be thick, and vascular calcifications within the

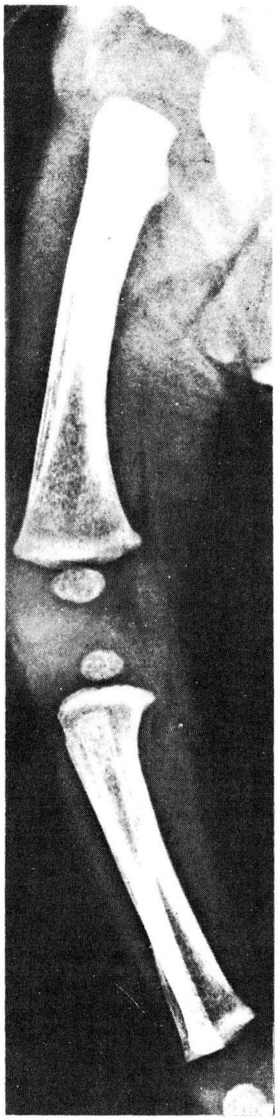

Fig. 5-13. Hypoparathyroidism in a 4-month-old infant. Note the double contour of the cortex. (Courtesy of S. Balsan)

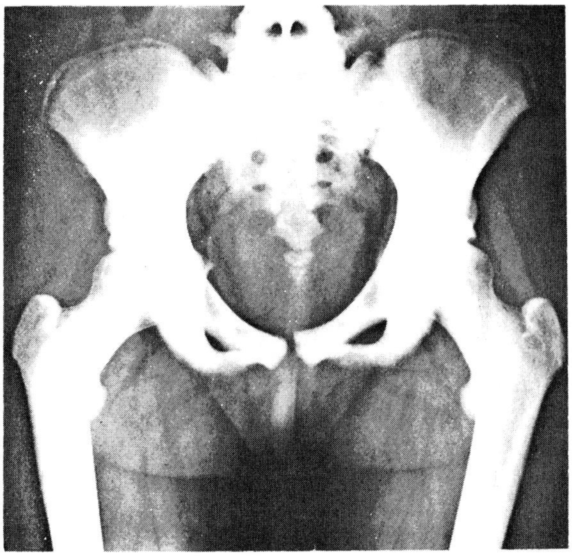

Fig. 5-14. Hypoparathyroidism in a 14-year-old girl with an unusually dense skeleton. (Courtesy of S. Balsan)

cerebellum and the basal ganglia have been reported. However, there are some unusual patients with a reduced bone density (Matthieu et al.).

Without therapy hypoparathyroidism may result in a reduced height and inefficient skeletal maturation, combined with an unusual facial appearance (Fig. 5-15).

We have already discussed the effect of parathormone on phosphorus and calcium metabolism (see p. 194). In many patients with hypothyroidism hypocalcemia is of a relatively mild degree, at the level of about 80 mg. This can, however, be much more marked, and there is always a strictly parallel alteration of the level of calcium and the occurrence of tetany. There is phosphoremia resulting from an increased tubular reabsorption of phosphorus. Calciuria is very low. It is not easy to understand the variations reported in the radiologic appearance of hypoparathyroidism. It would appear, experimentally, that parathyroidectomy reduces the fixation of calcium in bones and that it slows the liberation of fixed calcium. Depending on which of these factors predominates, bony density may be reduced or increased. On the other hand fixation of calcium depends in part on the product Ca × P. Its lowering would result in demineralization.

PSEUDO-HYPOPARATHYROIDISM

This disorder was defined in 1942 by Albright et al., after careful study of three patients suffering from a disorder somewhat similar to hypoparathyroidism, but unresponsive to parathormone.

This disorder is recognized during the first years of life because of mental retardation, tetany or convulsive crises.

The morphologically coarse appearance of these patients is quite characteristic. There is shortness of stature, a roundness of face, hypertelorism, and shortness of hands (Fig. 5-16). The trophic alterations of hypoparathyroidism are present in the form of cataracts.

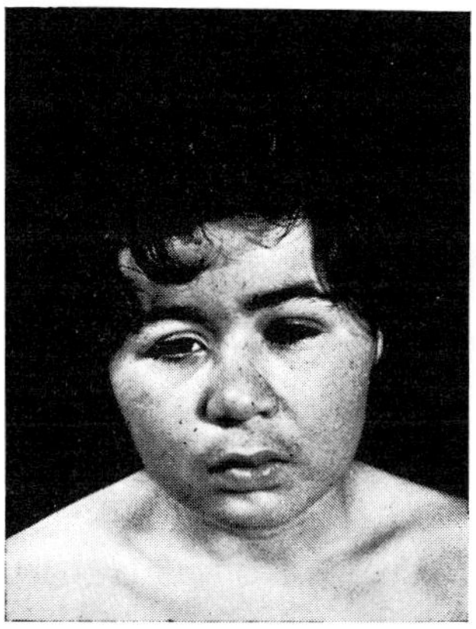

Fig. 5-15. Characteristic facial appearance in hypoparathyroidism. (Courtesy of S. Balsan)

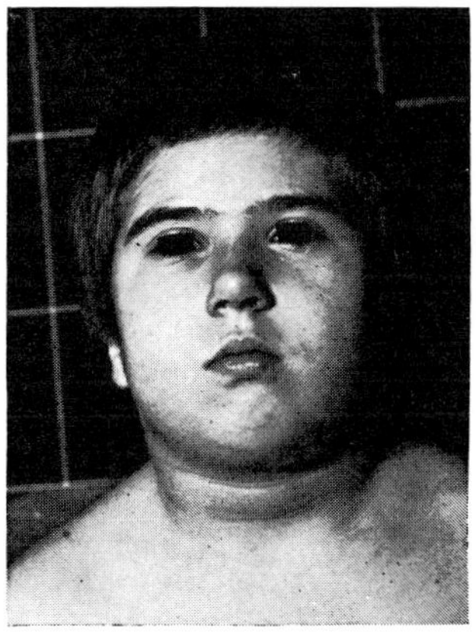

Fig. 5-16. Pseudo-hypoparathyroidism with the typical moon face. (Courtesy of P. Royer)

Radiologically, the most striking features involve the bones of the hand. These may be noted from the second year of life on (Fig. 5-17). The metacarpals, especially the 1st, 4th and 5th are shortened, the width of the growth cartilage is reduced and there is premature fusion of the epiphysis of these metacarpals. The diaphysis may be somewhat prominent, sometimes losing its normal modeling, especially during early infancy. Several phalanges may be similarly affected. Sometimes there is metaphyseal deformity, and frequently the epiphyses are coneshaped. These epiphyses may close prematurely or be totally absent. The foot may show similar abnormalities.

The long bones are frequently squat, with a relatively thin cortex and a somewhat increased radiolucency. There may be bowing of the radius. Some patients show signs of sub-periosteal resorption similar to that seen in hyperparathyroidism. This is considered a secondary phenomenon resulting from parathyroid stimulation by the low plasma calcium. Thickening of the skull has been noted. Teeth may be abnormal or of poor quality, and may erupt late. On radiographs the pulpa may be wide and the root narrow.

Calcifications of soft tissues occur frequently in pseudo-hypoparathyroidism. These are located peripherally, in the extremities under the skin near the joints. They are arranged in small heaps or small clusters of calcifications.

Serum values for calcium are low and for phosphorus are high. These values, however, do not respond to injections of parathormone.

In these patients an essential symptom, thus, is the resistance of the kidney to parathormone; it would appear that all the developmental anomalies are independent of this metabolic disturbance. It is quite possible that the primary lesion is a defect of the adenyl-cyclase-AMP cycle within the renal tubule. This system is necessary for the proper action of the hormone on phosphaturia. Possibly there are some cases in which the cyclic adenyl-cyclase-AMP system within the skeleton is defective, while its action is normal in the kidneys. This could help to explain the large number of different types of cases of pseudohypoparathyroidism (Frame et al.).

Pseudo-hypoparathyroidism follows a dominant mode of inheritance. There is, however, a markedly variable expressivity of the gene. Some individuals show only minor skeletal abnormalities.

Besides this type, Albright has further proposed a syndrome of pseudo-pseudo-hypoparathyroidism in which the morphologic anomalies are identical, but in which there is no abnormality of the phosphorus and calcium metabolism. In families with pseudo-hypoparathyroidism one can find such patients, which confirms this observation. Still, there are authors who have enlarged the definition and accepted under this heading a number of variable findings such as brachymetacarpy as the only common feature (Turner's syndrome, multiple exostoses, acrodysostosis). One should be very cautious when establishing this diagnosis.

HYPERPARATHYROIDISM

Hyperparathyroidism is an unusual disorder during infancy, and, like hypoparathyroidism, it is not diagnosed because of skeletal alterations, but because of GI symptoms, fatigability and/or hypotonia. During infancy this disorder can be responsible for marked dwarfism.

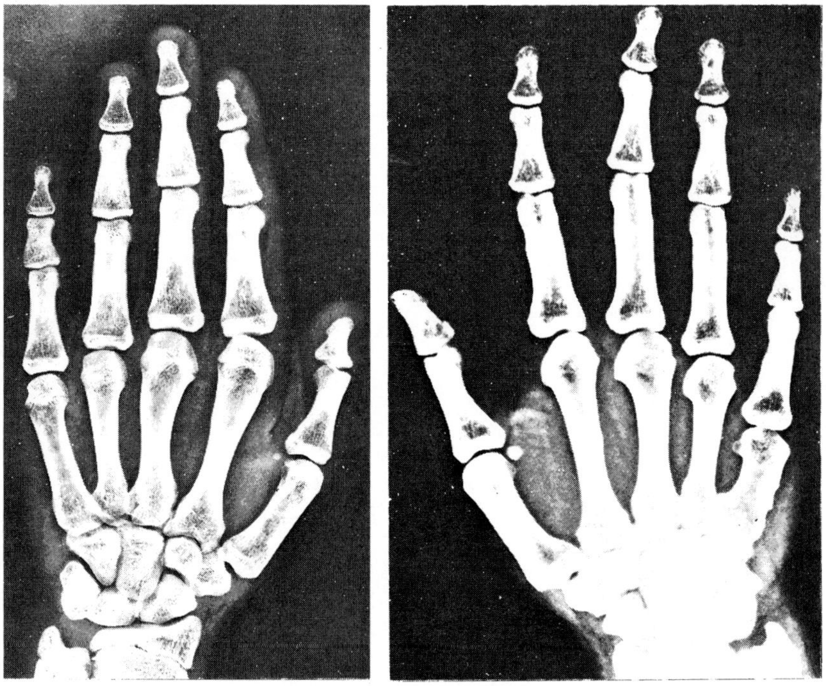

Fig. 5-17. Pseudo-hypoparathyroidism. (*Left*) in a 12-year-old boy, and (*Right*) in his mother. (Courtesy of C. Fauré)

A significantly diminished density of the entire skeleton is the most characteristic radiological finding. The cortex of long bones is narrow, trabeculation is markedly reduced, sometimes with a pseudo-cystic aspect in the metaphyseal or diaphyseal regions. Frequently there are spontaneous fractures and deformity of the diaphysis. Osteoclastic resorption can be noted, as evidenced by irregular contours of the lateral border of the metaphyses. This finding is most frequently noted at the upper end of the femur or humerus, the phalanges and metacarpals (Fig. 5-18). Epiphyses are abnormally radiolucent, as are vertebrae and the pelvis, in which the symphysis sometimes shows areas of resorption. Biconcave forms of vertebrae are seen, along with an abnormal spinal posture. The lamina dura loses its definition and may completely disappear (Fig. 5-19). The skull may lose its diploe, but during infancy we do not usually recognize the typical adult changes. Biochemical studies reveal an elevation of the level of calcium whereas there is lowering of phosphorus. Alkaline phosphatase is usually elevated in patients with marked skeletal involvement. Calciuria is little affected. The increased tubular reabsorption is actually compensated by the high serum concentration, especially the more complex citrate, which is not reabsorbed. Phosphorus excretion is normal or slightly increased in patients with skeletal involvement. Hydroxyprolinuria is also increased in these patients and we must stress that the presence of renal disorders is one of the feared complications of hyperparathyroidism, often seen in the presence of nephrocalcinosis.

Histologically, the bony anomalies are those of resorption of bony tissue, accompanied by osteoclastic proliferation. Bone is replaced by fibrous tissue. Dynamic studies have shown an acceleration of the bony metabolism with an increase in the exchangeable calcium reserve.

Hyperparathyroidism in the larger child is most frequently due to an adenoma. Healing is the rule after surgical removal, but therapy does not seem to have a direct connection to the cystic appearance, since this may not disappear after surgery. Multiple adenomatosis with pancreatic tumor or hypophyseal adenoma is very unusual but may be transmitted as a dominant disorder. In the newborn or small baby, and in addition to the very unusual intrauterine type of hyperparathyroidism resulting from unrecognized maternal hypoparathyroidism, we are faced most frequently by hypertrophy of the clear cells. In such a situation recurrence is the rule, and frequently there may be other signs and symptoms, such as multiple ulcera and pancreatic involvement, part of the Zollinger-Ellison syndrome.

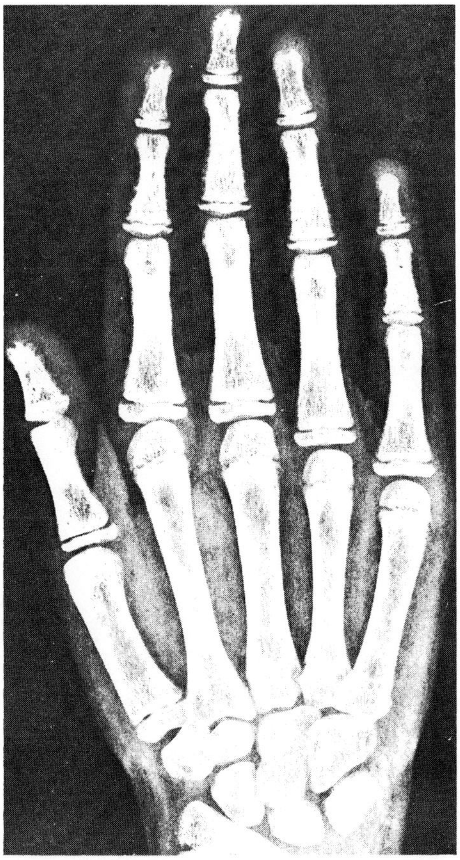

Fig. 5-18. Hyperparathyroidism in a 14-year-old girl. Notice the numerous areas of resorption, which are especially clear-cut on the second phalanx of the index and middle fingers. (Courtesy of P. Royer)

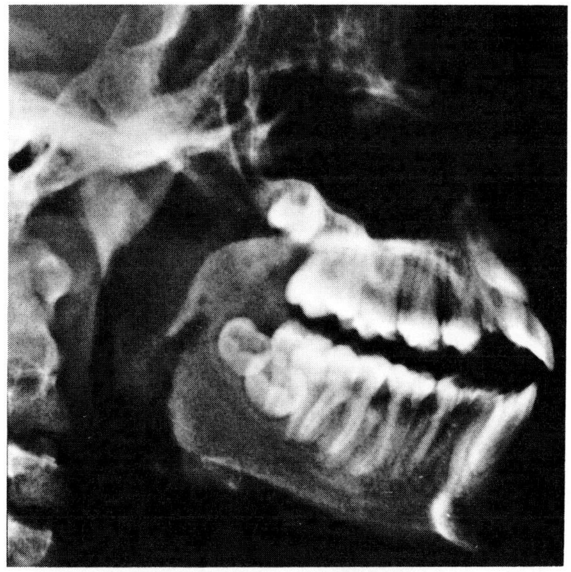

Fig. 5-19. Hyperparathyroidism. The lamina dura has completely disappeared. (Courtesy of S. Balsan)

We should remember that secondary hyperparathyroidism during infancy is much more frequent than primary types. We shall discuss its mechanism later with the renal osteopathies.

HYPOPHYSEAL INSUFFICIENCY

Isolated deficiency of somathormone, or its combination with other hormonal deficiencies, is responsible for severe dwarfism, which is rarely discovered before 1 to 3 years of age. Besides mild adiposity of the abdomen and the thighs, there may be a prematurely aged aspect of the skin, with early wrinkling in marked contrast to the infantile morphology of these patients. Puberty is delayed, but in some instances, especially in isolated hormonal deficiency (ateleiotic dwarfism = isolated deficiency of growth hormone), it may proceed normally at a later time. Secondary dentition appears markedly delayed.

Radiographically, growth of the bones is markedly retarded—the diaphyses are thin, as is their cortex. The development of the epiphyseal centers is also delayed. Still, the bone age is not considerably behind the height age, as is the case in hypothyroidism, except with an associated deficiency in thyreotropic hormone. In such a case there is a degree of epiphyseal dysgenesis, but this is always slight. Closure of the growth zones is excessively late, sometimes later than 30 or 40 years, and they may still be present at 70 years.

There are often fine irregularities at the metaphyseal end of the phalanges. They are predominantly noted in the first and second phalanges of each finger. The growth zone appears wavy as a result (Fig. 5-20). This feature can be seen in about one half of all cases, and is more marked than the irregularities which occur physiologically during growth. It is particularly pronounced after 5 years of age (Rappaport).

The basal angle of the skull is wide, the clivus short and the cranial vault thin. The frontal sinuses are small, and sometimes absent. A deformed sella turcica results from the presence of craniopharyngiomas. In ateleotic dwarfism, however, there is no increase of sellar size.

Somatropic hormone acts on the growth cartilage through the intermediary of somatomedine. This has

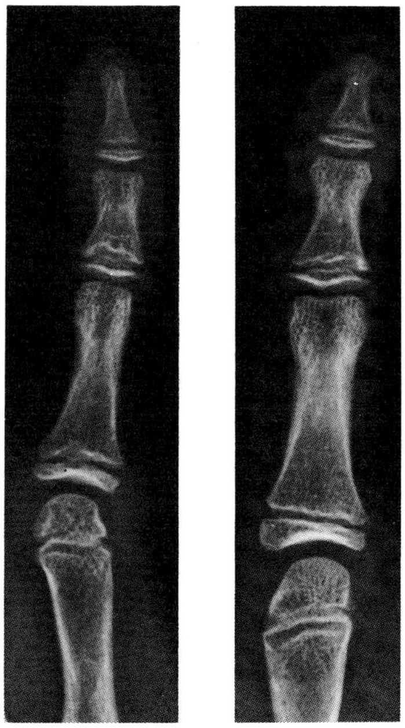

Fig. 5-20. Hypophyseal dwarfism in a 14-year-old girl. Note the abnormal metaphyseal outline of the phalanges. (Courtesy of R. Rappaport)

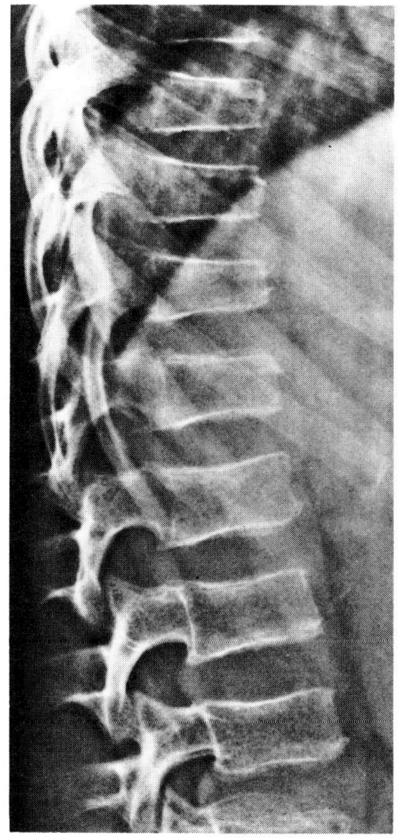

Fig. 5-21. Cushing's disease in a 7-year-old boy. Osteoporosis by concave deformity of the vertebral bodies. (Courtesy of R. Rappaport)

been proven by in vitro studies of cartilage of hypophysectomised rats after incubation. Somatomedine consists of a group of polypeptides of a relatively low molecular weight produced by several organs, especially the liver, under the influence of somatotropic hormone. This substance has an effect on the synthesis of nucleic acids, proteins and glycosaminoglycans. A special type of dwarfism with autosomal recessive transmission secondary to a deficit of this factor has been described. The symptomatology is identical to that already related, but the plasma concentration of growth hormone is increased and has no effect (Laron).

The etiology of the majority of patients with hypophyseal insufficiency is unknown. A number of isolated patients are encountered, however, there are some who suffer from dominant or autosomal recessively transmitted types with an isolated somathormone deficit (Rimoin).

HYPERPITUITARISM

With infants and children we must rarely deal with a patient with hypophyseal hyperactivity secondary to a tumor secreting somathormone (eosinophilic or chromophobic adenoma). The result, gigantism, usually has its onset around puberty. Growth may be prolonged up to the thirtieth year of life. The extremities are excessively long, especially the most distal portions. Sometimes the presence of Marfan's disease is suspected.

Besides the excessive length of the bones radiographic investigation will reveal the marked delay in closure of the growth zones, even in a young adult. Reduced density of the skeleton is not unusual, and is probably the result of hypercalciuria not compensated by an increased calcium resorption from the intestines. Contrary to this, plasma phosphorus is elevated because of the increased renal tubular reabsorption by growth hormone.

Study of the skull will show widening and deformity of the sella turcica as an expression of the hypophyseal tumor.

CUSHING'S DISEASE

Cushing's disease results from excessive production of cortisole. It is quite unusual during childhood. Growth retardation and bony lesions are keys to diagnosis, since, at this age, their visibility is certainly greater than that of obesity and facial alteration. Osteoporosis quite frequently results in back pain, may cause fractures, and is sometimes accompanied by kidney stones.

The cardinal radiologic features of Cushing's disease are osteoporosis of the spine and of the pelvis. The vertebral bodies are excessively radiolucent (Fig. 5-21). Often they are flattened and sometimes have the aspect of a biconcave lens. Vertebral compression secondary to a fracture is often noted. Ribs may be similarly affected, and they can be the site of fractures. The skull is sometimes demineralized. Bony maturation is delayed, and, in severely affected patients, comes to a complete stop. Correction of the radiologic findings, even after successful therapy, may take several years.

Prolonged therapy with cortisone or synthetic corticoids may have the same adverse effects as those just mentioned in Cushing's disease. This risk is particularly high in young patients treated for the nephrotic syndrome, but there may be additional factors: hypoproteinemia, and defective intestinal calcium absorption leading to osteoporosis. Cortisone seems to have an effect on collagen synthesis, as has been shown by a reduction of marked glycine incorporation in experiments cited by Vaes and Nichols on incubated bone slices. The same disturbance of collagen synthesis seems well documented in vivo by an increased hydroxyproline-excretion in the rat under prolonged cortisone treatment. This also has an inhibiting action on glucosaminoglycansynthesis in human fibroblast cultures, as proven by Castor. Finally, cortisone directly acts on the metabolism of phosphorus and calcium by reducing intestinal calcium resorption and possibly by altering the exchange of phosphorus and calcium between bone and the interstitial space. Therefore we assume that there is good reason for therapy with calcium and vitamin D to prevent secondary bony pathology in prolonged treatment with corticoids.

OTHER DISORDERS OF CORTICOADRENAL ORIGIN

Addison's disease is only rarely seen during childhood. It may occasionally be accompanied by a mild skeletal rarefaction. However, in disturbed synthesis of virilizing hormones there is a significant effect on growth and skeletal maturation. Growth is temporarily accelerated and accompanied by a marked advance of the bone age over the height age. Untreated patients inevitably undergo premature closure of growth zones, and have a resulting lack of height. Calcification of the costal cartilage and of the tracheal rings may also appear precociously, towards the tenth year of life. Treatment with hydrocortisone may prevent these symptoms.

ANOMALIES OF SEXUAL HORMONES

Secreting tumors — thecomas, granulosa-cell tumors, or testicular tumors may lead to accelerated skeletal maturation and early closure of the growth zones. Similar findings are seen in sexual precocity. Hypogonadism, however, will have the opposite effect on the growth zones, with growth proceeding for a longer period than normal.

In vivo experiments by Silberberg and Silberberg have demonstrated that estrogens and to a small degree testosterone exert a stimulating action on osteogenesis and that they reduce the resorption of metaphyseal spongy bone. This is a rather variable affect, and depends on the species studied. The action on collagen synthesis appears to be yet more variable.

In the rat testosterone given in small dosage will stimulate a proliferation of cells of the growth zone, but in high dosage it will inhibit this proliferation and actually result in the disappearance of cartilage. The same has been noted of estradiol, which in high dosage will result in a degeneration of chondrocytes and proliferation of the connective tissue vascular axes.

SECONDARY DISORDERS RESULTING FROM GENETICALLY DETERMINED ANOMALIES OF THE METABOLISM OF PHOSPHORUS AND CALCIUM

Vitamin D resistant rickets will be discussed together with hypercalciuria, hypophosphatasia and idiopathic hypocalcemia.

VITAMIN D RESISTANT RICKETS

There are several types of vitamin D resistant rickets and we shall successively investigate familial hypophosphatemic rickets, precocious pseudodeficiency rickets and late rickets. Rickets may also be

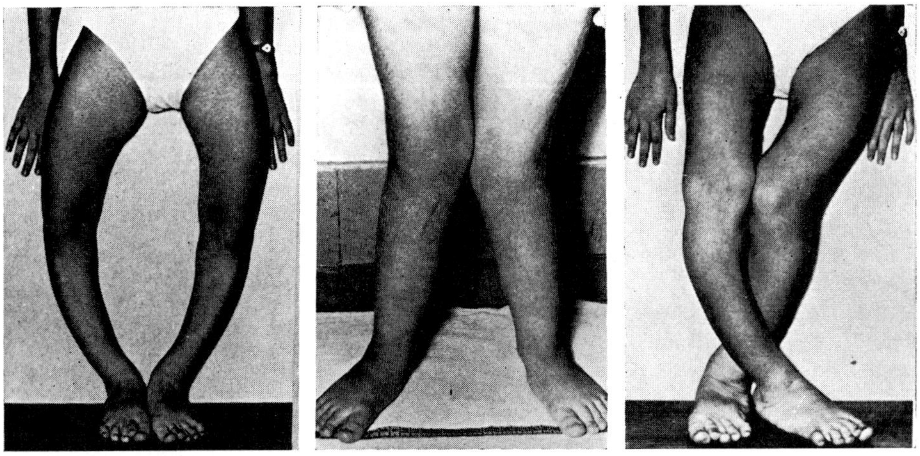

Fig. 5-22. Pictured here are different types of bowing which are seen in familial hypophosphatemic vitamin D resistant rickets. (Courtesy of S. Balsan)

caused by a series of hereditary metabolic disorders, such as cystinosis, tyrosinosis, the De Toni-Debré-Fanconi syndrome, and sometimes the syndrome of Lowe (see p. 224).

Familial Hypophosphatemic Vitamin D Resistant Rickets

This is the most frequently encountered type of vitamin D resistant rickets. It was described by Albright in 1937. The condition was noted much earlier, but was confused with achondroplasia.

Clinical Findings

The disorder is recognized most frequently around the second year of life, because of abnormal gait. Sometimes, however, discovery happens much later after a mild degree of bowing of the legs has occurred.

Hypophosphatemic familial rickets leads to a type of dwarfism with skeletal manifestations (Fig. 5-22). There is a progressive growth deficit during the growth period with a definitive height of 1.40 to 1.45 m. Skeletal deformity is most marked, involving the legs with bowing or occasionally genu valgum.

In most cases the metaphyses are palpable and there will typically be a rosary. Accentuation of the lumbar lordosis can be accompanied by dorsal kyphoscoliosis. Frontal bossing may be prominent and scaphocephaly is not exceptional. Teeth are of poor quality, because abnormal dentine formation, resulting in early shedding of the primary teeth.

Walking may be waddling, difficult, and painful, resulting in easy fatigability. The muscle tonus, however, is normal and there is no tetany in the course of vitamin D resistant rickets. Fractures are only rarely seen.

The development of the disease is progressive up to 20 years. From this age on there is no further progression of the deformities. Still, it is possible to have a further deterioration in the pathology at about 14 years of age and somewhat later.

Radiographic Findings

The findings seen during the course of vitamin D resistant rickets do not appreciably differ from those discussed in the chapter on deficiency rickets. Sometimes there are alternating denser and radiolucent bands, exactly following the outline of the metaphysis. The suggestion is that there are more or less active phases of this disease. The epiphyses and their ossification centers may have a somewhat irregular structure and their maturation may be delayed. A more characteristic appearance is that of a lacy structure of the bone, sometimes with pseudo-cystic images. This is best observed in the pelvis or in the distal end of the femur, where the bony structure appears ill defined (Fig. 5-23). The diaphyses are bowed and the cortex is widened at the concave side. Usually there is also coxa vara. Bony resorption or pseudofracture, and the development of tiny exostoses (Fig. 5-24) or ossification within the interosseous membrane, can also be noted.

The vertebrae often have a double contour analogous to that described in deficiency rickets, but the bony structure may be as irregular as that of long bones. Premature closure of cranial sutures is not un-

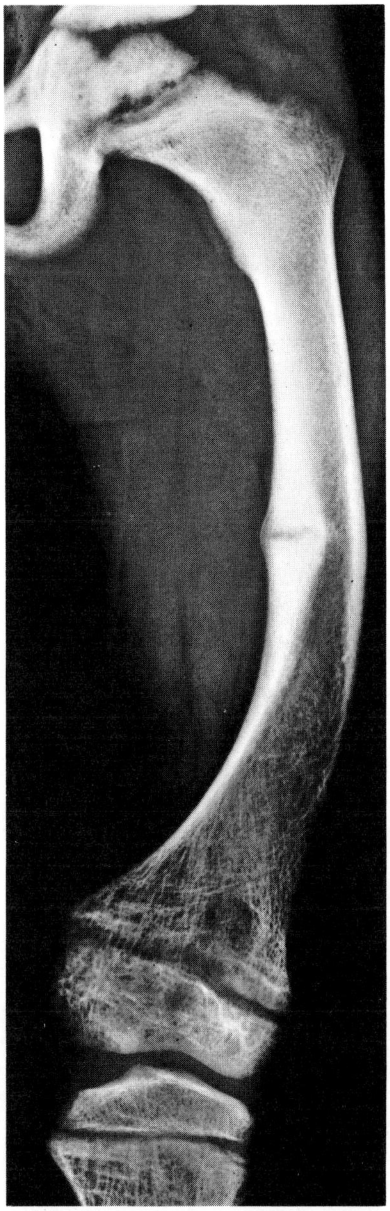

Fig. 5-23. Familial hypophosphatemic vitamin D resistant rickets in a 7-year-old boy. Notice the diaphyseal bowing of the femur with a fracture and the streaky appearance of the bony structure and metaphyseal pathology. (Courtesy of S. Balsan)

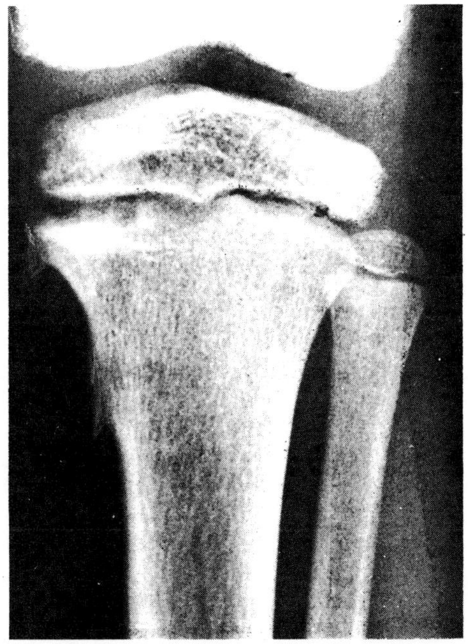

Fig. 5-24. Familial hypophosphatemic vitamin D resistant rickets in a 6-year-old boy. Note the tiny exostoses at the proximal end of the tibia. (Courtesy of S. Balsan)

usual, especially that of the sagittal suture, leading to scaphocephaly (Fig. 5-25). Occasionally there is absence of the lamina dura and the cavity of the pulpa may be of abnormal size with a horn extending all the way to the juncture of the dentine and enamel.

Biochemical Findings

The most characteristic finding is a low level of plasma phosphorus, between 15 and 25 mg/1. Calcium, however, is normal or only slightly low. The alkaline phosphatases are elevated.

Calciuria is low and renal tubular reabsorption of phosphorus is low. Renal function is normal. Intestinal reabsorption is low and the calcium balance is either negative or just slightly positive. The defect of phosphorus resorption is secondary to that of the calcium.

Histology of the bone shows identical lesions to those of deficiency rickets. Abnormal lamellar bone structure has also been described with a defect of mineralization around osteocytes, which may be secondary to alterations of the bony matrix.

Genetic Data and Pathogenesis

The pathogenesis of hypophosphatemic vitamin D resistant rickets has been studied repeatedly and discussed by many authors. A defective intestinal calcium absorption, anomaly of renal tubular phosphorus resorption and a primary bony defect have successively been discussed to explain this disorder. The renal theory is presently the strongest, and Glorieux and Scriver have suggested that the anomaly is the

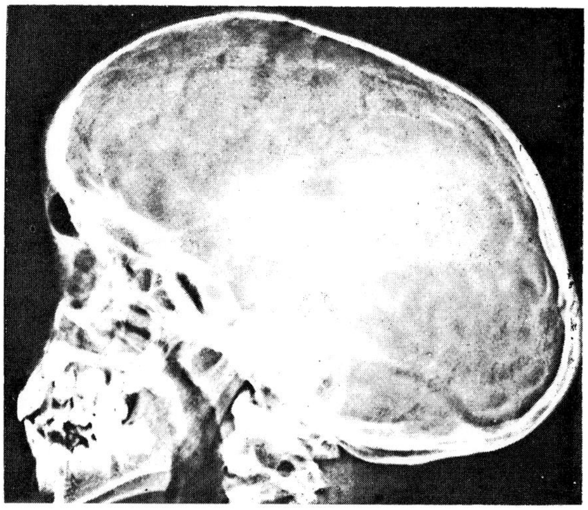

Fig. 5-25. Familial hypophosphatemic vitamin D resistant rickets in an 8-year-old girl. The scaphocephaly results from premature closure of the sagittal suture. (Courtesy of S. Balsan)

result of a primary defect of the renal tubules from the action of parathormone. It results from a loss of an inorganic phosphorus transport-mechanism sensible to that hormone. Still, this theory can not adequately explain the spectrum of observed facts.

Some have also suggested the possibility of a blockage of the movement of cellular phosphorus towards the interstitial space (Rey and Frézal). However, secondary hyperparathyroidism, as postulated by this theory, has never been verified by a determination of the content of parathormone.

Whatever the pathophysiology, it can be accepted that the disorder is genetically determined by dominant sex-linked transmission. The expression of the gene is not always complete in females, where it sometimes is limited to a simple hypophosphatemia without skeletal impact. The existence of an autosomal dominant type has been discussed, but so far is not fully proven.

Treatment

Treatment of vitamin D resistant rickets requires high dosages of vitamin D, in the order of 1 mg/day and sometimes even more. 25-hydroxycholecalciferol has proven itself five to eight times more effective at dosages of 0.10 to 0.50 mg/day. The effect of 1-25-dihydroxycholecalciferol is still greater. Follow-up of patients under treatment must be very careful, because of the risk of intoxication. If calcium goes beyond 105 mg or if there is a sudden increase in calciuria, interruption of therapy is mandatory. Similarly, if a patient must be immobilized for a prolonged period of time, such as after corrective orthopaedic measures, therapy must be interrupted. It is often necessary to perform corrective osteotomies. However, such an intervention is best begun towards the end of the growth period, in order to avoid recurrence of the deformity.

It is necessary to add to the vitamin therapy supplemental phosphorus, 1-1.5 g/day to be administered in four equal doses over each 24-hour period.

It is important to know the limits of the action of vitamin D therapy, since the results, especially the effect on skeletal growth, can be disappointing. Since there may be exacerbations of the disorder, cessation of therapy in the adult may not be final in patients 40, or even 50 years old.

Precocious Pseudo-Deficiency Rickets

The manifestations of this type have been carefully studied by Prader and Royer. This disorder is much more severe and precocious in nature than the preceding one. There is marked disturbance of growth, and deformities of the extremities and of the thorax are impressive. Fractures occur frequently. The general condition of the patient is markedly affected. Such children are often confined to their bed.

Radiologic findings are those of severe rickets, dramatic demineralization, multiple fractures that are often not recognized clinically, and Looser-Milkman zones (Fig. 5-26).

Even though this disorder is strikingly more severe than the preceding type, it responds much more readily to high doses of vitamin D. The growth and integrity of the skeleton will probably progress very well, but therapy must be carefully controlled and followed for years, since an interruption may lead to a rapid recurrence.

Biochemical study reveals the presence of hypocalcemia. Serum phosphorus, however, is practically normal or only slightly low. Hyperamino-aciduria is present, as in deficiency rickets. The genetic analysis of this disorder, frequently called pseudo-deficiency type, suggests the possibility of an autosomal recessive transmission. There is the possibility of sensibility on a multifactorial basis.

Recent studies (Balsan) would seem to indicate that this type could be due to a conversion defect of 25-hydroxy-cholecalciferol to 1-25-dihydroxycholecalciferol.

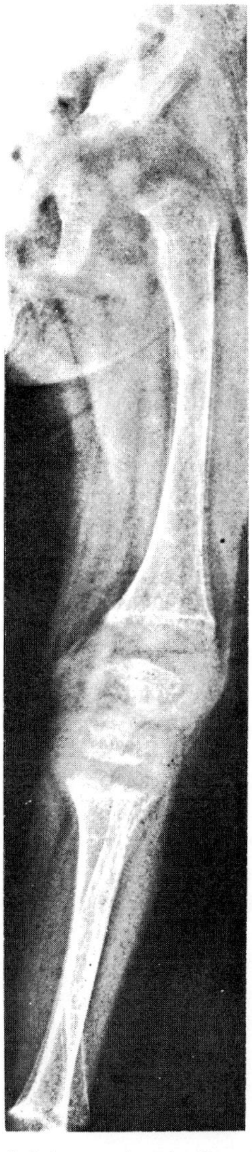

Fig. 5-26. Pseudodeficiency vitamin D resistant rickets in a 22-month-old infant. (Courtesy of S. Balsan)

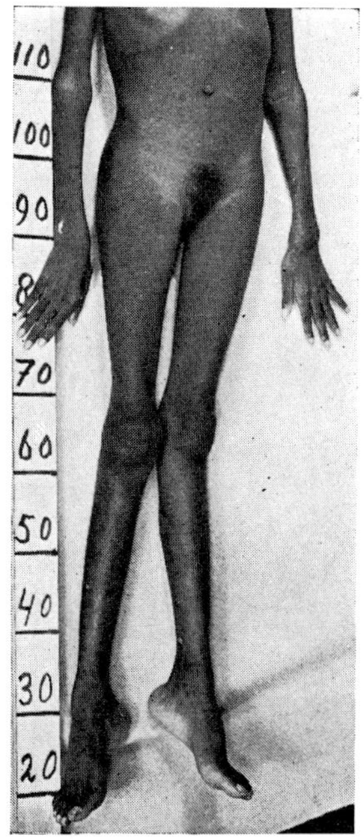

Fig. 5-27. Late form of vitamin D resistant rickets with marked muscular atrophy. (Courtesy of S. Balsan)

Delayed Type of Mac Cance

This type has its onset during the second part of infancy, in adolescence or sometimes even in adults. Clinically, these patients have pain, easy fatigability, and considerable deformity of extremities and spine. In the most severely affected patient there is marked bowing of the extremities. The patient is bedridden and incapable of getting up without help (Fig. 5-27).

The bones may lose their resistance to palpation and seem flexible. The trunk is short and deformed by scoliosis or kyphoscoliosis. Radiologic investigations reveal a high degree of skeletal demineralization. Bones can sometimes hardly be recognized within their surrounding soft tissue structures (Fig. 5-28). The cortex of the long bones becomes paper thin. Multiple fractures are frequently present and result in abnormal angulation. There are numerous Looser-Milkman zones. Severe scoliosis is virtually always present.

Biochemical study reveals severe hypophosphatemia. The value for serum phosphorus may be somewhere between 5 and 7 mg and sometimes is 3 mg. Serum calcium is normal or only slightly elevated and alkaline phosphatase values are high. Calcium- and phosphorus balance are negative, with the percentage of retained calcium during calcium perfusion relatively low. This is contrary to what is seen in other types of vitamin D resistant rickets. There is marked urinary glycine or glycylproline elimination. This is not, however, constant, and the name hyperglycinuric rickets proposed for this type does not appear to be justified for all such cases.

Therapy requires high doses of vitamin D, 10 to 20 mg/day, since the daily dose of 1 to 2 mg does not increase intestinal calcium resorption in these patients. Therapy leads to rapid improvement and definitive healing. Spontaneous recovery of the disorder has

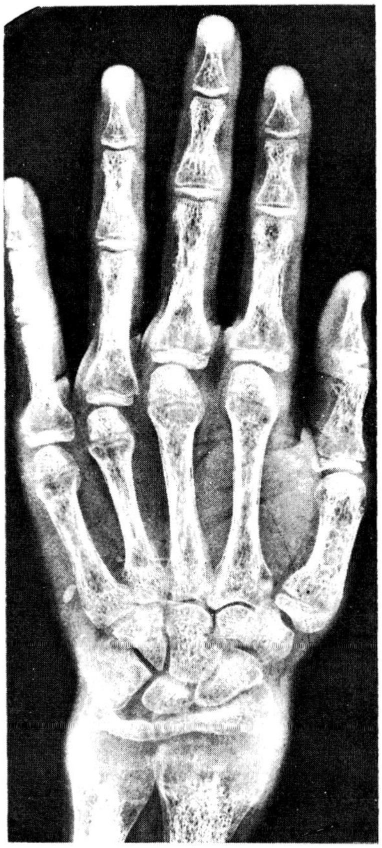

Fig. 5-28. Vitamin D resistant rickets, late form in a 13-year-old girl. There is marked demineralization of all the bones. (Courtesy of S. Balsan)

been reported after a number of years by Dent and by S. Balsan. Patients with the late type always occur isolated within a family, and it is therefore impossible to ascertain a genetic origin.

IDIOPATHIC HYPERCALCIURIA

This children's disorder has been described for the first time by Royer et al. It may be recognized at a variable age, sometimes from the second year on.

The disorder is recognized either because of disturbed growth, because of a polakisuria, or because of abdominal pain. Some very early cases were recognized during a workup for tetany secondary to hypocalcemia.

Dwarfism, often of a severe degree, is usually present, but it is harmonious, and there are no further skeletal deformities. There is no mental retardation or obesity. The severity of the growth disturbance is pronounced and may respond only poorly to therapeutic trials. Sometimes there is an associated nephrocalcinosis and also renal stone formation. Cataracts have been reported.

Radiographically, these patients show all the signs of severe osteoporosis. The cortical bone is thin and the bone on the whole is markedly radiolucent. In some cases there may be signs of associated rickets. The bone age is severely retarded and corresponds to, or may even be superior to, the height age. The polakisuria is resistant to pitressine, as in the significant hypercalciuria in the order of 20 mg/kg/24 h. This calciuria is not influenced by vitamin D in doses of 0.25 mg/day, nor by sodium bicarbonate. There is, however, a decrease if the patient is put on a regimen poor in calcium or sodium chlorate, or is administered sodium phytate and hydrochlorothiazide. Renal function study does not reveal glomerular pathology. Proteinuria of tubular origin can sometimes be recognized. A test with calcium perfusion which fails to completely block the reabsorption of phosphorus suggests the possibility of a mild degree of phosphate diabetes.

Serum calcium as a rule is normal, although an occasional observation of hypocalcemia has been reported with an early onset. Alkaline phosphatase is normal except with coexisting rickets.

The pathophysiology of this disorder is not known. If hypercalciuria seems to be responsible for the spectrum of signs and symptoms its origin is still unknown. The mild tubular affection, which may be secondary, and the excessive absorption of calcium, not always seen, cannot offer an explanation for this disorder.

The finding of hypercalciuria in the father and brothers of one patient is evidence of a possible genetic factor involved here. But this has not been clearly defined. Also, there is a marked male preponderance, and so far there have been only some exceptional observations in girls.

Two forms of therapy may help to improve the calcium balance in hypercalciuria. Hydrochlorothiazide will often only have a temporary effect, but a regimen poor in sodium chloride is more reliable. Under this form of therapy there is improved growth in some cases. It is necessary to add potassium chloride to the daily diet, in order to avoid a K-depletion, and the therapy plan should be interrupted for one month every six months.

HYPOPHOSPHATASIA

This disorder was described in 1948 by Rathburn, but in all likelihood it was seen earlier.

The age at discovery and the symptomatology can

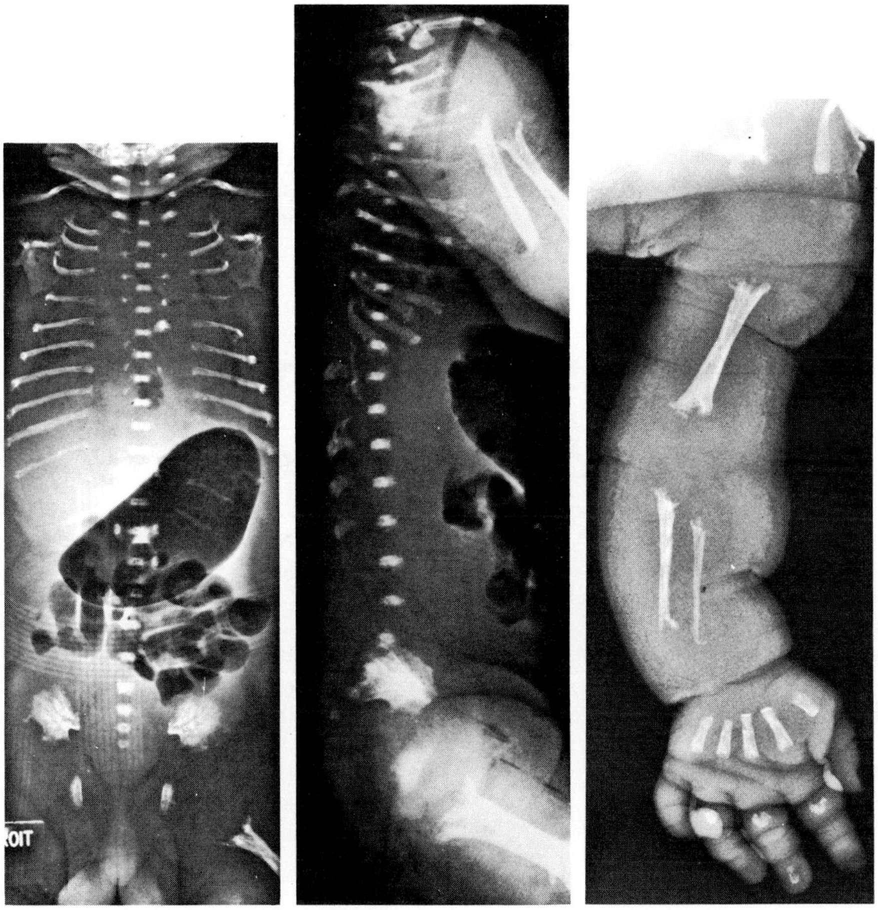

Fig. 5-29. Fatal type of hypophosphatasia. (Courtesy of J. Channarond)

be quite variable. Sometimes newborns are affected by this disease, and some do not survive. In other cases the diagnosis is made during later childhood, and sometimes only in adulthood.

In the neonatal types leading to early death, patients may show signs of micromelia and a lack of ossification of the cranial vault. Death results from respiratory distress. The ossification defect does not only involve the skull, but also the majority of the skeleton. The diaphysis of long bones is only partly visible, the ribs are filiform, the bones are short and poorly or not at all mineralized, and the vertebral bodies may be reduced to thin lines. Some islands of ossification are present in the region of the base of the skull, the face, the pelvis and the scapula (Fig. 5-28).

In the baby attention is focused on the disturbed general condition, digestive problems, moderate fever and sometimes on early shedding of teeth. Clinical study will show severe rachitic deformities, such as metaphyseal bulging, rosary of the chest wall, bowing of the lower part of the leg or angulation subsequent to a fracture. Palpation of the skull reveals a severe ossification defect. This is easily felt close to the sutures. The anterior fontanelle is excessively large and sometimes under pressure. Growth retardation is marked, as is hypotonia.

The radiologic appearance is somewhat reminiscent of severe rickets. There is widening, irregularity and poor definition of the metaphyseal borders. The height of the growth line is abnormal, and sometimes transparent zones are superimposed on the metaphysis, giving it the appearance of a "calix" or a "tulip" (Fig. 5-29). The cortex of the diaphysis seems to have a double contour, because of a poorly calcified layer around it. The epiphyseal centers appear late and they may be very small. The same goes for the carpal and tarsal bony elements. In the skull, clear areas in the vicinity of sutures simulate local enlargement. It is not unusual for these patients to develop a craniosynostosis.

The evolution of this type is severe and there may

be death of the patient in about two out of three cases from renal failure or pulmonary pathology. In surviving patients, however, progressive disappearance of the changes is possible.

In the late forms the symptoms are much less characteristic. Early shedding of teeth, an asymmetry of the extremities and genu valgum may be the only findings. In some patients the disorder is only recognized during adulthood following a fracture, or because of shortness. Radiographically there may be some mild metaphyseal irregularities, or sometimes only osteoporosis.

Biochemical tests will reveal a low alkaline phosphatase level, at 1 or 2 Bodansky units. This lack of alkaline phosphatase is also present in viscera, bone and leukocytes. Serum calcium is elevated 120 to 130 mg/l, this, at least, in early infancy. Serum phosphorus is normal and sometimes elevated. Signs for renal failure may be associated. Elevated urinary phospho-ethanolamine excretion seems to be a constant finding.

Histologic studies show a highly abnormal structure of the growth cartilage with irregular columns, only a few visible areas of calcification, and an excessive proliferation of osteoid tissue sometimes with persisting cartilaginous islands. The structure of the bony tissue is immature in the newborn as was shown by Engfeldt and Zetterström. Patients with a fatal course usually have signs of nephrocalcinosis.

If the findings in this disorder seem to prove an important role played by the phosphatases during osteogenesis, its pathophysiology is still poorly understood. It is by no means certain that the defect of ossification is the direct result of an excess of pyrophosphates, as some have suggested (Fleisch and Neuman).

Transmission follows an autosomal recessive mode. A slight reduction of the value for phosphatase or an excretion of phospho-ethanolamine can often be found in heterozygote individuals.

IDIOPATHIC HYPERCALCEMIA

This disorder was orginally described by Fanconi, and a large number of observations have confirmed its characteristics.

Clinical Findings

Idiopathic hypercalcemia is most often discovered during the first months of life because of digestive problems. There is loss of appetite and vomiting, associated with delayed growth and development of the baby. Clinical investigation reveals a characteristic appearance of the face, which will facilitate diagnosis for an experienced investigator. The nose is tipped up and its root is flat. The eyes are globular, and have an epicantus. The cheeks are round and pudgy, and the upper lip is prominent, contrasting somewhat with the relatively small, retracted chin (Fig. 5-30). Microcephaly, together with a psycho-motor retardation, is usually seen. This can be the most serious element in this disorder. Auscultation may show a systolic cardiac murmur of variable location, which most frequently results from pulmonary or aortic stenosis. Hypertension may be a reflection of renal failure secondary to nephrocalcinosis.

The prognosis of this disorder is variable. Certain types have a rapidly fatal course, despite therapeutic attempts. Death most frequently results from renal failure. In other instances, however, hypercalcemia will normalize, and if there is not too much mental retardation, the prognosis may even be good.

Radiographic Findings

Radiologically abnormal bony density affects the entire skeleton. The cortex of the long bones is thick, and sometimes there may no longer be a recognizable medullary space in the center of the diaphysis. Dense bands next to the growth cartilage are visible at the metaphyses. The epiphyseal centers have a darker central area surrounded by hyperlucent, dense rings (Fig. 5-31). The carpal and tarsal bones as well as the vertebral bodies can have a similar appearance. There may be dense endplates. Calcification of the intervertebral disks has been noted in several patients. The base of the skull, the periorbital region and sometimes even the vault itself may be unusually dense. There may be early closure of fontanelles. Soft tissue calcification can sometimes be recognized with or without nephrocalcinosis.

Biochemical Findings, Histology and Pathogenesis

Serum calcium is elevated above 115 mg and may be as high as 180 mg. Serum phosphorus is normal or only slightly elevated. Alkaline phosphatase is normal or low. Excretion of calcium is normal or increased, and phosphaturia is variable. Intestinal resorption of calcium may be increased, as was shown by a number of calcium balance studies. Signs of renal failure may be present, especially after prolonged hypercalcemia. Hypercholesterolemia above 2 g has been found in more than half of the patients.

Histology confirms the presence of osteosclerosis of all the bones. The bony structure is normal, but the bony lamellae are thick, compact, and poor in cells.

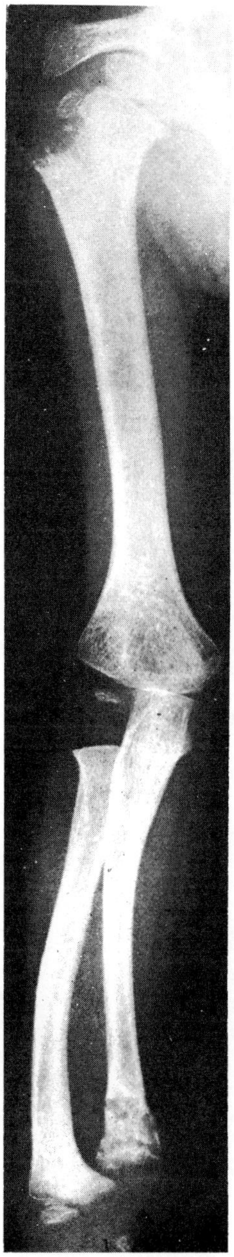

Fig. 5-30. Late type of hypophosphatasia in a 2½-year-old child. (Courtesy of J. Lefebvre)

Some observations refer to brothers and sisters, which makes a genetic origin of this disease likely. Still, a number of authors insist on the possibility of a fetopathy. Maternal intoxication by vitamin D during pregnancy was a suspected cause for a number of years, but this theory can now be formally discarded.

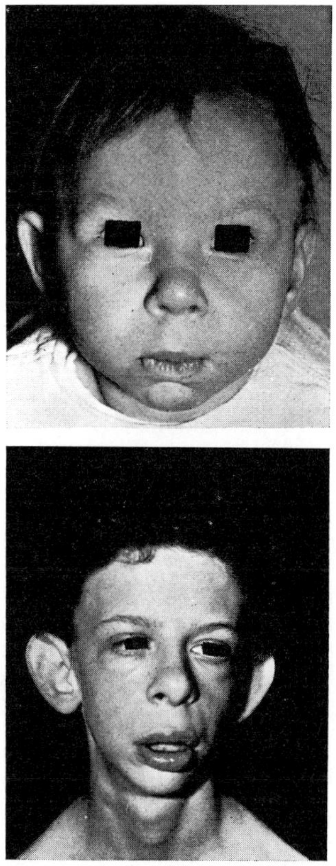

Fig. 5-31. Idiopathic hypercalcemia. Both the infant and the older child present characteristics facial appearances. (Courtesy of S. Balsan)

The pathophysiology of the disorder is still unknown. Hypersensitivity to vitamin D has been proposed, but idiopathic hypercalcemia shows considerable differences from hypervitaminosis D. Markedly high values for serum calcium cannot explain the facial dysmorphism, and even more importantly, the mental retardation. It would appear possible that a constitutional disturbance of vitamin D metabolism, or of the related steroids, is a prime cause of this disease. Still this has not been formally shown.

Clinical Types

There is marked variation in the clinical expression of this disorder. In some patients there is actually absence of hypercalcemia and the skeletal changes may only be minor. Similarly, Williams has described a disorder in the adult combining aortic or pulmonary stenosis with facial changes similar to those of hypercalcemia. It suggests that this is the same disorder in spite of the fact that all the calcium values tested have been normal. The so-called benign hypercalcemia described by Lightwood in reality is a simple hypersensitivity to vitamin D. It was observed in certain infants who were routinely given this vitamin, especially following its addition to milk as has been tried in England.

Treatment

Therapeutic efforts are directed towards lowering serum calcium. Thyroid extract is hardly used any more. There is some merit in attempting a regimen with low calcium intake combined with corticotherapy. The effect on the skeleton can be good, but mental retardation and the vascular lesions will not respond, nor will the renal failure, if already present.

RENAL AND INTESTINAL OSTEOPATHIES

Skeletal disorders resulting from severe and chronic renal or intestinal disorders are of considerable clinical importance. Their main manifestations are local bone pain, general fatigue, and disturbed growth. Therapy of such lesions is quite successful. Since the introduction of hemodialysis there is renewed interest in this type of pathology.

RENAL OSTEOPATHIES

The abnormal skeletal findings seen during different functional disorders of the kidneys during childhood will be reviewed.

Clinical Findings

As a prototype we shall describe the findings in uremic osteopathy.

The symptoms of renal failure usually precede those of skeletal involvement: polakisuria, thirst, and disturbed intestinal functioning. Growth cessation and dwarfism are important signs. They vary somewhat in their onset, depending on the severity and time of onset of the renal pathology. Bone pain and disturbed gait is not unusual. The onset of puberty is delayed, remaining almost parallel with the bony maturation.

It is not unusual to discover the skeletal manifestations by palpating metaphyseal flaring and a typical rosary during a careful physical examination, before fully appreciating the chronic renal disorder, which underlies all of these changes. During the later stage deformity of the legs will appear in valgus or varus position, and there may be functional difficulties. Excessive maxillary growth in some cases results in an unusually protruding, "simian" looking midfacial area.

Radiographic Findings

Four findings can be recognized on the radiograph. Most frequently there is a *reduction of bone density* with thin cortices and a low cortico-diaphyseal ratio. Growth arrestlines and bony trabeculations may be very prominent. Epiphyseal centers are insufficiently developed and their radiolucent centers contrast with the denser periphery (Fig. 5-32).

In other instances there may be signs of rickets, with irregular metaphyseal borders. There are characteristic features differentiating this disorder from rickets. The border of the growth cartilage is not always cup shaped, but is frequently oblique, and the metaphysis may appear asymmetrical. Epiphyseal separation, especially of the hip, the knee, and of the tibio-tarsal region is not unusual. Double contour of the periosteum is also noted (Fig. 5-33).

A third type of finding is that of *osteoclasia,* recognizable by subperiosteal zones of resorption along the cortex of long bones or close to metaphyses. This sign is most frequently located in the areas of the femoral neck, the proximal tibia and the metacarpals, but can be more widespread (Fig. 5-32).

Finally, *osteosclerosis* has been noted in a number of adult patients but does not often appear in children (Fig. 5-34). This finding is most often noted at the base of the skull and in vertebral bodies, usually appearing as transverse bands on lateral films.

Quite often all of these findings can be found in one patient and their combination is suggestive of the presence of renal osteopathy. Fibro-osteoclasia is a sign rather of chronic renal failure, than of renal tubular disorders. Extra-skeletal calcifications are seen only exceptionally in children. In spite of severe nephropathy the skeleton may still be radiographically normal.

Under therapy with calcium and vitamin D there is rapid improvement of the lesions. Rachitic changes will disappear at a somewhat slower rate.

Biochemical Findings

Serum calcium is usually low. During renal failure of slow onset serum phosphorus is high, except in the early phase. Urinary calcium output is low.

The most constant finding is an elevation of the values for alkaline phosphatases, up two to six times from the normal.

Parathormone determination reveals early increase of this substance. Hyperparathyroidism plays an important role in the metabolic disturbance resulting from renal failure. There is also a marked elevation of the content of stable vitamin D in the plasma.

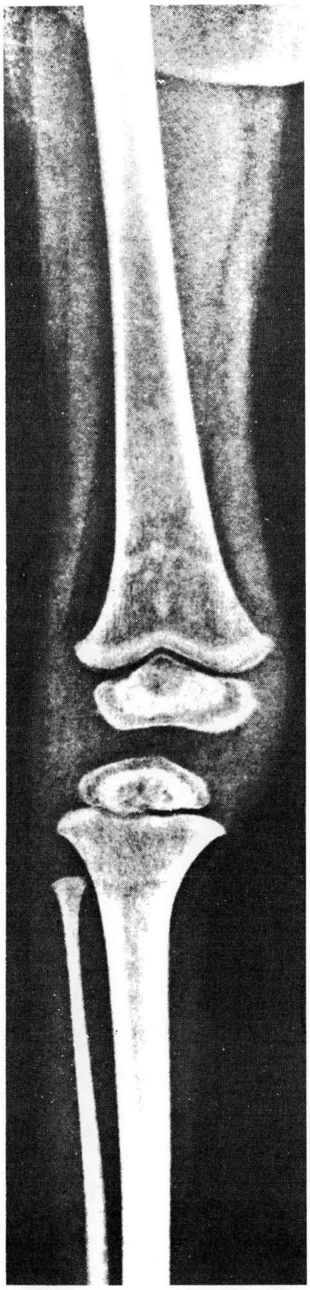

Fig. 5-32. Idiopathic hypercalcemia in a 3½-year-old girl. Note the dense metaphyseal lines and rings within the epiphyses along with widening of the diaphyseal cortex. (Courtesy of S. Balsan)

Etiology

It is not possible to clearly distinguish the renotubular pathology from tubular disorders. Still, some distinguishing features do exist.

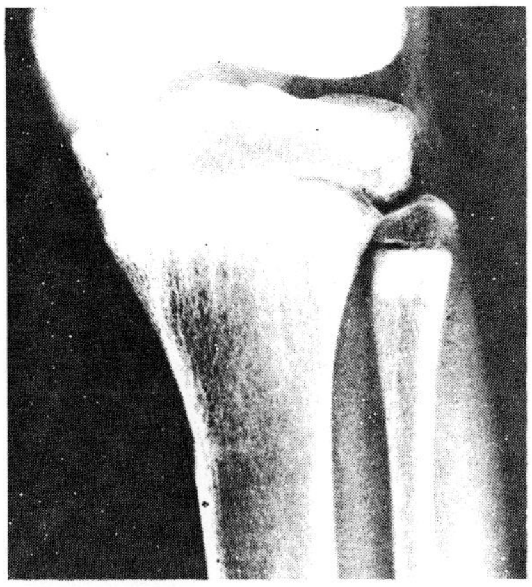

Fig. 5-33. Renal osteopathy in a 14-year-old girl. Notice the thin cortices, the prominent bony trabeculation, and the metaphyseal changes. There is resorption on the medial side. (Courtesy of P. Royer)

RENAL TUBULAR DISTURBANCES

In these disorders the patients lose excessive amounts of phosphorus or calcium. The lowering of the tubular phosphorus reabsorption coefficient may depend on the degree of secondary hyperparathyroidism and on the severity of the tubular pathology, or on both. In the pure types of renal tubular pathology there seems to be a normal intestinal calcium resorption and correction of acidosis will improve the calcium balance by reducing the renal calcium loss.

Idiopathic Hypercalciuria.

This disorder has been discussed in a preceding chapter. Its radiologic characteristics—marked osteoporosis—is attributed to a heavy loss of urinary calcium.

Renal Tubular Acidosis

This condition also results in osteoporosis, which is a sign of rickets. Fibro-osteoclasia is rarely seen and is the result of chronic uremia. Two chemical alterations, acidosis and hypercalciuria, appear to be responsible for the pathology, which includes growth arrest.

Normalization of the skeletal involvement can be achieved by giving sufficient amounts of bicarbonate to correct the calciuria. Urinary calcium loss must be regularly measured during therapy. Vitamin D must be

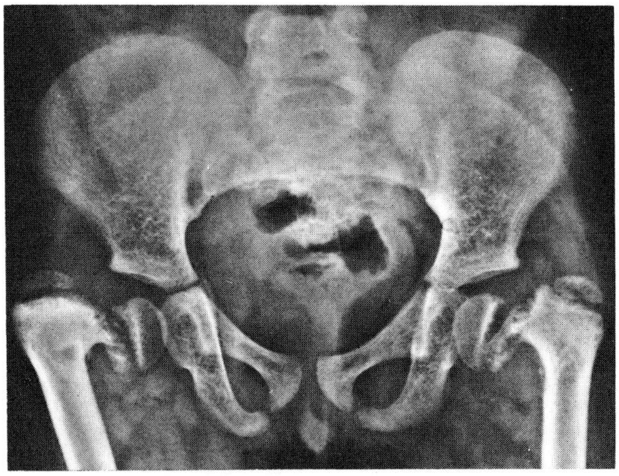

Fig. 5-34. Renal osteopathy in a 6-year-old boy. There is epiphyseolysis and displacement of the femoral head. Note the fracture of the femoral neck on the right with marked osteoclastic activity and abnormal bony structure. (Courtesy of S. Balsan)

given only in physiologic amounts. Large doses are not necessary, and may actually be dangerous.

The De Toni-Debre-Fanconi Syndrome

This may be an idiopathic disorder or a secondary condition during the course of several metabolic disturbances, such as tyrosinosis, Wilson's disease, or particularly cystinosis.

The latter disorder, in its early phase, manifests frequently the characteristics of severe rickets with fractures (Fig. 5-35). In the intermediary phase these patients suffer from glomerular failure, which may result in a temporary equilibrium with healing of rickets and remission of hyperaminoaciduria and phosphaturia. When the glomerular failure becomes more severe, signs of fibro-osteoclasia will appear.

Wilson's disease may radiographically manifest itself in osteoporosis and sometimes in rickets (see p. 21).

During the course of the unusual type of idiopathic De Toni-Debré-Fanconi syndrome there is a confirmation of severe rickets and osteoporosis in parallel with a chronic phosphorus depletion, which can respond to diuretics (Fig. 5-36).

During the course of a Lowe syndrome we may also encounter rickets. Chronic hypercalcemia may result in metaphyseal changes reminiscent of rickets, and sometimes also in isolated osteoporosis. Such lesions are somewhat similar to those seen in experimental potassium depletion.

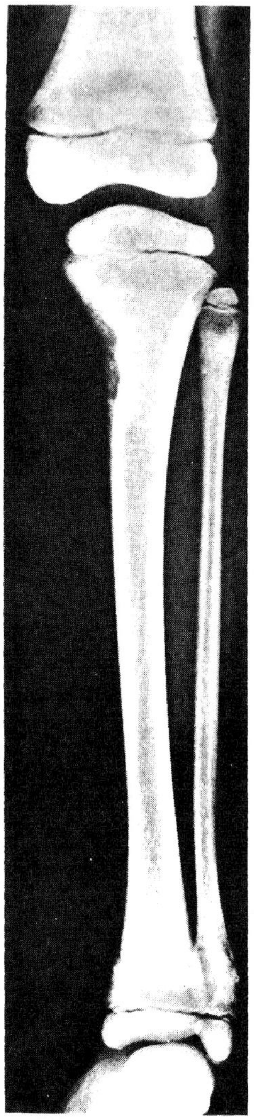

Fig. 5-35. Renal osteopathy in a 7-year-old girl who is suffering from oxalosis. Note the increased skeletal density. (Courtesy of P. Royer)

Total Renal Failure

The skeletal involvement is particularly severe in chronic and slowly developing renal failure. The reference is to oligonephronic hypoplasia and urinary malformations with renal hypoplasia. In nephronophthisis, which has a more rapid development, the bony lesions will be less serious. In the Alport syndrome we only rarely see skeletal involvement.

Renal failure will mainly lead to fibro-osteoclasia, which can be occasionally associated with rickets. An isolated occurrence of rickets is more rare than that which occurs with renal tubular disorders.

Treatment by hemodialysis leads to osteopathy of a

different type, radiologically characterized by osteoporosis, which will not respond to vitamin D. This lesion is more likely the result of marked calcium loss by dialysis and may also be a negative effect of certain other constituents, part of the dialysis solution.

Pathology

Until recently retention of phosphates secondary to renal failure was considered to be the major factor responsible for the skeletal changes (Bricker). An associated defect is disturbed calcium resorption. Hyperparathyroidism can be explained by the elevation of serum phosphorus accompanied by the low value for calcium. Sometimes hyperparathyroidism may become autonomous by developing an adenoma or diffuse hyperplasia.

The synthesis of the active form of vitamin D, 1-25-dihydroxycholecalciferol, by the kidney suggests another metabolism. This synthesis is in part under the influence of the phosphate content of the renal cortex. An elevation of this substance within the remaining functional nephrons would result in defective synthesis of this metabolite with its effect on bones and on the kidneys.

Treatment

Therapy for uremic osteopathy can be highly effective and should always be attempted, since there may be considerable improvement of the general condition of affected children. It consists of a combined intake of vitamin D in high dosage, 0.1 to 1 mg/day, combined with calcium 0.5 to 1 g, if serum calcium values are low. If phosphorus is high, the administration of aluminum hydroxide is recommended in order to maintain the phosphorus concentration between 30 and 50 mg/l. This type of therapy requires careful supervision and follow-up of serum calcium values. The intake should be reduced once radiologic healing has been achieved or as soon as the serum calcium is close to the normal level. Preventive therapy is of considerable value, and a dosage of 0.1 to 0.2 mg of vitamin D per day may completely prevent the appearance of skeletal changes in uremia.

If a patient is submitted to prolonged hemodialysis, a normal equilibrium of calcium should be maintained and the concentration of calcium within the dialysis solution should be close to 70 mg/l. Higher dosage will eventually lead to extra-skeletal calcifications.

In patients having undergone renal transplant, there is a risk of tertiary hyperparathyroidism with the possibility of severe hypercalcemia. This could justify subtotal parathyroidectomy.

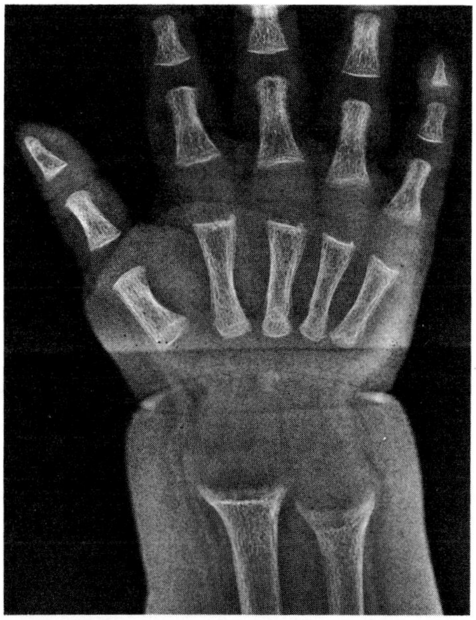

Fig. 5-36. Severe rickets and osteoporosis in this 1-year-old patient with markedly delayed bony maturation, suffering from De Toni-Debré-Fanconi syndrome. (Courtesy of J. Lefebvre)

Therapy of renal tubular disorders, especially of cystinosis and tyrosinosis is considerably less rewarding. In the chronic tubular acidosis of Albright, healing can be obtained by simply correcting the existing acidosis by giving sodium bicarbonate.

OSTEOPATHIES OF INTESTINAL ORIGIN

During childhood such skeletal complications are only seen in the course of severe chronic malabsorption syndromes with steatorrhea and severe atrophy of the intestinal mucosa. The main disorders having such a risk are celiac disease and the different types of intolerance to disaccharides. Only rarely does this complication occur in a patient with intolerance to carbohydrates or during mucoviscidosis. Better familiarity with the pathogenesis and logical therapy of these disorders has helped considerably in reducing the risk and severity of developing such skeletal changes. Digestive problems, together with growth arrest, are the key findings in these disorders. Skeletal changes rarely have a clinical consequence outside of growth failure.

Radiologically, the bones are slender with thin cortices. The bones are of reduced density, especially the metaphyseal regions. Often there are numerous lines of growth arrest. Trabeculation is irregular or poorly seen, and the skeleton has a washed out appearance.

Bowing of long bones and an occasional fracture may be noted. The metaphyseal borders are clearcut, slightly denser than the rest of the skeleton, and have the same aspect as the peripheral region of the epiphyseal centers.

Serum calcium is usually normal, but phosphatases are low. If there is a low calcium concentration phosphorus may be normal or elevated. Urinary calcium output is low, phosphaturia variable. In some cases serum magnesium is low. Skeletal findings of abnormal intestinal absorption are most frequently attributed to a lack of protein. However the lowering of total protein is usually much too mild to result in such a severe alteration of bones, and the increased fecal calcium loss must also play a role here. Together with fatty acids, calcium will form insoluble and nonabsorbable complexes (saponification), and disturbed resorption of vitamin D will further aggravate this defective calcium resorption.

Therapy will be directed against the underlying disorder. Calcium should be supplemented, but it is important to avoid too high a dosage, since this might aggravate steatorrhea. Finally vitamin D should be given parenterally in physiologic amounts.

REFERENCES

Metabolism and Homeostasis of Calcium

ARNAUD (C. D.), RASMUSSEN (H.) et ANAST (C.). Further studies on the interrelationship between parathyroid hormone and vitamin D. *J. clin. Invest., 1966,* **45**, *1955-1964.*

AVIOLI (L. V.) et HADDAD (J. G.). Vitamin D : current concepts. *Metabolism, 1973,* **22**, *507-531.*

BELANGER (L. F.) et MIGIGOVSKY (B. B.). Extra-trabecular crystallization in rickets. Effect of vitamin D · calcium and norethandrolone. *Proc. Soc. exp. Biol., 1961,* **106**, *19-21.*

BOURNE (G. H.). The biochemistry and physiology of bone. *New York, 1956, Academic Press, éd.*

BRICKER (N. S.), SLATOPOLSKY (E.), REISS (E.) et AVIOLI (L. V.). Calcium, phosphorus and bone in renal disease and transplantation. *Arch. intern. Med., 1969,* **123**, *543-553.*

CIBA FOUNDATION SYMPOSIUM 11 (new series). Hard tissue growth, repair and mineralization. *1 vol., Amsterdam, 1973, Elsevier-Excerpta Medica, éd.*

COMAR (C. L.) et BRONNER (F.). Mineral metabolism. An advanced treatise. Volume III, Calcium physiology. *New York and London, 1969, Academic Press, éd.*

COPP (D. H.), CAMERON (E. C.), CHENEY (B. A.), DAVIDSON (A. G. F.) et HENZE (K. G.). Evidence for calcitonin, a new hormone from the parathyroid that lowers blood calcium. *Endocrinology, 1962,* **70**, *638-649.*

CUISINIER-GLEIZES (P.), MATHIEU (H.) et ROYER (P.). Physiologie de l'excrétion rénale du calcium. *Pathol. et Biol., 1963,* **11**, *222-239.*

DE LUCA (H. F.). The kidney as an endocrine organ involved in calcium homeostasis. *Kidney intern., 1973,* **4**, *80-88.*

EISENBERG (E.). Effects of serum calcium level and parathyroid extracts on phosphate and calcium excretion in hypoparathyroid patients. *J. clin Invest., 1965,* **44**, *942-946.*

FOURMAN (P.) et ROYER (P.). Calcium et tissu osseux. Biologie et pathologie. *1 vol., Paris, 1970, Flammarion, éd.*

GAILLARD (P. J.), TALMAGE (R. V.) et BUDY (A. M.). The parathyroid glands, ultrastructure, secretion and function (Noordwijk, 1964). *Chicago, 1965, University of Chicago Press, éd.*

GAILLARD (P. J.). Bone culture studies with thyrocalcitonin. *Proc. Kon. Ned. Akad. Wet. Series C, 1967,* **70**, *309-320.*

HALLICK (R. B.) et HARRISON (H. C.). Metabolism of dihydrotachysterol in target tissues. *J. biol. Chem., 1972,* **247**, *91-92.*

KODICEK (E.). The intermediary metabolism of vitamin D : 1-25 dihydro-cholecalciferol, a kidney hormone affecting calcium metabolism. *In* Endocrinology 71. Proceeding Third International Symposium. *London, 1972, William Heinemann Medical Books, éd., p. 444-451.*

KRANE (S. M.), HARRIS (E. D., Jr.), SINGER (F. R.) et POTTS (J. T., Jr.). Acute effects of calcitonin on bone formation in man. *Metabolism, 1973,* **22**, *51-58.*

LICHTWITZ (A.) et PARLIER (R.). Calcium et maladies métaboliques de l'os. Vol. I : Os et métabolisme du calcium à l'état normal. Vol. II : Os et métabolisme du calcium à l'état pathologique. Vol. III : Intestin, rein et métabolisme du calcium. *Paris, 1964, Expansion scient. franç., éd.*

MALM (O. J.). Calcium requirement and adaptation in adult men. *1 vol., 290 p., Oslo, 1958, University Press, éd.*

MALM (O. J.). Calcium requirement and adaptation in adult men. *Scand. J. clin. Lab. Invest., 1958,* **10**, *suppl. 36.*

MILHAUD (G.). La thyrocalcitonine. *Presse méd., 1967,* **75**, *71-74.*

NEUMAN (W. F.), FIRSCHEIN (H.), CHEN (P. S.), MURLYAN (B. J.) et DISTEFANO (V.). On the mechanism of action of parathormone. *J. Amer. chem. Soc., 1956,* **78**, *3863-3864.*

NORDIN (B. E. C.) et SMITH (D. A.). Diagnostic procedures in disorders of calcium metabolism. *London, 1965, Churchill, éd.*

NORDIN (B. E. C.), SMITH (D. A.) et NISBET (J.). Bone mineralization and destruction rates determined by continuous feeding of radiocalcium. *Clin. Sci., 1964,* **27**, *111-122.*

NORDIO (S.). Attualità in campo di fisiopatologia del transporto organico del calcio. 1. tre aspetti fondamentali dell'azione della vitamina D. *Minerva pediat., 1967,* **19**, *1611-1615.*

NORDIO (S.). Attualità in campo di fisiopatologia del transporto organico del calcio. 2. Fisiopatologia della produzione del paratormone e della tirocalcitonina. *Minerva pediat., 1968,* **20**, *1119-1127.*

OMDAHL (J. L.) et DE LUCA (H. F.). Regulation of vitamin D metabolism and function. *Physiol. Rev., 1973,* **53**, *327.*

RASMUSSEN (H.). Ionic and hormonal control of calcium homeostasis. *Amer. J. Med., 1971,* **50**, *567.*

RASMUSSEN (H.), WONG (M.), BIKLE (D.) et GOODMAN (D. B. P.). Hormonal control of the renal conversion of 25-hydroxycholecalciferol to 1-25-dihydroxycholecalciferol. *J. clin. Invest., 1972,* **51**, *2502-2504.*

SACHS (C.), BOURDEAU (A.) et MALICHECQ (M.). Dosages des fractions de la calcémie. *Vie médicale, 1968,* **49**, *1745-1759.*

TALMAGE (R. V.) et ELLIOT (J. R.). Removal of calcium from bone as influenced by the parathyroids. *Endocrinology, 1958,* **62**, *717-722.*

THOMPSON (J. S.), PALMIERI (G. M. A.), ELIEL (L. P.) et CUTLER (G. A.). Effects of cortisone and adrenalectomy on the responses to thyrocalcitonin. *Endocrinology, 1968,* **83**, *470-474.*

VAES (G.). La résorption osseuse et l'hormone parathyroïdienne. *Bruxelles, 1967, Albert De Visscher, éd.*

WASSERMAN (R. H.), CORRADINO (R. A.) et TAYLOR (A. N.). Vitamin D-dependent calcium-binding protein. Purification and some properties. *J. biol. Chem., 1968,* **243**, *3978-3986.*

Avitaminoses. Hypervitaminoses

ALAVI (S. M.) et KEATS (T. E.). Toxopachyostéose diaphysaire tibiopéronière, syndrome de Weismann-Netter. *Amer. J. Roentgenol., 1973,* **118**, *314-317.*

AMMANN (P.). Beitrag zur A-Hypervitaminose. *Helv. paediat. Acta, 1968,* **23**, *137-146.*

BARR (C. E.). Osteogenic activity in acute ascorbic acid deficiency. *J. oral Ther. Pharmacol., 1967,* **4**, *5-24.*

BENEDETTI (G. B.), CANEPA (G.) et PELIZZA (A.). La malattia di Moeller-Barlow. Considerazioni clinico-radiografiche ed anatomo-patologiche su 12 casi di scorbuto infantile. *Chir. Organi Mov., 1963,* **53**, *112-159.*

BOISSIÈRE (H.), CAGNAT (R.), POISSONNIER (M.) et ANGÉLY (S. d'). Dystrophie ostéomalacique du prématuré. *Ann. Pédiat., 1964,* **40**, *367-383.*

BONUCCI (E.). Fine structure of epiphyseal cartilage in experimental scurvy. *J. Pathol., 1970,* **102**, *219-227.*

CASTANIER (J.) et BLOCH (J.). Réflexions à propos du poumon rachitique. *Rev. Pédiat., 1967,* **3**, *177-182.*

CHRISTIAENS (L.), FARRIAUX (J. P.), FONTAINE (G.) et DELECOUR (M.). La dystrophie ostéomalacique du prématuré. *Lille méd., 1965,* **10**, *617-623.*

DEBRÉ (R.) et BRISSAUD (H. E.). Action toxique de la vitamine D2 administrée à doses trop fortes chez l'enfant. *Ann. Méd., 1949,* **50**, *417-489.*

DENT (C. E.), RICHENS (A.), ROWE (D. J. F.) et STAMP (T. C. B.). Osteomalacia with long-term anticonvulsivant therapy in epilepsy. *Brit. Med. J., 1970,* **2**, *69-72.*

EPITALBRA-SCHNEBELEN (M. J.). Les séquelles du rachitisme carentiel. Etude clinique et radiologique. *Thèse Méd., Paris, 1970.*

FRAME (B.), JACKSON (C. E.), REYNOLDS (W. A.) et UMPHREY (J. E.). Hypercalcemia and skeletal effects in chronic hypervitaminosis A. *Ann. intern. Med., 1974,* **80**, *44-48.*

FRASER (D.), KOOH (S. W.) et SCRIVER (C. R.). Hyperparathyroidism as the cause of hyperaminoaciduria and phosphaturia in human vitamin D deficiency. *Pediat. Res., 1967,* **1**, *425-435.*

FRIIS-HANSEN (B.). Neonatal hepatitis with osteomalacia. *Acta paediat., 1956,* **45**, *376-381.*

JOWSEY (J.) et RIGGS (B. L.). Bone changes in a patient with hypervitaminosis A. *J. clin. Endocrin., 1968,* **28**, *1833-1835.*

KRAUER-MAYER (B.), OLAFSSON (A.), KNÜSEL (E.) et KAUFMANN (H. J.). Skorbut im Kindesalter. Eine in Vergessenheit geratene Krankheit. *Schweiz. med. Wschr., 1968,* **98**, *789-795.*

LAMY (M.), JAMMET (M. L.), NÉZELOFF (C.), AUSSANAIRE (M.) et RICORDEAU (G.). Ictère viral cirrhogène chez un nouveau-né. Lésions osseuses et pulmonaires. *Arch. franç. Pédiat., 1960,* **17**, *96-101.*

LAMY (M.), FRÉZAL (J.), REY (J.) et CAMUS (J. L.). Etude métabolique d'un cas de rachitisme tardif sensible à la vitamine D. *Arch. franç. Pédiat., 1966,* **23**, *15-21.*

LEFEBVRE (J.) et GUY (E.). Scorbut infantile. Maladie de Barlow. Avitaminose C. *Encyclopédie méd.-chir., 1956, 31134 C 10.*

LEFEBVRE (J.) et GUY (E.). Rachitisme. *Encyclopédie méd.-chir., 1959, 31135 A10.*

LEONIDAS (J. C.), BRILL (P. W.) et WALDMAN (N.). Antiepileptic therapy and rickets in children. *Radiology, 1973,* **109**, *409-412.*

MANKIN (H. J.). Rickets, osteomalacia, and renal osteodystrophy. *J. Bone Jt Surg., 1974,* **56**-*A, 101-128 et 352-386.*

MITCHELL (R. G.). Modern views on rickets and hypercalcaemia in infancy. *Wld Rev. Nutr. Diet., 1967,* **8**, *207-243.*

PAUPE (J.) et VIALATTE (J.). Le rachitisme carentiel tardif (à propos de 12 observations). *Thérapeutique (Sem. Hôp.), 1969,* **45**, *859-863.*

PEASE (C. N.). Focal retardation and arrestment of growth of bones due to vitamin A intoxication. *J. Amer. med. Ass., 1962,* **182**, *980-985.*

PERSSON (B.), TUNELL (R.) et EKENGREN (K.). Chronic vitamin A intoxication during first half year of life : description of five cases. *Acta paediat. (Uppsala), 1965,* **54**, *49-60.*

ROSSIER (A.), PAUPE (J.), MICHELIN (J.) et LARNAUDIE (J.). Dystrophie osseuse ostéomalacique chez d'extrêmes prématurés. *Arch. franç. Pédiat., 1958,* **15**, *477-498.*

ROYER (P.). Actualité du rachitisme commun. *J. Pédiat., 1957,* **1**, *185-192.*

ROYER (P.) et FRÉDÉRICH (A.). Le rein de l'hypervitaminose D et des hypercalcémies idiopathiques chez l'enfant. *Path. et Biol., 1960,* **8**, *783-789.*

ROYER (P.), SPAHR (A.) et GERBRAUX (S.). L'aminoacidurie du rachitisme commun et de la tétanie du nourrisson. *Sem. Hôp. Paris, 1956,* **32**, *254-258.*

ROYER (P.) et ARSANE (A.). Résistance à la vitamine D induite par les anticonvulsivants. *In* Journées parisiennes de Pédiatrie, 1973. *Paris, 1973, Flammarion, éd., p. 273-282.*

STEENDIJK (R.). Vitamin D and the pathogenesis of rickets and osteomalacia. *Folia med. neerl., 1968,* **11**, *178-186.*

WEISMANN-NETTER (R.) et STUHL (L.). Toxopachyostéose diaphysaire tibio-péronière. *Presse méd., 1956,* **64**, *790-791.*

WIND (L. T. de). Hypervitaminosis D with osteosclerosis. *Arch. Dis. Childh., 1961,* **36**, *373-380.*

Endocrine Diseases

ADAMS (P. H.), JOWSEY (J.) et KELLY (P. J.). Effects of

hyperthyroidism on bone and mineral metabolism in man. *Quart. J. Med., 1967,* **36**, *1-15.*

Albright (F.), Burnett (C. H.), Smith (P. H.) et Parson (W.). Pseudo-hypoparathyroidism, an example of « Seabright-Bantam » syndrome. Report of three cases. *Endocrinology, 1942,* **30**, *922-932.*

Albright (F.), Forbes (A. P.) et Henneman (P. H.). Pseudo-pseudohypoparathyroidism. *Trans. Ass. amer. Phycns, 1952,* **65**, *337-350.*

Bader (J.-Cl.), Canlorbe (P.), Lambertz (J.), Poitout (M.) et Lelong (M.). L'ostéo-dystrophie héréditaire d'Albright. Trois observations nouvelles avec épreuve à la thyrocalcitonine et au calcium 45. *Ann. Pédiat., 1968,* **44**, *269-280.*

Baud (C. A.) et Dupont (D. H.). Action des hormones sur le tissu osseux. *Rev. franç. Et. clin. biol., 1964,* **9**, *224-231.*

Bonakdarpour (A.), Kirkpatrick (J. A.), Renzi (A.) et Kendall (N.). Skeletal changes in neonatal thyrotoxicosis. *Radiology, 1972,* **102**, *149-150.*

Bronsky (D.), Kiamko (R. T.), Moncada (R.) et Rosenthal (I. M.). Intra-uterine hyperparathyroidism secondary to maternal hypoparathyroidism. *Pediatrics, 1968,* **42**, *606-613.*

Bronsky (D.). Hyperparathyroidism with Albright's osteodystrophy : case report and a proposed new classification of parathyroid disease. *J. clin. Endocrin., 1970,* **31**, *271-276.*

Castor (C. W.). Adrenocortical suppression of mucopolysaccharide formation in human connective tissue cell cultures. *J. Lab. clin. Med., 1962,* **60**, *788-798.*

Chigot (P. L.) et Ficat (C.). Anomalies de la main dans l'hyperparathyroïdie. *Rev. Chir. orthop., 1973,* **59**, *309-320.*

Dearden (L. C.) et Mosier (H. D., Jr.). Long-term recovery of chondrocytes in the tibial epiphyseal plate in rats after cortisone treatment. An electron microscopic study. *Clin. Orthop., 1972,* **87**, *322-331.*

Ehrig (U.) et Wilson (D. R.). Fibrous dysplasia of bone and primary hyperparathyroidism. *Ann. intern. Med., 1972,* **77**, *234-238.*

Eisenberg (E.) et Gordan (G. S.). Skeletal dynamics in man measured by non-radioactive strontium. *J. clin. Invest., 1961,* **40**, *1809-1825.*

Elders (M. J.), Garland (J. T.), Daughaday (W. A.), Fisher (D. A.), Whitney (J. E.) et Hughes (E. R.). Laron's dwarfism : studies on the nature of the defect. *J. Pediat., 1973,* **83**, *253-263.*

Fahmy (A.), Talley (P.), Frazier (H. M.) et Hillman (J. W.). Ultrastructural effects of estrogen on epiphyseal cartilage. *Calc. Tiss. Res., 1971,* **7**, *139-149.*

Farriaux (J. P.), Maillard (E.), Tahon (A.), Bois (R. du), Dupont (A.) et Fontaine (G.). Etude d'une nouvelle observation d'hyperparathyroïdie primitive par hyperplasie chez une enfant de un mois. *Ann. Pédiat., 1968,* **44**, *716-723.*

Frame (B.), Hanson (C. A.), Frost (H. M.), Block (M.) et Arnstein (A. R.). Renal resistance to parathyroid hormone with osteitis fibrosa « pseudo-hypohyperparathyroidism ». *Amer. J. Med., 1972,* **52**, *311-321.*

Greinacher (I.). Pseudo-Perthes. *Radiologe (Berl.), 1971,* **11**, *300-302.*

Job (J. C.), Milhaud (G.), Antener (I.) et Rossier (A.). Les anomalies du métabolisme calcique chez les enfants hypothyroïdiens. *Sem. Hôp. Paris, 1967,* **63**, *2412-2417.*

Job (J. C.), Lejeune (C.), Canlorbe (P.) et Rossier (A.). Le nanisme par insuffisance hypophysaire sporadique et idiopathique. Etude d'une série de 31 cas. *Arch. franç. Pédiat., 1972,* **29**, *117-133.*

Kunin (A. S.) et Meyer (W. L.). The effect of cortisone on the intermediary metabolism of epiphyseal cartilage from rats. *Arch. Biochem. Biophys., 1969,* **129**, *421-430.*

Laron (Z. V. I.), Pertzelan (A.) et Mannheimer (S.). Genetic pituitary dwarfism with high serum concentration of growth hormone; a new inborn error of metabolism. *Israel J. med. Sci., 1966,* **2**, *152-155.*

Lefebvre (J.) et Capdeville (R.). Aspects radiologiques des affections endocriniennes de l'enfant. *Encyclopédie méd.-chir., 1967, 31134 T10.*

Lelong (M.), Joseph (R.), Canlorbe (P.) et Scholler (R.). L'aspect cerclé des noyaux d'ossification chez l'enfant myxœdémateux. *Ann. Pédiat., 1955,* **31**, *73-76.*

Lindenfelser (R.), Schoenmackers (J.), Haubert (P.) et Kronert (W.). Der spongiöse Knochen beim primären Hyperparathyreoidismus. Strukturanalyse mit dem Raster-Elektronenmikroskop. *Virchows Arch. Abt. B, Zellpath., 1971,* **9**, *333-342.*

Lintermans (J. P.) et Seyhnaeve (V.). Hypothyroidism and vertebral anomalies. A new syndrom ? *Amer. J. Roentgenol., 1970,* **109**, *294-298.*

Loening (W. E. K.) et Vinik (A. I.). The association of growth hormone deficiency and pituitary myxoedema. *Helv. paediat. Acta, 1970,* **25**, *114-118.*

Matthieu (H.), Menibus (Cl. H. de), Frédérich (A.), Lestradet (H.) et Royer (P.). L'hypoparathyroïdie chronique primitive avec lésions d'ostéomalacie. *Ann. Pédiat., 1961,* **17**, *153-161.*

Mégevand (A.), Matthieu (H.) et Royer (P.). Anomalies squelettiques et troubles du métabolisme du calcium dans les insuffisances thyroïdiennes de l'enfant. XVIIIe Congrès Ass. Pédiat. langue franç., Genève, 1961, Vol. 1. *Basel - New York, 1961, Karger, éd. p. 205-248.*

Menking (M.), Wiebel (J.), Schmid (W. U.), Schmidt (W. T.), Ebel (K. D.) et Ritter (R.). Premature craniosynostosis associated with hyperthyroidism in 4 children. With reference to 5 further cases in the literature. *Mschr. Kinderheilk., 1972,* **120**, *106-110.*

Noble (H. M.) et Matty (A. J.). The effects of thyroxine on the movement of calcium and inorganic phosphate through the small intestine of the rat. *J. Endocrin., 1967,* **37**, *111-117.*

Rappaport (R.) et Rybak (M.). Aspects radiologiques irréguliers des métaphyses des doigts chez des enfants atteints d'insuffisance hypothalamo - hypophysaire. *Arch. franç. Pédiat., 1969,* **26**, *1135-1144.*

Rimoin (D.), Merimee (T. J.) et McKusick (V. A.). Sexual ateliotic dwarfism : a recessively inherited isolated deficiency of growth hormone. *Trans. Ass. amer. Phycns, 1966,* **79**, *297-310.*

Ritchie (G. MacL.). Dental manifestations of pseudohypoparathyroidism. *Arch. Dis. Childh., 1965,* **40**, *565-572.*

Royer (P.). La dysgénésie métaphysaire et la périostose localisée au cours de l'hypothyroïdie infantile. *Ann. Pédiat., 1961,* **37**, *149-152.*

Royer (P.), Matthieu (H.) et Balsan (S.). Troubles du métabolisme calcique dans l'insuffisance thyroïdienne de l'enfant. *Ann. Endocrin. (Paris), 1968,* **29**, *610-623.*

Silberberg (R.) et Hasler (M.). Stimulation of articular cartilage of young adult mice by hormones. *Path. Microbiol., 1971,* **37**, *23-36.*

SIMMONS (D. J.) et KUNIN (A. S.). Autoradiographic and biochemical investigations of the effect of cortisone on the bones of the rat. *Clin. Orthop., 1967,* **55**, *201-215.*

STANESCU (V.), BONA (C.) et IONESCU (V.). Histochemical and histoenzymological studies of tibial growing cartilage in pituitary dwarfism. *Acta histochem., 1967,* **26**, *169-184.*

STANESCU (V.), BONA (C.) et IONESCU (V.). Histochemical and histoenzymological investigations of growing cartilage in pseudo-hypoparathyroidism. *Acta endocrin. (Buc.), 1969,* **60**, *433-445.*

STEINBACH (H. L.), RUDHE (U.), JONSSON (M.) et YOUNG (D. A.). Evolution of skeletal lesions in pseudo-hypoparathyroidism. *Radiology, 1965,* **85**, *670-676.*

STEINBACH (H. L.) et YOUNG (D. A.). The roentgen appearance of pseudo-hypoparathyroidism (PH) and pseudo-pseudohypoparathyroidism (PPH). Differentiation from other syndromes associated with short metacarpals, metatarsals, and phalanges. *Amer. J. Roentgenol., 1966,* **97**, *49-66.*

VAES (G.) et NICHOLS (G. Jr.). Oxygen tension and the control of bone cell metabolism. *Nature (Lond.), 1962,* **193**, *379-380.*

Genetically Determined Diseases

ALBRIGHT (F.), BUTLER (A. M.) et BLOOMBERG (E.). Rickets resistant to vitamin D therapy. *Amer. J. Dis. Child., 1937,* **54**, *529-547.*

BALSAN (S.). Les hypercalcémies du nourrisson. *Vie médicale, 1968,* **49**, *1705-1712.*

BALSAN (S.) et GARABEDIAN (M.). 25-hydroxycholecalciferol, a comparative study in deficiency rickets and different types of resistant rickets. *J. clin. Invest., 1972,* **51**, *749-759.*

BESSLER (W. von) et FANCONI (A.). Die Röntgensymptome der Hypophosphatasie. Beobachtungen bei zwei Brüdern mit maligner neonataler Verlaufsform. *Fortschr. Röntgenstr., 1972,* **117**, *58-65.*

BÉTHENOD (M.), COTTE (M.-F.), COLLOMBEL (C.), FRÉDÉRICH (A.) et COTTE (J.). Hypophosphatasie à révélation néo-natale. Amélioration osseuse. Encéphalopathie convulsivante fatale. *Ann. Pédiat., 1967,* **14**, *835-841.*

BRIARD-GUILLEMOT (M.-L.), RAVERDY (E.), BALSAN (S.), REY (J.) et FRÉZAL (J.). Etude critique de l'hypophosphatémie pour l'étude génétique du rachitisme vitamino - résistant hypophosphatémique familial. *Arch. franç. Pédiat., 1972,* **29**, *1059-1068.*

BRICKMAN (H. S.), COBURN (J. W.), KUROKAWA (K.), BETHUNE (J. E.), HARRISSON (H. E.) et NORMAN (A. W.). 1-25-dihydroxycholecalciferol in hypophosphatemic vitamin D resistant rickets. *New Engl. J. Med., 1973,* **289**, *495-499.*

CHANNAROND (J.) et VERGER (P.). A propos d'un cas d'hypophosphatasie à forme majeure néo-natale. *Ann. Pédiat., 1961,* **8**, *263-268.*

ENGFELDT (R.) et ZETTERSTRÖM (R.). Osteodysmetamorphosis foetalis. *J. Pediat., 1954,* **45**, *125.*

FANCONI (G.), GIRARDET (P.), SCHLESINGER (B.), BUTLER (N.) et BLACK (J.). Chronische Hypercalcämie, kombiniert mit Osteosklerose, Hyperazotämie, Minderwuchs und congenitalen Missbildungen. *Helv. paediat. Acta, 1957,* **7**, *314-349.*

FANCONI (A.) et PRADER (A.). Die hereditäre Pseudomangelrachitis. *Helv. paediat. Acta, 1969,* **24**, *423-447.*

FLEISCH (H.) et NEUMAN (W. F.). Mechanisms of calcification : role of collagen, polyphosphates, and phosphatase. *Amer. J. Physiol., 1961,* **200**, *1296-1300.*

FOVET-POINGT (O.) et TOURSEL (F.). Une observation d'hypercalciurie idiopathique. *Pédiatrie, 1972,* **27**, *295-302.*

FRASER (D.), LANGFORD KIDD (B. S.) KOOH (S. W.) et PAUNIER (L.). A new look at infantile hypercalcemia. *Pediat. Clin. N. Amer., 1966,* **13**, *503-525.*

FRASER (D.), KOOH (S. W.), KIND (H. P.), HOLICK (M. F.), TANAKA (Y.) et DE LUCA (H. F.). Vitamin D dependant rickets : an inborn error of vitamin D metabolism. *New Engl. J. Med., 1973,* **289**, *817-822.*

GEIGER (H.). Röntgenologische Befunde bei Cystinose. *Fortschr. Röntgenstr., 1970,* **113**, *711-717.*

GENTIL (C.), PAUPE (J.), SCHEPENS (G.), ANTENER (I.), COLIN (J.), SATGÉ (P.), CANLORBE (P.) et LELONG (M.). Le rachitisme vitamino-résistant idiopathique. 5 observations avec dosage de l'activité vitaminique D du sérum. Revue critique de la littérature. *Ann. Pédiat., 1963,* **39**, *213-244.*

GLORIEUX (F.) et SCRIVER (C. R.). Loss of a parathyroid hormone sensitive component of phosphate transport in X-linked hypophosphatemia. *Science, 1972,* **175**, *997-1000.*

GUIBAUD (P.) et LARBRE (F.). A propos d'un cas d'hypophosphatasie à forme bénigne traitée par le phosphore. *Pédiatrie, 1970,* **25**, *319-330.*

HADDAD (J. G., Jr.), CHYU (K. J.), HAHN (T. J.) et STAMP (T. C. B.). Serum concentration of 25-hydroxyvitamin D in sex-linked hypophosphatemic vitamin D-resistant rickets. *J. Lab. clin. Med., 1973,* **81**, *22-27.*

KALLMEYER (J.), DUNEA (G.) et SCHWARTZ (F. D.). Hypophosphatemic osteomalacia with hyperglycinuria. *Ann. intern. Med., 1967,* **66**, *136-141.*

LAMY (M.), ROYER (P.), FRÉZAL (J.) et LESTRADET (H.). Le rachitisme vitamino-résistant familial hypophosphatémique primitif. *Arch. franç. Pédiat., 1958,* **15**, *1-24.*

LAMY (M.), NÉZELOFF (C.), FAURÉ (C.), JAMMET (M. L.) et AUSSANAIRE (M.). La forme sévère de l'hypercalcémie idiopathique. *Arch. franç. Pédiat., 1958,* **15**, *1001-1024.*

LEFEBVRE (J.), MICHEL (J. R.) et ROYER (P.). Les aspects radiologiques des altérations métaphysaires au cours de troubles métaboliques phosphocalciques. *Ann. Radiol., 1960,* **3**, *213-240.*

LIGHTWOOD (R.). Idiopathic hypercalcaemia in infants with failure to thrive. *Arch. Dis. Childh., 1952,* **27**, *302-303.*

MCPHERSON (R. I.), KROEKER (M.) et HOUSTON (C. S.). Hypophosphatasia. *J. canad. Ass. Radiol., 1972,* **23**, *16-26.*

MCCANCE (R. A.). Osteomalacia with Looser's nodes (Milkman's syndrome) due to a raised resistance to vitamin D acquired about the age of 15 years. *Quart. J. Med., 1947,* **16**, *33-46.*

NORDIO (S.), GATTI (R.) et TAMBUSSI (M.). Il nanismo ipercalciurico. *Minerva pediat., 1966,* **18**, *3-16.*

PAK (C. Y. C.), DELUCA (H. F.), BARTTER (F. C.), HENNEMAN (D. H.), FRAME (B.), SIMOPOULOS (A.) et DELEA (C. S.). Treatment of vitamin D-resistant rickets with 25-hydroxycholecalciferol. *Arch. intern. Med., 1972,* **129**, *894-899.*

PIMSTONE (B.), EISENBERG (E.) et SILVERMAN (S.). Hypophosphatasia : genetic and dental studies. *Ann. intern. Med., 1966,* **65**, *722-729.*

Prader (A.), Illig (R.) et Heierli (E.). Eine besondere Form der primären vitamin D-resistenten Rachitis mit Hypocalcamie und autosomal - dominantem Erbgang : die hereditäre Pseudo-Mangelrachitis. *Helv. paediat. Acta, 1961,* **16**, *452-468.*

Rasmussen (K.). Phosphorylethanolamine and hypophosphatasia. *Dan. med. Bull., 1968,* **15**, *suppl. 2, 1-*112.

Rathbun (J. C.). Hypophosphatasia. A new developmental anomaly. *Amer. J. Dis. Child., 1948,* **75**, *822-831.*

Rey (J.) et Frézal (J.). Pathogénie du rachitisme vitamino - résistant hypophosphatémique familial. *Rev. franç. Et. clin. biol., 1966,* **2**, *771-776.*

Royer (P.), Mathieu (H.), Gerbeaux (S.), Frederich (A.), Rodriguez-Soriano (J.), Dartois (A. M.) et Cuisinier (P.). Hypercalciurie idiopathique avec nanisme et atteinte rénale chez l'enfant. *Sem. Hôp. Paris, 1962,* **38**, *147-163.*

Royer (P.) et Gerbeaux-Balsan (S.). Les différents types de rachitisme vitamino-résistants idiopathiques. *Pédiatrie, 1966,* **21**, *352-354.*

Royer (P.). L'hypercalcémie idiopathique avec nanisme et atteinte rénale chez l'enfant. *Acta paediat. scand., 1967,* **172**, *186-191.*

Sereni (F.), Vaccari (A.), Carnelli (V.) et Principi (N.). Rachitisme vitamino-résistant type Prader. Etude métabolique de trois enfants d'une même fratrie. *Arch. franç. Pédiat., 1969,* **26**, *953-961.*

Silverman (F.) et Currarino (G.). Roentgen manifestations of hereditary metabolic diseases in childhood. *Metabolism, 1960,* **9**, *248-283.*

Sorel (R.), Dalous (A.), Fabre (J.), Rochiccioli (P.), Ghisolfi (J.) et Fabre (M. Th.). Hypercalciurie idiopathique avec nanisme. A propos d'une observation avec lésions rénales glomérulaires particulières en microscopie électronique. *Arch. franç. Pédiat., 1970,* **27**, *161-176.*

Steendijk (R.). Metabolic bone disease in children. *Clin. Orthop., 1971,* **77**, *247-275.*

Steendijk (R.) et Boyde (A.). Scanning electron microscopic observations on bone from patients with hypophosphataemic (vitamin D resistant) rickets. *Calc. Tiss. Res., 1973,* **11**, 242-250.

Williams (J. E. P.), Barratt-Boyes (B. G.) et Lowe (J. B.). Supravalvular aortic stenosis. *Circulation, 1961,* **24**, *1311-1318.*

Witmer (G.) et Balsan (S.). Biopsie osseuse dans quatre cas de rachitisme vitamino-résistant idiopathique. *Path. et Biol., 1968,* **16**, *421-429.*

Renal and Intestinal Osteodystrophies

Agus (Z. S.) et Goldberg (M.). Pathogenesis of uremic osteodystrophy. *Radiol. Clin. N. Amer., 1972,* **10**, *545-556.*

Balsan (S.), Royer (P.) et Mathieu (H.). Les rachitismes et les fibro-ostéoclasies des insuffisances rénales chroniques de l'enfant. *Arch. franç. Pédiat., 1966,* **23**, *769-794.*

Bricker (N.). Renal osteodystrophy. Therapy based on mechanism. *J. amer. med. Ass., 1970,* **211**, *97-101.*

Brickman (A. S.) et Norman (A. W.). Treatment of renal osteodystrophy with calciferol (vitamin D) and related steroids. *Kidney intern., 1973,* **4**, *161-167.*

De Luca (H.) et Avioli (L. V.). Treatment of renal osteodystrophy with 25-hydroxycholecalciferol. *Arch. intern. Med., 1970,* **126**, *896-899.*

Dittrich (J. K.). Zur Osteodystrophie infolge phenylalaninarmer Ernährung. I. Mitteilung. Klinische und röntgenologische Untersuchungen bei Kindern mit Phenylketonurie. *Z. Kinderheilk., 1965,* **93**, *1-11.*

Dittrich (J. K.) et Schott (H. J.). Zur Osteodystrophie infolge phenylalaninarmer Ernährung. II. Tierexperimentelle Untersuchungen. *Z. Kinderheilk., 1965,* **93**, *12-20.*

Eastwood (J. B.), Bordier (Ph. J.) et Wardener (H. E. de). Some biochemical histological radiological and clinical features of renal osteodystrophy. *Kidney intern., 1973,* **4**, *128-140.*

Greenfield (G. B.). Roentgen appearance of bone and soft tissue changes in chronic renal disease. *Amer. J. Roentgenol., 1972,* **116**, *749-757.*

Guibaud (P.), Larbre (F.), Freycon (M.-T.) et Genoud (J.). Ostéopétrose et acidose rénale tubulaire. Deux cas de cette association dans une fratrie. *Arch. franç. Pédiat., 1972,* **29**, *269-286.*

Hahn (T. J.) et Avioli (L. V.). Effect of chronic uremia on collagen metabolism in skin and bone. *Arch. intern. Med., 1970,* **126**, *882-886.*

Hall (M. C.) et Hume (D. M.). Bone changes in patients with renal transplants. *J. amer. med. Wom. Ass., 1968,* **23**, *1040-1047.*

Hall (M. C.), Elmore (S. M.), Bright (R. W.), Pierce (J. C.) et Hume (D. M.). Skeletal complications in a series of human renal allografts. *J. amer. med. Ass., 1969,* **208**, *1825-1829.*

Kirkwood (J. R.), Ozonoff (M. B.) et Steinbach (H.). Epiphyseal displacement after metaphyseal fracture in renal osteodystrophy. *Amer. J. Roentgenol., 1972,* **115**, *547-554.*

Kimberg (D. V.), Baerg (R. D.) et Gershon (E.). The nature of vitamin D resistance in experimental uremia. *Arch. intern. Med., 1970,* **126**, *891-895.*

Lamy (M.), Frézal (J.) et Rey (J.). Les stéatorrhées par troubles de l'absorption intestinale. *In* Rapport au XIXe Congrès Ass. Pédiat. langue franç., Paris, 1963. Vol. *1. Basel - New York, 1963, Karger, éd., p. 161-240.*

Meema (H. E.), Rabinovich (S.), Meema (S.) Lloyd (G. J.) et Oreopoulos (D. G.). Improved radiological diagnosis of azotemic osteodystrophy. *Radiology, 1972,* **102**, *1-10.*

Muldowney (F. P.). Metabolic bone disease secondary to renal and intestinal disorders. *Calif. Med., 1969,* **110**, *397-409.*

Rampini (S.), Fanconi (A.), Illig (R.) et Prader (A.). Effect of hydrochlorothiazide on proximal renal tubular acidosis in a patient with idiopathic « de Toni-Debré-Fanconi syndrome ». *Helv. paediat. Acta, 1968,* **23**, *13-21.*

Ritz (E.), Krempien (B.), Mehls (O.) et Malluche (H.). Skeletal abnormalities in chronic renal insufficiency before and during maintenance hemodialysis. *Kidney intern., 1973,* **4**, *116-127.*

Royer (P.), Lestradet (H.), Nordmann (R.), Mathieu (H.) et Rodriguez-Soriano (J.). Etudes sur quatre cas d'acidose tubulaire chronique idiopathique avec hypocitraturie. *Ann. Pédiat., 1962,* **38**, *188-209.*

Royer (P.), Habib (R.), Mathieu (H.) et Broyer (M.). Néphrologie pédiatrique. *Paris, 1972, Flammarion, éd.*

Stanbury (S. W.), Lumb (G. A.) et Mawer (E. B.). Osteodystrophy developing spontaneously in the course of chronic renal failure. *Arch. intern. Med., 1969,* **124**, *274-281.*

Villiaumey (J.) et Cerf (M.). Les altérations osseuses secondaires à l'entéropathie au gluten. *Rev. Méd., 1967,* **8**, *771-781.*

6 Disorders of the Metabolism of Glucides and Lipids

A large part of this section will be devoted to the study of the mucopolysaccharidoses and mucolipidoses. This will be followed by some comments on glycogenoses, and on Gaucher's and Niemann-Pick diseases.

THE MUCOPOLYSACCHARIDOSES

Mucopolysaccharidoses are skeletal disorders. They result from a defect in the degradation of acid mucopolysaccharides, which leads to visceral accumulation and severely disturbed enchondral growth. These patients show urinary excretion of these abnormal substances.

To identify these disorders we use the classification proposed by McKusick, which has been accepted by the International Committee on Nomenclature. It appears logical to study immediately after type I, mucopolysaccharidosis (Hurler's disease), all the clinically closely related syndromes such as type II, Hunter's disease (recessive sex-linked), type III, Sanfilippo's disease, type VI, polydystrophic dwarfism, and type V, Ullrich-Scheie disease or "Spät-Hurler."

Morquio's disease, or type IV, will be dealt with separately, since this is a considerably different disorder. Visceral storage of abnormal metabolites does not play a major role in its development. It is the result of severe skeletal involvement. Abnormal excretion of mucopolysaccharides has also been reported in other disorders, but this is an inconstant finding and its exact significance is still not fully appreciated.

MUCOPOLYSACCHARIDOSIS TYPE I (HURLER'S DISEASE)

This disorder had been seen prior to the thesis by G. Hurler, which was inspired by Pfaundler. Still, these authors gave the first exact description and definition of this disease. Hurler's disease is sometimes also referred to as the polydystrophy of Hurler, or dysostosis multiplex. The term gargoylism has been proposed by Ellis because of the facial dysmorphism faintly reminiscent of the aspect of gargoyles on cathedrals.

Clinical Findings

This disorder is recognized at a variable age, but most frequently during the second year of life. Morphologic changes recognizable at birth are most unusual.

Frequently parents will note a lumbar kyphosis, an unusually coarse facies or delayed psychomotor development. Limitation of motion or deformity of the flexed fingers may cause parents some anxiety. Physical examination will show striking cranio-facial alterations. In early infancy the facial features may only be somewhat coarse and there may be signs of scaphocephaly. Eventually, however, this abnormal appearance will become much more pronounced, the nose will be deep seated with excessively large nostrils, the lips and ears will be thick and the hair dry and coarse. The tongue becomes big and the teeth small and widely spaced (Fig. 6-1). The trunk is somewhat short and deformed by either a low thoracic or lumbar kyphosis (Fig. 6-1). A large umbilical hernia is usually present, often combined with inguinal hernias. The extremities are broad and held in slight flexion. Usually there is limitation of abduction of the shoulders and hips, together with limited extension of the elbows, the hips and the knees. Study of the hand shows the fingers to be very broad and slightly flexed. These changes will become progressively worse with the fingers held in irreducible flexion (Fig. 6-1).

The liver and spleen are enlarged, but splenomegaly may be a relatively late manifestation. There may be heart murmurs, usually best heard at the apex with a systolic or a diastolic murmur at the base. The heart is often large, and the ECG may show right or left strain.

In the very young infant there may not yet be a growth deficit. Actually, at this stage a patient may be bigger than the average, but eventually there is slowing of growth with a final height rarely above 1.30 to 1.40 m.

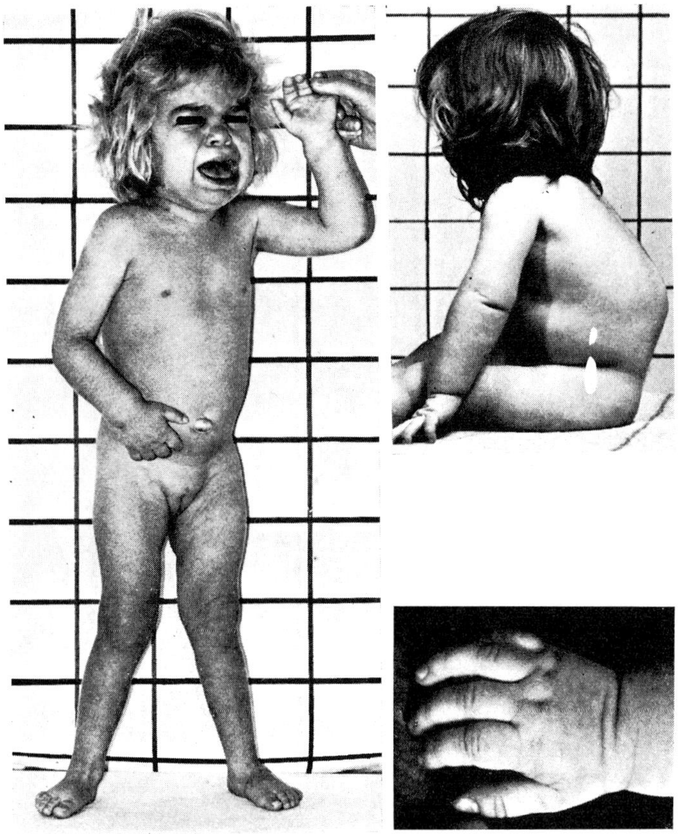

Fig. 6-1. Hurler's disease with its typical facial appearance, lumbar kyphosis, and claw hand deformity.

Psychomotor development appears almost normal during the first and second year of life, then comes to a stop. Mental deterioration will then set in. This may, however, occur at an earlier moment, and in some patients this may only happen much later and to a milder degree. The development slowly leads to eventual death, most frequently close to puberty. Heart failure and sometimes intercurrent infection are precipitating factors.

Hematologic study will show the presence of Gasser cells. These are lymphocytes containing cellular vacuoles usually grouped within a region of the cytoplasm, often having a somewhat darker center if studied by the May-Grunwald-Giemsa technique (Fig. 6-2, *Top, left*). These cells are not very prevalent and studying a number of smears is recommended in order to recognize one or two of them. In bone marrow smears there are plasma cells with numerous vacuoles in their cytoplasm. In the center of these there is a dark spot (Fig. 6-2, *Top, right*), referred to as cells of Buhot. Large reticular cells containing basophilic granulations can also be found (Fig. 6-2, *Bottom, left*). These Gasser II-cells are seen more frequently and show a greater variability than cells of Buhot.

Alder's anomaly, seen only rarely, is always mentioned with this type (Fig. 6-2, *Bottom, right*). Ophthalmologic study will show corneal opacities, which may sometimes be noted by the naked eye. Slit lamp study will fully confirm their presence. Other occular anomalies have been noted, such as congenital glaucoma, megalo-cornea, and optic atrophy towards the final stage of the disease. These findings are somewhat inconstant. Audiometry finally may show the frequent existence of a mixed type of transmission and perception deafness.

Radiographic Findings

In very young infants it is quite difficult to recognize radiologic features of this disorder. Still, anterior hypoplasia of a lumbar vertebra with a kyphosis are seen early along. During the second year of life, radiologic

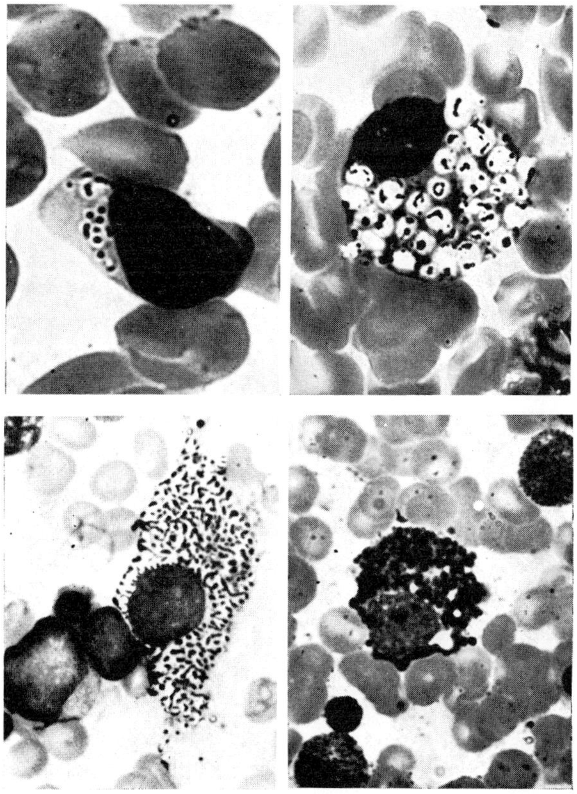

Fig. 6-2. Abnormal cells within the blood and bone marrow during the course of Hurler's disease (*Top, left*) Gasser cell. (*Top, right*) Buhot cell. (*Bottom, left*) Gasser Type II cell. (*Bottom, right*) Alder's granulation.

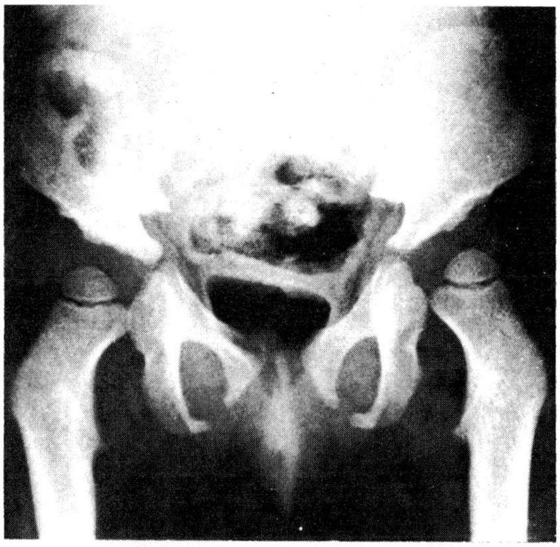

Fig. 6-3. Hurler's disease in a 3-year-old girl. Note the coxa valga and small femoral head, the massive appearance of the diaphysis, and the widening of the acetabulum.

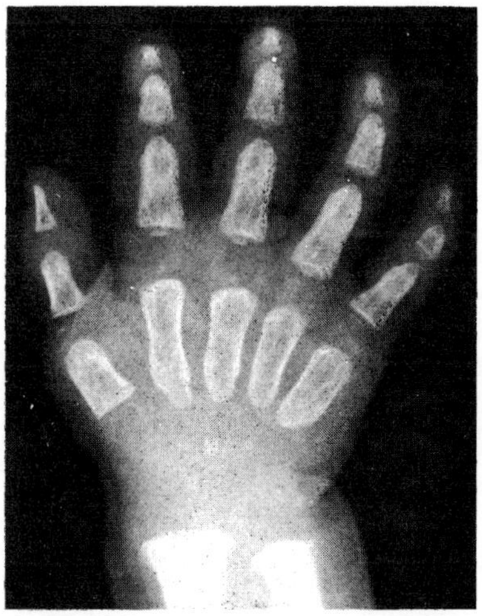

Fig. 6-4. Hurler's disease in an 18-month-old girl. At this age there are already recognizable changes involving the proximal metacarpals by local tapering. There is also generalized poor modeling.

changes become pronounced. The diaphysis of long bones may be large, and this aspect becomes even more pronounced during the further development. The metaphyseal border is sometimes uneven and may show a slight distal obliquity at radius and ulna. Coxa valga is almost the rule. The epiphyseal centers do not develop well, especially the femoral head (Fig. 6-3). The alterations of the hand are most striking (Fig. 6-4). The metacarpals lose their normal modeling and assume a form like a sucked sugar cone. The phalanges are also squat and trapezoidal. The ribs are broad and the pelvis is somewhat small. It flares laterally and the acetabular roof appears widened with a lateral obliquity. Frequently there is a lack of development of the antero-superior portion of a vertebral body, most frequently of the last thoracic or the 1st or 2nd lumbar vertebra. Sometimes the immediately adjacent vertebral body is somewhat similarly affected, but to a lesser degree. This finding is best appreciated on lateral films (Fig. 6-5). The skull can be increased in size and the sagittal suture may close prematurely. This results in the scaphocephalic aspect of some of the children. In some rare instances there may, however, be brachycephaly. The sella turcica is often deep and elongated with an excessive development of the clinoid apophyses (Fig. 6-6).

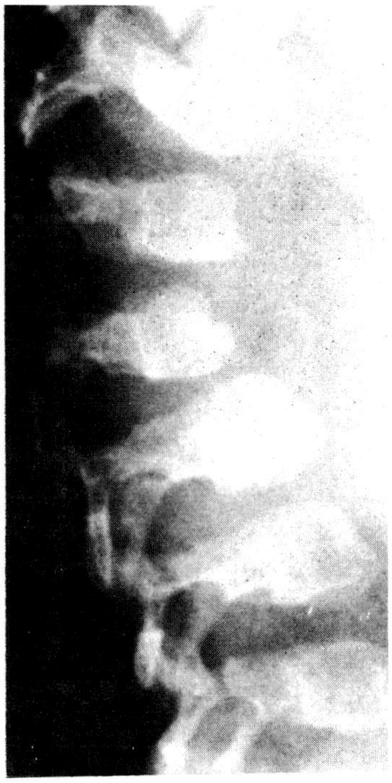

Fig. 6-5. Hurler's disease in an 8-year-old girl. Note the spurlike deformity of the 2nd lumbar vertebra.

Genetic Data

Hurler's disease is transmitted as an autosomal recessive disorder.

The detection of hetero-zygotes, and the recognition of the disorder *in utero,* has been proposed based on the presence of metachromatic granulations in cultured fibroblasts (Danes and Bearn), or by the uptake of ^{35}S. These methods have been replaced by the determination of the lack of the enzyme L-iduronidase.

Biochemical and Pathologic Findings

Internal organs reveal the presence of stored substances. Histochemical study has shown that these are mucopolysaccharides. It should be emphasized that these studies are exceedingly difficult because of the noted instability of mucopolysaccharides. Within the nervous system storage occurs only in the form of gangliosides. Chromatographic study of these demonstrates a relative increase in monosialo-gangliosides (G-5 and G-6). This finding has already been reported in other storage disorders such as Niemann-Pick disease and amaurotic idiocy.

The columnar arrangement is somewhat disorganized at the growth cartilage but there is no specific morphologic alteration. The matrix is strongly metachromatic and this metachromasia will not disappear following digestion by hyaluronidase.

Electron microscopy of hepatic cells has shown the presence of many round and variably sized intracytoplasmic inclusions. These contain a substance with a granular aspect and inclusions of varying size. Within nerve cells the most characteristic finding is the presence of corpuscles of 1 μ diameter which are composed of dense transverse bands, designated as "zebra bodies."

Urinary excretion of mucopolysaccharides is more than ten times the normally observed amount during infancy. Separation of these mucopolysaccharides by column-chromatography reveals the presence of two abnormal fractions in Hurler's disease. The prominent fraction is dermatan-sulfate and the less important one heparan sulfate.

Fibroblast culture will reveal the presence of metachromatic granulation, when studied by toluidine-blue staining. Biochemical studies of fibroblasts have led to the recognition of an accumulation of acid mucopolysaccharides. Still, it is critical to realize that the presence of granulations is not specific for mucopolysaccharidosis. They can also be seen in a large number of other disorders, such as lipidosis, and even mucoviscidosis and other cases.

Pathogenesis

Many theories have been proposed to define the pathogenesis of Hurler's disease. Recent studies, demonstrating a reciprocal correction of cultured fibroblasts by normal serum or serum from individuals afflicted by another type, have confirmed that the disease results from a defect of degradation of mucopolysaccharides. This has been suggested by Van Hoof and Hers based on ultrastructural studies. This metabolic defect is present in the mucopolysaccharidoses types II, III, V and VI. In mucopolysaccharidosis I it was already possible to identify the corrective factor. There is an enzymatic defect involving insufficient formation of L-iduronidase (Neufeld et al.). Still, many problems inherent in these disorders have not been resolved. It is very difficult to understand the mechanism of storage. Since the kidney is capable of eliminating the only partially broken down molecules, is there a defective cellular degradation? We also do not fully understand the accumulation of gangliosides in the CNS.

Treatment

Many different therapeutic approaches have been attempted and abandoned. The proof of the presence in normal serum of a factor inhibiting the occurrence

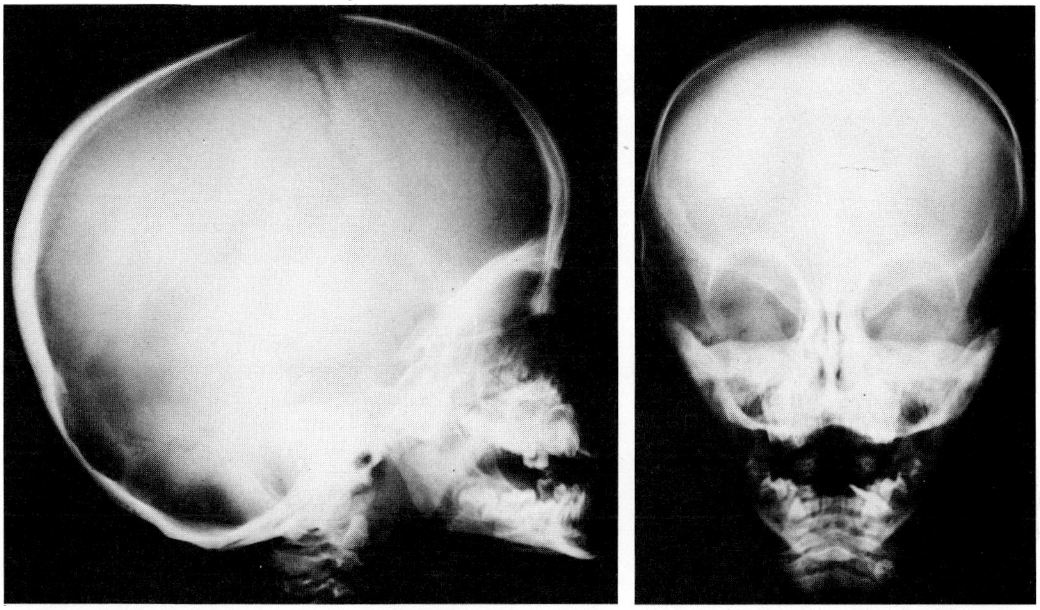

Fig. 6-6. Hurler's disease in a 16-month-old boy. The scaphocephaly is secondary to early closure of the coronal suture. Note the elongation of the sella turcica.

of metachromatic granulation in cultured fibroblasts (Hors-Cayla et al.) has led Di Ferante to propose plasma perfusion and then infusion of leukocytes. In spite of the high hopes put into these methods by their promoters, the results appear deceiving so far, and the methods are not without danger. A true form of therapy could only be the definition, manufacture and use of the deficient enzyme in a purified form. This can only be done, if this substance can be shown to be effective within the patient's organism. Attempts to extract the substance from urine are underway, but severe obstacles have been encountered.

MUCOPOLYSACCHARIDOSIS TYPE II (HUNTER'S DISEASE)

This disorder, having considerable similarities with the preceding one, was recognized as a distinct entity mainly on genetic grounds, since it has sex-linked recessive characteristics. Clinically, there are only mild differences from Hurler's disease (Fig. 6-7). A key difference is the lack of corneal opacities in slit lamp examination, and a somewhat slower general development, which, however, may be quite variable. Cardiac complications and deafness appear to be less frequently present. Radiologically, skeletal changes are less marked than in Hurler's disease (Fig. 6-8). Vertebral deformities are unusual and the metacarpals are much less severely involved (Fig. 6-9). Sagittal craniostenosis, however, is frequently present. The urinary excretion shows two abnormal fractions, heparan sulfate and dermatan sulfate. The heparan sulfate fraction is often higher than in Hurler's disease, but, more importantly, it contains two subfractions with a clearly different distribution. The hematologic findings are similar, and metachromatic granulations can be seen in cultured fibroblasts. An enzymatic defect is present, involving a sulfo-iduronate-sulfatase (Bach et al.).

The transmission of Hunter's disease occurs in a sex-linked recessive manner and the problem of the detection of transmitters is clearly indicated. Some authors have proposed the study of radioactive sulfur fixation on fibroblasts modified by prolonged culture or congealing. It would appear that thereby the enzyme deficient cells would be especially selected. The direct determination of sulfo-iduronate sulphatase would certainly give a more precise answer.

The development of the disease is quite variable from one family to another. This led some authors (Spranger, Lichtenstein et al.) to propose two types, one with a rapid evolution as in Hurler's disease, and another one, where the patients survive well beyond 20 years and do not show marked mental deterioration. The enzymatic defect seems to be identical, since there is no mutual correction of cultured fibroblasts. It is possible that these two types are due to allelic genes.

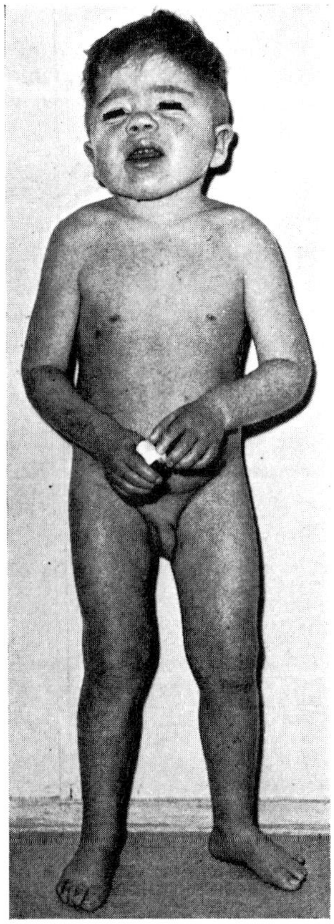

Fig. 6-7. Hunter's disease with a clinical appearance which is somewhat similar to that of patients with Hurler's disease. (see Fig. 6-1).

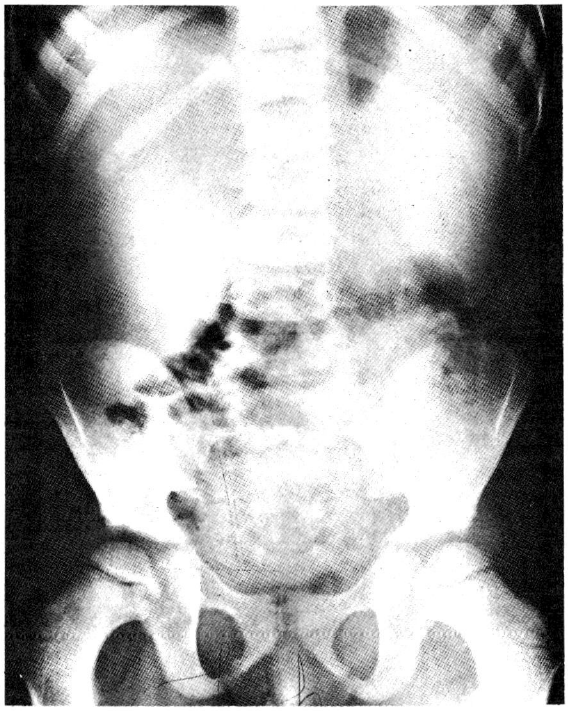

Fig. 6-8. Hunter's disease in a 4-year-old boy. There is widening of all the ribs.

MUCOPOLYSACCHARIDOSIS TYPE III (SANFILIPPO'S DISEASE, POLYDYSTROPHIC OLIGOPHRENIA)

This disorder is also recognized during the second year of life, mainly because of a psychomotor retardation and ensuing progressive mental deterioration.

Clinically, there is a somewhat coarse facial appearance reminiscent of the preceding disorders, but the final outcome of the facial appearance is always much less striking (Fig. 6-10). Growth is satisfactory, at least during the first few years. The extremities are normal. Usually there is hepatomegaly. The corneas are clear, but frequently these patients are deaf. The development is towards death with severe mental deterioration. This course is usually of longer duration than in Hurler's disease.

Frequently there are a large number of Gasser cells present in the peripheral blood. In the bone marrow Gasser II cells may also be found, together with Buhot's cells.

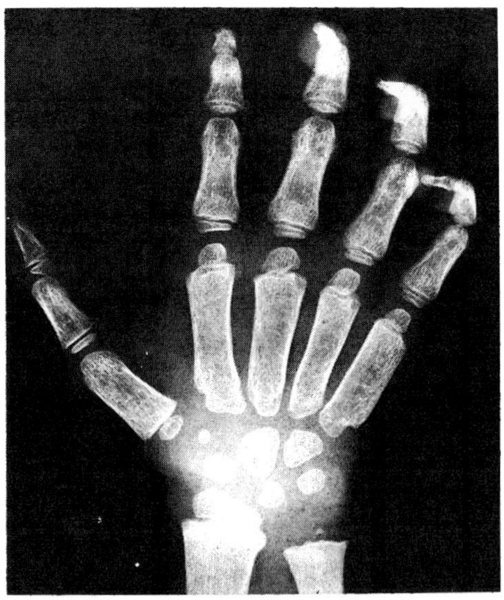

Fig. 6-9. Hunter's disease in a 5-year-old boy. The metacarpal alterations are somewhat less dramatic than those seen in Hurler's disease.

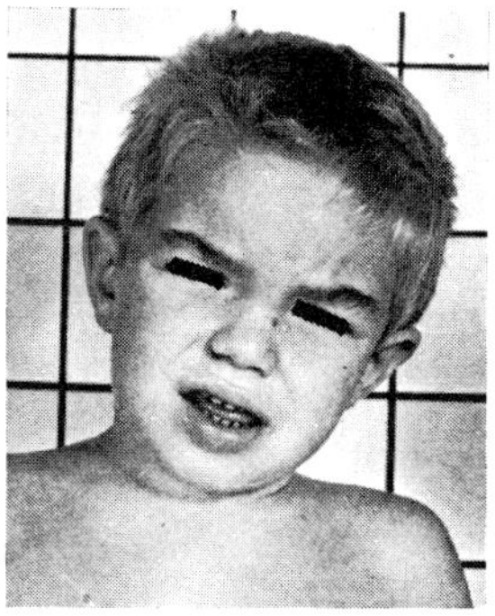

Fig. 6-10. Mucopolysaccharidosis Type III. The facial alterations are much less marked than those in the two preceding disorders.

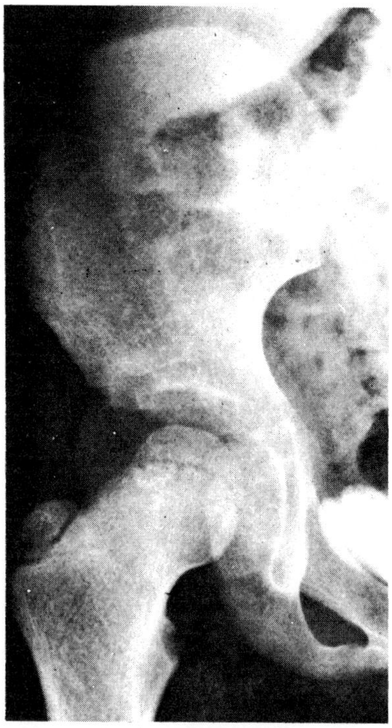

Fig. 6-12. Mucopolysaccharidosis Type III in a 4-year-old boy. Notice the small femoral head.

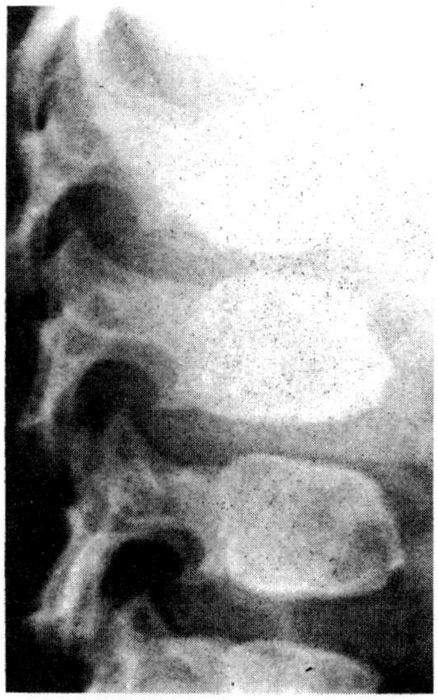

Fig. 6-11. Mucopolysaccharidosis Type III in a 4-year-old boy. Note the slight deformity and spur formation of vertebral bodies in the lower thoracic and lumbar regions.

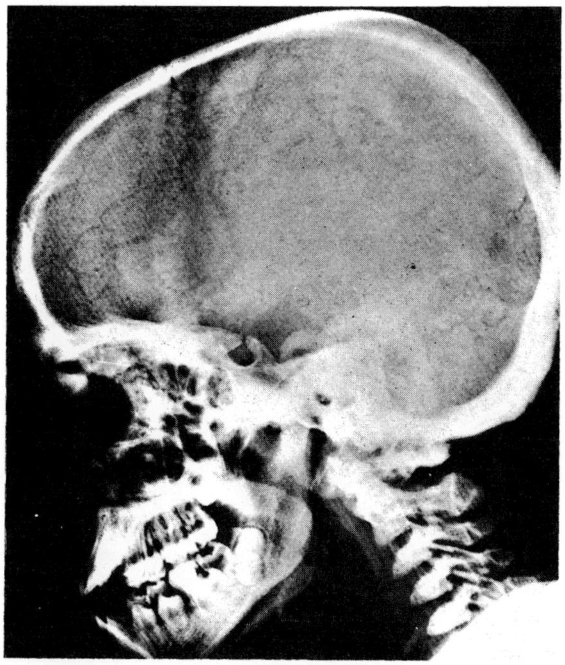

Fig. 6-13. Mucopolysaccharidosis Type III in a 12-year-old boy. There is thickening of the cranial vault and the base of the skull is somewhat dense.

The radiologic changes are mainly recognized when studying the spine, pelvis and skull. The vertebral bodies have a slightly ovoid aspect and may have an anterior spur formation (Fig. 6-11). The iliac wings may be square and the femoral head is small in relation to the acetabulum with a somewhat irregular roof and the tendency to become horizontal (Fig. 6-12). The cranial vault is often thick, sometimes there is a dense base and the sella turcica is normal (Fig. 6-13). There is no scaphocephaly present.

Transmission occurs as an autosomal recessive disorder. Heparan sulfate is always found in high concen-

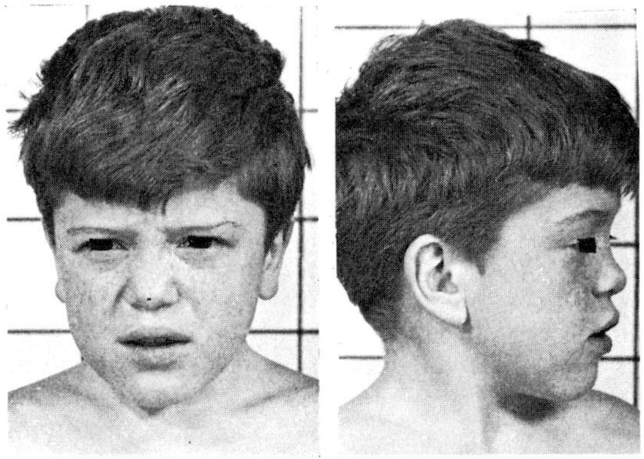

Fig. 6-14. Mucopolysaccharidosis Type VI. The facial features are made much less dramatic than in Type I and II.

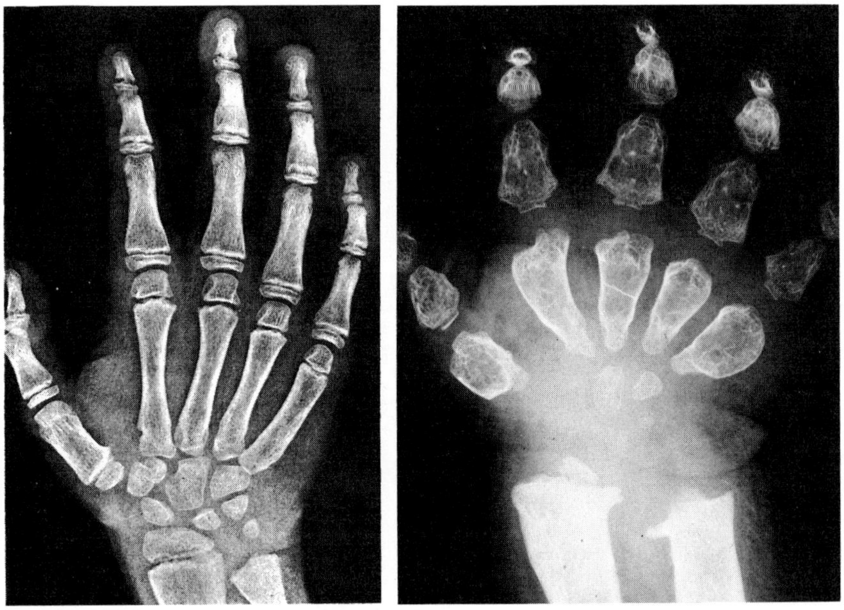

Fig. 6-15. Mucopolysaccharidosis Type VI. The markedly different appearance of the hands of two different boys at 13 years of age is evidence of the heterogeneity of this disorder.

tration in the urine, but dermatan sulfate may be only minimally present or even lacking.

Studying fibroblasts and their mutual correction in culture media, Neufeld et al. have shown that mucopolysaccharidosis type III actually refers to two distinct entities, possibly even three. Clinical and radiological criteria could not separate these properly. In one of these, type A, the enzymatic deficit is that of a herparan-sulfamidase (Von Figura and Kresse) and in the other, type B, it is N-acetyl-α-D-glucosaminidase.

MUCOPOLYSACCHARIDOSIS TYPE VI (POLYDYSTROPHIC DWARFISM)

This disorder is rare in comparison with the preceding one. Morphologic findings are in the foreground.

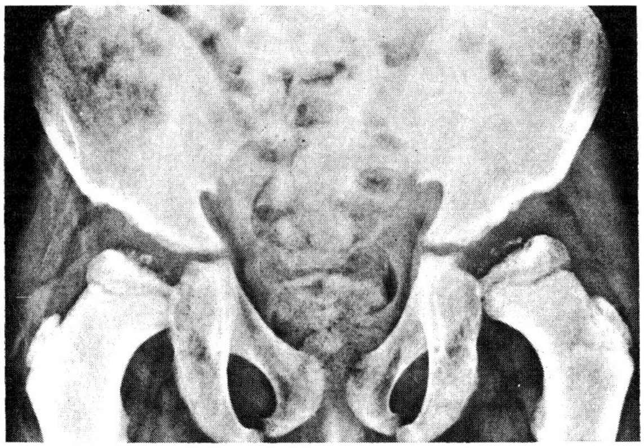

Fig. 6-16. Mucopolysaccharidosis Type VI in a 6-year-old boy. Note the markedly dysplastic femoral head and coxa valga along with the widened acetabula.

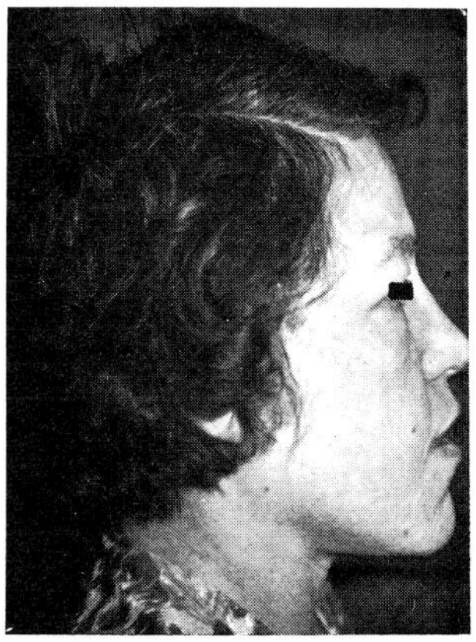

Fig. 6-17. Mucopolysaccharidosis Type V in a 32-year-old woman.

Growth retardation, involving the trunk and the extremities, is noted during the second or third year. A discrete sternal protrusion and lumbar kyphosis together with genu valgum are frequently present. Articular motion is minimally limited and the fingers are not fixed in position. The facial appearance is somewhat reminiscent of Hurler's disease, but the degree of involvement is much less severe (Fig. 6-13). Hepatosplenomegaly, corneal opacities, and deafness are usually part of this disorder. The psychomotor development, however, does not seem to be affected, at least during the first 20 years of life.

Alder's granulations are seen with a high incidence, in this type of mucopolysaccharidosis, and we have noted them in every patient. The radiologic findings are abnormal epiphyses, coxa valga, a slight radio-ulnar obliquity at the distal region and a pointed aspect of the metacarpal ends (Fig. 6-15 and Fig. 6-14). In the type of patients described here there is hardly any involvement of the diaphyses of the long bones. A cuneiform aspect of the first lumbar vertebra has been noted, and the sella turcica may be omega shaped.

Transmission is by an autosomal recessive mode. The urinary excretion of mucopolysaccharides is almost completely limited to dermatan sulfate.

It would appear that here again we can distinguish two different types. The one conforming to the initial description, which we have given above, and the other which manifests some degree of dwarfism and skeletal deformities of a more serious nature (Rampini). In this second type there are marked alterations of the diaphyses of long bones. They are short and square and particularly the phalanges and metacarpals are much more severely affected, somewhat reminiscent of their appearance in Hurler's disease (Fig. 6-14).

The enzymatic defect of this disease is not yet known. In the first form we have noted, together with M. C. Hors, a deficiency in arylsulfatase B within fibroblasts. But we are unaware of the exact significance of this finding. A similar observation was made in three patients by Strumpf et al.

MUCOPOLYSACCHARIDOSIS TYPE V (ULLRICH-SCHEIE DISEASE, "SPÄT-HURLER")

This disorder has a much slower course than the preceding types. It is often recognized only during adolescence, or in young adults, because of deformed fingers, corneal opacities or cardiac problems.

Height may only minimally be affected, since adults reach 1.50 m. The facial alterations are limited to prognathism with a somewhat massive development of the lower facial features (Fig. 6-16). The deformity of the hands is quite striking. There is a flexed position of the fingers, and the fingers are square. The corneal involvement may be severe, with a milky aspect. The disorder is compatible with prolonged survival and many of these patients will live more than 40 years.

Radiologically there is only mild skeletal involvement, such as coxa valga, slight distal radial and ulnar obliquity and phalangeal deformity (Fig. 6-17).

Biochemical study reveals that the urinary findings are identical with those seen in Hurler's disease. The transmission is by autosomal recessive inheritance. The enzymatic defect appears to be the same as in Hurler's disease – L-iduronidase. It would appear possible, however, that the disease is due to a different allelic gene and further research is needed to eliminate the possibility of heterogeneity in this group.

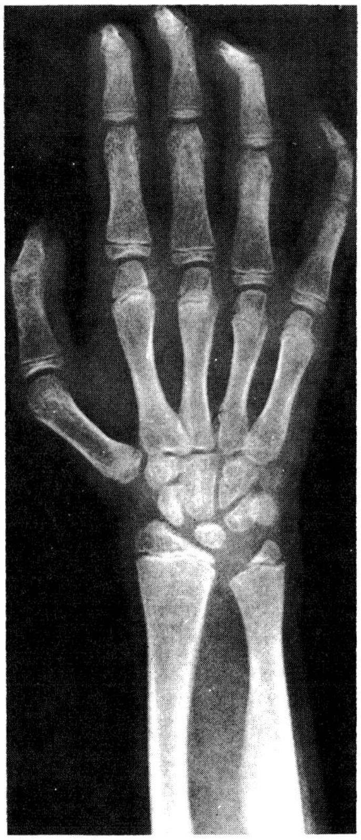

Fig. 6-18. Mucopolysaccharidosis Type V. This is the same patient as Fig. 6-17 at the age of 13 years when there was only mild skeletal involvement.

MORQUIO'S DISEASE (MUCOPOLYSACCHARIDOSIS TYPE IV)

This disorder was recognized by Morquio and Brailsford in 1929. The discovery of a metabolic defect of the mucopolysaccharides was only made in 1961.

Clinical Findings

This disease is usually recognized during the first and second year of life, because of a progressive deformity of the thorax, or difficulties with gait secondary to genu valgum and flat feet. At first examination there will be only a mild growth deficit, but this will become much more severe in the older child. Dwarfism is mainly limited to the severely abnormal trunk, with marked sternal protrusion. Sometimes there is also thoraco-lumbar kyphosis. The extremities may be somewhat short. Severe genu valgum is almost the rule, together with flat feet and a slight ulnar deviation of the hand (Fig. 6-18). Ligamentous hyperlaxity of the wrist and fingers contrasts with the limitation of movement of the proximal joints, particularly the hip. Facial dysmorphism is usually clear cut in the older child. The lower part of the face protudes. This is further emphasized by the striking posture of the head, which is held in posterior flexion. The teeth are abnormal. They have grayish enamel and abnormal calcification resulting in a punctate appearance. Slit lamp examination of the cornea will show the presence of fine opacities, which may be clincially disturbing. Loss of hearing is frequently present, but to a mild degree. It must be investigated by an audiogram. This a secondary manifestation of pathology involving the middle and inner ear.

Alder's granulations have occasionally, but not regularly, been noted in the peripheral blood. There are no Gasser or Buhot cells in the bone marrow.

The development of the disease is characterized by an almost complete growth stop at about ten years. Dwarfing is thus severe and the adult may not grow to a height of more than 1 m, or only rarely more than 1.20 m. The mental development of these patients is entirely normal and there are no signs of visceral storage during the later development. The skeletal deformities are sometimes responsible for complications, especially respiratory problems and medullary compression. These are most frequently localized in the cervical area, resulting from a hypoplastic dens. In those patients with a very short spine, it is also possible that the medulla descends lower than in the normal person and that there is lumbar compression.

Radiographic Findings

In early infancy there is hardly any radiologic manifestation. Prior to one year of age the vertebral bodies will show a practically normal form and height and the only possible finding on a lateral view is just a bare indication of the subsequent anterior hypoplasia of a lumbar vertebra (Fig. 6-19). The epiphyses are affected very little.

Progressively there will be more and more severe platyspondyly, and from the second or third year on this will become very clear. All vertebral bodies are reduced in height and on a lateral view they have an anterior "tongue." The last thoracic or the first or second lumbar vertebrae often shows anterior hypoplasia. The involved vertebral bodies are pushed in a posterior direction (Fig. 6-20 and 6-21). Tomographic study of the cranial base of the skull helps one to recognize hypoplasia of the dens, a finding not present in Hurler's disease (Fig. 6-22). The cranial vault and the area of the sella are only mildly abnormal. The diaphysis of the long bones is somewhat shortened and the metaphyses frequently appear irregular. There is also

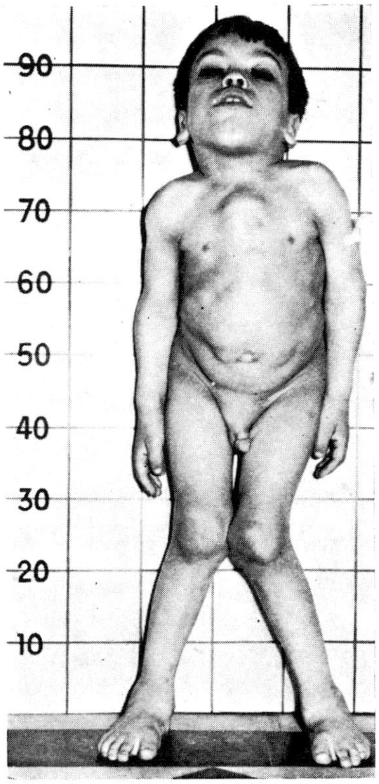

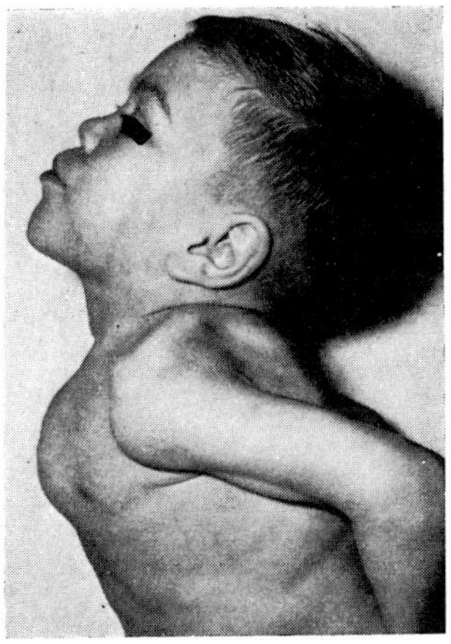

Fig. 6-19. Morquio's disease. Note the marked shortening of the trunk, the genu valgum, the anterior bulge of the sternum, and retroflexion of the head.

insufficient development of the epiphyses, and they are abnormal in outline and structure. These epiphyseometaphyseal changes become progressively more severe during growth. The femoral head may thus completely disappear, while the femoral neck becomes shorter. Pelvic films, besides widening of the acetabula, reveal a valgus deformity of the femoral necks. Eventually there will be subluxation and formation of a pseudoacetabulum (Fig. 6-23). The proximal ends of the metacarpals are conical or wavy, but these bones preserve normal modeling, which is quite different from the changes seen in Hurler's disease. The distal ends of radius and ulna may be oblique and almost facing one another (Fig. 6-24). The modifications of the wrist and of the metacarpals in combination with coxa valga, and anterior hypoplasia of the lower thoracic and upper lumbar vertebrae will help in recognizing Morquio's disease, and in avoiding confusion with other generalized types of platyspondyly.

In the adolescent or adult, there are serious deformities. The height of the spine is dramatically shortened, the long bones are short and the epiphyses markedly abnormal. The femoral neck is unusually short and dislocated. It is important to be familiar with the severe progressive characteristics of the epiphyseal changes, which is one of the characteristics of Morquio's disease. Actually, during early infancy and in young children with this disorder, the epiphyses are practically normal, whereas at the end of growth these are severely altered. This is particularly true of the femoral head, which may have completely disappeared in the adult.

Genetic, Biochemical, and Pathologic Findings

Morquio's disease is transmitted as an autosomal recessive lesion. Both sexes are equally affected and the incidence of paternal consanguinity is close to 20 per cent.

In the rare instances of anatomic studies (Einhorn et al., Schenk and Haggerty) no visceral storage could be found by microscopy. However, electron microscopy study by Tondeur and Loeb has shown that most Kupffer cells are distended by clear vacuoles of considerable size. Their aspect is reminiscent of those seen in Hurler's disease. Similar findings have been recorded in atypical cellular contents, the nature of which have not yet been elucidated. Involvement of liver cells, however, is much more discrete. Histologic and histochemical study of growth cartilage has resulted in the finding that these are extremely disorganized, totally lacking columnar alignment. The carti-

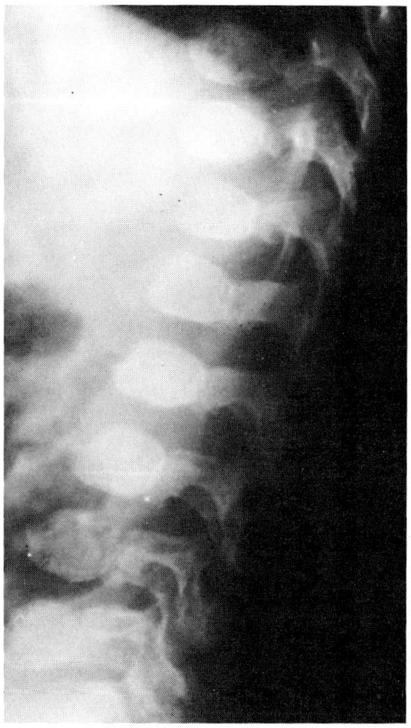

Fig. 6-20. Morquio's disease in a 9-month-old infant. The height loss of all vertebral bodies is of a moderate degree and the anterior changes are just becoming noticeable at this time. (Courtesy of F. Morvan)

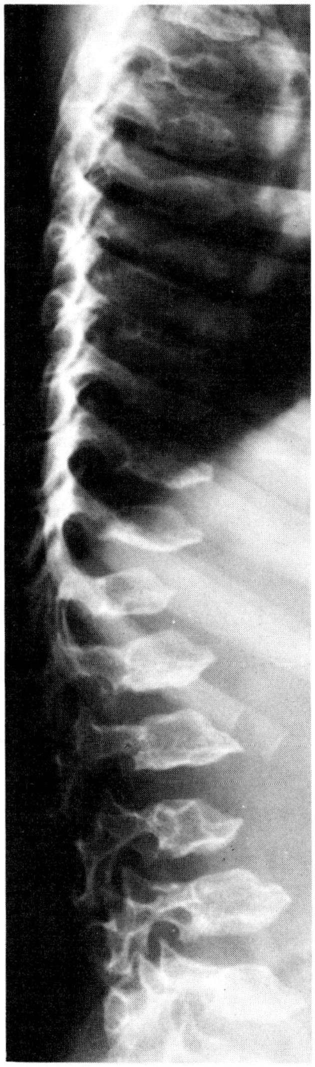

Fig. 6-21. Morquio's disease in a 5-year-old girl. There is generalized platyspondyly with an anterior tonguelike deformity, along with hypoplasia of LI, which is slightly displaced posteriorly.

laginous cells are large, even in the area that seems to correspond to the reserve zone (resting zone). The matrix is rich in fibrous tissue, and metachromasia as evidence of the presence of mucopolysaccharides is only visible at the periphery of these chondrocytes. Primary trabeculation is almost totally absent. Numerous vacuoles have been demonstrated within chondrocytes by electron microscopy (Sengel et al., Maynard et al.).

The urinary excretion of abnormal amounts of keratan sulfate has been fully confirmed. Sometimes there is also a slight increase of the normal fraction of chondroitine -4 or 6-sulfate. It appears, however, that in the adult this excretion is reduced, and it is, therefore, difficult to demonstrate this keratan-sulfate. Cultured fibroblasts will show metachromatic granulations. All this suggests a metabolic disorder of mucopolysaccharides with a serious effect on the growth and structure of several tissues, such as cartilage and cornea. Storage in the viscera is not the main problem.

The presence of corneal opacities and the abnormal excretion of keratan-sulfate in Morquio's disease have led certain authors to define a new entity called "Morquio-Ullrich" disease (Zellweger, Goidanich). This would be a disorder different from Morquio's disease, since visceral storage would be associated with skeletal findings. This approach, however, appears unnecessary. Actually, even though Morquio's publication did not mention corneal opacities, these have since been proven to be present in one of his original patients (Soto). It is therefore not at all necessary to add a subdivision to Morquio's disease, which is thus clearly defined.

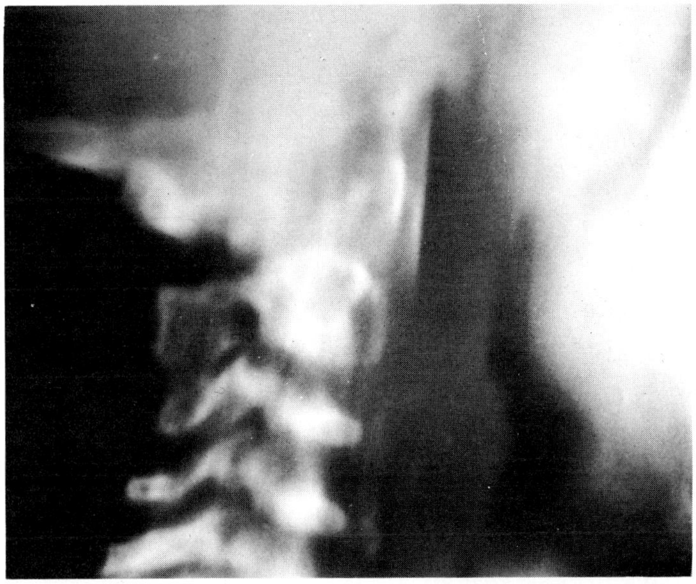

Fig. 6-22. Morquio's disease in a 7-year-old boy. A tomography of the atlantooccipital region demonstrates the hypoplasia of the dens.

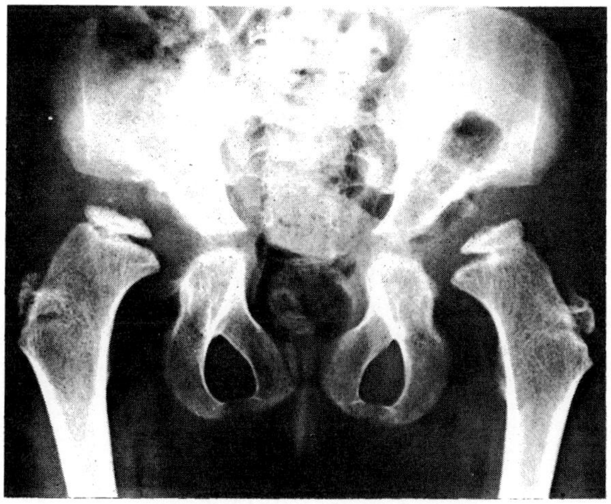

Fig. 6-23. Morquio's disease in a 7-year-old girl. Note the coxa valga with poorly developed femoral heads and marked widening of the acetabula.

Treatment

There is presently no therapy available against the basic disorder. Orthopedic surgery can offer help to these patients. In the younger patient it is necessary to treat lumbar kyphosis when this becomes marked. Later surgical correction of the genu valgum should be considered. The hip should be carefully followed, because of the high risk of dislocation, and varisation-osteotomy may be helpful. A hearing aid may also be beneficial to some of these patients. It is, however, unusual that the ophthalmologic condition requires keratoplasty.

Regular neurologic follow-up examinations are necessary, and some authors (Bailey), because of the high risk of neurologic complications, actually recommend systematically offering these patients fixation of the cervical spinal region. It is our personal policy not to suggest such a procedure to patients with Morquio's disease with the exception of those with early neurologic findings and a proven instability of the atlanto-occipital region who face a risk of dislocation C_1-C_2.

OTHER MUCOPOLYSACCHARIDOSES

Besides the six types described, there are other disorders with similar findings. They will be discussed now.

Mucopolysaccharidosis with an elimination of chondroitine-4-sulfate. This disorder seems to deserve its own place (Thomson, Philippart, Spranger). Clinically this disorder is highly reminiscent of mucopolysaccharidosis type I, but lacks the typical facial features

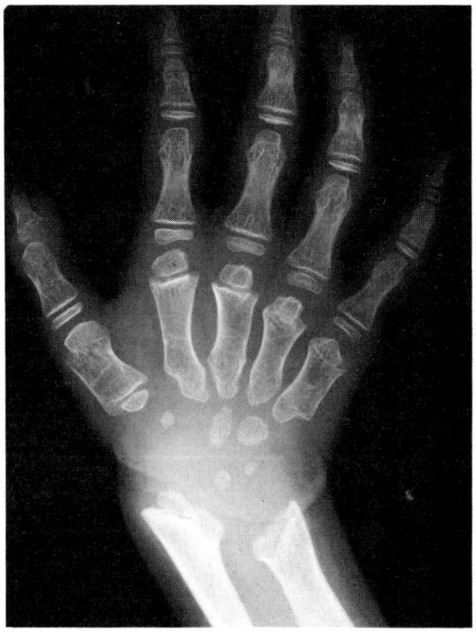

Fig. 6-24. Morquio's disease in a 5-year-old girl with marked tapering of the proximal ends of the metacarpals and forming a right angle at the distal end of the radius and ulna.

and mental retardation. Radiologically the bones are not impressive, but the typical alterations described for this mucopolysaccharidosis can be clearly recognized (coxa valga, radio-ulnar obliquity and conic metacarpal changes). There is an abnormal urinary excretion of chondroitine-4-sulfate. The disorder is probably inherited as an autosomal recessive lesion. It would appear that this disorder is not the result of a defect in β-glucuronidase as has been thought. The latter, however, is responsible for another mucopolysaccharidosis, mainly type VII, with a rather variable clinical manifestation (Sly, Beaudet, Gehler et al.) along with mild skeletal involvement (slight deformity of the iliac wings, coxa valga and a slight elongation of sella turcica). The polynuclear cells contain Alder's granulations and the urinary polysaccharides are elevated, but the nature of these has not been fully elucidated.

Another set of findings groups the disorders with an abnormal elimination of keratan-sulfate. Besides Morquio's disease, somewhat similar patients have been seen showing much less involvement (Fig. 6-25). There are no corneal opacities, but there is a moderate amount of keratan-sulfate in the urine. It appears impossible to decide whether this is an allelic variant or a minor form of Morquio's disease or an entirely different disorder.

Recently a disorder has been described associating abnormal enchondral growth with an extra-pyramidal syndrome consisting of athetosis and corneal opacities in the presence of urinary keratan-sulfate excretion (Fig. 6-26). Radiologically there is decreased height of vertebral bodies, frequently with aplasia of the 1st lumbar vertebra. The femoral heads are irregular and flattened and there is coxa valga with an oblique acetabular roof (Fig. 6-27). This disorder seems to have a slowly progressive course and is transmitted as an autosomal recessive lesion.

Other disorders such as Dyggve's syndrome, however, should not be confused with the mucopolysaccharidoses (see p. 231), and the one described by Winchester et al., (Hollister et al.). In the latter disorder of which we have observed a patient (patient of B. Le Marec), there is a serious involvement of the skeleton with changes at the wrist reminiscent of osteolysis, but there is no abnormal urinary excretion (Fig. 6-28).

A series of individual observations and a number of syndromes require considerable further study before they can be reliably classified. This is the case, for instance, in the geleophysic dwarfism of Spranger. There is a combination of an unusual facial appearance, hepatomegaly, the accumulation of dermatan-sulfate, and short bones of the hand, especially the 1st metacarpal.

THE MUCOLIPIDOSES

Besides the mucopolysaccharidoses it has been proposed to group together a number of other disorders, in which biochemical histochemical or ultramicroscopic studies have shown that there is a mixed storage disorder composed in part by lipids and mucopolysaccharides. The elimination in the urine of the latter substance is normal, with the exception of sulfatidosis with mucopolysacchariduria. The term mucolipidosis has been proposed to identify this group of disorders which are still poorly understood.

We shall limit the discussion to those types that have been adequately defined: mucolipidosis type I, mucolipidosis type II, mucolipidosis type III, sulfatidosis with mucopolysaccharidosis, fucosidosis and mannosidosis. To this group we shall add generalized gangliosidosis.

MUCOLIPIDOSIS TYPE I

This disorder has been defined by Spranger et al., 1968, under the term lipomucopolysaccharidosis.

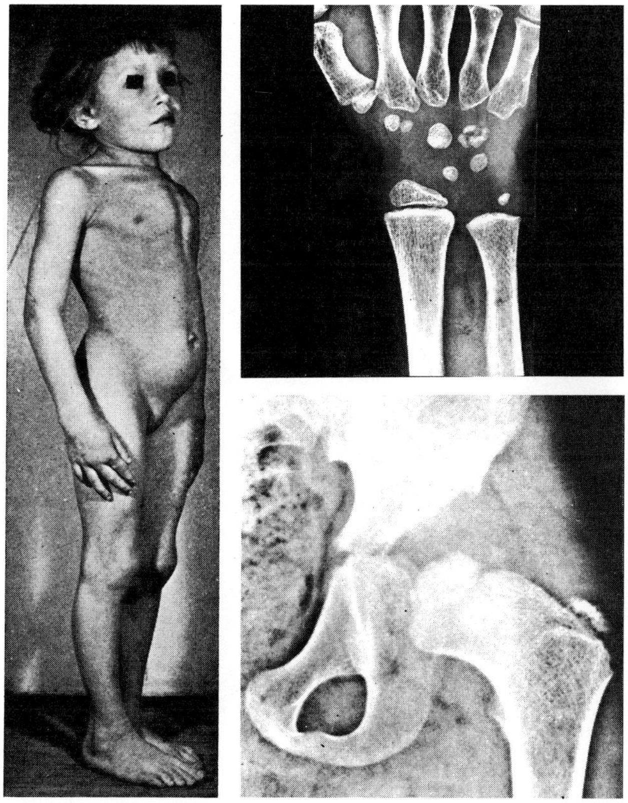

Fig. 6-25. Pseudo-Morquio disease in a 6-year-old girl. The deformity of the trunk, chest, and lower extremities is less severe than the classic appearance of a patient with Morquio's disease. The radiographic findings at wrist level, and at the hand and hip are also less severe.

Sometimes it is also referred to as mucopolysaccharidosis Gal+ because of an elevation of β-galactosidase present in the tissues, but this is not an entirely specific finding.

The disorder is discovered because of psychomotor retardation and deafness. Clinically there is a characteristic, heavy featured facial appearance. The liver and spleen are not always large. Examination of the eye ground will show the presence of a cherry red spot. In the circulating blood there are vacuolated lymphocytes, and in bone marrow large cells containing numerous vacuoles (Fig. 6-29). Cultured fibroblasts contain slightly metachromatic granulations. Radiographic study will show that the skeletal changes are quite similar to those seen in Hurler's disease (Fig. 6-30).

It is our feeling that the clinical and radiologic findings of this disorder, as well as its prognosis, are difficult to clearly define at this time, since there may be considerable confusion with mannosidosis. Neurologic difficulties with local motor ataxia may occur during later stages.

The transmission of this disease appears to be autosomal recessive, but there are still questions open as to the exact pathogenesis.

MUCOLIPIDOSIS TYPE II

Isolated by Leroy under the name of "I cell disease," this disorder can be recognized under different circumstances. At birth there may be a very narrow thorax with facial abnormalities, and articular limitations, sometimes secondary to dislocation. Respiratory tract infection may lead to the discovery of the underlying disease within the first few days. In other cases discovery may happen only later, towards 6 months of age or even later on, because of psychomo-

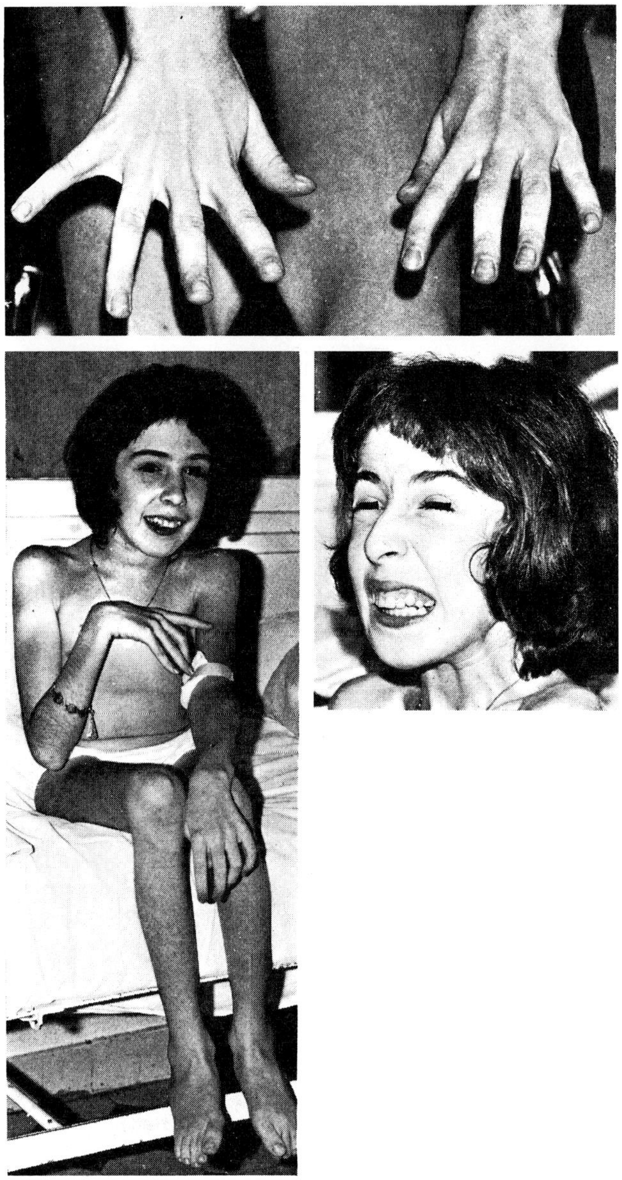

Fig. 6-26. Mucopolysaccharidosis with athetosis and the elimination of keratan-sulfate.

tor retardation. Clinical examination reveals a craniofacial appearance that may already be present at birth and will become more pronounced rapidly. Even though there is a close resemblance with gargoylism, there are some differences (Fig. 6-31). Most frequently there is brachycephaly. Besides a flattening of the bridge of the nose and the thick and anteverted nostrils, there is an excessive distance from the nose to the upper lip, a marked gingival hypertrophy, and sometimes a large tongue. The surface of the skin is thickened and infiltrated. Many joints show limitation of motion, which will become progressively more severe. The liver is often large. On the whole corneas are clear, but corneal opacities have been demonstrated by slit lamp examination.

Hematologic study shows that lymphocytes contain numerous empty vacuoles, some with a small dark area in their center. Urinary excretion of mucopoly-

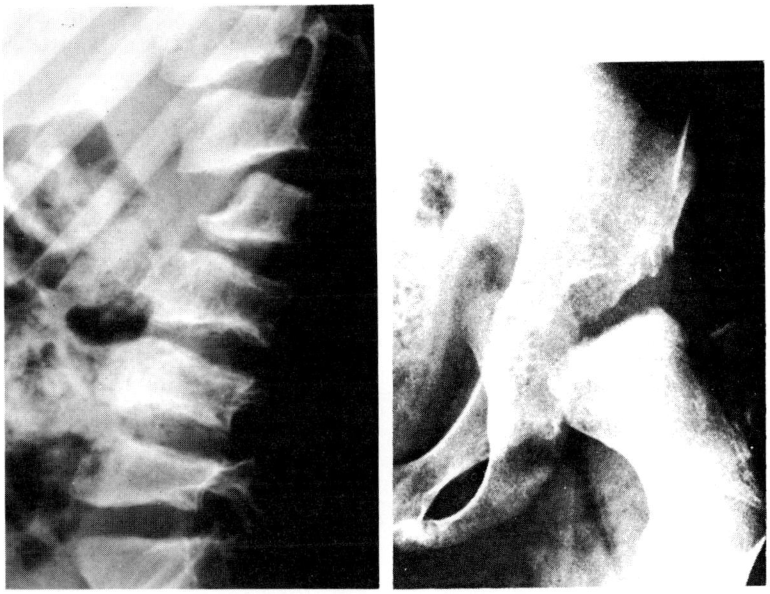

Fig. 6-27. Mucopolysaccharidosis with athetosis in a 12-year-old girl. (*Left*) Loss of vertebral height with hypoplasia of the 2nd lumbar vertebra. (*Right*) Coxa valga and marked hypoplasia of the femoral head.

saccharides is normal, and hydrolases in the serum show a considerable increase of their activity, whereas they are normal within cells (Thomas et al.).

The development of this disease is very serious, leading to death within the first years, usually before 3 years of age. There are patients with a form of this disease surviving somewhat longer.

Radiographic study shows a very peculiar development of the bony lesions. At birth and during the first few months the aspect is that of osteomalacia. The bones are excessively radiolucent, with a markedly irregular lacy trabeculation, and show widening of the metaphyses with a local uneven and irregularly dense border (Fig. 6-32). The immediately adjacent zones seem to be too transparent. A double contour of the cortex is frequently seen, sometimes there is a layered appearance, and occasionally the suggestion of a fracture. Dislocation of the hip or of the shoulder is not unusual. The metacarpal bones have a characteristic aspect in the form of an "olive." The ribs are also involved and the chest can be very narrow, so that there may be confusion with asphyxiating thoracic dysplasia. There is a progressive alteration of the bony changes. The abnormal radiolucency disappears and the bones then assume an aspect that is very close to that seen in Hurler's disease. The metacarpal bones are severely deformed like "sucked on sugar cones"

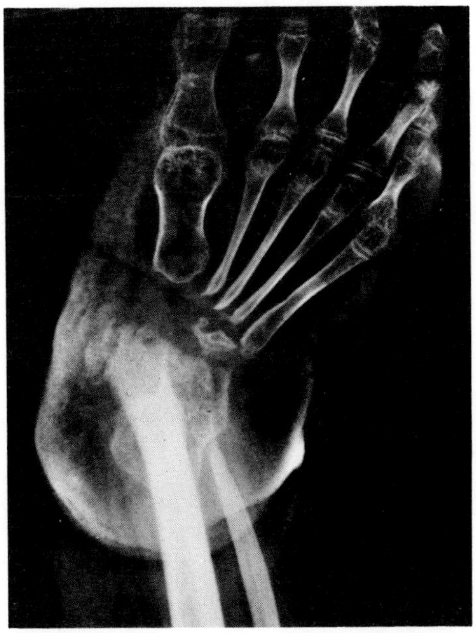

Fig. 6-28. Winchester's syndrome in a 12-year-old girl. The radiograph reveals multiple osteolytic lesions of the carpals and surrounding bones. (Courtesy of B. LeMarec)

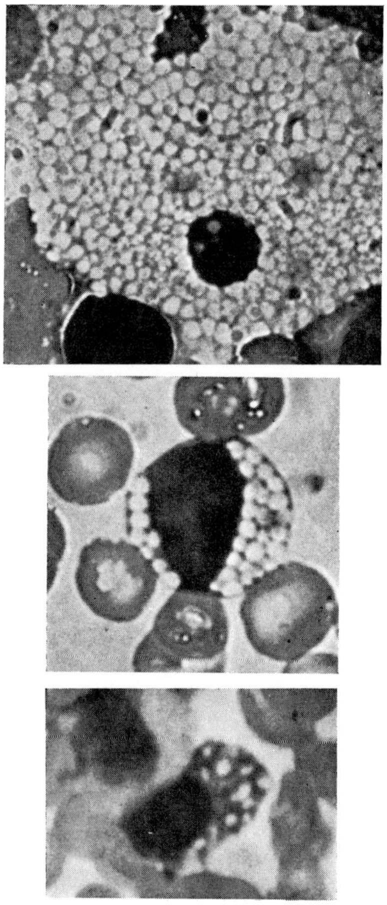

Fig. 6-29. Abnormal cells found in the blood and bone marrow of patients with mucolipidoses (*Top*) Mucolipidosis Type I with large foamy bone marrow cells. (*Center*) Mucolipidosis Type II with lymphocytes filled with many vacuoles. (*Bottom*) Mucolipidosis Type III, marrow cell with optically empty vacuoles.

(Fig. 6-33), and the vertebral bodies have a tendency to show anterior spur formation. Only the frequently brachycephalic skull differs from the findings in mucopolysaccharidosis type I.

The pathogenesis of this disorder is not yet fully understood, but it would appear that it is similar to an anomaly of hydrolase-synthesis in the otherwise normal cell. Might this be a defect of a transferase or of a sialidase? This disorder leads to numerous errors and confusions, especially during the early phases, because of similarities with hyperparathyroidism, rickets osteomalacic rickets and syphilis. Hematologic study will be very helpful in resolving doubts.

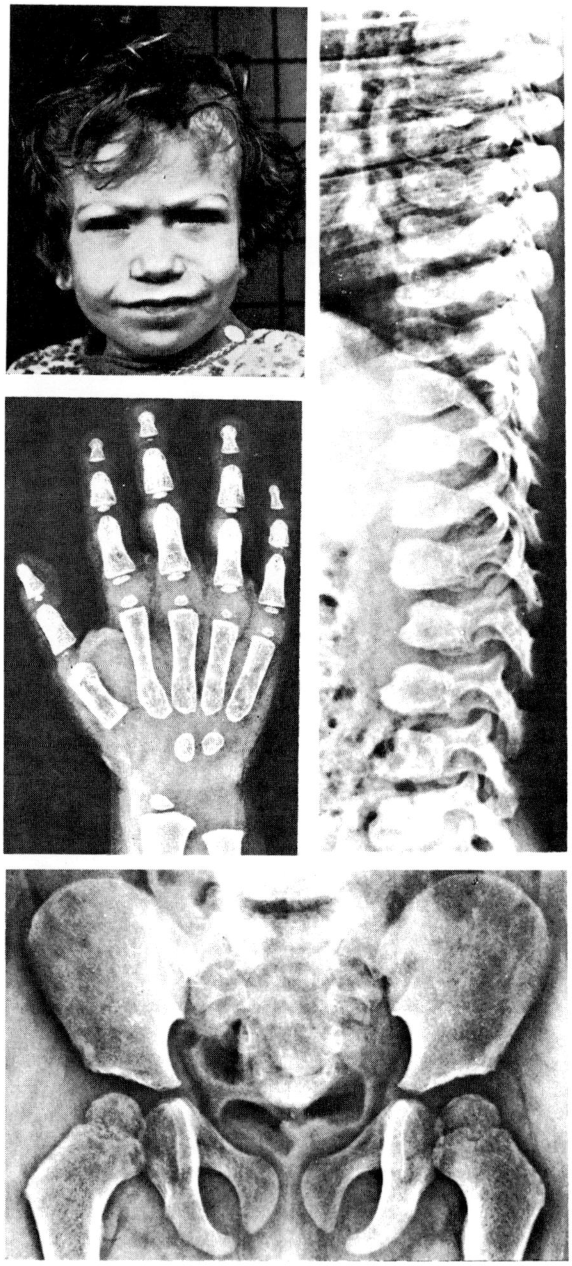

Fig. 6-30. Mucolipidosis Type I. The appearance of the vertebrae and the bones of the hand are similar to those seen in mucopolysaccharidosis Type I.

MUCOLIPIDOSIS TYPE III PSEUDO-POLYDYSTROPHY

This disorder is usually recognized around the second year of life because of a growth deficit, mild craniofacial disproportion, and limitation of movement

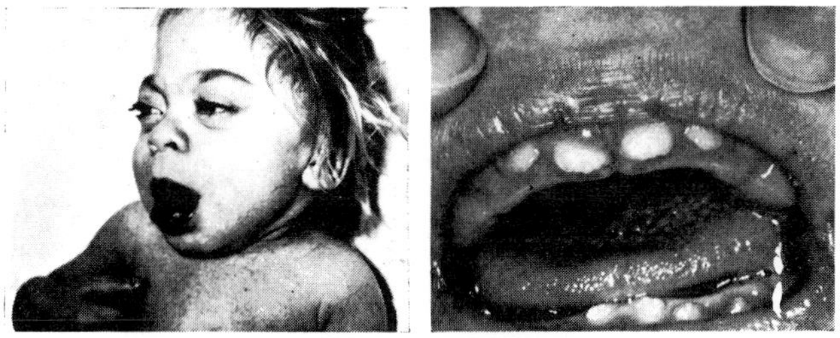

Fig. 6-31. Mucolipidosis Type II. Note the characteristic appearance of the face and gingival hypertrophy.

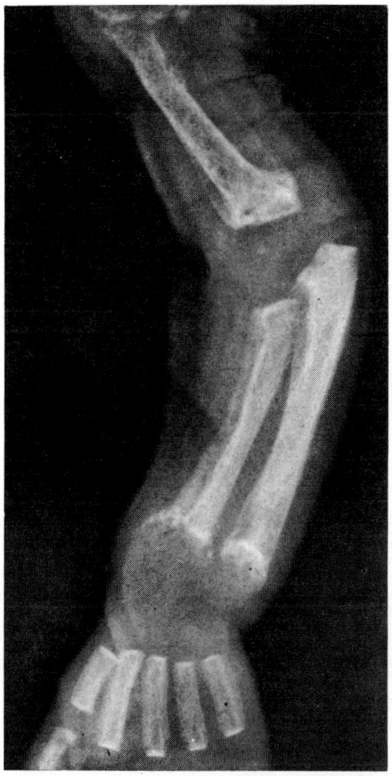

Fig. 6-32. Mucolipidosis Type II in a newborn baby. Notice the marked cupping and the irregularity in the metaphyseal outline and the cortical structures. (Courtesy of J. Pont)

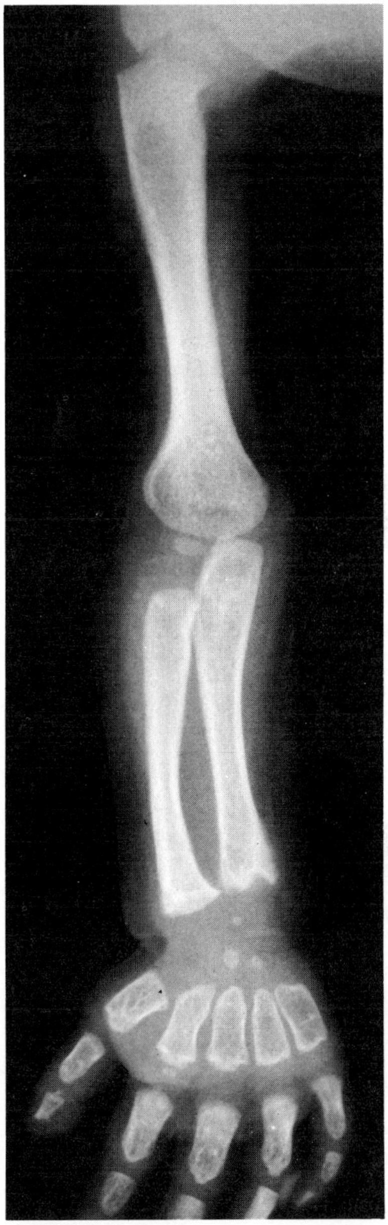

Fig. 6-33. Mucolipidosis Type II at 18 months. The radiographic changes are similar to those in mucopolysaccharidosis Type I. (Courtesy of A. Rossier)

in and clawing of the fingers (Fig. 6-34). Fine corneal opacities are always present. The development of the disease is slow, with late mental deterioration and relatively little progression. Growth disturbance may sometimes be severe.

Abnormal bone marrow cells, resembling those of Buhot, can be noted, but their vacuoles will appear optically empty. Urinary excretion of mucopolysaccharides is normal. Cultured fibroblasts will contain metachromatic granulations. There is an elevation of hydrolases in the serum (Humbel).

Radiologically, some findings are reminiscent of

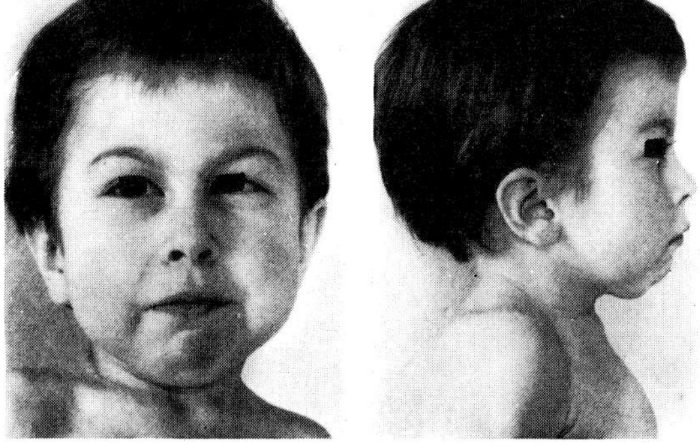

Fig. 6-34. Mucolipidosis Type III.

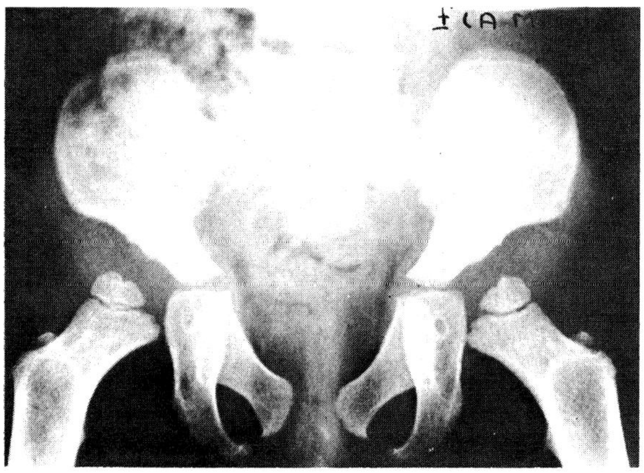

Fig. 6-35. Mucolipidosis Type III in a 5-year-old girl. The changes, particularly of the form of both iliac bones, are similar to those seen in Morquio's disease (see Fig. 6-23).

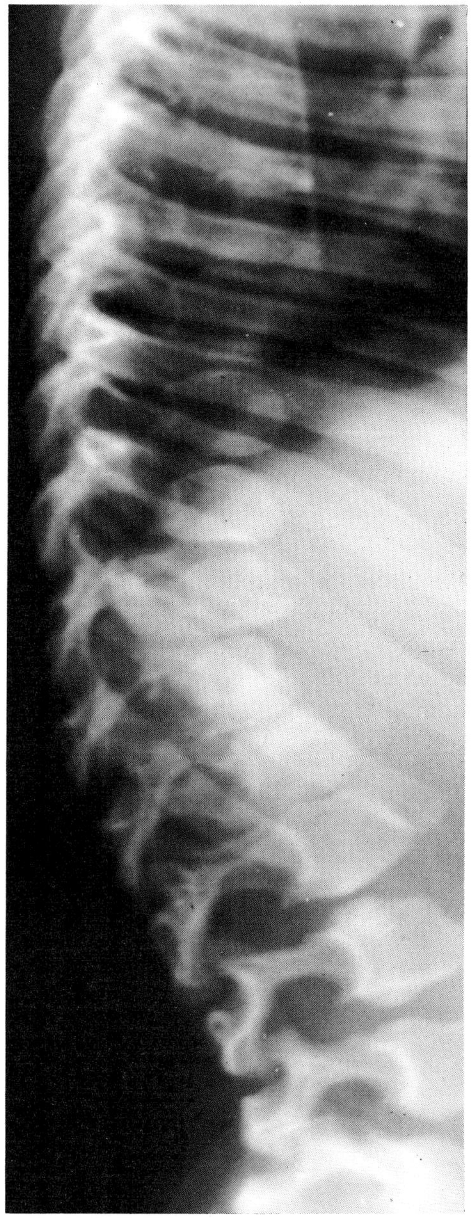

Fig. 6-36. Mucolipidosis Type III in a 5-year-old girl. The early changes of anterior tongue formation can be recognized in some vertebral bodies along with hypoplasia of Th12. The loss in height is less than in Morquio's disease.

Morquio's disease. These are obliquity of the acetabulum and coxa valga (Fig. 6-35), hypoplasia of the apophysis of the dens. There is only a mild reduction of vertebral height (Fig. 6-36). Irregularity of the plateau of vertebrae can appear during the course of a patient's disease, and in some, progressive scoliosis. The long bones are somewhat coarse, but they do not offer the massive aspect of Hurler's disease. The skull is only mildly affected.

The disorder is most likely inherited as an autosomal recessive trait, but its exact nature remains unknown.

Therapy should be directed against the progression of the scoliosis. Varisation osteotomy is sometimes indicated to prevent dislocation of the hip.

SULFATIDOSIS WITH MUCOPOLYSACCHARIDURIA

This is the only disorder of the group of mucolipidosis with an abnormal metabolite of mucopolysaccharides in the urine. Originally described by Austin,

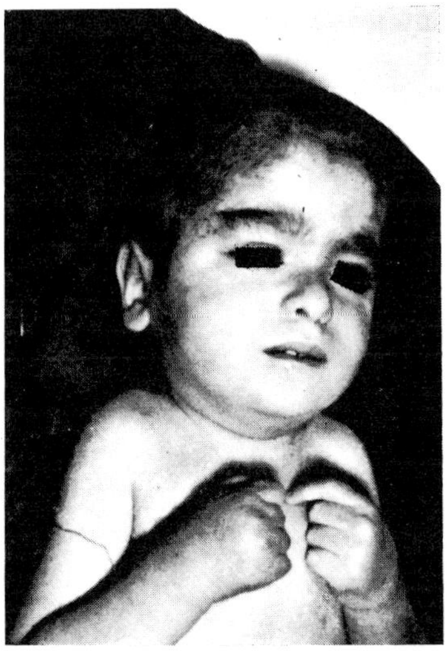

Fig. 6-37. Sulfatidosis with mucopolysacchariduria. (Courtesy of S. Thieffry)

this disorder has also been carefully studied by Thieffry et al.

Discovered during the first months of life, the clinical manifestations of this disorder are rapidly progressive mental deterioration accompanied by neurological difficulties. The latter are characterized by a total loss of all spontaneous motor activity and lively, hyperactive reflexes. The facial features are heavy (Fig. 6-37) but liver, spleen and cornea remain normal. The course is rapidly fatal.

Radiologically the vertebral bodies have an ovoid form. The metacarpals are widened and the sagittal suture seems to close early. The urinary excretion of mucopolysaccharides is identical to that of Hurler's disease, there may, however, be sulfatides found in the sediment after centrifugation. The blood and bone marrow contain Gasser and Buhot cells and Alder's granulations. A deficit in A, B and C aryl-sulfatases seems to be at the base of this disorder, which has, in all likelihood, an autosomal recessive transmission.

FUCOSIDOSIS

Since the skeletal changes are somewhat similar, we discuss this disorder isolated by Durand et al. here.

The clinical findings are variable. Mental deterioration is the most prominent finding, sometimes combined with neurologic problems. such as hypertonicity, spasticity or decerebrate rigidity. Skeletal involvement is always mild, with an ovoid aspect of vertebral bodies and widening of ribs or coxa valga. In some patients this disorder seems to be mainly an affliction of the skin (Epinette et al.). The cornea remains clear and lymphocytes contain optically empty vacuoles.

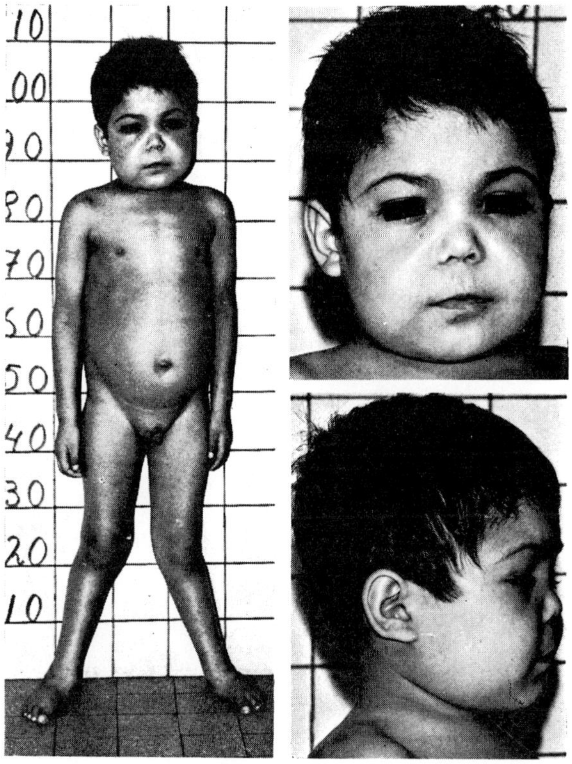

Fig. 6-38. Mannosidosis with a flat and round face.

The disorder is inherited as an autosomal recessive, and is the result of a deficit in α-fucosidase.

MANNOSIDOSIS

Defined by Ockerman et al., this disorder is recognized because of a sudden onset of psychomotor retardation, with only mild tendency to progression. The facial features are somewhat heavy, with a high forehead and a depressed root of the nose. The face is somewhat flat (Fig. 6-38). Hypotonicity and clumsy movements have been noted. The presence of an umbilical hernia, cataracts and deafness have been described.

Radiologically, the most striking finding is a somewhat coarse trabeculation with some irregularity at the metaphyseal ends, which are sometimes signs of rickets. The anterior border of the upper lumbar ver-

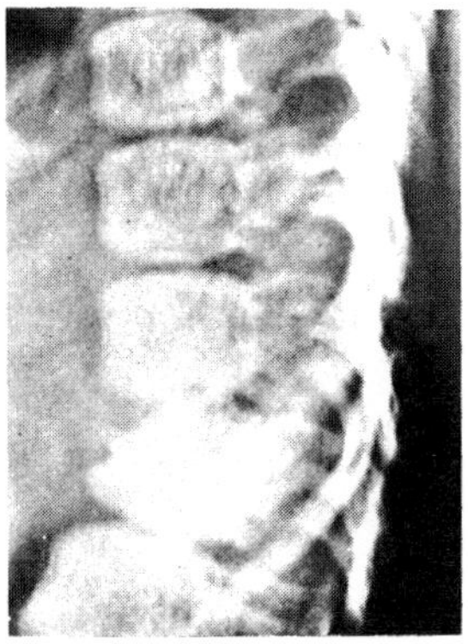

Fig. 6-39. Mannosidosis in a 9-year-old boy. There is spur formation of L1.

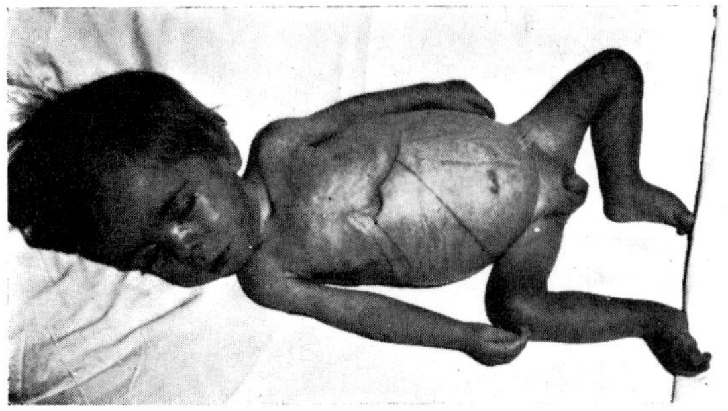

Fig. 6-40. Generalized gangliosidosis. (Courtesy of P. Royer)

tebrae is often oblique, so that its inferior portion has a tonguelike deformity (Fig. 6-39). The long bones are somewhat squat, slightly bent, and the cranial vault may be thickened. Lymphocytes are vacuolated and some polynuclear cells may contain granulations. The urine contains excessive amounts of oligosaccharides rich in mannose.

Transmission of this disorder is autosomal recessive and the disorder is due to a deficit in α-mannosidase. This finding can be substantiated by testing the liver or leukocytes.

The list of mucolipidoses is far from complete. One should consider the possibility of a disorder belonging to this group if an infant develops psycho-motor retardation or mental regression accompanied by facial dysmorphism, or simply a somewhat heavy facial appearance, combined with signs of visceral storage, especially hepatomegaly. Vacuolated lymphocytes may confirm this suspicion, whereas the bony involvement may be limited to a somewhat ovoid appearance of vertebral bodies, a coarse and squat aspect of long bones and sometimes mild changes of the forearm or thickening of the cranial vault.

GM_1 GANGLIOSIDOSIS

Sometimes referred to as Landing's disease, this disorder was first considered to be an atypical mucopolysaccharidosis.

The clinical findings are in evidence very early, sometimes in the first days or at least the first months. Neonatal edema may be noticed in half of the cases, involving the extremities and the face. Sometimes there is also ascites. In other patients there is a psychomotor retardation, or abnormal facial features are noticed by the family.

During clinical evaluation there is often noted a large head with coarse facial features, a flat bridge of the nose with hypertelorism and a big tongue (Fig. 6-34). Hypotonicity is usually present and may be responsible for kyphosis. This finding, however, may be replaced by hypertonicity towards the end of the course of the disease. There may be a large liver, and in half of the cases there has been a large spleen. Blindness and deafness are frequently seen. Slit lamp examination sometimes shows the presence of corneal opacities, and examination of the eyeground will occasionally reveal a cherry red spot. The circulating blood usually contains vacuolated lymphocytes.

This disorder has a particularly serious prognosis with frequent respiratory complications, and will lead to the patient's death within the first two or three years of life.

The most constant radiographic findings affect the spine, and they may be present very early. The finding of hypoplasia of the anterosuperior portion of one or two upper lumbar vertebrae with posterior displacement is typical. This aspect is quite similar to that seen in Hurler's disease (Fig. 6-40). Sometimes we only note an ovoid shape of the vertebrae. The long bones may be somewhat short and coarse as may be the metacarpals and the phalanges. Trabeculation may be prominent with a cortical double contour. These findings may lead to confusion with those seen in mucolipidosis type II. The ribs may also be somewhat wide. The skull frequently is large and dolichocephalic.

Gangliosidosis is transmitted as an autosomal recessive disorder. The storage essentially consists of normal GM_1 monosialoganglioside. Enzyme determination reveals a constant total lack of β-galactosidase, which, in all likelihood, is responsible for this disorder.

There is still another type of GM_1 gangliosidosis: GM_1 gangliosidosis type II. In this disorder we note rapid mental deterioration together with ataxia, spastic tetraplegia and signs of decerebration. Some skeletal findings may be reminiscent of the disorder just discussed. Within tissues there is a deficiency of isoenzymes B and C, and of β-galactosidase.

OTHER DISORDERS OF METABOLISM OF GLYCIDES AND LIPIDES

Some short comments should be added on the glycogenoses and two forms of lipidosis, with frequently noted skeletal involvement: Gaucher's and Niemann-Pick disease.

GLYCONGENOSES

No attempt is made to completely discuss the different types of glycogenosis. Their radiologic appearances are much milder than that of the disorders just presented.

The glycogenoses often lead to a global growth deficit, the mechanism of which is not well understood.

Radiographic findings are predominantly those of osteoporosis with a somewhat lacy aspect of the bony trabeculations and a reduction of the cortico-diaphyseal ratio of long bones or the bones of the hand. There is a high incidence of arrested growth lines. Bone maturation is frequently delayed. A defect of modeling of the distal end of the metacarpals has been noted in glycogenosis I (Preger et al.).

In some patients gouty changes have been noted. In spite of the fact that this has been seen at 6 years of age (Field), it is more often noted during adolescence. It is recognized by swelling of the soft tissues and only very mild bony involvement without destruction.

GAUCHER'S DISEASE

This disorder results from a defect of degradation of sphingolipides, because of a deficiency of β-glucosidase.

Most frequently this disorder is recognized because of the presence of marked splenomegaly. This condition leads to a bone marrow examination, which reveals the presence of characteristic storage cells. Radiologic study, if conducted systematically, will show typical skeletal findings in three out of four patients. The patients may complain about pain within bones or joints and marked functional disturbance. Functional disturbances may lead to the recognition of the disease in young infants. There may be inflammatory and febrile episodes. This may be seen in about one third of all patients.

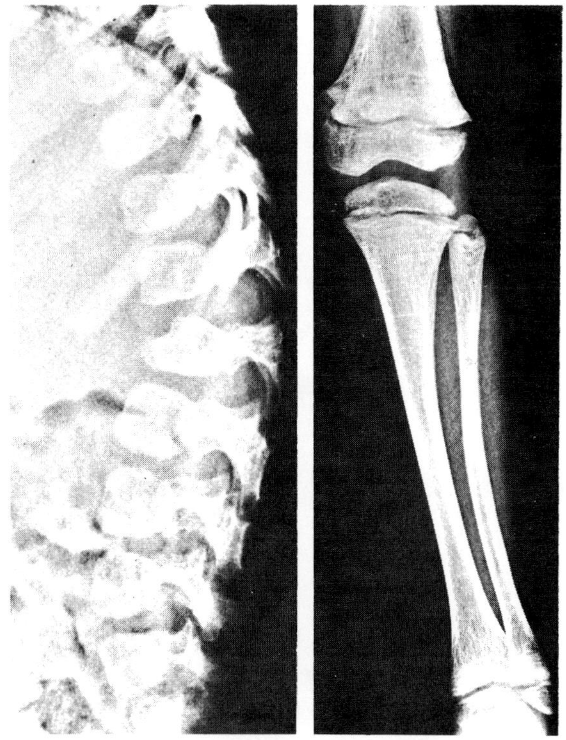

Fig. 6-41. Generalized gangliosidosis in an 8-month-old baby. The spinal appearance is similar to that of Hurler's disease. The findings, however, are present at a much earlier time. (Courtesy of P. Royer)

Radiologic investigation will show a normal skull, but marked involvement of the long bones, especially the femur (Fig. 6-41). The long bones lose their modeling and the most actively growing metaphyseal ends will have an Erlenmeyer-flask appearance. The cortex is thin and the spongiosa may not be visible because it is replaced by stored material. The density of the bone may be diminished, irregular, even micropolycystic. There may be areas of unusual density and a somewhat sclerotic region may be located around osteoporotic zones, especially close to the inner cortex. This may lead to a reduction of the medullary cavity. In spite of the fact that a periosteal reaction is unusual, the presence of severe pain may give the erroneous impression that the disease in question is osteomyelitis.

Quite often there is aseptic necrosis of the head of the humerus or of the femur. Its evolution is the same as in osteochondritis, and the necrotic phase is followed by local repair. A generalized reticular osteoporosis can be present with an uneven collapse of vertebrae, which retain normal intervertebral distances. Kyphosis may appear. Pathological fractures of long

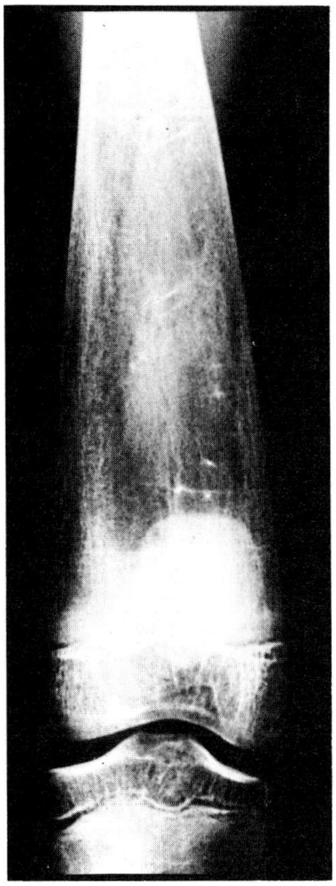

Fig. 6-42. Fourteen-year-old girl with Gaucher's disease resulting in the Erlenmeyer flask appearance of the distal femora due to lack of tubulation. (Courtesy of H. J. Kaufmann)

bones are not unusual. It is somewhat surprising that these bony lesions are seen with a high incidence in patients after splenectomy. This has led some authors to limit the indication for this procedure to the most severe hemorrhagic form of this disease.

NIEMANN-PICK DISEASE

This disorder is characterized by the accumulation of sphingomyelin and cholesterol, secondary to a metabolic disorder of phospholipides—a lack of sphingomyelinase.

In its most frequent form this disorder is recognized because of central nervous system involvement, by spleno- and hepatomegaly. Death occurs usually within the first two years.

It has been shown that besides this form there is another type of involvement of the central nervous system, but with a slower course. This form, called Nova Scotia type, is compatible with survival into adolescence and should not be referred to here, since it spares the skeleton.

Frequent involvement of the skeleton in Niemann-Pick disease can be expected, but this may be latent. There is widening of the medullary cavity and narrowing of the cortex. A modeling defect at the metaphyses can be recognized after a lengthy time of observation, especially in those patients where the central nervous system is not seriously involved. The local findings may then be reminiscent of those of Gaucher's disease. This is true of findings within the medullary cavity at the proximal end of the femur. Coxa valga is often present, and is present in all children who cannot walk. Widening of the metacarpals may be found in the type with slow development and may be accompanied by thinning of the cortex and a coarse lacy appearance of the bone. The aspect may even be similar to that of mucopolysaccharidoses (Lachman et al.). Wedging of vertebrae in the lumbar region has been noted (Swischuk).

Histologic study documents the presence of Niemann-Pick cells within the periosteum and helps to confirm the storage within and widening of the medullary cavity.

REFERENCES

Mucopolysaccharidoses

ALDER (A.). Ueber konstitutionell bedingte Granulationsveränderungen der Leukocyten. *Deut. Arch. Klin. Med., 1938,* **183**, *372-378.*

ALEU (F. P.), TERRY (R. D.) et ZELLWEGER (H.). Electron microscopy of two cerebral biopsies in gargoylism. *J. Neuropathol. exp. Neurol., 1965,* **24**, *304-317.*

AUTIO (S.), VISAKORPI (J. K.) et JARVINEN (H.). Aspartyglycosaminuria (AGU). Further aspects on its clinical picture, mode of inheritance and epidemiology based on a series of 57 patients. *Ann. clin. Res., 1973,* **5**, *149-155.*

BACH (G.), FRIEDMAN (R.), WEISSMAN (B.) et NEUFELD (E. F.). The defect in the Hurler and Scheie syndromes : deficiency of α-L-iduronidase. *Proc. nat. Acad. Sci. (Wash.), 1972,* **69**, *2048-2051.*

BACH (G.), EISENBERG (F., Jr.), CANTZ (M.) et NEUFELD (E. F.). The defect in the Hunter syndrome. Deficiency of sulfoiduronate sulfatase. *Proc. nat. Acad. Sci. (Wash.), 1973,* **70**, *2134-2138.*

BAILEY II (J. A.). Disproportionate short stature, diagnosis and management. *Philadelphia, 1973, Saunders, éd., p. 357-371.*

BARTON (R. W.) et NEUFELD (E. F.). The Hurler corrective factor, purification and some properties. *J. biol. Chem., 1971,* **246**, *7773-7779.*

BARTON (R. W.) et NEUFELD (E. F.). A distinct biochemical deficit in the Maroteaux-Lamy syndrome (mucopolysaccharidosis VI). *J. Pediat., 1972,* **80**, *114-116.*

BEAUDET (A. L.), DI-FERRANTE (N.), NICHOLS (D.) et FERRY (G. D.). β-glucuronidase deficiency : altered enzyme substrate recognition. *Amer. J. hum. Genet. (abstr.), 1972,* **24**, *259.*

BLAW (M. E.) et LANGER (L. O.). Spinal cord compression in Morquio Brailsford's disease. *J. Pediat., 1969,* **74**, *593-600.*

BOOTH (C. W.) et NADLER (H. L.). Plasma infusions in an infant with Hurler's syndrome. *J. Pediat., 1973,* **82**, *273-278.*

BOOTH (C. W.) et NADLER (H. L.). Demonstration of the heterozygous state in Hunter's syndrome. *J. Pediat., 1974,* **53**, *396-399.*

BRAILSFORD (J. F.). Chondro-osteodystrophy. *Amer. J. Surg., 1929,* **7**, *404-410.*

BROVELLI (A.), LATERZA (L.), LENZI (L.) et CASTELLANI (A. A.). Characterization of urinary peptoglycans in Morquio's disease. *Calcif. Tiss. Res., 1968,* **1**, *324-329.*

CAMPAILLA (E.) et MARTINELLI (B.). Morquio's disease : modification of mucopolysacchariduria with advancinq age : report of three cases. *Birth Defects Original Article Series, 1969,* V *n° 4, 172-173.*

CANTZ (M.), CHRAMBACH (A.), BACH (G.) et NEUFELD (E. F.). The Hunter corrective factor. Purification and preliminary characterization. *J. biol. Chem., 1972,* **247**, *5456-5462.*

COPPA (G. V.), SINGH (J.), NICHOLS (B. L.) et DI FERRANTE (N.). Urinary excretion of disulfated disaccharides in Hunter syndrome : correction by infusion of a serum fraction. *Analyt. Let., 1973,* **6**, *225-233.*

DANES (B. S.) et BEARN (A. G.). Hurler's syndrome : demonstration of an inherited disorder of connective tissue in cell culture. *Sciences, 1965,* **149**, *987-989.*

DANES (B. S.) et BEARN (A. G.). Cellular metachromasia, a genetic marker for studying the mucopolysaccharidoses. *Lancet, 1967,* **i**, *241-243.*

DEAN (M. F.), MUIR (H.) et EWINS (R. J. F.). Hurler's, Hunter's, and Morquio's syndromes. A biochemical study in the light of current views of the underlying defects. *Biochem. J., 1971,* **123**, *883-894.*

DEAN (M. F.), MUIR (H.) et BENSON (P. F.). Mobilization of glycosaminoglycans by plasma infusion in mucopolysaccharidosis type III. Two types of response. *Nature, 1973,* **243**, *143-146.*

DEKABAN (A. S.) et CONSTANTOPOULOS (G.). Mucopolysaccharidoses. Relation of elevated cerebral spinal fluid to mental retardation. *Arch. Neurol., 1973,* **28**, *385-388.*

DI FERRANTE (N.), NICHOLS (B. L.), DONNELLY (P. V.), NERI (G.), HERGOVCIC (R.) et BERGLUND (R. K.). Induced degradation of glycosaminoglycans in Hurler's and Hunter's syndromes by plasma infusion. *Proc. nat. Acad. Sci. (Wash.), 1971,* **68**, *303-307.*

DORFMAN (A.) et LORINCZ (A. E.). Occurrence of urinary acid mucopolysaccharides in the Hurler syndrome. *Proc. nat. Acad. Sci. (Wash.), 1957,* **43**, *443-446.*

EINHORN (N. H.), MOORE (J. R.) et ROWNTREE (L. G.). Osteochondrodystrophia deformans (Morquio's disease). Observation and autopsy in one case. *Amer. J. Dis. Child., 1946,* **72**, *536-544.*

ELLIS (R. W. B.), SHELDON (W.) et CAPON (N. B.). Gargoylism (chondro-osteo-dystrophy, corneal opacities, hepato-splenomegaly and mental deficiency). *Quart. J. Med., 1936,* **5**, *119-139.*

ESCOUROLLE (R.), BERGER (B.) et POIRIER (J.). Biopsie cérébrale d'un cas de mucopolysaccharidose H. S. (oligophrénie polydystrophique ou maladie de Sanfilippo). Etude histochimique et ultrastructurale. *Presse méd., 1966,* **74**, *2869-2874.*

FIGURA (K. von) et KRESSE (H.). The Sanfilippo B corrective factor : a N-acetyl-α-D-glucosaminidase. *Biochem. Biophys. Res. Commun., 1972,* **48**, *262-269.*

FRATANTONI (J. C.), HALL (C. W.) et NEUFELD (E. F.). The defect in Hurler's and Hunter's syndromes : faulty degradation of mucopolysaccharide. *Proc. nat. Acad. Sci. (Wash.), 1968,* **60**, *699-706.*

FRATANTONI (J. C.), HALL (C. W.) et NEUFELD (E. F.). Hurler and Hunter syndromes : mutual correction of the defect in cultured fibroblasts. *Science, 1968,* **162**, *570-572.*

FRATANTONI (J. C.), HALL (C. W.) et NEUFELD (E. F.). The defect in Hurler and Hunter syndromes. II. Deficiency of specific factors involved in mucopolysaccharide degradation. *Proc. nat. Acad. Sci. (Wash.), 1969,* **64**, *360-366.*

GASSER (C.). Diskussion zu Alder. *Schweiz. med. Wschr., 1950,* **80**, *1097-1098.*

GEHLER (J.), CANTZ (M.), TOLKSDORF (M.), SPRANGER (J.), GILBERT (E.) et DRUBE (H.). Mucopolysaccharidosis VII : β-Glucuronidase deficiency. *Hum. Genet., 1974,* **23**, *149-158.*

GOIDANICH (I. F.) et LENZI (L.). Morquio - Ullrich disease, a new mucopolysaccharidosis. *J. Bone Jt Surg., 1964,* **46-A**, *743-746.*

GRENET (P.), LESTRADET (H.), DUGAS (M.), SARRUT (S.), BADOUAL (J.) et ALIBERT (L.). Mucopolysaccharidose avec élimination d'héparitine-sulfate (oligophrénie polydystrophique). *Presse méd., 1966,* **74**, *2863-2868.*

HALL (C. W.), CANTZ (M.) et NEUFELD (E. F.). A β-glucuronidase deficiency mucopolysaccharidosis : studies in cultured fibroblasts. *Arch. Biochem. Biophys., 1973,* **155**, *32-38.*

HAUST (M. D.), GORDON (B. A.), BRYANS (A. M.), WOLLIN (D. G.) et BINNINGTON (V.). Heparitin sulfate mucopolysaccharidosis (Sanfilippo disease) : a case study with ultrastructural, biochemical and radiological findings. *Pediat. Res., 1971,* **5**, *137-150.*

HERS (H. G.) et VAN HOOF (F.). Lysosomes and mucopolysaccharidoses. *Biochem. J., 1969 c,* **115**, *34-36.*

HOLLISTER (D. W.), RIMOIN (D. L.), LACHMAN (R. S.), COHEN (A. H.), REED (W. B.) et WESTIN (G. W.). The Winchester syndrome : a non lysosomal connective tissue disease. *J. Pediat., 1974,* **84**, *701-709.*

HORS-CAYLA (M. C.), MAROTEAUX (P.) et GROUCHY (J. de). Fibroblastes en culture au cours des mucopolysaccharidoses : influence du sérum sur la métachromasie. *Ann. Génét., 1968,* **11**, *265-266.*

HUMBEL (R.), MARCHAL (C.) et FALL (M.). Diagnosis of Morquio's disease : a simple chromatographic method for the identification of keratosulfate in urine. *J. Pediat., 1972,* **81**, *107-108.*

HUNTER (C.). A rare disease in two brothers. *Proc. roy. Soc. Med., 1917,* **10**, *104-116.*

HURLER (G.). Ueber einen Typ multipler Abartungen, vorwiegend am Skelettsystem. *Z. Kinderheilk., 1919,* **24**, *220-234.*

JENKINS (P.), DAVIES (G. R.) et HARPER (P. S.). Morquio-Brailsford disease. A report of four affected sisters with absence of excessive keratan sulphate in the urine. *Brit. J. Radiol., 1973,* **46**, *668-675.*

Kint (J. A.), Dacremont (G.), Carton (D.), Urye (E.) et Hooft (C.). Mucopolysaccharidosis, secondarily induced abnormal distribution of lysosomal isoenzymes. *Sciences, 1973,* **181**, *352-354.*

Knudson (A. G.), Di Ferrante (N.) et Curtis (J. E.). Effect of leukocyte transfusion in a child with type II mucopolysaccharidosis. *Proc. nat. Acad. Sci. (Wash.), 1971,* **68**, *1738-1741.*

Konyar (E.), Tondeur (M.) et Resibois (A.). Histochemical demonstration of acid mucopolysaccharides in Sanfilippo's disease : an ultrastructural study of the liver. *Virchows Arch. Abt. B., 1972,* **11**, *224-233.*

Kresse (H.). Mucopolysaccharidosis III A (Sanfilippo A disease). Deficiency of a heparin sulfamidase in skin fibroblasts and leucocyte. *Biochem. Biophys. Res. Commun., 1973,* **54**, *1111-1118.*

Kresse (H.) et Neufeld (E. F.). The Sanfilippo A corrective factor. *J. Biol. Chem., 1972,* **247**, *2164-2170.*

Kresse (H.), Wiesman (U.), Cantz (M.), Hall (C. W.) et Neufeld (E. F.). Biochemical heterogeneity of the Sanfilippo syndrome : preliminary characterization of two deficient factors. *Biochem. Biophys. Res. Commun., 1971,* **42**, *892-898.*

Lafon (J.), Bérard-Badier (M.), Chamlian (A.), Mariani (R.), Casanova (P.) et Adéchy-Benkoel (L.). Etude ultrastructurale des cellules périsinusoïdales du foie dans trois cas de mucopolysaccharidoses. *Pathol. et Biol., 1972,* **15**, *15-21.*

Lambotte (C.), Winand (R.), Chantraine (J. M.), Biertho (G.) et Leruth-Fafchamps (Y.). Le traitement des mucopolysaccharidoses par des perfusions de plasma humain. Modification des mucopolysaccharides de haut et de faible poids moléculaire. *Acta paediat. belg., 1971,* **25**, *297-309.*

Lamy (M.), Maroteaux (P.) et Bader (J. P.). Etude génétique du gargoylisme. *J. Génét. hum., 1957,* **6**, *156-178.*

Langer (L. O., Jr.) et Carey (L. S.). The roentgenographic features of the KS mucopolysaccharidosis of Morquio (Morquio-Brailsford's disease). *Amer. J. Roentgenol., 1966,* **97**, *1-20.*

Lichtenstein (J. R.), Bilbrey (G. L.) et McKusick (V. A.). Clinical and probable genetic heterogeneity within mucopolysaccharidosis II, report of a family with a mild form. *Johns-Hopkins med. J., 1972,* **131**, *425-435.*

Linker (A.), Evans (L. R.) et Langer (L. O.). Morquio's disease and mucopolysaccharide excretion. *J. Pediat., 1970,* **70**, *1039-1047.*

Loeb (H.), Jonniaux (G.), Resibois (A.), Cremer (N.), Dodion (J.), Tondeur (M.), Grégoire (P. E.), Richard (J.) et Cieters (P.). Biochemical and ultrastructural studies in Hurler's syndrome. *J. Pediat., 1968,* **73**, *860-874.*

Lyon (G.), Rosemberg (S.) et Thieffry (St.). Une forme rare de mucopolysaccharidose chez l'enfant, à rapprocher du « Hurler tardif » et du « syndrome de Scheie ». *Arch. franç. Pédiat., 1971,* **28**, *83-94.*

Maroteaux (P.), Levêque (B.), Marie (J.), Lamy (M.) et Foucher (M.). Une nouvelle dysostose avec élimination urinaire de chondroïtine-sulfate B. *Presse méd., 1963,* **71**, *1849-1852.*

Maroteaux (P.), Lamy (M.) et Foucher (M.). La maladie de Morquio. Etude clinique, radiologique et biologique. *Presse méd., 1963,* **71**, *2091-2094.*

Maroteaux (P.) et Lamy (M.). Hurler's disease, Morquio's disease, and related mucopolysaccharidoses. *J. Pediat., 1965,* **67**, *312-323.*

Maroteaux (P.). Différenciation biochimique des maladies de Hurler et de Hunter par fractionnement de l'héparitine sulfate. *Rev. europ. Et clin. biol., 1970,* **15**, *203-205.*

Maroteaux (P.) et Hors-Cayla (M. C.). Le problème biologique des mucopolysaccharidoses. *Ann. Biol. clin., 1970,* **28**, *111-114.*

Maroteaux (P.) Un nouveau type de mucopolysaccharidose avec athétose et élimination urinaire de kératan-sulfate. *Nouv. Presse méd., 1973,* **2**, *975-979.*

Matalon (R.) et Dorfman (A.). The structure of acid mucopolysaccharides produced by Hurler fibroblasts in tissue culture. *Proc. nat. Acad. Sci. (Wash.), 1968,* **60**, *179-185.*

Matalon (R.) et Dorfman (A.). Hurler's syndrome, an α-L-iduronidase deficiency. *Biochem. Biophys. Res., Commun., 1972,* **47**, *959-964.*

McKusick (V. A.). Heritable disorders of connective tissue. *4e édit., St. Louis, 1972, Mosby, éd., p. 521-686.*

McKusick (V. A.). The nosology of the mucopolysaccharidoses. *Amer. J. Med., 1969,* **47**, *730-747.*

McKusick (V. A.), Howell (R. R.), Hussels (I. E.), Neufeld (E. F.) et Stevenson (R. E.). Allelism, non-allelism and genetic compounds among the mucopolysaccharidoses. *Lancet, 1972,* **i**, *993-996.*

Maynard (J. A.), Cooper (R. R.) et Ponseti (I. V.). Morquio's disease (mucopolysaccharidosis type IV). Ultrastructure of epiphyseal plates. *Lab. Invest., 1973,* **28**, *194-205.*

Mittwoch (U.). Abnormal lymphocytes in gargoylism. *Brit. J. Haemat., 1959,* **5**, *365-368.*

Morquio (L.). Sur une forme de dystrophie osseuse familiale. *Bull. Soc. pédiat., 1929,* **27**, *145-152.*

Morquio (L.). Sur une forme de dystrophie osseuse familiale. *Arch. Méd. Enf., 1935,* **38**, *5-24.*

Muir (H.). The structure and metabolism of mucopolysaccharides (glycosaminoglycans) and the problem of the mucopolysaccharidoses. *Amer. J. Med., 1969,* **47**, *673-690.*

Neufeld (E. F.) et Fratantoni (J. C.). Inborn errors of mucopolysaccharide metabolism. *Science, 1970,* **169**, *141-146.*

Nja (A.). A sex-linked type of gargoylism. *Acta paediat., 1946,* **33**, *267-286.*

O'Brien (J. S.). Sanfilippo's syndrome : profound deficiency of α-acetyl-glucosaminidase activity in organs and skin fibroblasts from type B patients. *Proc. nat. Acad. Sci. (Wash.), 1972,* **69**, *1720-1722.*

O'Brien (J. S.), Miller (A. L.), Loverde (A. W.) et Veath (M. L.). Sanfilippo's disease type B : enzyme replacement and metabolic correction in cultured fibroblasts. *Science, 1973,* **181**, *753-755.*

Philippart (M.) et Sugarman (G. I.). Chondroitin-4-sulphate mucopolysaccharidosis. A new variant of Hurler's syndrome. *Lancet, 1969,* **ii**, *854.*

Rampini (S.) et Maroteaux (P.). Ein ungewöhnlicher Phänotyp des Hurler-Syndroms. *Helv. paediat. Acta, 1966,* **21**, *376-386.*

Rampini (S.). Der Spät-Hurler. Ullrich-Scheie-Syndrom, Mukopolysaccharidose V. *Schweiz. med. Wschr., 1969,* **99**, *1769-1778.*

Sanfilippo (S. J.), Podosin (R.), Langer (L.) et Good

(R. A.). Mental retardation associated with acid mucopolysacchariduria (heparitin sulfate type). *J. Pediat., 1963,* **63**, *837-838.*

SCHEIE (H. G.), HAMBRICK (G. W., Jr.) et BARNESS (L. A.). A newly recognized forme fruste of Hurler's disease (gargoylism). *Amer. J. Ophthal., 1962,* **53**, *753-769.*

SCHENK (E. A.) et HAGGERTY (J.). Morquio's disease. A radiologic and morphologic study. *Pediatrics, 1964,* **34**, *839-850.*

SENGEL (A.), STOEBNER (P.) et JUIF (J.). Les chondrocytes de la maladie de Morquio. Vacuoles ergastoplasmiques à inclusions spécifiques. *Microscopie, 1971,* **10**, *33-40.*

SILBERBERG (R.), RIMOIN (D. L.), ROSENTHAL (R. E.) et HASLER (M. B.). Ultrastructure of cartilage in the Hurler and Sanfilippo syndromes. *Arch. Path., 1972,* **94**, *500-510.*

SLY (W. S.), QUINTON (B. A.), MCALISTER (W. H.) et RIMOIN (D. L.). Beta glucuronidase deficiency : report of clinical radiologic and biochemical features of a new mucopolysaccharidosis. *J. Pediat., 1973,* **82**, *249-257.*

SOTO (O.). Communication personnelle.

SPRANGER (J. W.), KOCH (F.), MCKUSICK (V. A.), NATZSCHKA (J.), WIEDEMANN (H. R.) et ZELLWEGER (H.). Mucopolysaccharidosis VI. *Helv. paediat. Acta, 1970,* **25**, *337-362.*

SPRANGER (J. W.), SCHUSTER (W.) et FREITAG (F.). Chondroitin-4-sulfate mucopolysaccharidosis. *Helv. paediat. Acta, 1971,* **26**, *387-396.*

SPRANGER (J. W.), GILBERT (E. F.), TUFFLI (G. A.), ROSSITER (F. P.) et OPITZ (J. M.). Geleophysic dwarfism : a « focal mucopolysaccharidosis ? ». *Lancet, 1971,* ii, *97-98.*

SPRANGER (J.). The systemic mucopolysaccharidoses. *Ergeb. inn. Med. Kinderheilk., 1972,* **32**, *166-246.*

STANESCU (V.), BONA (C.) et IONESCU (V.). The tibial growing cartilage biopsy in the study of growth disturbances. *Acta endocrin., 1970,* **64**, *577-601.*

STRUMPF (D. A.), AUSTIN (J. H.), CROCKER (A. C.) et LAFRANCE (M.). Mucopolysaccharidosis type VI (Maroteaux-Lamy syndrome). *Amer. J. Dis. Child., 1973,* **126**, *747-756.*

THOMPSON (G. R.), NELSON (N. A.), CASTOR (C. W.) et GROBELNY (S. L.). A mucopolysaccharidosis with increased urinary excretion of chondroitin-4-sulfate. *Ann. intern. Med., 1971,* **75**, *421-426.*

TONDEUR (M.) et LOEB (H.). Etude ultrastructurale du foie dans la maladie de Morquio. *Pediat. Res., 1969,* **3**, *19-26.*

TONDEUR (M.). Etude ultrastructurale des mucopolysaccharidoses et d'affections apparentées. *Thèse, Méd., Bruxelles, 1973.*

ULLRICH (O.). Die Pfaundler-Hurlersche Krankheit. Ein Beitrag zum Problem pleiotroper Genwirkung in der Erbpathologie des Menschen. *Ergebn. inn. Med. Kinderheilk., 1943,* **63**, *929-1000.*

VAN HOOF (F.) et HERS (H. G.). The abnormalities of lysosomal enzymes in mucopolysaccharidoses. *Europ. J. Biochem, 1968 a,* **7**, *34-44.*

VAN HOOF (F.). Les mucopolysaccharidoses en tant que thésaurismoses lysosomiales. *Thèse Méd., Louvain, 1972.*

WINCHESTER (P.), GROSSMAN (H.), WAN NGO LIM et DANES (B. S.). A new acid mucopolysaccharidosis with skeletal deformities simulating rheumatoid arthritis. *Amer. J. Roentgenol., 1969,* **106**, *121-128.*

ZELLWEGER (H.), PONSETI (I. V.), PEDRINI (V.), STAMLER (F. S.) et VON NOORDER (G. K.). Morquio-Ullrich's disease : report of two cases. *J. Pediat., 1961,* **59**, *549-561.*

Mucolipidoses

AUSTIN (J. H.). Mental retardation. Metachromatic leucodystrophy. *In* C. H. Carter, Medical aspects of mental retardation. *Springfield, Ill., 1965, Thomas, éd., p. 768-813.*

AUTIO (S.), NORDEN (N. E.), OCKERMAN (P. A.), RIEKKINEN (P.), RAPOLA (J.) et LOUHIMO (T.). Mannosidosis : clinical, fine-structural and biochemical findings in three cases. *Acta paediat. scand., 1973,* **62**, *555-565.*

DELIGNE (J.). La mucolipidose de type II ou I-cell disease. A propos de trois observations. *Thèse Méd., Lille, 1973.*

DURAND (P.), PHILLIPART (M.), BORRONE (C.), DELLA CELLA (G.) et BUGIANI (O.). Una nuova malattia da acumulo di glicolipidi. *Minerva pediat., 1967,* **19**, *2187-2196.*

DURAND (P.), BORRONE (C.) et DELLA CELLA (G.). Fucosidosis. *J. Pediat., 1969,* **75**, *665-674.*

EPINETTE (W. W.), NORINS (A. L.), DREW (A. L.), ZEMAN (W.) et PATEL (V.). Angiokeratoma corporis diffusum with L-fucosidase deficiency. *Arch Derm., 1973,* **107**, *754-757.*

GILBERT (E. F.), DAWSON (G.), ZU RHEIN (G. M.), OPITZ (J. M.) et SPRANGER (J. W.). I-cell disease, mucolipidosis II. Pathological, histochemical, ultrastructural and biochemical observations in four cases. *Z. Kinderheilk., 1973,* **114**, *259-292.*

GUIBAUD (P.), LEUNG-TACK-KI (A.), COTTOW (J. B.), MATHIEU (M.) et LARBRE (F.). Mucolipidose de type III. Deux observations dans une fratrie. Etude clinique et ultrastructurale. *Pédiatrie, 1973,* **28**, *485-494.*

HICKMAN (S.) et NEUFELD (E. F.). A hypothesis for I-cell disease : defective hydrolases that do not enter lysosomes. *Biochem. Biophys. Res. Commun., 1972,* **49**, *992-999.*

HUMBEL (R.). Communication personnelle.

KABACK (M. M.), SLOAN (H. R.), SONNEBORN (M.), HERNDON (R. M.) et PERCY (A. K.). GM1-gangliosidosis type I : in utero detection and fetal manifestations. *J. Pediat., 1973,* **82**, *1037-1041.*

KENYON (K. R.), SENSENBRENNER (J. A.) et WYLLIE (R. G.). Hepatic ultrastructure and histochemistry in mucolipidosis II (I-Cell disease). *Pediat. Res., 1973,* **7**, *560-568.*

LANDING (B. H.), SILVERMAN (F. N.), GRAIG (J. M.), JACOBY (M. D.), LAHEY (M. E.) et CHACWICK (D. L.). Familial neurovisceral lipidosis. *Amer. J. Dis. Child., 1964,* **108**, *503-522.*

LEROY (J. G.) et DE MARS (R. I.). Mutant enzymatic and cytological phenotypes in cultured human fibroblasts. *Science, 1967,* **157**, *804-806.*

LEROY (J. G.), SPRANGER (J. W.), FEINGOLD (M.), OPITZ (J. M.) et CROCKER (A. C.). I-cell disease. A clinical picture. *J. Pediat., 1971,* **79**, *360-365.*

LOEB (H.), TONDEUR (M.), JONNIAUX (G.), MOCKEL-POHL (S.) et VAMOS-HURWITZ (E.). Biochemical and ultrastructural studies in a case of mucopolysaccharidosis « F » (fucosidosis). *Helv. paediat. Acta, 1969,* **24**, *519-537.*

LOEB (H.), TONDEUR (M.), TOPPET (M.) et CREMER

(N.). Clinical biochemical and ultrastructural studies of an atypical form of mucopolysaccharidosis. *Acta paediat. scand., 1969,* **58**, *220-228.*

Maroteaux (P.) et Lamy (M.). La pseudo-polydystrophie de Hurler. *Presse méd., 1966,* **74**, *2889-2892.*

Maroteaux (P.), Hors-Cayla (M. C.) et Pont (J.). La mucolipidose de type II. *Presse méd., 1970,* **78**, *179-181.*

Melhem (R.), Dorst (J. P.), Scott (C. I., Jr.) et McKusick (V. A.). Roentgen findings in mucolipidosis III (pseudo-Hurler polydystrophy). *Radiology, 1973,* **106**, *153-160.*

O'Brien (J. S.), Stern (M. B.), Landing (B. H.), O'Brien (J. K.) et Donnell (G. N.). Generalized gangliosidosis. *Amer. J. Dis. Child., 1965,* **109**, *338-346.*

O'Brien (J. S.), Okada (S.), Ho (M. W.), Fillerup (D. L.), Veath (M. L.) et Adams (K.). Ganglioside storage diseases. *Fed. Proc., 1971,* **30**, *956-969.*

Öckerman (P. A.). A generalized storage disorder resembling Hurler's syndrome. *Lancet, 1967,* **ii**, *239-241.*

Öckerman (P. A.). Mannosidosis : isolation of oligosaccharide storage material form brain. *J. Pediat., 1969 b,* **75**, *360-365.*

Pfeiffer (R. A.), Diekmann (L.), Wierich (W.), Bassewitz (D. B.), Junemann (G.), Damaske (E.), Werries (E.) et Wassle (K.). Klinische, pathologische und biochemische Untersuchungen in cinem Fall von infantiler generalisierter Gangliosidose (GM1-Mucolipidose). *Z. Kinderheilk., 1972,* **112**, *23-42.*

Rampini (S.), Isler (W.), Baerlocher (K.), Bischoff (A.), Ulrich (J.) et Pluss (H. J.). Die Kombination von metachromatischer Leukodystrophie und Mukopolysaccharidose als selbständiges Krankheitsbild (Mukosulfatidose). *Helv. paediat. Acta, 1970,* **25**, *436-461.*

Sacrez (R.), Juif (J. G.), Gigonnet (J. M.) et Gruner (J. E.). La maladie de Landing ou idiotie amaurotique infantile précoce avec gangliosidose généralisée de type GM1. *Pédiatrie, 1967,* **22**, *143-162.*

Seringe (Ph.), Plainfossé (B.), Lautmann (F.), Loril-loux (J.), Calamy (G.), Berry (J. P.) et Watchi (J. M.). Gangliosidose généralisée du type Norman-Landing, à GM1 (étude à propos d'un cas diagnostiqué du vivant du malade). *Sem. Hôp. Paris, 1968,* **44**, *685-704.*

Spranger (J. W.), Wiedemann (H. R.), Tolksdorf (M.), Graucob (E.) et Caesar (R.). Lipomucopolysaccharidose. *Z. Kinderheilk., 1968,* **103**, *285-306.*

Spranger (J. W.) et Wiedemann (H. R.). The genetic mucolipidoses. Diagnosis and differential diagnosis. *Humangenetik, 1970,* **9**, *113-139.*

Suzuki (K.), Suzuki (K.) et Kamoshita (S.). Chemical pathology of GM1-gangliosidosis (generalized gangliosidosis). *J. Neuropath., 1969,* **28**, *25-73.*

Taber (P.), Gyepes (M. T.), Philippart (M.) et Ling (S.). Roentgenographic manifestations of Leroy's I-cell disease. *Amer. J. Roentgenol., 1973,* **118**, *213-221.*

Taylor (H. A.), Thomas (G. H.), Miller (C. S.), Kelly (T. E.) et Siggers (D.). Mucolipidosis III (pseudo-Hurler polydystrophy). Cytological and ultrastructural observations of cultured fibroblast cells. *Clin. Genet., 1973,* **4**, *388-397.*

Thieffry (S.), Lyon (G.) et Maroteaux (P.). Encéphalopathie métabolique associant une mucopolysaccharidose et une sulfatidose. *Arch. franç. Pédiat., 1967,* **24**, *425-432.*

Thomas (G. H.), Taylor (H. A.), Reynolds (L. W.) et Miller (C. S.). Mucolipicosis III (Pseudo-fibroblasts cells). *Ped. Res., 1973,* **7**, *751-756.*

Voelz (C.), Tolksdorf (M.), Freitag (F.) et Spranger (J.). Fucosidose. *Mschr. Kinderheilk., 1971,* **119**, *352-355.*

Wolfe (L. S.), Callahan (J.), Fawcett (J. S.), Andermann (F.) et Scriver (C. R.). GM1-gangliosidosis without chondrodystrophy or visceromegaly. Galactosidase deficiency with gangliosidosis and the excessive excretion of a keratan sulfate. *Neurology, 1970,* **20**, *23-44.*

Glycogenoses. Lipidoses

Battaglia (L.) et Chiandussi (D.). Manifestazioni ossee della lipoidosi cerebrosidica di Gaucher. *Chir. Organi Mov., 1965,* **54**, *151-160.*

Field (R. A.). Glycogénoses : Von Gierke's disease, acid maltase deficiency and liver glycogen phosphorylase deficiency. *Amer. J. clin. Path., 1968,* **50**, *20-28.*

Kamoshita (S.), et Suzuki (K.). Infantile Niemann-Pick disease. A chemical study with isolation and characterization of membranous cytoplasmic bodies and myelin. *Amer. J. Dis. Child., 1969,* **117**, *379-394.*

Klumper (A.), Strey (M.), Willing (W.) et Hohmann (B.). Das Krankheitsbild des Morbus Gaucher mit besonderer Berücksichtigung der ossären Form. *Fortschr. Röntgenstr., 1968,* **109**, *640-646.*

Lachman (R.), Crocker (A.), Schulman (J.) et Strand (R.). Radiological findings in Niemann-Pick disease. *Radiology, 1973,* **108**, *659-664.*

Preger (L.), Sanders (G. W.), Gold (R. H.), Steinbach (H. L.) et Pitman (P.). Roentgenographic skeletal changes in the glycogen storage diseases. *Amer. J. Roentgenol., 1969,* **107**, *840-847.*

Silverstein (M. N.) et Kelly (P. J.). Osteoarticular manifestations of Gaucher's disease. *Amer. J. med. Sci., 1967,* **253**, *569-576.*

Part Four:

Secondary Skeletal Diseases

Most chronic visceral disorders can have an affect on the skeleton. Renal and intestinal disorders of long standing have a metabolic effect on it, and have therefore already been discussed. In this third part we shall limit our discussion to four large groups of factors under which bony disorders of other than primary importance have definite significance for the diagnosis. These are: Anomalies of growth (either dwarfism or excessive growth), chromosomal aberrations, hematologic disorders and neurologic diseases.

7 Essentially Disturbed Growth

Aside from the disorders we have investigated in the first part, there are congenital or hereditary disorders where abnormal growth does not appear to be the direct result of bony involvement. The importance of these alterations should not be overlooked.

In this chapter we will successively study both deficient and excessive growth. A large number of complex syndromes have been omitted here, either because they are not clearly defined or because, as a rule, there is no skeletal involvement.

INSUFFICIENT GROWTH

In this first subsection we group together, in a somewhat contrived fashion, the following disorders: essential dwarfism, Bloom's syndrome, the syndrome of brachymorphy spherophakia (Weill-Marchesani), osteodysplastic gerodermia, the oto-palato-digital syndrome, Larsen's syndrome, and Ehlers-Danlos disease.

ESSENTIAL TYPES OF DWARFISM

Our knowledge of these disorders is still quite rudimentary and their isolation and definition is based on peculiarities of facial morphology, and appearance of the extremities or genital organs. Ocular or cutaneous anomalies and precocious aging are characteristically seen in some of these cases.

Classification is difficult and sometimes arbitrary. Usually we distinguish dwarfism with intrauterine onset and those types with late development. Such a division may be faulty, since in the same syndrome dwarfism may sometimes only appear after birth, whereas in some patients it is fully present in the newborn (Pashayan et al.).

We feel that it is preferable to differentiate dwarfism with mental retardation as a key element having significant prognostic importance from those without this finding. We shall not discuss idiopathic intrauterine dwarfism, since it does not have characteristic skeletal findings.

Dwarfism With Mental Retardation

In this group we identify the typus amstelodamensis of Cornelia de Lange, the Rubinstein-Taybi syndrome, birdheaded dwarfism, leprechaunism, the syndrome of Smith, Lemli and Opitz, and Coffin's syndrome.

The Typus Amstelodamensis or the Syndrome of Cornelia de Lange

This syndrome is most frequently recognized during the first few days of life, because of morphologic signs and difficulty in feeding. There can be regurgitation, even respiratory distress and cyanosis during the newborn period.

Clinically, there are typical facial changes combined with abnormal development of extremities and a disturbed mental development. The facial appearance is quite particular, so that affected children look strikingly similar (Fig. 7-1). The eyebrows are thick and meet in the midline, the eyelashes are abnormally long and curved, the bridge of the nose is flat and the nostrils are oriented anteriorly. There may be an excessive distance between the internal angle of the eyelids. The mouth has the form of an inverted V with both sides pulled downwards, and the chin is small and receding. The palate is frequently high and may be divided. Teeth are small and widely spaced. Microcephaly can be accompanied by brachycephaly. The hair line may be abnormally low in the neck and there may be hypertrichosis of the forehead, the region of the lower back and sometimes of the forearms. These babies have a peculiar cry, somewhat weak and coarse. Familiarity with this may help with the diagnosis. Frequently there is also cyanosis of the face or a somewhat marbled appearance of the skin.

The hands are short and square. Usually there is

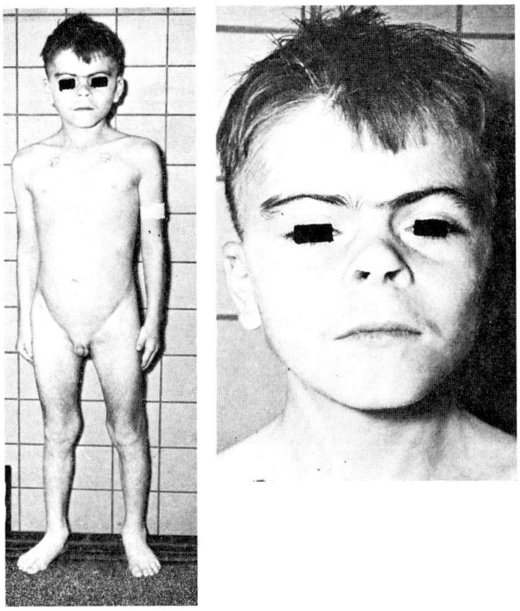

Fig. 7-1. Cornelia de Lange syndrome. (Taken from Rossier, A.: Pédiatrie, CMC, Flammarion)

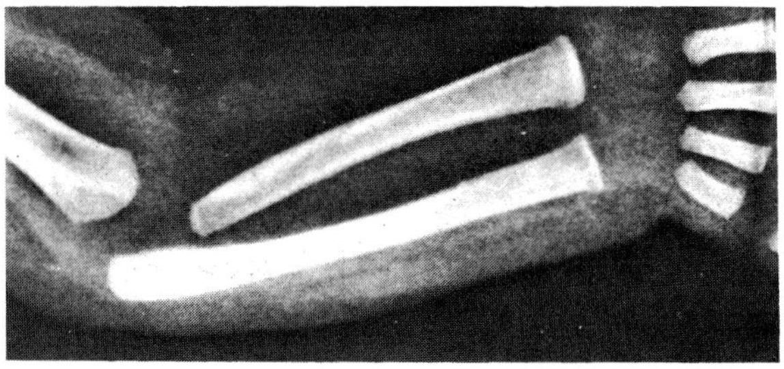

Fig. 7-2. Cornelia de Lange syndrome in an infant. (Courtesy of J. Sauvegrain)

clinodactyly of the 5th finger together with limitation of movements of the elbow. Sometimes the humeri are somewhat short. A single palmar crease and alterations of dermatoglyphics, especially in the region of the hypothenar, have been reported repeatedly. The feet are small, the toes short, and frequently there is syndactyly between the second and third toes. More severe anomalies of the extremities have been seen, such as complete syndactyly, oligodactyly and even phocomelia.

The growth deficit is variable, but there is a general weakness of these infants and a frequently low birthweight. Mental retardation is severe (IQ usually below 50), which explains the poor prognosis of children with this disease.

The most characteristic radiologic finding is a somewhat inconstant hypoplasia of the radial head, often subluxed anteriorly, accompanied by a short and square first metacarpal (Fig. 7-2). Cone-shaped epiphyses, carpal fusion, and more rarely a small exostosis of the lower third of the humerus have also been noted. A low acetabular angle described by Lee and Kenney seems to have a high incidence. The metatarsal can be short. The ribs are horizontal, the thorax is wide in its midportion and the sternum is short with advanced bone maturation, whereas the bone age itself of these patients is usually delayed. Besides microcephaly, the skull is unremarkable.

The high incidence of a reduced urinary excretion of aminoacids would seem to suggest a disturbed renal filtration; hypogammaglobulinemia has also been reported.

Histologic and histochemical studies of the growth cartilage (Stanescu et al.) have revealed an abnormal local arrangement, and its composition of ground substance, which seems to contain abnormal glycoproteins in combination with a weak activity of several lysosomal enzymes.

The etiology of the typus amstelodamensis is unclear. Familial observations are unusual (Beratis et al.), and an autosomal recessive transmission does not seem to be very likely. There are patients on record with chromosomal aberrations in which translocation has been reported because of the presence of an extra chromosomal fragment, these are inconstant and almost uncharacteristic findings. As in a number of syndromes studied later, it is possible that a chromosomal disturbance undetectable with our present day methods could be at the basis of this syndrome. It should be noted that the short head mutation of the mouse does have a certain analogy with this disorder (Ptacek et al.).

The Rubinstein-Taybi Syndrome

Discovered at a variable age, this syndrome is characterized by peculiar anomalies of the fingers and of the face in combination with mental and physical growth retardation.

The hands are short and wide, with, most characteristically, broad thumbs. The unusually impressive thumb is often implanted somewhat high. The distal phalanx is deviated laterally; sometimes even subluxed, and opposition may become impossible. The distal part of other fingers may also be large, but much less strikingly so. Interdigital webs have been described and also anomalies of dermatoglyphics. A simian crease may be present. The feet are flat and wide with a large big toe, sometimes subluxed. The distal phalanx of the other toes may also be somewhat large. A sixth toe can be present, as can dystrophy of the nails.

Facial alterations are another key feature of this disorder. The forehead is low; the palpebral fissures are oblique towards the inferior and lateral side and they may be excessively separated from one another. Frequently there is epicantus, and the thick eyebrows may meet in the midline. Ptosis, refraction-anomalies and cataracts have been described. The nose is narrow, prominent, more or less beakshaped and the nasal septum is often deviated. The mouth is small, the upper lip narrow and the commissures somewhat prominent. The chin is small and triangular in shape. The palate is highly arched, the teeth may be irregularly arranged and of poor quality. The cranial volume is low and the neck short (Fig. 7-3).

Growth retardation is of variable degree, often moderate, but may suddenly become more pronounced after birth. The mental retardation is serious, with an IQ usually below 50. A number of other anomalies have also been mentioned, such as ocular, cardiac, urinary and genital anomalies. Ectopic testicles are a frequent finding in boys.

Radiologic study confirms the widening and deformity of the thumb (Fig. 7-4). The distal phalanx, which is most prominently involved, has a grossly triangular form and is unusually wide at its base. There may even be an incomplete duplication and dislocation. The bony structure may be irregular. The proximal phalanx, sometimes hardly affected, may, however, assume the form of a regular triangle, with its wide angle in the superior-lateral position. The metacarpals may be coarse with a slight modeling defect, and the distal phalanges quite often are also widened. Camptodactyly of the fifth finger has been reported. These anomalies are not always symmetrically present. Radiographs of the feet may show practically the same findings (Fig. 7-4). Study of the skull and of the face will confirm its reduced volume, hypertelorism, and sometimes a flattening of the occipital region together with a large foramen magnum. Some costal or vertebral anomalies, such as fusion of the first ribs and fusion of the arches of the occipital vertebrae, have also been noted in individual patients. Sternal anomalies are frequently present, such as premature fusion of the ossification centers (and doubling). The long bones are usually normal with the exception that the short and square femoral necks are in valgus position. Skeletal maturation is delayed, and in one observation by Brandner and Saur, this was exacerbated by multiple epiphyseal dysplasia and a proximal fibular exostosis.

The pathophysiology of the Rubinstein-Taybi syndrome is unknown. This disorder appears in isolated instances, and even though there have been patients with abnormal caryotype, there is no generally acceptable chromosomal abnormality present. The theory of a reciprocal 14-15 translocation suggested by Simpson has not been proven. Still, it is not entirely excluded that this disease could be due to a so far unrecognized complex chromosomal rearrangement.

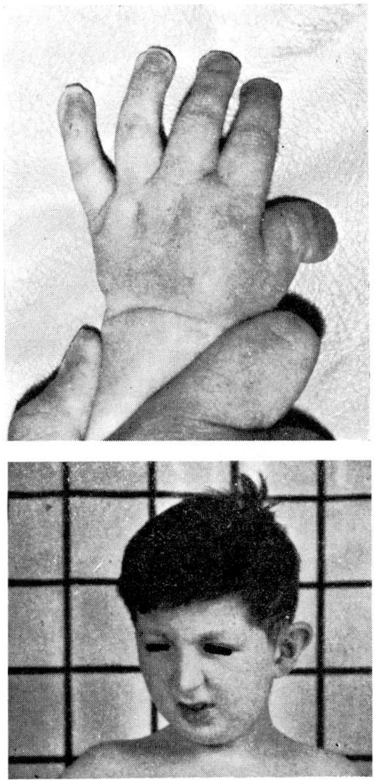

Fig. 7-3. Rubinstein-Taybi syndrome. (Courtesy of M. Lamy)

Birdheaded Dwarfs

Initially described by Virchow, this type of dwarfism has been particularly well studied by Seckel. Facial alterations are the hallmark of this disorder, together with delayed mental and statural growth.

The disorder is usually recognized from birth because of low birthweight dwarfism. The facial appearance at this time is already suggestive, combining a more or less significant degree of microcephaly with a low forehead, an arched beaklike nose contrasting with deep-set facial structures, and marked retrognathia. The profile of the face thus is reminiscent of a bird (Fig. 7-5). Dwarfism is usually very marked and may be accompanied by minor anomalies of the extremities – syndactyly and shortness of the fifth finger.

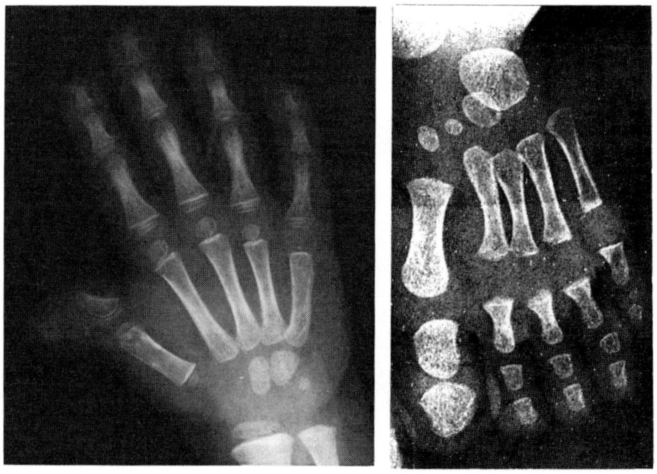

Fig. 7-4. Rubinstein-Taybi syndrome in a 3-month-old infant. (Courtesy of M. Lamy)

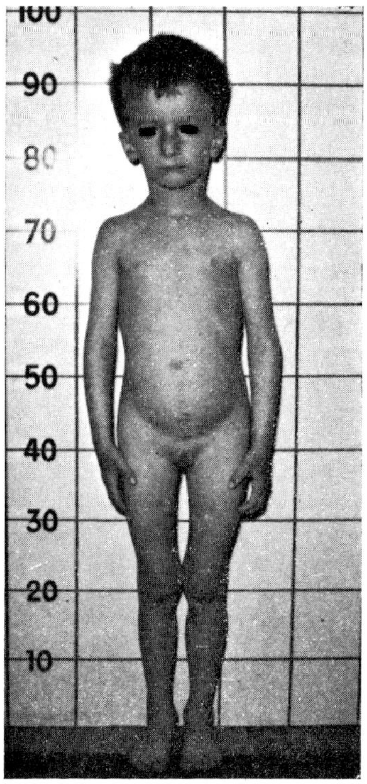

Fig. 7-5. Birdheaded dwarf. (Courtesy of A. Rossier)

The degree of mental retardation can be variable, but is usually severe. The testes are frequently in an ectopic location.

Radiographic study shows microcephaly. Sometimes there is early closure of sutures and facial asymmetry. Bowing of the distal phalanges and shortening of the fifth finger is not rare. Hypoplasia of the radial head with subluxation at the elbow has been noted several times, as has shortening of the proximal portion of the fibula and the absence of articulation with the tibia. Shortness of the femoral necks, even dislocated hips or a defect of the development of the ischiopubic segments may also be present. Sometimes there are costal and vertebral anomalies, such as cervical ribs and sacralisation of the last lumbar vertebra. The delay of the bone age may be severe, but it always corresponds to the height age. One of the most impressive findings is the anarchic formation of different ossification centers, some appearing precociously, and others appearing very late.

The possible occurrence of this disease in brothers and sisters suggests a recessive transmission. The craniofacial appearance of this type of dwarfism, in spite of certain analogies, clearly differs from the changes seen in the Hallermann-Streiff-François syndrome which has been discussed on p. 267. In the latter there is always dwarfism present, and in addition there is usually cataract formation, microphthalmia, and other ocular anomalies, as well as hypotrichosis, cutaneous atrophy and dental anamalies.

Leprechaunism

The name of this disorder results from the resemblance of these infants to the gnomes of Irish folklore.

The aspect in these patients is indeed most unusual. Dwarfing to a severe degree has its onset at birth or in

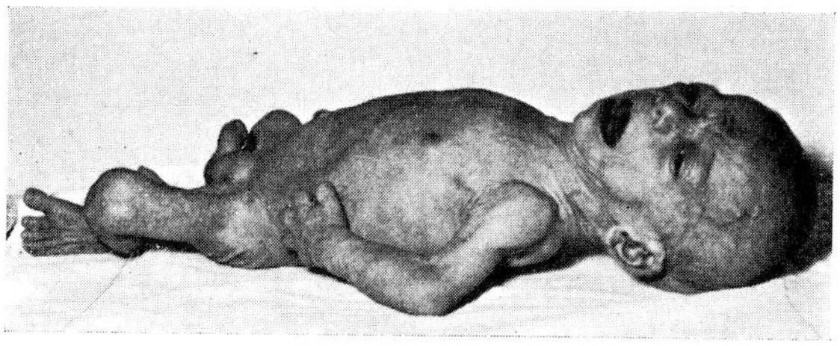

Fig. 7-6. Leprechaunism. (Courtesy of P. Canlorbe)

the first few months thereafter. The eyes protrude and are widely spaced, the nose is large and flat, the ears often are big and low set (Fig. 7-6). These patients often are malnourished, because of severe feeding difficulties. Their subcutaneous and muscular tissues may be atrophic. There is frequent hirsutism and hypertrophy of the mammary glands, external genital organs and the gonads. Widening of the distal portions of the extremities has been noted several times. Mental retardation is observed.

Radiologic study shows diffuse osteoporosis, severely delayed bone age, and sometimes irregularly formed epiphyses and metaphyses. These changes may become more severe as these children grow (Patterson).

The development of this disease is particularly unhappy, since most of the babies will die during the first year of life. Prolonged survival is however possible in patients with the onset of symptoms after birth.

Anatomic study has so far resulted in contradictory findings. Consanguinity of parents and the observation of several such patients in a family suggest an autosomal recessive transmission of this disease, at least in some families.

The Smith-Lemli-Opitz Syndrome

This syndrome, described in 1964, combines dwarfism and anomalies of the face and of the extremities with those of the genital organs. There is also mental retardation.

Usually the disorder is discovered during the first weeks of life because of the morphologic changes, or because of vomiting or delayed development. Pyloric stenosis has been noted several times in these patients. Growth retardation may be in evidence from birth or have its onset somewhat later, resulting in a marked growth deficit. The craniofacial anomalies are most striking. Besides microcephaly there is widening of the bridge of the nose and anterior orientation of the nostrils. Epicantus, ptosis and internal strabism are also present, together with a small and retracted chin (Fig. 7-7). Inspection of the mouth will show widening of the alveolar ridges, a highly arched palate, and sometimes even a cleft or bifid uvula. The hands may show shortening of the middle fingers or of the thumb, possibly with a mild degree of polydactyly or clinodactyly of the fifth finger. The feet are often involved by syndactyly of the second and third toe. Sometimes there is pes varus or metatarsus adductus. Abnormal dermatoglyphics are the rule. Genital anomalies may include hypospasiadias, a small penis, a hypoplastic or incompletely fused scrotum, and often cryptorchidism. Sometimes there is a deep coccygeal fossa. In one-third of the patients there is congenital heart disease.

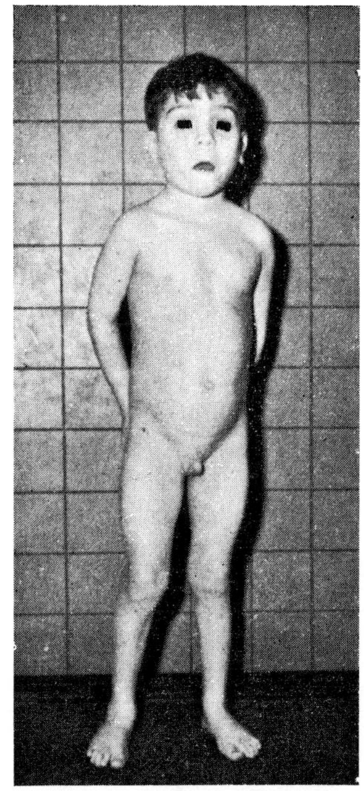

Fig. 7-7. Smith-Lemli-Opitz syndrome. (Courtesy of A. Rossier)

Radiographic study will not reveal any specific findings, and the bone age stays abreast of the height age. The size of the skull is small. Some changes can be noted at the level of the hand and feet: shortening of the first phalanx of the thumb and large toe or of the middle phalanx of the index finger, and shortening of the first metacarpal bone. The long bones are rather slender. Coxa valga is of no great importance in these infants, since they will never walk. A punctate epiphyseal appearance has only been noted once.

The caryotype is normal, but involvement of several children in the same family, and of direct cousins, suggest the possibility of an autosomal recessive transmission with a relatively high incidence of the genes.

Lowry et al. have proposed to bring together the

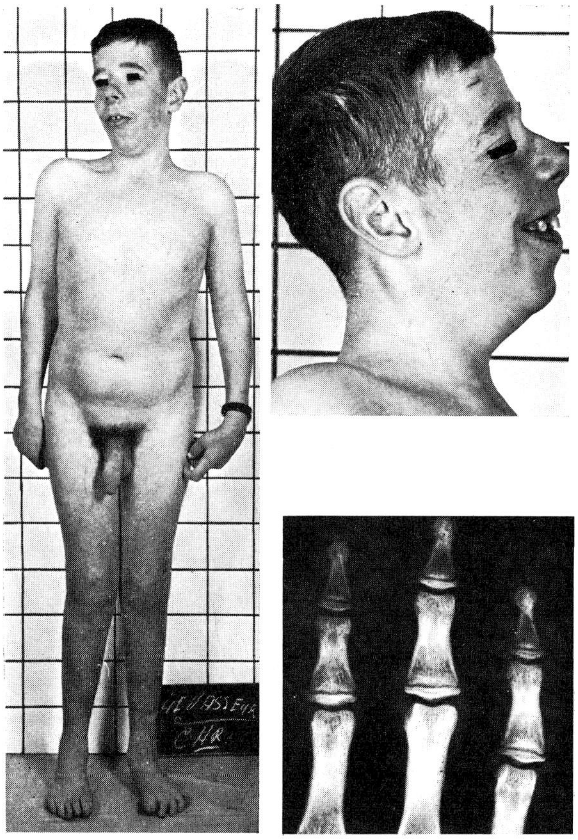

Fig. 7-8. Coffin's syndrome in a 16-year-old boy. Note the marked hypertrophy at the tuberculum of the end phalanges.

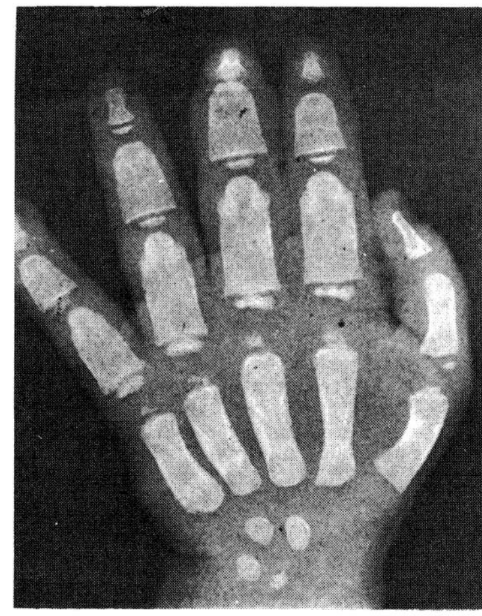

Fig. 7-9. Marshall's syndrome with clearly advanced bone age in this newborn. There is an unusual widening of practically all the phalangeal bones. (Courtesy of R. Rappaport)

Smith-Lemli-Opitz syndrome and the typus Rostockiensis of Ullrich-Feichtiger. The latter disorder, however, besides micrognathia and genital anomalies also includes anomalies of the ears and polydactyly (see p. 174). Such a polydactyly, usually lacking or only minimally suggested here, did indeed exist in Lowry's patient. The categorization of the typus Rostockiensis appears to us still very difficult to clearly define. In some older observations, without, however, having recourse to the actual caryotype, it seems possible to group them with trisomy 13.

Coffin's Syndrome

This syndrome can be differentiated from the preceding one because of only minimal growth disturbance in the presence of marked mental retardation, and because of an unusually grotesque facial appearance reminiscent of gargoylism. This appearance is only fully developed in the older child, or at adolescence. It is characterized by acromegaloid features, wide-set eyes, a pugilistic nose and large ears. There frequently is mandibular prognathism (Fig. 7-8). The hands are large and flabby with tapering fingers. Flat feet, limitation of motion at the elbow and kyphoscoliosis with a mild degree of sternal protrusion complete the signs and symptoms of this syndrome. The growth deficit is only mild.

Radiographic findings are those of a small head and hyperostosis frontalis interna or excessive development of the frontal sinus. The facial bones are hypoplastic and the mandibular angle is large. The vertebral end plates are irregularly formed with intraspongy herniation as is typical in Scheuermann's disease. The terminal phalanges of the fingers may be drumstick shaped (Fig. 7-8, *Bottom, right*).

This disorder seems to affect boys electively and the recognition of individuals in families of patients with some milder signs of this disorder would seem to suggest the possibility of a genetic transmission. This is, however, not yet entirely accepted. There could be autosomal dominant transmission with a variable expressivity or sex-linked characteristic.

Marshall et al. have described a syndrome in babies which is accompanied by characteristic facial features such as a high forehead and protruding eyes. Involved babies have respiratory difficulties and mental retardation. There is early death. Radiologic findings are particularly striking. There is an unusually advanced bone age, often present at birth. The carpal bones are impressively widened and reminiscent of the changes in mucopolysaccharidoses, whereas the long bones are rather slender (Fig. 7-9).

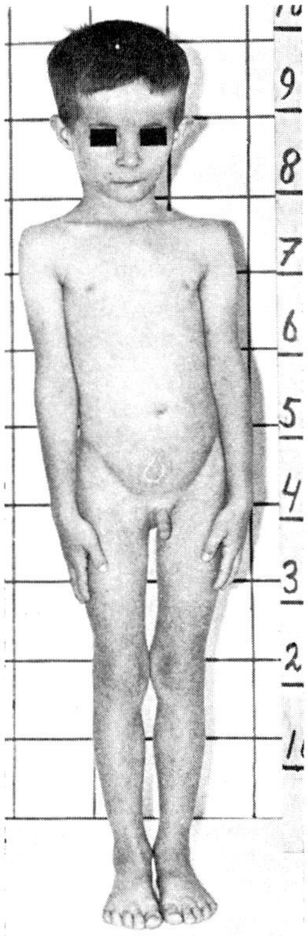

Fig. 7-10. Silver's syndrome with easily recognizable asymmetry of the extremities. (Courtesy of R. Rappaport)

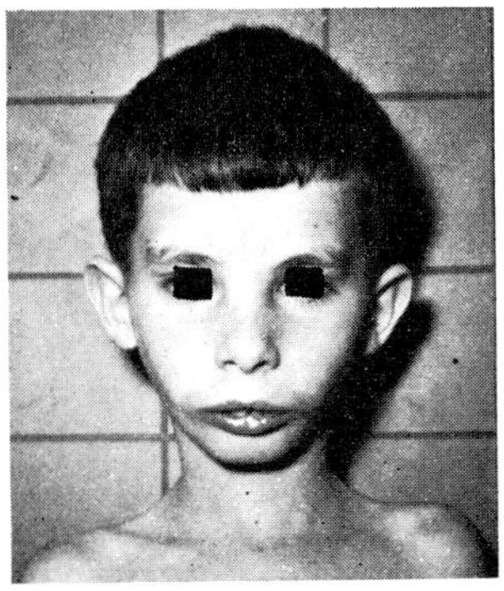

Fig. 7-11. Russell's syndrome. (Courtesy of A. Rossier)

Dwarfism Without Mental Retardation

We will review here the Silver syndrome, the Russell syndrome, progeria and progeroid conditions, and the Freeman-Sheldon syndrome. The so-called pug nosed dwarfism of Black, which often seems the result of somathormone deficit, is discussed on p. 211.

Silver Syndrome

The Silver syndrome associates a form of dwarfism with hemihypertrophy and genital developmental anomalies.

Dwarfism is frequently already present at birth, but may be only moderate in degree. Hemihypertrophy may also be present, but moderate. A discrete facial dysproportion is frequently noted, since the face itself may be triangular and both sides of the mouth may droop (Fig. 7-10). "Café au lait" spots, a syndactyly of toes and incurving of the fifth finger are frequently present.

The genital anomalies are characterized by precocious puberty or by elevated urinary gonadotrophines. Cryptorchidism and hypospadia have also been described (Rimoin).

The radiologic findings will confirm hemihypertrophy, which is not limited to the soft tissues, but which may well involve the long bones and epiphyses. Sometimes this hypertrophy is only segmental or partial, and may be limited to the spine or a single extremity. The development of the epiphyses and the bone age are usually symmetrically retarded corresponding to the heightage. In rare patients there is a maturation delay of the smaller side only. Besides hemihypertrophy, skeletal investigation will reveal hypoplasia and incurving of the middle phalanx of the fifth finger. Rarely, there is hypoplasia of a thoracic vertebra or an irregularity of the end plates of several vertebrae.

The etiology remains unresolved. Silver claims that he has seen this condition in a mother and daughter (quoted by Fuleihan et al.). The characteristics of this condition have been considerably widened in concept by a number of authors, particularly by Silver himself, incurring the inherent risk of watering down the individuality of the syndrome. Many authors confuse this condition with the Russell syndrome, which we shall now discuss.

Russell's Syndrome

This syndrome is characterized by a severe craniofacial disproportion, which is combined with a growth deficit and low weight (Fig. 7-11).

Dwarfism is noted at birth, but the gracility of such patients is deceptive, since they may appear taller than they really are. The weight deficit is eventually proportionally even more significant. Muscles are underdeveloped. The length of the lower extremity may be relatively excessive, while the arms may be somewhat short. Sometimes there is a degree of asymmetry, occasionally also lordosis and a narrow thorax. Bowing

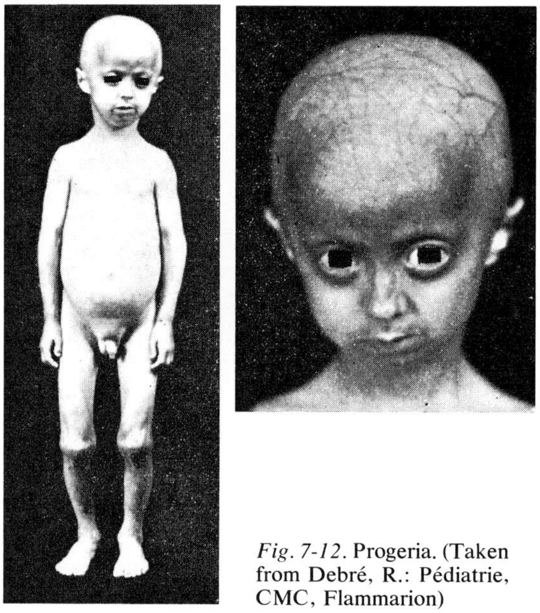

Fig. 7-12. Progeria. (Taken from Debré, R.: Pédiatrie, CMC, Flammarion)

of the fifth finger and a deformed calcaneus in valgus were described in the initial patients of Russell.

The craniofacial disproportion is present at birth with a pseudo-hydrocephalic appearance of the skull (Szalay). This is one of the differentiating features from the Silver syndrome. The anterior fontanelle closes late, but the head circumference is no larger than in age-matched normal infants. The mandible is underdeveloped and the face has a triangular aspect with a wide mouth in the form of an inverted V and lowset corners. The profile of the face with the markedly bulging forehead, the small face, and the tiny mandible is entirely characteristic (Fitch and Pinsky). Mental development is, on the whole, normal.

Radiologic findings of the skeleton are: delayed maturation, a large skull, an underdeveloped mandible and clinodactyly.

The etiology is unknown. Fuleihan et al. have described three brothers and sisters of a mother, who was also unusually small. Russell was certain of abnormal findings of the placenta – in several of his cases the size was small and areas of infarction were present.

Progeria and Progeroid Conditions

These conditions, including Werner's syndrome, Cockayne's syndrome, and Rothmund's syndrome are discussed next. Progeria is a condition in which the patients age prematurely, and in which there is a growth deficit with beginning manifestation usually in the second year of life.

These children are typical in appearance. They lose their hair, develop atrophic skin with many brown pigmented spots, protruding veins, especially of the head, and waste their subcutaneous tissue and musculature (Fig. 7-12). Severe arteriosclerosis often leads to death from coronary or cerebral incidents.

Even though several longitudinal studies of lipids and lipoproteins have shown an elevation, which seems largely under the influence of the regimen (McNamara et al.), this elevation is not always present.

Radiology will show an excessive skeletal radiolucency, the slenderness of the diaphyses of long bones is in marked contrast with the relatively protruding epiphyses. Growth arrest lines are sometimes quite prominent (Reichel et al.). Coxa valga is usually present, and also valgus of the femoral head. The elbows are deformed by widening of the condyle and flattening of the radial head. The terminal phalanges of fingers and toes are slender and pointed. Acroosteolysis has frequently been reported. The clavicles are short and thin, the thorax is narrow. Vertebrae are often ovoid with frequent persistence of the anterior vascular channel (Schwartz). The development of the skull appears adequate, but the anterior fontanelle closes late. The bony facial structures are small as is the mandible, which has a large angle. The bone age is usually normal, but epiphyseal closure may be delayed. Early arthrotic changes can be present.

Certain publications suggest that an abnormal collagen is responsible for this disorder. Villée. et al. have shown that within skin there is an increase of insoluble collagen and an elevated temperature for retraction. A regimen high in poly-unsaturated fats does not seem to have an effect on the course of this disease.

The pathophysiology is unknown. A single observation of an affected brother and sister, whose parents are first cousins, suggests the possibility of an autosomal recessive transmission. Besides progeria there are other syndromes accompanied by precocious aging. Werner's syndrome usually has its onset in adults. Juvenile cataracts are combined with sclerodermia, atrophy of the skin, an atheroma and arterial calcifications. Growth is delayed. The development of this disorder is slowly progressive with death around 50 years. The bones are slender and usually show osteoporosis. Often there are calcifications of the tissues.

Even though mental retardation, with its onset around 18 months, is usually part of this condition, we would like to include here the Cockayne syndrome. This condition, with an onset soon after birth, results in severe dwarfism with cachexia, retinal atrophy with blindness, partial deafness, and an abnormal sensitivity to light.

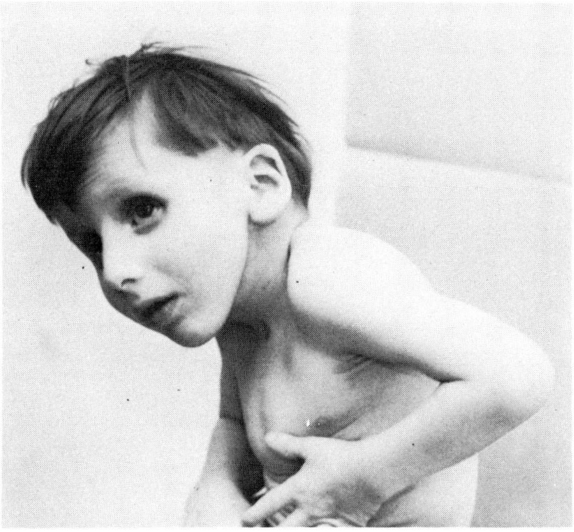

Fig. 7-13. Cockayne's syndrome. (Taken from Debré, R.: Pédiatrie, CMC, Flammarion)

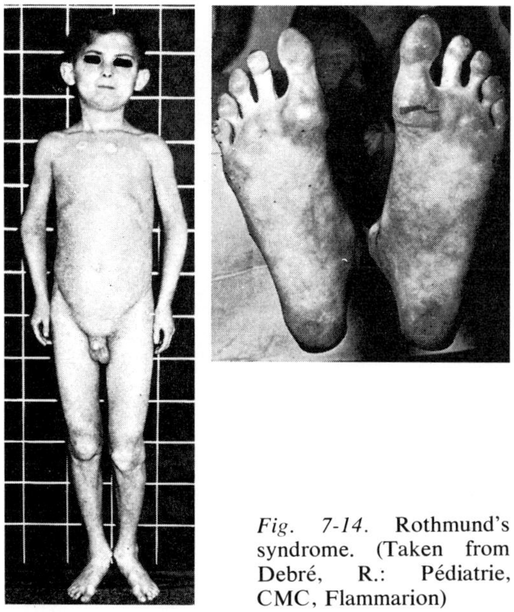

Fig. 7-14. Rothmund's syndrome. (Taken from Debré, R.: Pédiatrie, CMC, Flammarion)

Besides the growth deficit there is a lack of subcutaneous tissue, especially in the area of the face, resulting in a narrow nose and deeply sunken eyes. The mandible is small (Fig. 7-13), the second toe sometimes short. The joints are all too large, often with limitation of movement. Kyphosis is frequently present, and the following neurologic disturbances can often be found: nystagmus, intention tremor and ataxia.

Radiologic study, besides generalized osteoporosis, will show, towards the second and third year (Riggs and Seibert), that diaphyses of the long bones are slender, with prominent epiphyses of the elbow, the knee and the tibio-tarsal region. The immediately adjacent metaphyses are also prominent. Frequently there is coxa valga. An unusually dense appearance of phalangeal epiphyses and those at the distal end of the ulna and the trochanter major may be noted, sometimes there will also be early closure of the phalangeal epiphyses. The size of the carpal and tarsal bones may be excessive. Clavicles and ribs are slender. The height of the posterior vertebral border may be reduced. The iliac wings are narrow and high, leading to an open, large iliac angle, whereas the acetabular roof remains low and can be almost horizontal. Microcephaly is usually present and there may be subsequent intracranial calcifications. In some cases the skull appears to be enlarged.

Rothmund's syndrome has its onset during the first few months in a reticulated erythema of the face followed by atrophy, poikilodermia, and telangiectasia. Abnormal development of hair and nails is the rule. Bilateral cataract may be noted towards four years of age, and hypogonadism has been reported (Fig. 7-14).

These patients usually are short with slender extremities and markedly short hands. Shortening of the fingers is predominantly located at the most peripheral segment. There may also be syndactyly, aplasia of the thumb, a cleft of the hand or foot and even more severe hypoplasia of the bones of the forearm. Dental anomalies may also be noted.

Radiographic studies confirm the different malformations of the hands. In addition, osteolysis of the terminal phalanges has been described (Maurer et al.). Other observations referred to a bipartite patella, an unusual bony density, and an appearance reminiscent of fibrous displasia (Taylor).

This disorder is inherited as an autosomal recessive and appears to have a higher incidence in girls.

The Freemann-Sheldon Syndrome

This disorder was described by Freemann and Sheldon in 1938, and is also known under the term "whistling face syndrome" as suggested by Burian, 1963. The facial appearance is very striking, because of the small size of the mouth, which can hardly be opened. These patients have a very poor mimic, the eyes are deeply set within the orbits and there seems to be an excessive amount of orbital soft tissues. Strabism, blepharophimosis, and slanting of the palpebral fissures laterally, may be present together with a vertical or V-shaped groove of the chin (Fig. 7-15). Growth is re-

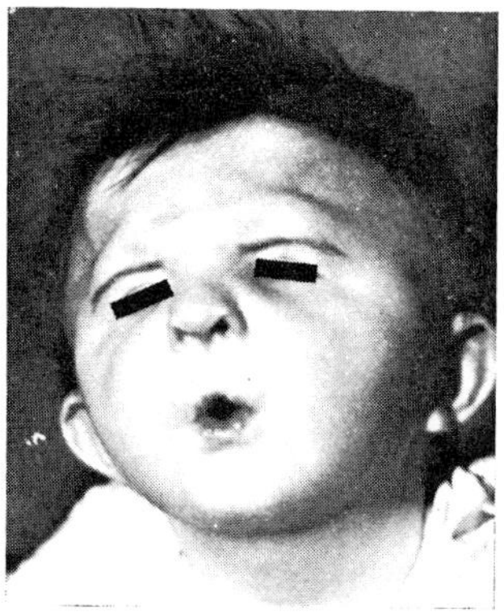

Fig. 7-15. Freeman-Sheldon syndrome. (Courtesy of R. Walbaum)

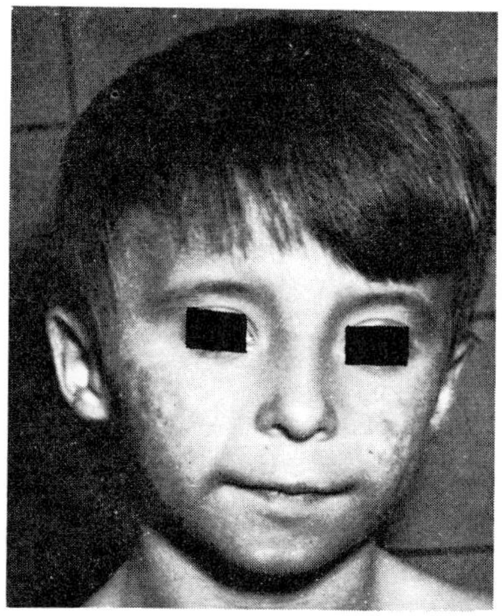

Fig. 7-16. Bloom's syndrome. Note the prominent skin changes over both cheeks. (Courtesy of A. Rossier)

tarded, and irreducible flexion deformity of the fingers with ulnar deviation are always present. Bilateral clubfoot is an almost constant finding. The intelligence is normal.

Radiologically, the skull and face have a square appearance with a reduced AP diameter. The occipital groove is deep and the foramen magnum oriented posteriorly. The tip of the mandible is protruding. The bones of the hands do not show anything significant besides their abnormal relationship. The bone age is markedly retarded in comparison with the chronological age. Curvature of the spine and spina bifida occulta have been noted.

The disorder follows a dominant mode of transmission.

This condition should not be confused with ulnar deviation of the "windmill" fingers, which is also transmitted as a dominant disorder, but does not have any facial alterations (Jaquemain).

BLOOM'S SYNDROME

This is characterized by multiple chromosomal anomalies, such as chromatid or chromosomal breaks and recombinations. Anomalies also found in Fanconi's anemia are discussed on page 295.

The clinical findings are those of intrauterine dwarfism associated with teleangiectasia. This condition, which has an early onset, is mainly limited to the face, where it has a butterfly distribution and only rarely affects the hands and forearms (Fig. 7-16). These lesions are very sensitive to light and exposure to the sun. Exposure will result in the appearance of blisters. The definitive height is around 1.40 m (Germann), and there are some skeletal anomalies that may be present, such as syndactyly, clinodactyly, extra fingers, pes equinus and an absence of the metatarsal bones. Dislocation of the left hip was noted in the patient of Sizonenko. Abnormal formation of teeth—lack of lateral incisors—is not unusual.

The seriousness of this disease is emphasized, since quite often a malignancy, especially leukemia, will later be part of this disorder.

Bloom's syndrome is more frequently seen in boys, and it is transmitted as an autosomal recessive disorder. The gene has a particularly high incidence amongst Ashkenasi Jews. It is possible that the cause of intrauterine dwarfing may be a disturbance of cellular division, since these cells do contain abnormal chromosomes.

Therapy, besides precautionary measures to protect from skin lesions, consists of a constant and careful supervision in order to detect malignancy at the earliest possible moment.

THE SPHEROPHAKIA-BRACHYMORPHIA SYNDROME (WEILL-MARCHESANI)

This syndrome is a combination of ocular anomalies and disturbed growth. Weill, in 1932, described the association of ectopia of the lens, and poor growth. Marchesani, in 1939, emphasized the simultaneous presence of spherophakia and brachydactyly in affected individuals.

The disorder is usually recognized because of eye symptoms. These may however go unnoticed until adolescence or well into adulthood.

Clinically, these patients are somewhat short, but only slightly, however, there is more marked shortening of their hands and feet, where the joints may be slightly prominent. The skull is brachycephalic, the face round, the neck short and the trunk may be wide. Discrete limitation of movements of several joints, especially of the fingers is not unusual. Ocular findings, not present at birth, are a combination of myopia and subluxation of the lens and a secondary lesion. Glaucoma frequently complicates the condition. The disorder is compatible with an almost normal life. Still, the danger of coronary thrombosis has been mentioned.

Radiologically, the long bones are somewhat coarse, but shortening only involves the metacarpals, the metatarsals and the phalanges. Besides cone-shaped epiphyses there are no further anomalies.

The Weill-Marchesani syndrome seems to be due to an autosomal recessive gene manifesting in the heterozygote state resulting in reduced height.

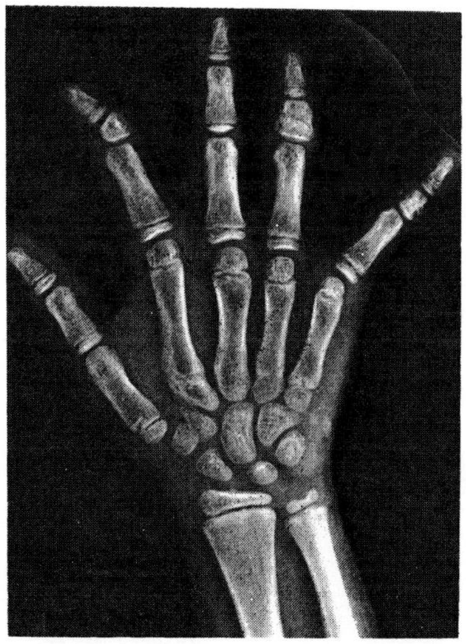

Fig. 7-17. Otopalatodigital syndrome. Characteristic changes of the proximal portion of the 2nd metacarpal and the phalanges.

HEREDITARY OSTEODYSPLASTIC GERODERMIA

This disorder has been well described by Bamatter et al. It is transmitted as an incompletely recessive sex-linked disorder, since the gene only manifests itself in a woman, who is a transmitter. The cutaneous lesions are localized mainly on the backs of hands and feet, where local atrophy and hyperlaxity of the skin is evident. A growth deficit is frequently noted, together with a mild degree of facial dysmorphism, that is: a somewhat senile facial expression, prognatism of the mandible and abnormally spaced teeth. Patients also show a mild degree of bony fragility and articular and ligamentous hyperlaxity. The feet are flat.

Radiologically, osteoporosis is most characteristically present, involving mainly the spine, and, in young infants, vertebral bodies (double contour). Platyspondyly, with a biconcave lens-shape, is not unusual, but sometimes there is wedging of several vertebrae. Dislocation of the hip has been seen several times.

THE OTO-PALATO-DIGITAL SYNDROME

Defined by Langer, this complex of malformations does, indeed, deserve its own place. This disorder is, in its complete form, only seen in boys, whereas girls may show it only partially.

The changes of the hand and of the face, with a hearing defect, sometimes a cleft palate, and a mild growth deficit, hardly ever start before 2 years of age. The thumb and big toe are short and spatula-shaped. The distal phalanx of the three middle fingers is widened, whereas the fifth finger is laterally curved. Frontal bossing, hypertelorism, widening of the bridge of the nose, lateral slanting of the palpebral fissures and a small mouth with low set corners, all result in a rather typical facial appearance. A cleft palate is frequently also present. The thorax may be narrow below the nipples. There may also be limitation of movements of the elbows. Deafness appears secondary to anomalies and repeated infections of the middle ear. A mild degree of mental retardation reported by several authors may at least in part be the result of disturbed hearing.

The most striking radiologic findings, in our opinion, are those of the metacarpals and metatarsals (Fig. 7-17). There is a supernumerary epiphysis or a pseudoepiphysis, which has a conical or pointed proximal end. The 2nd metacarpals and metatarsals are the most strikingly involved bones with the 3rd also frequently affected. A mild defect in tubulation can be also present. The distal epiphyses of these bones may also be somewhat unusually shaped. The distal phalanx of the thumb may be unusually large, with a cone-shaped epiphysis. The other fingers are often mildly curved towards the midline of the hand. A high incidence of carpal changes has been recorded—comma shaped trapezoid, a transverse aspect of the capitatum, fusion of the trapezium and scaphoid, and duplication of the semilunar and an extra distal bone. The carpal angle is larger than normal (Poznanski et al.). Tarsal bones are equally involved.

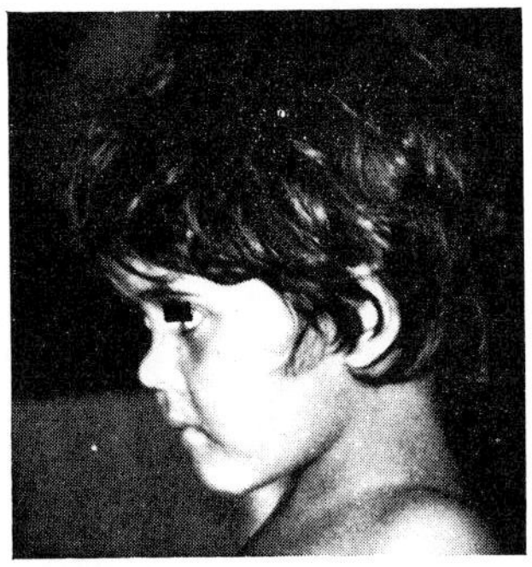

Fig. 7-18. Larsen's syndrome with its characteristic facial appearance. (Courtesy of G. Payet)

Hypoplasia of the proximal end of the radius is not unusual with posterior dislocation. There may be coxa valga and slight diaphyseal bowing. Pneumatization of facial bones and of the mastoids may be poor. The base of the skull can be thick in its anterior region and the clivus may be abnormally vertical. Delayed fusion of the vertebral arches has been recorded. This syndrome does seem to be genetically determined, but its exact transmission is not yet clear, since the following modes are possible: dominant, autosomal recessive, sex-linked, with intermediary manifestation in heterozygote females.

LARSEN'S SYNDROME

Larsen's syndrome was isolated in 1950, because of abnormal joint laxity with severe multiple dislocations, combined with unusual facial appearance and sometimes with a cleft palate. This disorder is recognized at birth because of the very striking dislocations.

The facial disproportion of these patients results from insufficient development of the midportion of the face, which seems to be receding in relation to the prominent forehead and the somewhat prominent mandible. The bridge of the nose is flat and the eyes seem to be widely spaced. A cleft palate has been reported several times (Fig. 7-18).

The extremities are prominently involved, and, as a result of the articular laxity, there are different dislocations present, such as dislocated hips, anterior dislocation of the tibia, dislocation of the elbows and clubbed feet. Walking can be especially difficult, if not entirely impossible, for these children. Only repeated orthopaedic measures and interventions will eventually bring about a somewhat less than satisfactory result. Growth of these patients is disturbed, and affected adults reach a height of around 1.20 m.

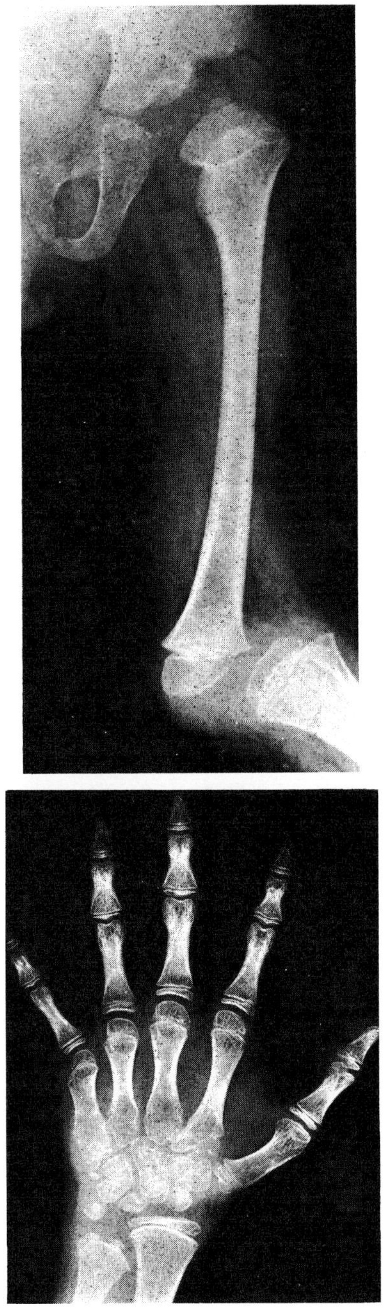

Fig. 7-19. Larsen's syndrome. (*Top*) Dislocated hip and knee in a 5-year-old. (*Bottom*) At 12 years of age with extra carpal bone. (Courtesy of D. Nusslé)

Radiographically, we note abnormal epiphyseal development of the epiphyses. These appear to be flattened, irregular, and unusually radiolucent. They may have an aspect similar to the immediately adjacent metaphysis. The thickness of the cortex, however, is normal.

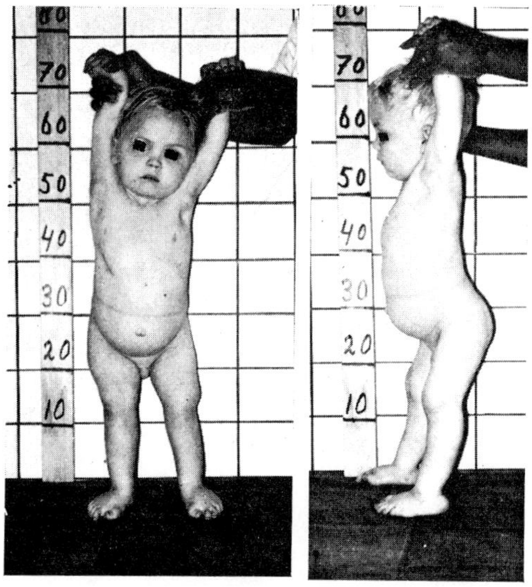

Fig. 7-20. Desbuquois-type dwarfism. (Courtesy of P. Royer)

Among the most characteristic findings is an abnormal shape of carpal bones with extra bony elements present (Fig. 7-19). The tarsal bones are also markedly abnormal and the ossification of the calcaneus can be from two separate centers with ulterior fusion. There are also deformed spurs of the metacarpals. This finding is most strikingly present on the second metacarpals, where an extra epiphysis or pseudoepiphysis at the proximal end can be noted. The metatarsals can be similarly involved. These findings are reminiscent of those of the oto-palato-digital syndrome.

Vertebral changes are not unusual, and consist of irregular end plates, and reduced height, sometimes accompanied by spinal deviation. More complex malformations of the cervical spine have been occasionally reported. In these there was a serious risk of a dislocation of the neck. This disorder, it has been noted, affects brothers and sisters in a number of families. This would suggest an autosomal recessive transmission. In other familial observations, however (Latta et al.), an irregular dominant transmission has been noted (discrete facial anomaly in the mother). The syndrome, therefore, must be considered to be heterogeneous in some instances. In spite of the presence of the findings described here, total growth has been only mildly affected and radiographic changes are mild. In others, however, a particularly severe type of dwarfism is noted (Fig. 7-20). Ligamentous laxity, even though present, is much less serious. Radiologic study shows a mild deviation of fingers and generalized osteoporosis (Fig. 7-21). This unquestionably autosomal recessive type was described originally by Desbuquois et al.

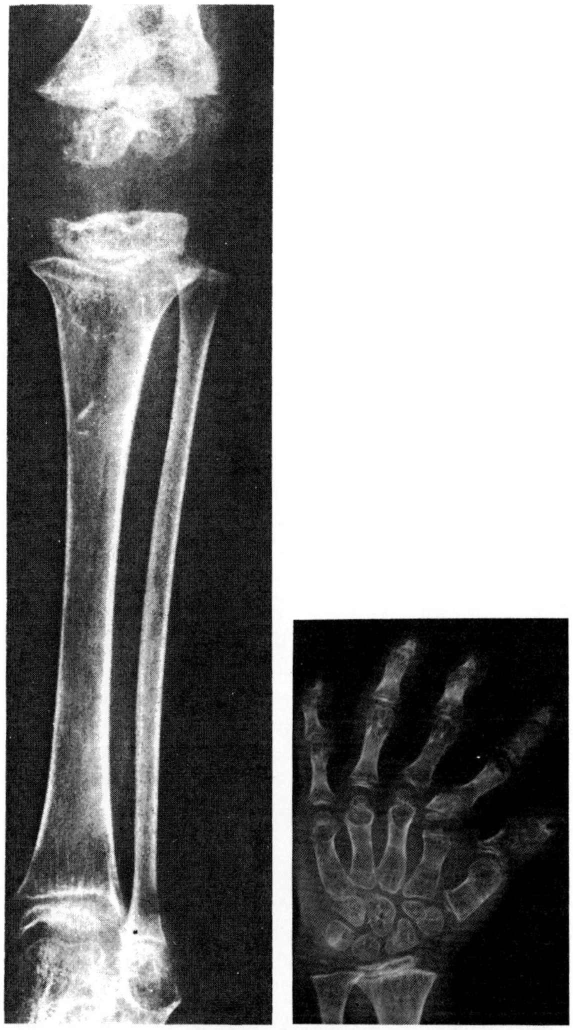

Fig. 7-21. Desbuquois-type dwarfism in 6-year-old boy. Note the characteristic severe deformity of the metacarpal bones and the very short bones of the hand. (Courtesy of P. Royer)

EHLERS-DANLOS DISEASE

In spite of the fact that this disorder is mainly one of the skin and the periarticular tissues, it may occasionally result in somewhat disturbed growth, especially of the spine. We therefore mention this problem in this chapter.

The hyperelasticity of the skin is accompanied by papyraceous scars or molluscoid pseudo-tumors located in the main pressure zones: the elbows, the knees and the heels (Fig. 7-22).

Hypermobility of the joints helps to explain the disturbance of gait and also the difficulties of posture in severely affected patients. They have flat feet and genu

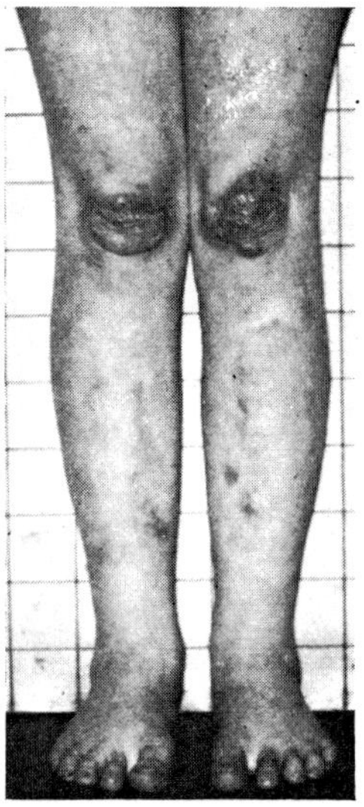

Fig. 7-22. Ehlers-Danlos disease. Typical scar formation over both knees and shins. (Courtesy of M. Lamy)

recurvatum. Frequently there is also kyphoscoliosis. These patients are of short stature. Dental anomalies can also be noted—small teeth which are widely spaced.

Radiographic study will show that in addition to the kyphoscoliosis there may be several deformed, usually wedged, vertebrae. A serious degree of spondylolisthesis has been reported by McKusick. The long bones are hardly affected, with the exception of slight bowing. In severely affected patients there may, however, be dislocations of the hip, the patella or of the radial head. Radioulnar synostosis and bony bridging between the acetabulum and the trochanter are only rarely present. The latter finding may be the result of a bleeding tendency, which may be part of this syndrome.

Ehlers-Danlos disease is a heterogeneous disorder. Six different types have so far been identified. Transmission is most frequently dominant. There is, however, a recessive sex-linked form and another one type VI, which is transmitted as an autosomal recessive lesion. The anomaly of collagen, which is its underlying cause, has been carefully studied in the latter form and proven to result from a deficiency in lysylhydroxylase.

EXCESSIVE GROWTH

Discussed here will be Marfan's disease, cerebral gigantism, the Wiedemann-Beckwith syndrome, hemihypertrophy, and the Klippel-Trenaunay syndrome.

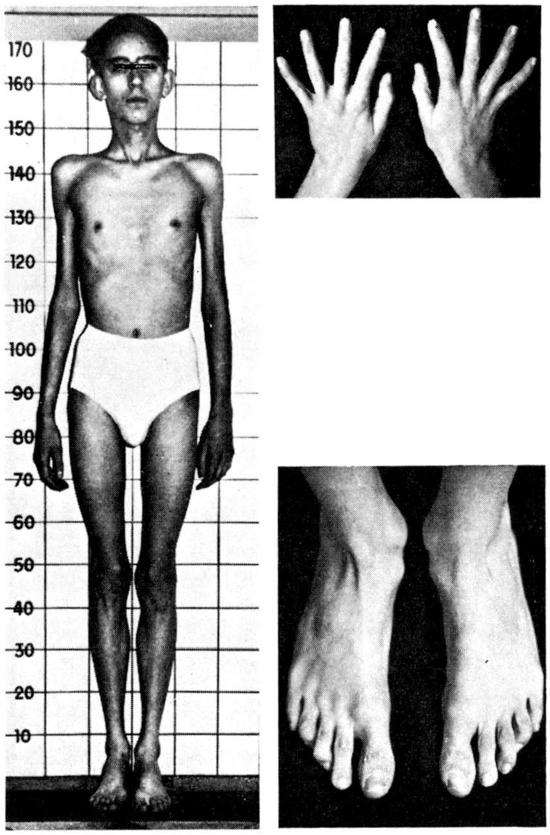

Fig. 7-23. Marfan's disease. Note the slender and elongated appearance along with arachnodactyly.

MARFAN'S DISEASE

This disorder was described by Marfan in 1896, under the name dolichostenomelia (δολιχος = long, μελος = limb), because of the abnormal aspect of the limbs. An excellent study of this disease is contained in McKusick's book.

Clinical Findings

The age of the patient and the actual circumstances leading to the discovery of this disease are quite variable. During infancy it is most frequently a problem of abnormal growth or disturbed vision, which will lead to a physical examination. In adults, however, the main presenting symptom will be cardiac in nature. The disorder leads to physical, ocular and cardiovascular changes. Clinical study will show a most striking relatively increased length of the limbs in relation to the size of the trunk. The lower segment (distance pubis to ground) is bigger than the upper segment (pubis to vertex) (Fig. 7-23). The excessive length of the extremities is somewhat exaggerated by their slenderness. The most peripheral parts are the most severely affected. This implies that the fingers and toes are especially long and narrow, which has led to the designation of the disease as arachnodactyly, as proposed by Achard. The big toe may be especially prominent. The height of affected children is often considerably above the mean for the age. Adults may be quite tall, but they are not to be considered as giants.

Ligamentous hyperlaxity usually leads to flat feet, genu recurvatum, and sometimes true dislocation of the hip or of the knee. The muscular development is poor, as is the subcutaneous tissue. Inguinal hernias are frequently present.

The thorax is narrow, with a funnel shape. Quite frequently patients suffer from early scoliosis, since in about half of the patients there is onset before 6 years of age. These frequently painful scolioses are most often thoracic in location with a rightsided convexity or a double curvature, thoracic right and lumbar left.

The skull is often dolichocephalic and the face long and narrow with a slight anterior bulge of the mandible and a high arched palate. The voice may be high pitched with a peculiar sound.

In spite of the fact that this is not an absolutely constant finding ectopy of the lens is one of the most characteristic findings in Marfan's disease. Most frequently bilateral, this may result in a complete dislocation of the lens—either into the anterior chamber or into the aqueus—with the serious risk of blindness. Often there are anomalies of the irido-corneal angle resulting in ocular hypertension. Retinal detachment also presents a real risk.

A final group of potentially dangerous complications are those resulting from aortic lesions. Almost half of the patients develop dilatation of the aorta or a desecting aneurysm with a variable onset as a result of necrosis of the aortic media. Such lesions can already be present during early childhood.

There may also be pulmonary manifestations, as studied by several authors (Boland, Morère et al.). These are secondary not only to the thoracic and spinal alterations, but also to anomalies of the bronchi and the parenchyma. The latter have a tendency to form atelectasis or diffuse or cystic emphysema. Spontaneous pneumothorax may be one of the complications occurring quite frequently in patients with Marfan's disease.

The prognosis is based on the degree of cardioaortic involvement, which may often lead to early death and also to blindness. Respiratory complications should not be overlooked, since they may lead to serious complications during surgery or orthopedic problems.

Radiographic Findings

The bones of the extremities and the ribs appear to be excessively long and slender. They do have normal cortical thickness. The form of the metaphyses and of the epiphyses are normal. The bone age is sometimes slightly advanced, particularly in unusually tall individuals. Sometimes there is a somewhat striated appearance of the metaphyses. Radiographs of the foot will confirm the abnormal size of the 1st toe and may show spur-formation of the calcaneus (Fig. 7-24). Sinclair has proposed to measure the metacarpal index: mean of the ratio of the length over the width as measured in the middle of the diaphysis of the second to the fifth metacarpals of the right hand. This index, equal to or below eight in normal children, is clearly much higher in patients with Marafan's disease, where it is above ten. Spinal films may show abnormally high vertebral bodies, usually with a reduced AP diameter. The anterior and posterior borders may be concave, leading to the "diabolo aspect." The spinal canal may have excessively wide foramina. These findings are similar to those seen in patients with a scoliosis as part of Von Recklinghausen's disease. Wedging of vertebral bodies and epiphysitis during growth have been reported. The pelvis occasionally has the typical aspect of protrusio acetabuli and sometimes there is a dislocated hip. The skull is dolichocephalic with an abnormally long base. Thickness of the vault is normal. The facial structures appear unusually narrow and mandibular prognathism can be noted.

Anatomic and Biochemical Findings

An increased urinary output of hydroxyproline, repeatedly reported in Marfan's disease, is not a specific finding. It is inconstant, especially in the adult. A lowering of the value for seromucoids, reported by Bacchus, could not be verified (Leeming and McKusick). The same must be stated for urinary excretion of mucopolysaccharides (Tortorolo et al.). Our own studies of patients with Marfan's disease did not reveal any quantitative or qualitative anomaly of urinary excretion.

Anatomic study did not result in any specific findings either. When studying the aorta, the most striking findings are the involvement of the media by fragmentation and dissociation of the elastic fibers, and the decreased presence of collagen. Sometimes there is a metachromatic interstitial substance (Bolande). In the skin, Laitinen has been able to demonstrate an increase of soluble collagen. Le Coulant and Broustet mention a high content in orceinophilic material, reminiscent of the finding in early infancy.

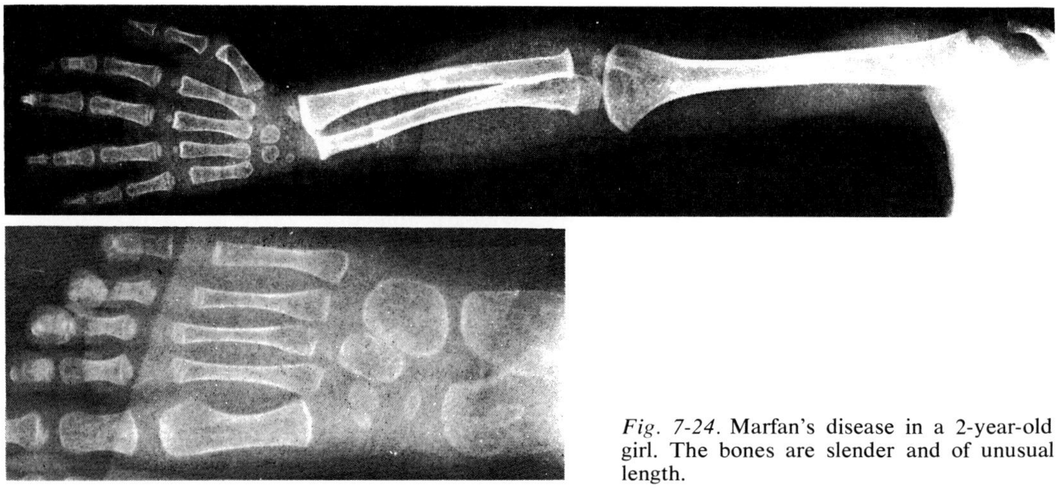

Fig. 7-24. Marfan's disease in a 2-year-old girl. The bones are slender and of unusual length.

Genetic Data and Pathogenesis

Marfan's disease has been recognized in all races and has an equal instance in both sexes. Numerous pedigrees have been carefully analyzed and this study supports dominant transmission of the disorder. In one family some individuals have only minor involvement limited to ocular or morphologic anomalies. An estimation of the incidence of mutation is highly difficult, but there is an elevation of paternal age, in some isolated instances (Murdoch et al.).

Pathogenesis has been repeatedly discussed, but is not yet fully understood. The histologic lesions of the aortic media initially suggested that the primary anomaly might be one of the elastic fibers. The fully maintained normal characteristics of these, however, in a number of tissues such as the trachea or the intervertebral disks (Roark), together with the observation that the suspending ligaments of the lens do not contain elastic fibers, are strong arguments against this theory.

A primary pathology of collagen fibers, due to synthesis of an abnormal constituent, is presently the favored hypothesis. The fact of a dominant transmission would seem to exclude an enzymetic defect as proposed by some authors (Nenci and Beltrami). Such a primary involvement could explain the aortic lesion; on the other hand analogies between Marfan's disease and experimental lathyrism in the rat are well known. The latter condition leads to kyphoscoliosis and aortic aneurysm by way of a direct action of amino-nitriles on aggregates of collagen fibers (Gross). Studies by Laitinen even suggest that in Marfan's disease there is an acceleration of collagen metabolism demonstrated by an elevation of incorporation of radioactive proline and hydroxyproline into the skin.

The presence of a metachromatic substance does not necessarily argue against this theory, since an increase of tissue-mucopolysaccharides has been recognized also in lathyrism. Still, by electron microscopy Bolande was unable to demonstrate structural anomalies of collagen fibers. In addition, there is still no explanation of the abnormal bony growth. It is not excluded that a reduction of tension of the periosteum might have an effect on bone growth as was experimentally the result of partial removal (Lacroix).

Clinical Types and Diagnosis

Several authors, especially Grenier, have emphasized the frequent association of contractures or muscular retractions in children with arachnodactyly (Fig. 7-25). This finding can be present from birth and by preference involves the elbows, the knees and the fingers, which may be in constant flexion. The facial expression of these individuals can be somewhat unusual with a small open mouth, micrognathia, and a deformed antihelix. Transmission is dominant. Sometimes these patients have a kyphoscoliosis. Ocular findings, however, seem to be always lacking, just as cardiac changes, so that this association probably represents a somewhat different disorder from Marfan's disease. For this reason the term arachnodactyly with congenital contractures has been proposed (Beals and Hecht).

Marfan's disease, furthermore, should not be confused with homocystinuria (see p. 315). If there is mental retardation this will help in the diagnostic approach and chromotography of urinary amino acids will bring full confirmation of this diagnosis.

Confusion is also possible with the syndrome of pheochromecytoma, thyroid carcinoma and multiple

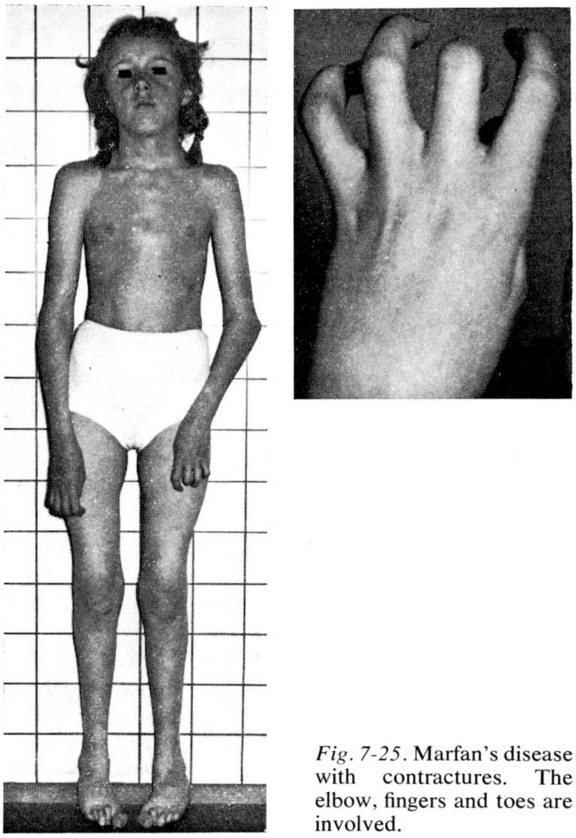

Fig. 7-25. Marfan's disease with contractures. The elbow, fingers and toes are involved.

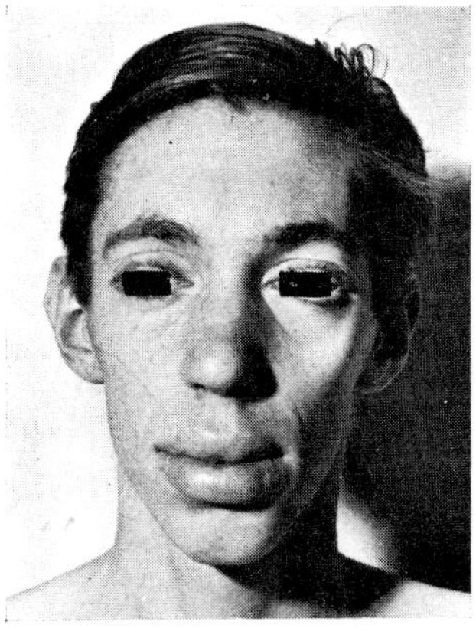

Fig. 7-26. Syndrome of pheochromocytoma, thyroid carcinoma and multiple neuromas. Typical facial appearance with prominent lips. (Courtesy of M. Lévi)

neuromas (Levy et al.). The disease can be recognized by the peculiar facial aspect with thick heavy lips, and by multiple neuromas electively located on the lips and the anterior portion of the tongue (Fig. 7-26). Early diagnosis is critical because of the coincidental or later presence of thyroid carcinoma and pheochromocytoma, which must be treated as rapidly as possible.

The most difficult problem in differential diagnosis exists in children, where height appearance and arachnodactyly suggest a possibility of Marfan's disease. There are no signs of ocular or cardiac involvement. In the absence of such findings, it is strictly impossible to predict whether these changes may not appear later. Careful supervision of such patients is mandatory, because their incidence is by no means rare.

Treatment

In children and during adolescence all possible measures directed against the thoracic and spinal deformity should be offered to affected patients. Physiotherapy and, whenever necessary, surgical fusion should be properly timed. Protrusio acetabuli can offer considerable orthopaedic problems. The idea of advancing puberty has been entertained, especially in girls with excessive growth. This approach, giving estrogen and methroxyprogesterone (Depoprovera), might possibly stop the evolution of severe types of scoliosis (McKusick). Surgical intervention to prevent the complete dislocation of the lens might be necessary, together with regular careful follow-up of the intraocular pressure.

We review here some of the therapeutic measures attempted to prevent rupture of a dissecting aneurysm. Besides vascular surgery, vascular homotransplants, or aortic prosthesis, there has been the proposal to use drugs to reduce the contractibility of the myocardium, especially propanolol (Halpern et al.). Reserpin seems to have a beneficial effect. Operative risks mentioned earlier must always be remembered if a surgical intervention is attempted in an individual suffering from Marfan's disease.

CEREBRAL GIGANTISM

Brief mention should be given to this syndrome described by Sotos et al. Besides the unusual size of such infants, there is an advanced bone age parallel to the height age. There are however no skeletal malformations. The craniofacial appearance is unusual with a voluminous skull, marked frontal bossing and a very prominent brow ridge. Frequently there is also hypertelorism with slightly slanted palpebral fissures laterally and also a slight degree of prognathism (Fig. 7-27).

Radiologic study will demonstrate the excessive size of the skull and the somewhat oversized mandible. The orbital roof is in a high position and the dorsum

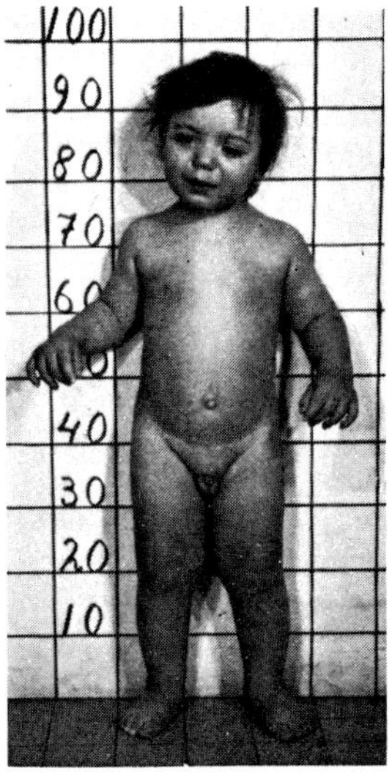

Fig. 7-27. Cerebral gigantism. (Courtesy of R. Rappaport)

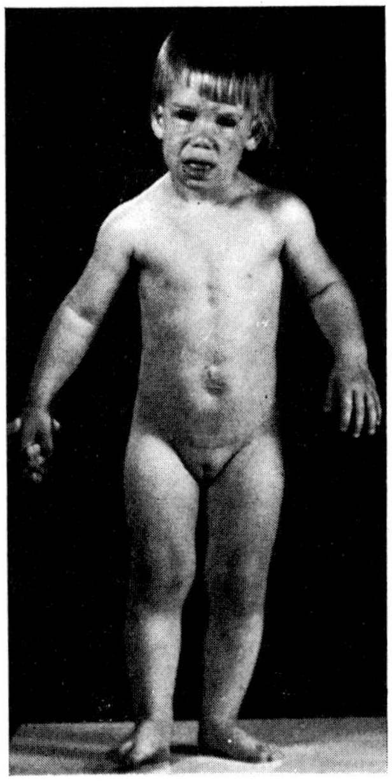

Fig. 7-28. Beckwith-Wiedemann syndrome. (Courtesy of H. R. Wiedemann)

sellae often inclined posteriorly. The sutures may be wide with persistence of wormian bones in the anterior fontanelle (Poznanski and Stevenson). Syndactyly (Mikulowski, Guihard) and vertebral anomalies – vertebra-plana, anterior hypoplasia of a vertebral body –

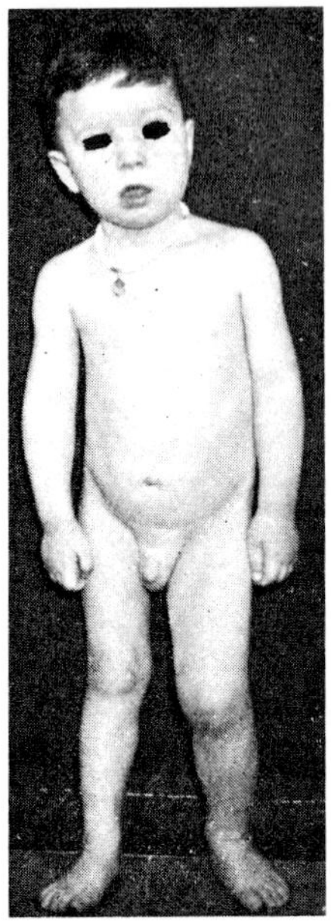

Fig. 7-29. Hemihypertrophy. (Taken from: Pédiatrie, CMC, Flammarion)

have also been seen. The bone age corresponds to the height age. Encephalopathy and mental retardation, often of severe degree, accompany gigantism. Several familial cases would seem to suggest the possibility of a genetic factor at the base of this syndrome. Its pathophysiology is completely unknown. The possibility of a growth factor so far unidentified could be entertained.

THE BECKWITH-WIEDEMANN SYNDROME

This disorder is also characterized by gigantism, which does not always seem to be present at birth, but may become evident during the first months of life. The syndrome combines macroglossia, and an omphalocele or umbilical hernia with visceromegaly. Frequently there is also an additional facial naevus flammeus, a groove of the earlobe and also microcephaly (Fig. 7-28). An abnormal glucose metabolism is frequently found, especially severe hypoglycemia in the young infant. Eventually there is a high risk of these patients developing intraabdominal neoplasia, especially Wilms tumor, and hepatoblastoma or adrenal carcinoma.

Radiologically, microcephaly is combined with an occipital prominence, an increased mandibular angle and prognathism. A mild spurlike deformity of the lumbar vertebrae seems to be frequently present (Lee). Besides the advanced bone age, and sometimes hemihypertrophy, we note a mild degree of abnormal metaphyseal modelling of the long bones. This finding may persist in the proximal humerus. The hands may be short with cone-shaped phalangeal epiphyses.

The mode of transmission of the Beckwith-Wiedemann syndrome is still under discussion (a dominant gene with a variable expressivity or a recessive gene?).

Cytomegaly and other cellular anomalies have been described in many tissues—gonades, adrenal cortex, renal cortex—but the exact nature of the disorder is not known.

There are further syndromes with excessive growth. Among those we would like to refer to the syndrome of lipodystrophy of Beradinelli. In this disorder in bigger children there is a lipodystrophy with hyperlipemia and sometimes diabetes, in combination with accelerated growth and muscular hypertrophy. The hands may have a somewhat massive aspect and the feet may also be large. Radiologic study shows an advanced bone age, sometimes widened cortices, and a reduced medullary cavity.

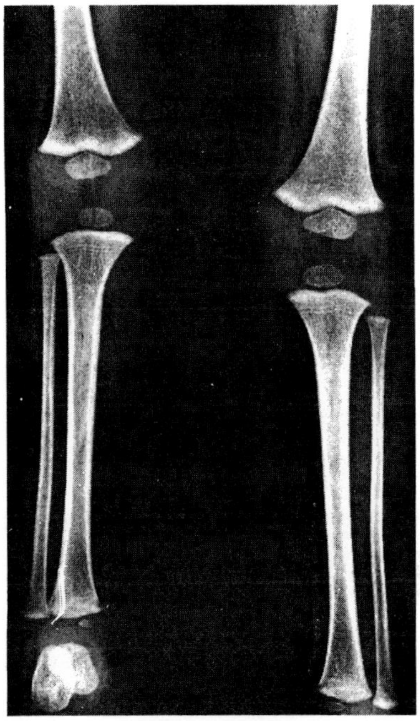

Fig. 7-30. Hemihypertrophy. There is asymmetry of the long bones and epiphyses.

HEMIHYPERTROPHY

This unusual anomaly is defined as hypertrophy of one half of the body. This may be clinically evident in the first months of life, but may go unnoticed until late in the first year, when the patient starts to walk. An uneven size of the legs may then be noted.

The hypertrophy is particularly marked if one compares the size of the leg, but the difference in length is usually moderate, within 2 to 5 cm. The diameter of the different segments is also increased. Hemihypertrophy also affects the arms, the trunk, the abdomen and sometimes the external genital organs. In the face there may be unilateral enlargement with hyperplasia of the external ear, sometimes of the tongue and the gingiva (Fig. 7-29). On the hypertrophied side there may be hypertrichosis, early eruption of teeth, teleangiectasias, café au lait spots and flat angiomas. The last three conditions need not be on the hypertrophied side.

Radiographic study reveals that the hypertrophy involves the skeleton to the same degree that it affects the soft tissues (Fig. 7-30). Length and width of the bone is increased. The epiphyses are larger and develop more rapidly. This also refers to the carpal and tarsal bones. There may, in addition, be several anomalies of the hands and feet: syndactyly, polydactyly, clinodactyly or brachydactyly and clubbed feet. Films of the skull and face can reveal local asymmetry, which may also affect the mandible. The spine frequently shows scoliotic changes, most frequently the result of an asymmetry of the pelvis. Hemihypertrophy of vertebrae has also been reported.

The reasons for hemihypertrophy are completely unknown. The frequent association with vascular anomalies could indicate a possible relationship with the Klippel-Trenaunay syndrome. These anomalies, however, are not limited to only one side of the body.

Some authors have reported the finding of chromosomal mosaics (Ellis, Ferrier, Hook), but this is far from a constant finding. Several familial observations are on record which would suggest a genetic factor.

Therapy to compensate for the difference in length, especially of the legs, may require surgical interventions. Repeatedly, the association of this condition with Wilms tumor has been reported. Intravenous urography should be performed whenever hemihypertrophy is discovered.

Before one can entertain the diagnosis of hemihypertrophy or other possible causes for asymmetric growth of the extremities, neurofibromatosis (see p. 323), congenital elefantiasis, the trophedema of Meige (which does not involve the skeleton), and the Klippel-Trenaunay syndrome must be ruled out.

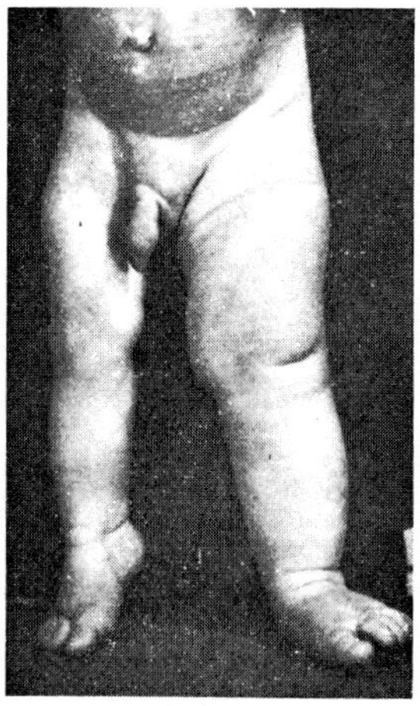

Fig. 7-31. Klippel-Trenaunay syndrome.

THE KLIPPEL-TRENAUNAY SYNDROME

This syndrome was described in 1900 and is characterized by hypertrophy of one extremity which results from vascular anomalies presenting also as a cutaneous angioma or venous dilatation. This type of hypertrophy resulting from vascular anomalies was later described by Parkes-Weber in the English literature, so that both eponyms are used.

Clinically, abnormal developments and the size of the affected limbs may be recognized either from birth, or later. Most frequently one leg has an increased length and size (Fig. 7-31). Besides the hypertrophy there is a unilateral flat angioma of variable extent, which may reach the trunk, and varicose dilatations, sometimes already noted at birth.

Radiographic study will show that the hypertrophy involves the skeleton and the soft tissues. On the affected side there is an increased size and length of bones and the volume of the epiphyses is also larger than on the other side. The difference in length is variable and may increase during growth.

The Klippel-Trenaunay syndrome results from venous congenital anomalies blocking the return of blood (stenoses, agenesis, fibrous bands located most frequently in the popliteal fossa). Rarely, there is an arterio-venous fistula. Phlebography is an indispensable examination to evaluate this condition. This information should be obtained with the aim of removing the obstacle to the venous circulation. Successful management can stop the excessive growth of the lower extremity. It is necessary to attempt surgery early. Furthermore, one should compensate for the difference in length of both legs with an elevator shoe or surgical elongation of the healthy side. Osteotomy with reduction of the involved side can also be considered. Both of these surgical approaches may have to be combined.

The Klippel-Trenaunay syndrome must be clearly distinguished from varicose angiomatosis, which radiologically is recognizable only by the presence of phlebolithes, but never leads to hypertrophy of a limb.

REFERENCES

Dwarfism With Mental Retardation

Abraham (J. M.) et Russell (A.). De Lange syndrome. A study of nine examples. *Acta paediat. scand., 1968,* **57**, *339-353.*

Beck (B.). Familial occurrence of Cornelia de Lange's syndrome. *Acta paediat. Scand., 1974,* **63**, *225-231.*

Beratis (N. G.), Hsu (L. Y. F.) et Hirschhorn (K.). Familial de Lange syndrome. Report of three cases in a sibship. *Clin. Genet., 1971,* **2**, *170-176.*

Brandner (M.) et Saur (G.). Generalisierte Dysplasie der Epiphysen und metaphysäre Exostosen beim Rubinstein-Taybi-Syndrom. *Fortschr. Röntgenstr., 1972,* **117**, *317-323.*

Canlorbe (P.), Allaire (Y.) et Lelong (M.). Le léprechaunisme. Nouvelle observation et revue de la littérature. *Sem. Hôp. Paris, 1968,* **44**, *1074-1083.*

Coffin (G. S.), Siris (E.) et Wegienka (L. C.). Mental retardation with osteocartilaginous anomalies. *Amer. J. Dis. Child., 1966,* **112**, *205-213.*

Dallaire (L.). Syndrome of retardation with urogenital and skeletal anomalies (Smith-Lemli-Opitz syndrome) : clinical features and mode of inheritance. *J. med. Genet., 1969,* **6**, *113-120.*

Decobert (G.), Berranger (P. de) et Gillot (F.). Problèmes nosologiques posés par le syndrome de Cornelia de Lange. A propos de trois observations. *Ann. Pédiat., 1973,* **20**, *755-762.*

Donohue (W. L.) et Uchida (I.). Leprechaunism, a euphuism for a rare familial disorder. *J. Pediat., 1954,* **45**, *505-519.*

Filippi (G.). The Rubinstein-Taybi syndrome. Report of 7 cases. *Clin. Genet., 1972,* **3**, *303-318.*

Fitch (N.). A mutation in mice producing dwarfism, brachycephaly, cleft palate and micromelia. *J. Morph., 1961,* **109**, *141-149.*

Germain (M.). Le syndrome de Coffin. *Thèse Méd., Paris, 1972.*

Gross-Kieselstein (E.), Ben Galim (E.), Amir (N.) et Abrahamov (A.). Leprechaunism (Donohue's syndrome). *Amer. J. Dis. Child., 1973,* **126**, *500-503.*

Hariga (J.), Koulischer (L.) et Dantine (R.). Aberrations chromosomiques et syndrome de Cornelia de Lange (à propos d'une nouvelle observation clinique). *Presse méd., 1968,* **76**, *2107-2108.*

Hayem (F.), Boisse (J.), Réthoré (M. O.), Labrune (M.), Hambourg (M.) et Mozziconacci (P.). Le syndrome de Rubinstein-Taybi. Discussion des formes incomplètes et familiales. *Pédiatrie, 1970,* **25**, *89-102.*

Harper (R. G.), Orti (E.) et Baker (R. K.). Bird-headed dwarfs (Seckel's syndrome). *J. Pediat., 1967,* **70**, *799-804.*

JOB (J.-C.), ROSSIER (A.) et GRANDPREY (J. DE). Etudes sur les nanismes constitutionnels. II. Le syndrome de Rubinstein et Taybi. *Sem. Hôp. Paris, 1964,* **40,** *2826-2830.*

KALLO (A.), LAKATOS (I.) et SZIJARTO (L.). Leprechaunism (Donohue's syndrome). *J. Pediat., 1965,* **66,** *372-379.*

LANGE (C. DE). Sur un type nouveau de dégénération (Typus amstelodamensis). *Arch. Méd. Enf., 1933,* **36,** *713-719.*

LEE (F. A.) et KENNY (F. M.). Skeletal changes in the Cornelia de Lange syndrome. *Amer. J. Roentgenol., 1967,* **100,** *27-39.*

LEGRAND (J.) et MAURAT (J.-CL.). Contribution à l'étude du syndrome de Rubinstein-Taybi. A propos de deux nouvelles observations. *Arch. Ophtal. (Paris), 1973,* **33,** *641-656.*

LEVY-LEBLOND (E.), D'OELSNITZ (M.), VAILLANT (J.-M.) et MAROTEAUX (P.). Le syndrome de Rubinstein et Taybi (à propos de quatre observations). *Arch. franç. Pédiat., 1969,* **26,** *523-535.*

LIEBER (E.), GLASER (J. H.) et JHAVERI (R.). Brachmann - de Lange syndrome. Report ot two cases in a sibship. *Amer. J. Dis. Child., 1973,* **125,** *717-718.*

LOWRY (R. B.), MILLER (J. R.) et MACLEAN (J. R.). Micrognathia, polydactyly and cleft palate. *J. Pediat., 1968,* **72,** *859-861.*

MAROTEAUX (P.). Une observation du syndrome de Coffin. *Arch. franç. Pédiat., 1968,* **25,** *116-117.*

MARSHALL (R. E.), GRAHAM (C. B.), SCOTT (C. R.) et SMITH (D. W.). Syndrome of accelerated skeletal maturation and relative failure to thrive : a newly recognized clinical growth disorder. *J. Pediat., 1971,* **78,** *95-101.*

MCKUSICK (V. A.), MAHLOUDJI (M.), ABBOTT (M. R.), LINDENBERG (R.) et KEPAS (D.). Seckel's bird-headed dwarfism. *New Engl. J. Med., 1967,* **277,** *279-286.*

METZK (H.), LÄSSIG (W.) et KÖHLER (H.). Das Smith-Lemli-Opitz-Syndrom. *Pädiat. Pädol., 1972,* **7,** *259-266.*

NEVO (S.), BENDERLY (A.), LEVY (J.) et KATZNELSON (M. B. M.). Smith-Lemli-Opitz syndrom in an inbred family. *Amer. J. Dis. Child., 1972,* **124,** *431-433.*

PASHAYAN (H.), WHELAN (D.), GUTTMAN (S.) et FRASER (F. C.). Variability of the de Lange syndrome : report of 3 cases and genetic analysis of 54 families. *J. Pediat., 1969,* **75,** *853-858.*

PATTERSON (J. H.) et WATKINS (W. L.). Leprechaunism in a male infant. *J. Pediat., 1962,* **60,** *730-739.*

PATTERSON (J. H.). Presentation of a patient with leprechaunism. *Birth Defects, Original Article Series, 1969, V n° 4, 117-121.*

PROCOPIS (P. G.) et TURNER (B.). Mental retardation, abnormal fingers, and skeletal anomalies : Coffin's syndrome. *Amer. J. Dis. Child., 1972,* **124,** *258-261.*

PTACEK (L. J.), OPITZ (J. M.), SMITH (D. W.), GERRITSEN (T.) et WAISMAN (H. A.). The Cornelia de Lange syndrome. *J. Pediat., 1963,* **63,** *1000-1020.*

ROBINSON (C. D.), PERRY (L. W.), BARLEE (A.) et MELLA (G. W.). Smith-Lemli-Opitz syndrome with cardiovascular abnormality. *Pediatrics, 1971,* **47,** *844-847.*

RUBINSTEIN (J. H.) et TAYBI (H.). Broad thumbs and toes and facial abnormalities. A possible mental retardation syndrome. *Amer. J. Dis. Child., 1963,* **105,** *588-608.*

RUBINSTEIN (J. H.). The broad thumbs syndrome. Progress report 1968. *Birth Defects, Original Articles Series, 1969, V n° 2, 25-41.*

SAUK (J. J.), LITT (R.), ESPIRITU (C. E.) et DELANEY (J. R.). Case report familial bird-headed dwarfism (Seckel's syndrome). *J. med. Genet., 1973,* **10,** *196-198.*

SCHUMACHER (H.). Das Smith-Lemli-Opitz-Syndrom. *Z. Kinderheilk., 1969,* **105,** *88-98.*

SECKEL (H. P. G.). Bird-headed dwarfs : studies in developmental anthropology including human proportions. *Springfield, Ill., 1960, C. C. Thomas Publ., éd.*

SÉE (G.), DAYRA (J. Cl.), BRODIN (M.) et LLEWELLYN (D.). Syndrome de Cockayne et encéphalopathie évolutive. *Ann. Pédiat., 1974,* **21,** *215-221.*

SIMPSON (N. E.). The Rubinstein-Taybi syndrome : chromosomal studies. *Amer. J. hum. Genet., 1973,* **25,** *230-236.*

SMITH (D. W.), LEMLI (L.) et OPITZ (J. M.). A newly recognized syndrome of multiple congenital anomalies. *J. Pediat., 1964,* **64,** *210-217.*

SMITH (G. F.), JUSTICE (P.) et HSIA (D. Y. Y.). Blood enzymes in the de Lange syndrome. *J. med. Genet., 1972,* **9,** *172-173.*

SRSEN (S.). Smith-Lemli-Opitz syndrome : report of a new case and review of the literature. *Acta paediat. Acad. Sci. hung., 1972,* **13,** *301-308.*

STANESCU (V.), BONA (C.) et IONESCU (V.). Histochemical and cytoenzymological studies on the growing cartilage in de Lange syndrome. *Acta histochem., 1968,* **30,** *1-18.*

SUMMITT (R. L.) et FAVARA (B. E.). Leprechaunism (Donohue's syndrome) : A case report. *J. Pediat., 1969,* **74,** *601-610.*

TAYBI (H.) et RUBINSTEIN (J. H.). Broad thumbs and toes and unusual facial features. A probable mental retardation syndrome. *Amer. J. Roentgenol., 1965,* **93,** *362-366.*

VISVESHWARA (N.), RUDOLPH (N.) et DRAGUTSKY (D.). Syndrome of accelerated skeletal maturation in infancy, peculiar facies and multiple congenital anomalies. *J. Ped., 1974,* **84,** *553-556.*

WEISSENWASSER (W. H.), HALL (B. D.), DELAVAN (G. W.) et SMITH (D. W.). Coffin-Siris syndrome. *Amer. J. Dis. Child., 1973,* **125,** *838-847.*

WILSON (M. G.). Rubinstein-Taybi and D1 trisomy syndromes. *J. Pediat., 1968,* **73,** *404-408.*

Dwarfism Without Mental Retardation

BARTA (O.), BELLYEI (A.) et KRANICZ (J.). Ueber das Freeman-Sheldonsche Syndrom. *Arch. orthop. Unfall-Chir., 1973,* **75,** *69-75.*

BELLAFIORE (V.), GIUFFRE (L.) et SCIALFA (A.). La sindrome di Rothmund (studio istologico cutaneo-lenticolare e citogenetico). *Ann. Ottal., 1966,* **92,** *394-407.*

BLACK (J.). Low birth weight dwarfism. *Arch. Dis. Childh., 1961,* **36,** *633-644.*

BURIAN (F.). The « whistling face » characteristic in a compound cranio-facio-corporal syndrome. *Brit. J. plast. Surg., 1963,* **16,** *140-142.*

CURI (J. F. J.), VANUCCI (R. C.), GROSSMAN (H.) et NEW (M.). Elevated serum gonadotrophins in Silver's syndrome. *Amer. J. Dis. Child., 1967,* **114,** *658-661.*

DI MATTEO (J.), CANLORBE (P.), BERKMAN (M.), AUDOIN (J.) et BOUSQUET (O.). Syndrome de Werner ou progeria de l'adulte. Manifestations cardio-vasculaires. *Bull. Soc. méd. Hôp. Paris, 1967,* **118,** *477-490.*

FERRIER (P. E.) et FERRIER (S. A.). Silver's syndrome : report of a case with chromosomal and dermatoglyphic study. *J. Pediat., 1967,* **70**, *438-440.*

FITCH (N.) et PINSKY (L.). The lateral facial profile of the Silver-Russell dwarf. *J. Pediat., 1972,* **80**, *827-829.*

FREEMAN (E. A.) et SHELDON (J. H.). Cranio-carpotarsal dystrophy. An undescribed congenital malformation. *Arch. Dis. Childh., 1938,* **13**, *277-283.*

FULEIHAN (D. S.), DER KALOUSTIAN (V. M.) et NAJJAR (S. S.). The Russell-Silver syndrome : report of three siblings. *J. Pediat., 1971,* **78**, *654-657.*

GAREIS (F. J.), SMITH (D. W.) et SUMMITT (R. L.). The Russell-Silver syndrome with asymmetry. *J. Pediat., 1971,* **79**, *775-781.*

GERMAN (J.). Bloom's syndrome. I. Genetical and clinical observations in the first twenty-seven patients. *Amer. J. hum. Genet., 1969,* **21**, *196-227.*

JACQUEMAIN (B.). Die angeborene Windmühlenflugelstellung als erbliche Kombinationsmissbildung. *Z. Orthop., 1966,* **102**, *146-154.*

KIRCHNER (M.) et HESSE (V.). Beitrag zum Bloom-syndrom. *Hum. Genet., 1972,* **15**, *25-32.*

MARGOLIN (F. R.) et STEINBACH (H. L.). Progeria. Hutchinson-Gilford syndrome. *Amer. J. Roentgenol., 1968,* **103**, *173-178.*

MAURER (R. M.) et LANGFORD (O. L.). Rothmund's syndrome. A cause of resorption of phalangeal tufts and dystrophic calcification. *Radiology, 1967,* **89**, *706-708.*

MC DOWELL et SPROLES (T.). The Russel-Silver Syndrome. *Amer. J. Dis. Child., 1973,* **126**, *794-796.*

MOSELEY (J. E.), MOLOSHOK (R. E.) et FREIBERGER (R. H.). The silver syndrome : congenital asymmetry, short stature and variations in sexual development. *Amer. J. Roentgenol., 1966,* **97**, *74-81.*

OZONOFF (M. B.) et CLEMETT (A. R.). Progressive osteolysis in progeria. *Amer. J. Roentgenol., 1967,* **100**, *75-79.*

PFEIFFER (R. A.) et AMMERMANN (M.). Das Syndrom von Freeman und Sheldon. 3 neue Beobachtungen. *Z. Kinderheilk., 1972,* **112**, *43-53.*

REICHEL (W.), BAILEY II (J. A.), ZIGEL (S.), GARCIA-BUNUEL (R.) et KNOX (G.). Radiological findings in progeria. *J. amer. Geriat. Soc., 1971,* **19**, *657-674.*

RIGGS (W., Jr.) et SEIBERT (J.). Cockayne's syndrome. Roentgen findings. *Amer. J. Roentgenol., 1972,* **116**, *623-633.*

RIMOIN (D. L.). The Silver syndrome in twins. *Birth Defects, Original Article Series, 1969,* III *n° 2, 183-197.*

ROSEN (R. S.), CIMINI (R.) et COBLENTZ (D.). Werner's syndrome. *Brit. J. Radiol., 1970,* **43**, *193-198.*

ROSSIER (A.) et JOB (J. C.). Etudes sur les nanismes constitutionnels. I. Le nanisme congénital : syndrome de Russell, syndrome de Silver. *Sem. Hôp. Paris, 1964,* **40**, *2819-2825.*

ROSSIER (A.) et PINAUD (M. F.). Le nanisme intra-utérin idiopathique. *Sem. Hôp. Paris, 1967,* **43**, *2399-2404.*

RUSSELL (A.). A syndrome of « intra-uterine » dwarfism recognizable at birth with cranio-facial dysostosis, disproportionately short arms, and other anomalies (5 examples). *Proc. roy. Soc. Med., 1954,* **47**, *1040-1044.*

SCHUMACHER (K.), RODERMUND (O. E.) et DOEPFMER (R.). Das Werner-syndrom. Beitrag zur Symptomatologie und Ätiologie. *Arch. klin. Med., 1969,* **216**, *116-147.*

SCHWARZ (E.). Roentgen findings in progeria. *Radiology, 1962,* **79**, *411-414.*

SILVER (H. K.), KIYASU (W.), GEORGE (J.) et DEAMER (W. C.). Syndrome of congenital hemihypertrophy, shortness of stature and elevated urinary gonadotropins. *Pediatrics, 1953,* **12**, *368-376.*

SILVER (H. K.). Asymmetry, short stature, and variations in sexual development. A syndrome of congenital malformations. *Amer. J. Dis. Child., 1964,* **107**, *495-515.*

SILVER (H. K.). Rothmund-Thomson. An oculo-cutaneous disorder. *Amer. J. Dis. Child., 1966,* **111**, *182-190.*

SIZONENKO (P.), JOB (J. C.), KREISLER (L.) et ROSSIER (A.). Etudes sur les nanismes constitutionnels. III. Nanisme intra-utérin avec érythème télangiectasique et anomalies chromosomiques : syndrome de Bloom. *Sem. Hôp. Paris, 1967,* **43**, *2404-2411.*

SZALAY (G. C.). Pseudohydrocephalus in dwarfs : the Russell dwarf. *J. Pediat., 1963,* **63**, *622-633.*

SZALAY (G. C.). Intra-uterine growth retardation versus Silver's syndrome. *J. Pediat., 1964,* **64**, *234-240.*

SZALAY (G. C.). Russell dwarf versus Silver syndrome. *J. Pediat., 1972,* **80**, *1066-1068.*

TAYLOR (W. B.). Rothmund's syndrome, Thomson's syndrome : congenital poikeiloderma with or without juvenile cataracts : a review of the literature. Report of a case and discussion of the relationship of the two syndromes. *Arch. Derm., 1963,* **75**, *236-244.*

VILLEE (D. B.), NICHOLS (G.) et TALBOT (N. R.). Metabolic studies in two boys with classical progeria. *Pediatrics, 1969,* **43**, *207-216.*

WALBAUM (R.), LEJEUNE (M.), POUPARD (B.), LACHERETZ (M.) et FONTAINE (G.). Le syndrome de Freeman-Sheldon (syndrome du siffleur). *Ann. Pédiat., 1973,* **20**, *357-364.*

WEINSTEIN (S.) et GORLIN (R. J.). Cranio-carpo-tarsal dysplasia or the whistling face syndrome. I. Clinical considerations. *Amer. J. Dis. Child., 1969,* **117**, *427-433.*

WIEDEMANN (H. R.). Ueber einige progeroide Krankheitsbilder und deren diagnostiche Einordnung. *Z. Kinderheilk., 1969,* **107**, *91-106.*

ZUCKER-FRANKLIN (D.), RIFKIN (H.) et JACOBSON (H. G.). Werner's syndrome. An analysis of ten cases. *Geriatrics, 1968,* **23**, *123-135.*

Weill-Marchesani Syndrome. Osteodysplastic Gerodermia. Oto-palato-digital Syndrome. Larsen Syndrome. Ehlers-Danlos Syndrome

AASE (J. M.). Oto-palato-digital syndrome. *Birth Defects, Original Article Series, 1969,* V *n° 3, 43-44.*

BAMATTER (F.), FRANCESCHETTI (A.), KLEIN (D.) et SIERRO (A.). Gérodermie ostéodysplasique héréditaire. Un nouveau biotype de la « progeria ». *Ann. Paediat. (Basel), 1950,* **174**, *126-127.*

BEIGHTON (P.) et HORAN (F.). Orthopaedic aspects of the Ehlers-Danlos syndrome. *J. Bone Jt Surg., 1969,* **51-B**, *444-453.*

BROCHER (J. E. W.), KLEIN (D.), BAMATTER (F.), FRANCESCHETTI (A.) et BOREUX (G.). Röntgenologische Befunde bei Geroderma osteodysplastica hereditaria. *Fortschr. Röntgenstr., 1968,* **109**, *185-198.*

COVENTRY (M. B.). Some skeletal changes in the Ehlers-Danlos syndrome. *J. Bone Jt Surg., 1961,* **43-A**, *855-860.*

DESBUQUOIS (G.), GRENIER (B.), MICHEL (J.) et ROSSIGNOL (C.). Nanisme chondrodystrophique avec ossification anarchique et polymalformations chez deux sœurs. *Arch. franç. Pédiat., 1966,* **23**, *573-587.*

DUDDING (B. A.), GORLIN (R. J.) et LANGER (L. O.). The oto-palato-digital syndrome. A new symptom-complex consisting of deafness, dwarfism, cleft palate, characteristic facies, and a generalized bone dysplasia. *Amer. J. Dis. Child., 1967,* **113**, *214-221.*

FEILER-OFRY (V.), STEIN (R.) et GODEL (V.). Marchesani's syndrome and chamber angle anomalies. *Amer. J. Ophthal., 1968,* **65**, *862-866.*

FEINBERG (S. B.). Congenital mesodermal dysmorphodystrophy. *Radiology, 1960,* **74**, *218-224.*

HEILMANN (K.), NEMETSCHEK (TH.) et VÖLKL (A.). Das Ehlers-Danlos-Syndrom aus morphologischer und chemischer Sicht. *Virchows Arch., Abt. A, 1971,* **354**, *268-284.*

KRANE (S.), PINNELL (S. R.) et ERBE (R. W.). Decreased lysyl-protocollagen-hydroxylase activity in fibroblasts from a family with a newly recognized disorder : hydroxylysine-deficient collagen *(abstract). J. clin. Invest., 1972,* **51**, *52a.*

LANGER (L. O., Jr.). The roentgenographic features of the oto-palato-digital (OPD) syndrome. *Amer. J. Roentgenol., 1967,* **100**, *63-70.*

LARSEN (L. J.), SCHOTTSTAEDT (E. R.) et BOST (F. C.). Multiple congenital dislocations associated with characteristic facial abnormality. *J. Pediat., 1950,* **37**, *574-581.*

LATTA (R. J.), GRAHAM (C. B.), AASE (J.), SCHAM (S.) et SMITH (D. W.). Larsen's syndrome : a skeletal dysplasia with multiple joint dislocations and unusual facies. *J. Pediat., 1971,* **78**, *291-298.*

MARCHESANI (O.). Brachydaktylie und angeborene Kugellinse als Systemerkrankung. *Klin. Mbl. Augenheilk., 1939,* **103**, *392-406.*

MCKUSICK (V.). Heritable disorders of connective tissue. *St Louis, 1966, C. V. Mosby Co., éd., p. 120.*

POZNANSKI (A. K.), MACPHERSON (R. I.), GORLIN (R. J.), GARN (S. M.), NAGY (J. M.), GALL (J. C., Jr.), STERN (A. M.) et DIJKMAN (D. J.). The hand in the oto-palato-digital syndrome. *Ann. Radiol., 1973,* **16**, *203-209.*

RENNERT (O. M.). The Marchesani syndrome. A brief review. *Amer. J. Dis. Child., 1969,* **117**, *703-705.*

SILVERMAN (F. N.). Larsen's syndrome : congenital dislocation of the knees and other joints, distinctive facies, and, frequently, cleft palate. *Ann. Radiol., 1972,* **15**, *297-328.*

STEEL (H. H.) et KOHL (E. J.). Multiple congenital dislocations associated with other skeletal anomalies (Larsen's syndrome) in three siblings. *J. Bone Jt Surg., 1972,* **54-A**, *75-82.*

SVANE (S.). Ehlers-Danlos syndrome. A case with some skeletal changes. *Acta orthop. scand., 1966,* **37**, *49-57.*

THIEMANN (H. H.). Zapfenepiphysen in Kombination mit Teilsymptomen des Marchesani-Syndroms. *Fortschr. Röntgenstr., 1960,* **93**, *367-370.*

WEILL (G.). Ectopie des cristallins et malformations générales. *Ann. Oculist. (Paris), 1932,* **169**, *21-44.*

ZABRISKIE (J.) et REIMAN (M.). Marchesani syndrome. *J. Pediat., 1958,* **52**, *158-169.*

Marfan's Disease

ACHARD (C.). Arachnodactylie. *Bull. Soc. méd. Hôp. Paris, 1902,* **19**, *834.*

BEALS (R. K.) et HECHT (F.). Congenital contractural arachnodactyly. A heritable disorder of connective tissue. *J. Bone Jt Surg., 1971,* **53-A**, *987-993.*

BOLANDE (R. P.). The nature of the connective tissue abiotrophy in the Marfan syndrome. *Lab. Invest., 1963,* **12**, *1087-1093.*

BOLANDE (R. P.) et TUCKER (A. S.). Pulmonary emphysema and other cardiorespiratory lesions as part of the Marfan's abiotrophy. *Pediatrics, 1964,* **33**, *356-366.*

FULEIHAN (F. J. D.), SUH (S. K.) et SHEPARD (R. H.). Some aspects of pulmonary function in the Marfan syndrome. *Bull. Johns-Hopk. Hosp., 1963,* **113**, *320-329.*

GRENIER (B.), LAUGIER (J.), SOUTOUL (J.) et DESBUQUOIS (G.). Maladie de Marfan et arthrogrypose. A propos d'un cas chez un nouveau-né. *Ann. Pédiat., 1969,* **45**, *182-186.*

GROSS (J.). An intermolecular defect of collagen in experimental lathyrism. *Biochim. biophys. Acta, 1963,* **71**, *250.*

HALPERN (B. L.), CHAR (F.), LAMONT MURDOCH (J.), HORTON (W. B.) et MCKUSICK (V. A.). A prospectus on the prevention of aortic rupture in the Marfan syndrome with data on survivorship without treatment. *Johns-Hopk. med. J., 1971,* **129**, *123-129.*

HELDRICH (F. J., Jr.) et WRIGHT (C. E.). Marfan's syndrome. Diagnosis in the neonate. *Amer. J. Dis. Child., 1967,* **114**, *419-423.*

JONES (C. R.), BERGMAN (M. W.), KITTNER (P. J.) et PIGMAN (W.). Urinary hydroxyproline excretion in Marfan's syndrome as compared with age matched controls. *Proc. Soc. exp. Biol. (N. Y.), 1964,* **116**, *931-933.*

LAITINEN (O.), UITTO (J.), IIVANAINEN (M.), HANNUKSELA (M.) et KIVIRIKKO (K. I.). Collagen metabolism of the skin in Marfan's syndrome. *Clin. chim. Acta, 1968,* **21**, *321-326.*

LACROIX (P.). L'organisation des os. *Paris, 1949, Masson, éd.*

LAMY (M.), JAMMET (M. L.) et DEJOULX (B.). La maladie de Marfan (dolichosténomélie). *Pédiatrie, 1964,* **19**, *61-70.*

LE COULANT (P.) et BROUSTET (A.). La maladie de Marfan. *In* « Maladies du tissu élastique cutané ». *Paris, 1968, Masson et Cie, éd., p. 265-280.*

LEEMING (J. T.) et MCKUSICK (V. A.). Serum seromucoide levels in the Marfan syndrome. *Bull. Johns-Hopk. Hosp., 1962,* **110**, *38-48.*

LÉVY (M.), HABIB (H.), LYON (G.), SCHWEISGUTH (O.), LEMERLE (J.) et ROYER (P.). Neuromatose et épithélioma à stroma amyloïde de la thyroïde chez l'enfant. *Arch. franç. Pédiat., 1970,* **27**, *561-583.*

LOWRY (R. B.) et GUICHON (V. C.). Congenital contractural arachnodactyly : a syndrome simulating Marfan's syndrome. *Canad. med. Ass. J., 1972,* **107**, *532-533.*

MACLEOD (P. M.) et FRASER (C.). Congenital contractural arachnodactyly. *Amer. J. Dis. Child., 1973,* **126**, *810-813.*

MARFAN (A. B.). Un cas de déformation congénitale des quatre membres, plus prononcée aux extrémités, caractérisée par l'allongement des os avec un certain degré d'amincissement. *Bull. Soc. méd. Hôp. Paris, 1896,* **13**, *220-226.*

MATALON (R.) et DORFMAN (A.). The accumulation of hyaluronic acid in cultured fibroblasts of the Marfan syndrome. *Biochem. biophys. Res. Commun., 1968,* **32**, *150-154.*

MORÈRE (P.), STAIN (J. P.), PARIS (P.), DORDAIN (M.), DUBOIS (T.) et BOQUET (J.). Les manifestations thoraco-pulmonaires de la maladie de Marfan. *Sem. Hôp. Paris, 1972,* **48**, *2807-2812.*

MCKUSICK (V. A.). The Marfan syndrome. *In* « Heritable disorders of connective tissue ». *4e édit., St. Louis, 1972, C. V. Mosby Co., éd., p. 61-223.*

MURDOCH (J. L.), WALKER (B. A.) et MCKUSICK (V. A.). Parental age effects on the occurrence of new mutations for the Marfan syndrome. *Ann. hum. Genet., 1972,* **35**, *331-336.*

NENCI (I.) et BELTRAMI (C. A.). Marfan's syndrome, a hereditary enzymopenia (letter). *Lancet, 1968,* **ii**, *1302.*

PRIEST (R. E.), MOINUDDIN (J. F.) et PRIEST (J. H.). Collagen of Marfan syndrome is abnormally soluble. *Nature, 1973,* **245**, *264-266.*

ROARK (J. W.). Marfan's syndrome; report of one case with autopsy, special histological study and review of the literature. *Arch. intern. Med., 1959,* **103**, *123-132.*

SINCLAIR (R. J. G.), KITCHIN (A. H.) et TURNER (R. W. D.). The Marfan syndrome. *Quart. J. Med., 1960,* **29**, *19-46.*

TORTOROLO (G.), ROMANO (C.) et SEGNI (G.). Mucopolisaccariduria e sindrome di Marfan. *Minerva pediat., 1965,* **17**, *1897-1903.*

Cerebral Gigantism. Beckwith-Widemann Syndrome. Hemi-hypertrophy. Klippel-Trénaunay Syndrome

BECKWITH (J. B.). Macroglossia, omphalocele, adrenal cytomegaly, gigantism, and hyperplastic visceromegaly. *Birth Defects, Original article series V, 1969, n° 2, 188-196.*

BERARDINELLI (W.). An undiagnosed endocrino-metabolic syndrome. Report of two cases. *J. clin. Endocr., 1954,* **14**, *193-204.*

COHEN (M. M., Jr.), GORLIN (R. J.), FEINGOLD (M.) et BENSEL (R. W. ten). The Beckwith-Wiedemann syndrome. Seven new cases. *Amer. J. Dis. Child., 1971,* **122**, *515-519.*

COSTIL (J.) et RICHARDET (J. M.). Le gigantisme cérébral. *Journées Parisiennes de Pédiatrie, Paris, 1973, Flammarion, éd., p. 321-334.*

ELLIS (J. R.). A girl with triploïd cells. *Nature (Lond.), 1963,* **198**, *411-413.*

FERRIER (D.). Congenital asymetry associated with diploid-triploid asymetry and large satellites. *Lancet, 1964,* **1**, *80-82.*

FRAUMENI (J. F.), GEISER (C. F.) et MANNING (M. D.). Wilms' tumor and congenital hemi-hypertrophy. Report of five new cases and review of literature. *Pediatrics, 1967,* **40**, *886-899.*

GOLD (R. H.) et STEINBACH (H. L.). Lipoatrophic diabetes mellitus (generalized lipodystrophy) : roentgen findings in two brothers with congenital disease. *Amer. J. Roentgenol., 1967,* **101**, *884-896.*

GUIHARD (J.), VELOT-LEROU (A.) et L'HIRONDEL (J.). Le gigantisme cérébral (observation de deux cas familiaux). *J. Méd. Caen, 1971,* **6**, *1-11.*

HENRY (M.), LOUIS (J. P.), HOEFFEL (J. C.) et PERNOT (C.). Hémihypertrophie congénitale associée à une anomalie des arcs aortiques et à diverses malformations squelettiques, cutanées, oculaires. *Ann. méd. Nancy, 1972,* **11**, *1111-1120.*

HOOFT (C.), BOEDTS (F.) et VAN ACKER (K.). Le syndrome de Wiedemann et Beckwith (omphalocèle, macroglossie, gigantisme). *Ann. Pédiat., 1969,* **16**, *49-55.*

HOOK (B. E.) et YONIS (J. J.). Congenital asymetry associated with trisomy 18 mosaicism. *Amer. J. Dis. Child., 1965,* **110**, *551-555.*

JAEKEN (J.), SCHUEREN-LODEWEYCKX (M. van der) et EECKELS (R.). Cerebral gigantism syndrome. A report of 4 cases and review of the literature. *Z. Kinderheilk., 1972,* **112**, *332-346.*

KLIPPEL (M.) et TRÉNAUNAY (P.). Du nævus variqueux ostéo-hypertrophique. *Arch. gén. Méd., 1900,* **77**, *641-672.*

LEE (F. A.). Radiology of the Beckwith-Wiedemann syndrome. *Radiol. Clin. N. Amer., 1972,* **10**, *261-276.*

LELONG (M.), CANLORBE (P.), MATHIEU (H.), BERKMANN et DROUET. Un cas d'hémi-hypertrophie congénitale avec anomalies du développement osseux. *Arch. franç. Pédiat., 1956,* **33**, *301-303.*

MARIE (J.), ROYER (P.), LEVÊQUE (B.), DEBAUCHEZ (C.) et RAPPAPORT (R.). Gigantisme avec encéphalopathie et dysmorphie cranio-faciale. *Ann. Pédiat., 1965,* **12**, *682-691.*

MCNAMARA (T. O.), GOODING (C. A.), KAPLAN (S. L.) et CLARK (R. E.). Exomphalos-macroglossia-gigantism (Visceromegaly) syndrome (the Beckwith-Wiedemann syndrome). *Amer. J. Roentgenol., 1972,* **114**, *264-267.*

MIKULOWSKI (W.), STOPYROWA (J.) et MEDVEY (K.). Gigantism and acromegaly in a six years old boy. *Endokr. pol., 1962,* **13**, *407-412.*

PARKES-WEBER (F.). Haemangiectasic hypertrophy of limbs. Congenital phlebarteriectasis and so-called congenital varicose veins. *Brit. J. Child. Dis., 1918,* **15**, *13-17.*

POZNANSKI (A. K.) et STEPHENSON (J. M.). Radiographic findings in hypothalamic acceleration of growth associated with cerebral atrophy and mental retardation (cerebral gigantism). *Radiology, 1967,* **88**, *446-456.*

RIET (F. M. S.). Association d'un gigantisme congénital (type Sotos) et d'une hémihypertrophie corporelle totale. *Thèse Méd., Paris, 1973.*

SEIP (M.) et TRYGSTAD (O.). Generalized lipodystrophy. *Arch. Dis. Child., 1963,* **38**, *447-453.*

SERVELLE (M.), CORNU (C.), LAURENS (P.), FORMAN (J.), BOUCHARD (F.) et THEPOT (Y.). L'hypertrophie veineuse des membres. *Sem. Hôp. Paris, 1960,* **36**, *2580-2586.*

SOTOS (J. F.), DODGE (P. R.), MUIRHEAD (D.), CRAWFORD (J. D.) et TALBOT (N. B.). Cerebral gigantism in childhood. A syndrome of excessively rapid growth with acromegalic features and non-progressive neurologic disorder. *New Engl. J. Med., 1964,* **271**, *109-116.*

WEILL (J.), BONNET (G.) et LEVEAU (H.). Syndrome de Klippel-Trenaunay. *Arch. franç. Pédiat., 1949,* **6**, *24-34.*

WIEDEMANN (H. R.). Complexe malformatif familial avec hernie ombilicale et macroglossie : Un syndrome nouveau ? *J. Génét. hum., 1964,* **13**, *223-232.*

WIEDEMANN (H. R.). Ueber das, « Kerbenohr » beim Exomphalos - Makroglossie - Gigantismus - Syndrom, Ohrläppchen-Fisteln und über das Vorkommen entsprechender Erschneinungen bei anderweitigen Syndromen sowie bei Gesunden. *Z. Kinderheilk., 1973,* **115**, *95-110.*

8 Chromosomal Aberrations

It is difficult to present a discussion of bony anomalies in chromosomal aberrations, since this list of disorders is still incomplete and under constant revision. Also, skeletal studies are often not systematically performed, especially when such patients die at a very early age. We can, therefore, only refer to the most important aberrations without attempting to describe their complete clinical or dermatoglyphic characteristics.

We will approach these disorders by first describing the chromosomal aberrations of the sex chromosomes X and Y followed by those of the autosomes.

ABERRATIONS OF THE SEX CHROMOSOMES

TURNER'S SYNDROME

The most frequently encountered caryotype in this disorder is a single X chromosome found among 45 chromsomes – 45X. There are a number of other aberrations capable of causing this syndrome which include mosaic 46XX-45X, isochromosome X, and partial deletion of the X chromosome. Some of these aberrations may result in a somewhat abnormal clinical appearance.

Besides a lack of development of secondary sexual characteristics, these patients have a markedly disturbed growth. There are several other malformations present in the Turner syndrome.

At birth these patients are small, and their definitive adult height is between 1.40 m and 1.50 m. They have a coarse and massive appearance with a wide shield-like thorax and widely spaced mamillae. A pterygium colli is often associated with a short neck and abnormal facial features: epicanthus, ratrognathism, low hairline and lowset ears. An increased carrying angle is typically noted. In the newborn period there may be edema of the back of the hands and feet combined with cutis laxa, which can be noted in about one third of all patients. This clinical picture has also been referred to as the Bonnevie-Ullrich syndrome.

Radiographically, the most characteristic skeletal findings are those of the knees, the wrists and the hands. The diameter of the proximal tibial epiphysis is reduced in its medial portion – Kosowicz sign, and the tibial plateau is concave medially and slightly slanted, overlapping the adjacent metaphysis. The latter is widened and poorly modeled. Quite frequently there is a tiny exostosis in exactly this location. We frequently note an asymmetry of the femoral condyles (Fig. 8-1). These findings, however, are not seen in young girls, since they are hardly ever present before the seventh year of life. The carpal bones are arranged in a gothic curve, because of the high position of the semilunar. The carpal angle formed by a tangent from the semilunar to the triquetrum and the tangent from the semilunar to the scaphoid is less than 130°, the normal. The distal end of the radius has a high degree of obliquity resulting, sometimes, in Madelung's deformity. The fourth, and sometimes the fifth, metacarpal are often characteristically short. This shortening may be minimal, and in some patients it is necessary to actually measure the corresponding phalanges to fully evaluate this sign. Normally the sum of the length of the ground and middle phalanx is equal to the length of the metacarpal. Here this value is much larger (Fig. 8-2). Occasionally, there is also some anomaly of the middle and end phalanx of the fifth finger. The foot may also show shortening of the fifth metatarsal. Patients with Turner's syndrome also have a significantly retarded bone age, especially after puberty. There may be a small sella turcica with prominent posterior clinoid processes and sometimes hypoplasia of the 1st cervical vertebra. The thoracolumbar vertebrae may have irregular endplates during growth. The skeletal elements may appear less dense than normally. There are no signs of a serious degree of osteoporosis or fractures. This increased radiolucency can be recognized in young patients. It is accompanied by a coarse trabecular pattern of the epiphyses, and sometimes by the

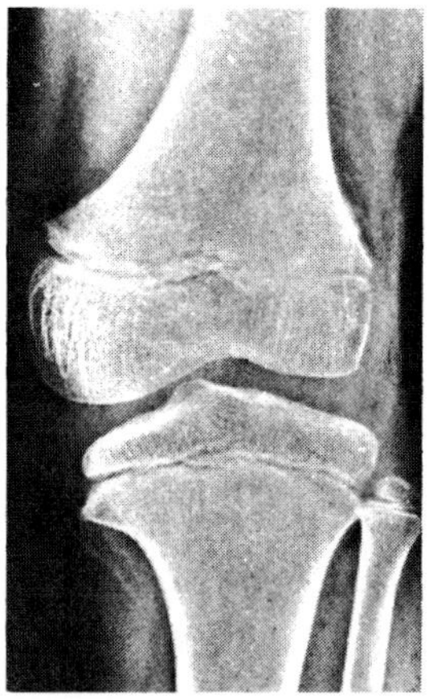

Fig. 8-1. Turner's syndrome at 9 years of age. There is partial collapse of the medial tibial plateau. (Courtesy of R. Rappaport)

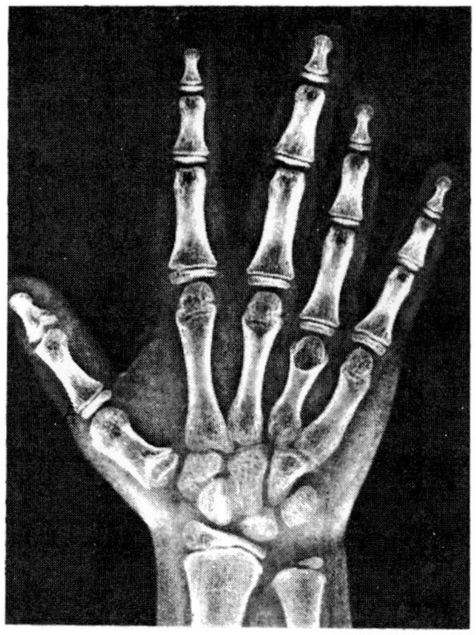

Fig. 8-2. Turner's syndrome in a 9-year-old girl. Note the prominence of the bony trabeculation of the carpus and the metacarpal epiphyses. Also to be noted is wedging of the epiphysis of the 1st metatarsal bone and the marked shortening of the 4th metacarpal. (Courtesy of R. Rappaport)

presence of small geodes. This aspect can be well recognized in the metacarpal epiphyses, and even the carpal bones. This finding seems to have considerable significance in establishing the diagnosis of the Turner syndrome (Fig. 8-2).

Histologic and histochemical study of the growth zone reveals significantly abnormal findings. The zones of basal cartilage and of serial cartilage are markedly reduced, with widely spaced cells within the matrix and within the columnar cartilage. They often have the tendency to cluster in islands. The hypertrophic cartilage is markedly developed, containing swollen cells. Enzymatic anomalies are present, together with alterations of the ground substance, especially the distribution of acid mucopolysaccharides (Stanescu).

These findings suggest that the hormonal deficit resulting from ovarian agenesis cannot alone be responsible for the ensuing growth disturbance. This could have been concluded from a careful radiologic study.

The phenotype of the Turner syndrome can also appear in boys or in girls with no recognizable anomaly of the X chromosome in Noonan's syndrome. The characteristic facial appearance, the pterygium colli and the increased carrying angle are present. Mental retardation is frequently noted. Noonan emphasizes the presence of a malformation of the pulmonary artery in such patients. Mental retardation is quite rare in Turner's syndrome. The same goes for the funnel chest. The incidence of genital anomalies is variable in boys as well as girls and fertility may be normal (Heller). Radiologic study may also show brachymetacarpy, osteoporosis and coarsely lacy bony structure. Some vertebral anomalies, for example, wedged vertebra, spina bifida are also on record.

The origin of this syndrome is still not understood. Some authors suggest a rearrangement of an X chromosome, which seems unlikely in view of the clinical findings (Summit) and also in view of the method of transmission, which seems to follow an autosomal dominant mode (Bolton).

THE KLINEFELTER SYNDROME

In this syndrome the most frequently noted caryotype comprises 47 chromosomes among which there are 2 X and 1 Y : 47 XXY. Still, as in Turner's syndrome, other chromosomal anomalies of the sex chromosomes can be found : 48 XXYY, 48 XXXY, 49 XXXYY, 49 XXXXY.

The diagnosis may be difficult to make before puberty. The only help may come from a careful study of the genital anomalies, cryptorchidism or hypospadias, which are found in association with a psychomotor retardation. The symptoms may justify the study of the caryotype. In the adolescent excessive height with underdeveloped musculature, or a tender skin, may be the result of an insufficient development of the sexual characteristics. Frequently there is also gynecomastia and the testicles are small and soft. One should not

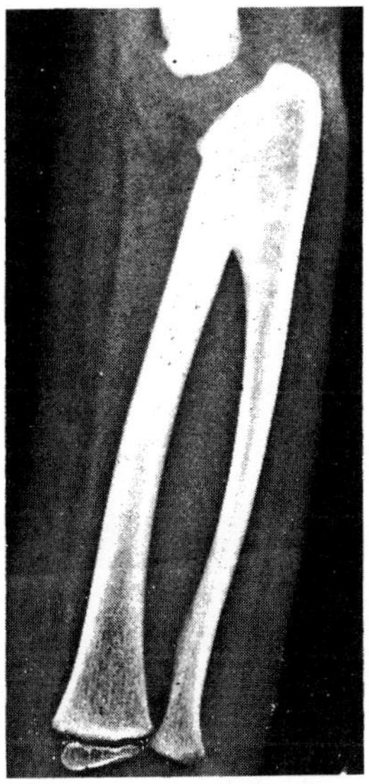

Fig. 8-3. XXXXY syndrome at 2½-years of age. Note the radio-ulnar synostosis. (Courtesy of M. O. Réthoré)

overlook that the clinical aspect may be quite variable and that not all affected patients are unusually tall.

Radiologically, there is no characteristic skeletal finding. Smallness of the sella turcica has sometimes been referred to. Shortening of the 4th metacarpal and a lack of modeling of several phalanges, which assume a somewhat trapezoid aspect, have occasionally been noted. Disappearance of the tuberculum of the distal phalanx leads to a pointed or square shape at its end, as reported by Ohsawa et al.

There are numerous other aberrations of the sex chromosomes, but they do not seem to have a clearly defined corresponding clinical expression. Still, we would like to insist on the high incidence of radio-ulnar synostosis in individuals who have an excessive amount of X chromsomes, especially patients with XXYY (Fig. 8-3). Some authors report a high incidence of epiphyseal involvement in the XXXY syndrome (Pajewski et al.). XYY men are often very tall. There may be an increased aggressivity. These patients often look somewhat like those with Marfan's disease.

AUTOSOMAL ANOMALIES

The most characteristic chromosomal aberrations involving autosomes are trisomies, the presence of three chromosomes of the same pair; deletions—lack

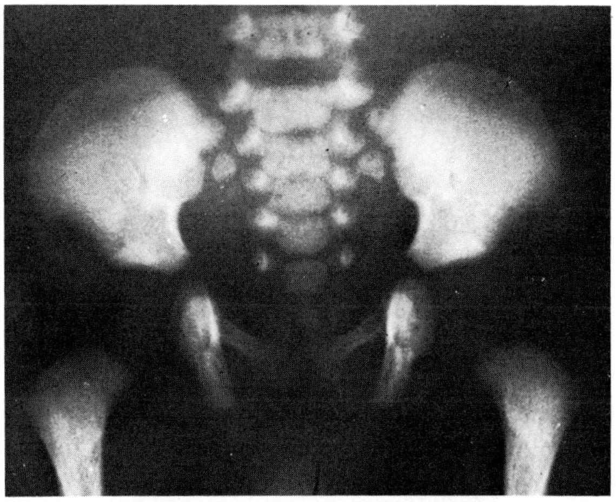

Fig. 8-4. Trisomy 21 in a newborn boy. Note the low acetabular and iliac angles with the low position of the anterior superior iliac spine. The iliac wings look like "elephant's ears." (Courtesy of H. J. Kaufmann)

of an autosome or of parts of a chromosome; and translocations—transfer of the portion of one chromosome onto a chromosome of another or of the same pair.

TRISOMY 21

By far the most frequently seen chromosomal aberration is trisomy 21 (mongolism).

Radiologically, the pelvic changes occur most frequently and have a characteristic appearance. They are, however, not constant, and Caffey, who has described them well, only noticed them in 13 out of 19 patients. The iliac wings are wide, sometimes comparable to an elephant's ear, and the roof of the acetabulum is horizontal. The acetabular angle formed by Hilgenreiner's line and the tangent through the acetabulum can be close to 4° during the first month of life, whereas the normal value at birth is 25°. The iliac angle formed by Hilgenreiner's line and the tangent through the anterior superior iliac spine and the lateral edge of the acetabulum is also low, with a mean of 45°, compared to the normal of 55° in the newborn (Fig. 8-4).

Skull films, besides occasionally revealing microcephaly, may show flattening of the occiput, an abnormal convexity of the frontal region (Roche et al.), and may also show persisting widening of sutures, especially of the metopic suture, sometimes beyond the tenth year. Pneumatization of the frontal sinus may be lacking.

The second phalanx of the 5th finger is often short and the distal phalanx occasionally widened. Currarino and Jary emphasize the high incidence of two ossification centers for the sternum. The bone age is as a rule retarded.

TRISOMY 13

This trisomy leads to severe anomalies recognized at birth, consisting of microcephaly, microphthalmia, bilateral harelip, anomalies of the external ear, hemangiomas. A constantly present polydactyly is accompanied by flexion deformity of the fingers and a "jumping" thumb. The feet show a "rocker bottom" anomaly. Mental retardation is always present and severe. Study of the brain frequently will reveal arhinencephaly. Many patients, in addition, have a heart lesion and numerous other visceral anomalies. A slowly downhill course with death around 3 months of age is the rule.

Radiologically, the skull is small with a low forehead, there are often increased convolutional markings, sometimes appearing like a lacunar skull. Frequently there is hypertelorism. The mandible is small. Skeletal maturation is always delayed. Study of the fingers is difficult, but does not seem to show anomalies of the bony elements other than the frequent polydactyly and a narrow aspect of the distal phalanges. The astragalus is frequently abnormally placed between calcaneus and cuboid, which results in the "rocker bottom" deformity. Malformed ribs and hypoplasia of the 1st pair as well as absence of the 11th and 12th rib are frequent findings. Ribs may appear like ribbons. An increased interpedicular distance of cervical vertebrae has been noted (James et al.).

TRISOMY 18

This type of trisomy is also clinically noted at birth. Some babies are underweight and show a small head with a prominent occiput. The external ears are obliquely oriented and have a triangular shape of the superior portion, which gives them the aspect of a faun. The mandible is hypoplastic, sometimes as in the Pierre Robin syndrome. The neck is short, the thorax small and protruding, the pelvis is narrow. The fingers are held in a flexed position and the abnormally long thumb is obliquely overlying the middle finger. Pes equino-varus is usually also noted. Severe mental retardation is always present as are, usually, heart lesions and other visceral anomalies. A progressive downhill course with death during the first trimester can be expected.

Radiographic study will reveal scaphocephaly with an occipital prominence and a narrow forehead, small orbits and a small mandible. The ribs are thin and poorly shaped. The sternum is short, and the clavicles are sometimes fragmented. Vertebral anomalies—hemivertebra, vertebral fusion—have been reported, together with an exaggerated rotation of the iliac wings resulting in an unusually narrow pelvis. The long bones are somewhat reduced in size and there is a severe retardation of bony maturation, sometimes evidenced by the total absence of ossification centers for several phalanges or the 1st metacarpal. The 1st phalanx of the big toe is often smaller than that of the 2nd toe.

TRISOMY 8

This more recently described trisomy involves mainly the skeleton and leads only to a mild degree of mental retardation.

Clinically, these patients have a large head with a prominent forehead and abnormal ears, a short neck. The trunk appears long and narrow and has a sternal depression. Rigidity of joints is regularly present, involving a number of joints of the extremities to a varying degree. The feet are in equino-varus and sometimes have flexion deformity of the big toe. Camptodactyly or clinodactyly may be present. The flexor creases are unusually deep. Height is normal.

Radiographically, there may be vertebral anomalies, such as wedged vertebra and widened posterior arches. Ribs are short and broad. A thirteenth pair is often noted. The iliac wings are narrow and the femoral neck is in valgus position (Fig. 8-5). The metacarpal and carpals can be plump.

There is also the possibility of only a partial trisomy 8. If there is trisomy of the long arm, the clinical picture is close to the one described, without joint involvement and with normal ribs. If there is trisomy of the short arm, there is microcephaly, and also articular, vertebral and costal involvement (Lejeune and Réthoré).

TRISOMY 9

Trisomy of the short arms of chromosome 9 (9p-) has been well defined by M. O. Réthoré et al. Such patients suffer from multiple malformations, combined with a severe degree of mental retardation. The clinical aspect is that of mild microcephaly with enophthalmus, a lateral slant of the palpebral fissures, hypertelorism, batears, a fleshy nose and drooping corners of the mouth. The most characteristic radiologic finding is marked shortening of the middle phalanx of several fingers. Sometimes there is also a smallness of the pelvis or of the patella.

CRI-DU-CHAT SYNDROME

Recognized by Lejeune et al., this disorder results from a partial deletion of the short arm of chromosome 5. It is usually recognized in somewhat underdeveloped babies, who also show psychomotor retardation. The craniofacial anomalies are quite characteristic. There is a round face, laterally slanting palpebral fissures and often significant hypertelorism and epicanthus. The chin is small and retracted. These patients always have a microcephalus and a very prominent forehead. The unusual whining cry of these babies has led to the name of this disorder.

Radiographic study will confirm the presence of microcephaly and hypertelorism. It will also show an increased iliac angle, whereas the acetabular angle remains normal. The iliac wings are poorly developed and almost rectangular. Bony maturation is not delayed and in some patients may even be advanced. Several authors have reported on the presence of supernumerary ribs or vertebrae.

In patients with deletion of the short arm of chromosome 4—Wolf-Hirschhorn syndrome—there are slender bones, narrow iliac wings and brachycephaly. Sometimes the forearm may be somewhat short and the distal phalanges may be poorly developed. Also there may be a scoliosis and premature fusion of sternal elements (Coffin).

The other autosomal lesions do not lead to significant skeletal anomalies. Supernumerary ribs have been noted in patients with deletions of long arms of chromosome 18 (18q-), and cebocephaly has been recorded in deletions of the short arms of the same chromosome (18p-). In the former disorder there may be long fingers and the 1st metacarpal can be short.

Under the name polydyspondyly, Turpin and Lejeune have described spinal anomalies accompanied by the translocation of a chromosome 13-15 to a chromosome 21-22. De Grouchy and Mlynarsky report on similar anomalies, but with a translocation between two chromosomes of the group 13-15. These alterations, however, have remained isolated, and it is still difficult to fully appreciate the role of translocations for the formation of skeletal lesions. Such skeletal involvement may be by the formation of cervical blockvertebrae or by the fusion of the posterior arches of two bodies—C_2C_3 or C_3C_4. Rachischisis and riblike deformity of apophyses have also been reported. A dorsal scoliosis is usually present, and hemivertebra formation is recorded in Turpin's case. The interpedicular distance of the 1st thoracic vertebra may be smaller than usual. Partial or total lumbalisation of S_1 has also been seen.

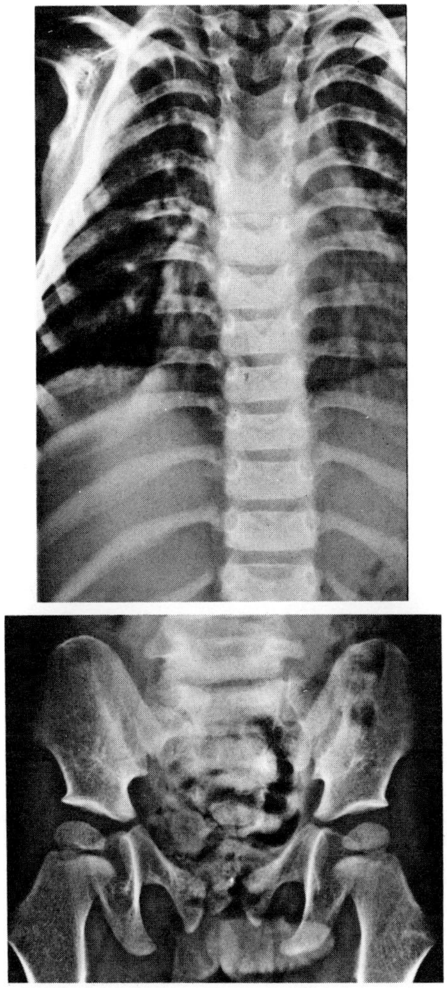

Fig. 8-5. Trisomy 8 in a 2½-year-old boy. Note the spinal anomalies of the cervical area and the extra thoracic vertebra. The ribs are broad and there is a 13th pair. (Courtesy of M. O. Réthoré)

Hemivertebrae, malformations of the ribs and dislocated hips, combined with anal atresia and the presence of a small extra chromosome, have been reported in the syndrome of coloboma. With the exception of trisomy 8 and polydyspondyly it is remarkable how little the skeleton is really affected in these chromosomal aberrations. In Turner's syndrome, and especially in newborns with trisomy 21, it is important to remember that radiographic study of skeletal elements can be very useful to confirm the diagnosis.

REFERENCES

BEALS (R. K.). Orthopaedic aspects of the XO (Turner's) syndrome. *Clin. Orthop., 1973,* **97**, *19-30.*

BOLTON (M. R.), PUGH (D. M.), MATTIOLI (L. F.), DUNN (M. I.) et SCHIMKE (N. R.). The Noonan syndrome : A family study. *Ann. intern. med., 1974,* **80**, *626-629.*

CASPERSSON (T.), LINDSTEN (J.), ZECH (L.), BUCKTON (K. E.) et PRICE (W. H.). Four patients with trisomy 8 identified by the fluorescence and Giemsa handing technique. *J. Med. Genet., 1972,* **9**, *1-7.*

CLEVELAND (W. W.), ARIAS (D.) et SMITH (G. F.). Radioulnar synostosis, behavioral disturbance, and XYY chromosomes. *J. Pediat., 1969,* **74**, *103-106.*

COFFIN (G. S.). A syndrome of retarded development. *Amer. J. Dis. Child., 1968,* **115**, *698-702.*

COFFIN (G. S.) et WILSON (M. G.). Wolf-Hirschhorn syndrome. *Amer. J. Dis. Child., 1971,* **121**, *265.*

COLLINS (E.) et TURNER (G.). The Noonan syndrome, a review of the clinical and genetic features of 27 cases. *J. Pediat., 1973,* **83**, *941-950.*

CURRARINO (G.) et GARY (E.). A developmental variant of ossification of the manubrium sterni in mongolism. *Radiology, 1964,* **82**, *916.*

GARN (S. M.), GALL (J. C., Jr.) et NAGY (J. M.). Brachymesophalangia-5 without cone-epiphysis mid-5 Down's syndrome. *Amer. J. phys. Anthrop., 1972,* **36**, *253-255.*

GERMAN (J.). Chromosomal breakage syndrome. *Birth Defects, Original Article Series, 1969,* V *n° 5, 117-131.*

GROUCHY (J. DE), LAMY (M.), THIEFFRY (S.), ARTHUIS (M.) et SALMON (CH.). Dysmorphie complexe avec oligophrénie : délétion des bras courts d'un chromosome 17-18. *C. R. Acad. Sci., 1963,* **256**, *1028-1029.*

GROUCHY (J. DE), MLYNARSKI (J.-C.), MAROTEAUX (P.), LAMY (M.), DESHAIES (G.), BENICHOU (C.) et SALMON (CH.). Syndrome polydysspondylique par translocation 14-15 et dyschondrostéose chez un même sujet. Ségrégation familiale. *C. R. Acad. Sci. (Paris), 1963,* **256**, *1614-1616.*

GROUCHY (J. DE), ROYER (P.), SALMON (CH.) et LAMY (M.). Délétion partielle des bras longs du chromosome 18. *Path. et Biol., 1964,* **12**, *579-582.*

GROUCHY (J. DE). The 18 p−, 18 q− and 18 r syndromes. *Birth Defects, Original Article Series, 1969,* V *n° 5, 74-87.*

HAMERTON (J. L.). Human cytogenetics. General cytogenetics. *2 vol., New York et London, 1971, Academic Press, éd.*

HELLER (R. H.). The Turner phenotype in the male. *J. Pediat., 1965,* **66**, *48-63.*

HIRSCHHORN (K.), COOPER (H. L.) et FIRSCHEIN (I. L.). Deletion of short arms of chromosome 4-5 in a child with defects of midline fusion. *Hum. Genet., 1965,* **1**, *479-482.*

JACOBSEN (P.), MIKKELSEN (M.) et ROSLEFF (F.). The trisomy 8 syndrome : report of two further cases. *Ann. Génét., 1974,* **17**, *87-94.*

JAMES (A. E., Jr.), BELCOURT (C. L.), ATKINS (L.) et JANOWER (M. L.). Trisomy 18. *Radiology, 1969,* **92**, *37-43.*

JAMES (A. E., Jr.), BELCOURT (C. L.), ATKINS (L.) et JANOWER (M. L.). Trisomy 13-15. *Radiology, 1969,* **92**, *44-49.*

JAMES (A. E., Jr.), ATKINS (L.), FEINGOLD (M.) et JANOWER (M. L.). The « cri du chat » syndrome. *Radiology, 1969,* **92**, *50-52.*

JANCU (J.). Radioulnar synostosis. A common occurrence in sex chromosomal abnormalities. *Amer. J. Dis. Child., 1971,* **122**, *10-11.*

KEATS (Th. E.) et BURNS (Th.). The radiologic manifestations of gonadal dysgenesis. *Radiol. clin. N. Amer., 1964* **II**, *2.*

KLINEFELTER (H. F., Jr.), REIFENSTEIN (E. C., Jr.) et ALBRIGHT (F.). Syndrome characterized by gynecomastia, aspermatogenesis whithout aleydigism and increased of follicules stimulating hormone. *J. clin. Endocr., 1942,* **2**, *615-627.*

KOSOWICZ (J.). Skeletal changes in Turner's syndrome and their significance in differential diagnosis. *Polish Med. Hist. Sci. Bull., 1959,* **2**, *n° 3-4, 23-26.*

LABRUNE-COGIS (M.). Contribution à l'étude des signes radiologiques osseux au cours des aberrations chromosomiques (à propos de 80 observations personnelles). *Thèse Méd., Paris, 1965.*

LAMY (M.). Le syndrome de Klinefelter de l'enfant. *Pathol. Biol, 1963,* **11**, *1301-1309.*

LEJEUNE (J.), GAUTIER (M.) et TURPIN (R.). Etude des chromosomes somatiques de neuf enfants mongoliens. *C. R. Acad. Sci. (Paris), 1959,* **248**, *1721-1722.*

LEJEUNE (J.), LAFOURCADE (J.), BERGER (R.) et RETHORÉ (M.-O.). Maladie du cri du chat et sa réciproque. *Ann. génét. Sem. Hôp., 1965,* **8**, *11-15.*

LEJEUNE (J.), BERGER (R.), LAFOURCADE (J.) et RETHORÉ (M.-O.). La délétion partielle du bras long du chromosome 18. Individualisation d'un nouvel état morbide. *Ann. génét., 1966,* **9**, *32-38.*

LEJEUNE (J.), DUTRILLAUX (B.), RETHORÉ (M.-O.), BERGER (R.), DEBRAY (H.), VÉRON (P.), GORCE (F.) et GROSSIORD (A.). Sur trois cas de trisomie C. *Ann. Génét., 1969,* **12**, *28-35.*

LEJEUNE (J.) et RETHORÉ (M.-O.). Trisomies of chromosome n° 8. *Nobel 23, Chromosome identification, 1973, 214-216.*

LEVY (E. P.), PASHAYAN (H.), FRASER (F. C.) et PINSKY (L.). XX and XY Turner phenotypes in a family. *Amer. J. Dis. Child., 1970,* **120**, *36-43.*

MALLET (R.) et LABRUNE (B.). Le mongolisme, trisomie 21. *Paris, 1967, J. B. Baillière et Fils, éd.*

MALPUECH (G.), DUTRILLAUX (B.), FONCK (Y.), GAULME (J.) et BOUCHE (B.). Trisomie 8 en mosaïque. *Arch. franç. Pédiat., 1972,* **29**, *853-859.*

MAMELLE (J. C.), DUTRUGE (J.) et GILLY (R.). Syndrome de Klinefelter. A propos de 18 cas. *Pédiatrie, 1972,* **27**, *851-876.*

MEYERSON (L.) et GWINUP (G.). Turner's syndrome in the male. *Arch. intern. Med., 1965,* **116**, *125-130.*

MLYNARSKI (J.-C.). Dyschondrostéose, polydysspondylie, aberration chromosomique par translocation 14/15, syndrome de Klippel-Trenaunay, et troubles mentaux chez un même sujet : transmission et ségrégation familiales. *Thèse Méd., Paris, 1963.*

NICOLINO (J.). Le squelette dans les dysgénésies gonadales. *Thèse Méd., Marseille, 1961.*

NIELSEN (J.), FRIEDRICH (U.), HÖLM (V.), PETERSEN (G. B.), STABELL (I.), SIMONSEN (H.) et JOHANSEN (K.). Turner-phenotype in males. *Clin. Genet., 1973,* **4**, *58-63.*

NOONAN (J. A.) et EHMKE (D. A.). Associated noncardiac malformations in children with congenital heart disease. *J. Pediat., 1963,* **63**, *468-470.*

OHSAWA (T.), FURUSE (M.), KIKUCHI (Y.), SUDA (Y.), TAMIYA (T.) et HIKITA (M.). Roentgenographic manifestations of Klinefelter's syndrome. *Amer. J. Roentgenol., 1971,* **112**, *178-184.*

PAJEWSKI (M.), SCHMIDT (R.) et ROSENBLATT (M.). Epiphyseal dysplasia a constant finding in the XXXXY syndrome. *The Annual leo G. Rigler Lecture, skeletal Radiogenetics, Tel Aviv, 1974.*

RÉTHORÉ (M.-O.), HŒHN (N.), ROTT (H. D.), COUTURIER (J.), DUTRILLAUX (D.) et LEJEUNE (J.). Analyse de la trisomie 9 p— par dénaturation ménagée. A propos d'un nouveau cas. *Humangenetik, 1973,* **18**, *129-138.*

ROSENBERG (D.) et TELL (G.). Syndrome de Turner à propos d'une statistique de 60 observations. *Pédiatrie, 1972,* **27**, *831-850.*

SAINT-ROME (G.), DAVIGNON (A.) et KRATZ (C.). A propos du syndrome de Noonan. Etude génétique et cardiologique de deux observations. *Un. méd. Can., 1970,* **99**, *1602-1613.*

SINGLETON (E. B.), ROSENBERG (H. S.) et YANG (S. J.). The radiographic manifestations of chromosomal abnormalities. *Radiol. clin. N. Amer., 1964,* **2**, *281-295.*

STANESCU (V.), PITIS (M.), IONESCU (V.) et BONA (C.). Histochemical and cytoenzymological studies on the growing cartilage in Turner's syndrom. *Acta histochem. (Jena), 1965,* **20**, *309-330.*

STOLL (Cl.), SACREZ (R.), WILLARD (D.) et FREYSZ (H.). Un cas de trisomie 18 avec aplasie bilatérale du radius et thrombopénie. *Pédiatrie, 1972,* **27**, *537-542.*

SUMMIT (R. L.). Noonan syndrome. *Birth Defects, Original Article Series, 1969,* V *n° 5, 39-41.*

TURNER (H. H.). A syndrome of infantilism, congenital webbed neck and cubitus valgus. *Endocrinology, 1938,* **23**, *566-574.*

WEBER (F. M.), DOOLEY (R. R.) et SPARKES (R. S.). Anal atresia, eye anomalies and an additional small abnormal acrocentric chromosome (47 XX, mart) : report of a case. *J. Pediat., 1970,* **76**, *594-597.*

WOLF (U.), REINWEIN (H.), PORSCH (R.) et coll. Defizienz an den kurzen Armen eines Chromosoms nr. 4. *Humangenetik, 1965,* **1**, *397-413.*

9 Hematologic Disorders

C. Fessard

This chapter offers a review of the skeletal manifestations of anemias, blood dyscrasias, reticuloses, and bleeding disorders.

ANEMIAS

We will review the congenital anemias and Fanconi's anemia. Other types do not have an effect on the skeleton.

THE HEMOLYTIC ANEMIAS

The incidence and severity of bony lesions is a direct expression of the time of onset, the intensity, and the chronicity of hemolysis. Most striking involvement can be expected during the course of hemoglobinopathies: thalassemia or hemoglobin A or C disease. Spherocytosis, however, will only lead to very mild skeletal changes. These anemias are hereditary disorders of either the hemoglobin or of the membrane of the erythrocytes. Hemoglobinopathies usually are transmitted as an autosomal recessive disorder, and the gene may manifest itself in heterozygotes. Defects of the membrane of erythrocytes are inherited as autosomal dominant disorders manifesting clinically as chronic normochromic anemia of variable severity, accompanied by mild icterus and sometimes severe splenomegaly. Usually there are also findings of an elevated reticulocyte count and the peripheral presence of erythroblasts.

These anemias result in a considerable hyperplasia of the erythropoetic bone marrow of a child in the majority of skeletal elements. This compensatory hyperplasia leads to an enlargement of the medullary cavity and an atrophy of the spongy bone and of cortical thickness. The bony changes are not always strictly parallel to the severity of the hematologic disorder and the involvement of the skull is not always in keeping with that of the rest of the skeleton.

Thalassemia

The main underlying anomaly is the presence of a high proportion of fetal hemoglobin. The aspect of the erythrocytes is that of "target cells." They have an increased resistance to hypotonic solutions. There is marked medullary hyperplasia. Homozygote patients show the most striking radiologic findings. Patients with the severe type of this disorder—Cooley's anemia—do not survive long. Heterozygotes, however, show far less severe chronic changes. These are seen most frequently.

Clinically these patients have a growth deficit and an abnormal facial appearance. Marked hypotelorism and prominent cheeks can give these patients a "mongoloid aspect." In some instances there is displacement of the upper incisors anteriorly, resulting in abnormal occlusion.

The radiologic changes of the skull and face are the most characteristic findings, developing fully during the second part of childhood (Fig. 9-1). The widening of the diploe has its onset in the frontal region and will subsequently extend to the rest of the cranial vault, with the exception, however, of the lower occipital squama. This progressive widening leads to a very thin external table and the reduction of the cortico-diploid ratio. The vault assumes a ground glass appearance. Bony trabeculation will develop perpendicular to the internal table radially, resulting in the classicial "hair on end" appearance. The facial bones are also involved. Medullary hyperplasia results in bony expansion and delayed pneumatization. Only the sphenoid sinus and the ethmoid cells are pneumatized. The long bones and the spine often are also involved to a variable degree. The long bones may be somewhat plump and poorly modeled, and the vertebral bodies may be slightly large. Usually there is delayed growth and maturation. Early and uneven fusion of epiphyses is present in about 15% of these patients. Osteoporosis is on the whole generalized, but of variable intensity with wide lacy trabeculation throughout the diaphyses. The cortex is thin as a result of massive internal resorp-

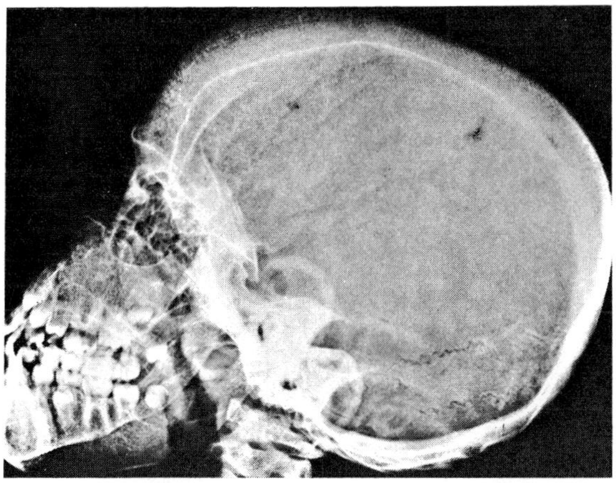

Fig. 9-1. Thalassemia with the characteristic skull and face changes in a young woman. (Courtesy of M. Laval-Jeantet)

tion. The remaining bony trabeculae appear thick, giving the spongiosa a more or less trabeculated aspect like a net, predominantly visible throughout the bones of the hands and feet (Fig. 9-2). In spite of this somewhat fragile appearance, there is no unusual incidence of pathological fractures or vertebral deformity.

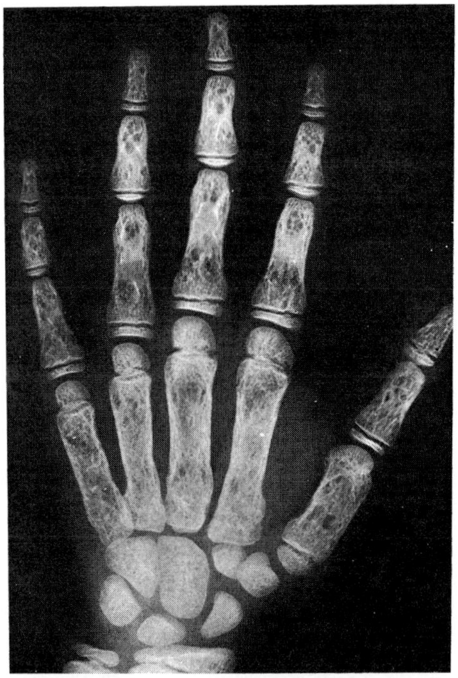

Fig. 9-2. Thalassemia in an 8-year-old boy. Note the lacy appearance of the bony structure. (Courtesy of M. Laval-Jeantet)

Sickle Cell Disease

Due to the presence of a significant amount of hemoglobin S, affected patients have a high incidence of hemolytic crises. Thrombotic visceral or bony involvement results in local pain and fever. Relative hypoxia is a precipitating factor, since this will bring about the unusual form of the red cells, the typical sickle cells. The ischemic foci are especially prone to local infection, which explains the high incidence of salmonella osteomyelitis. Homozygote patients show the most characteristic skeletal involvement at an early age, even during the first year. Heterozygote patients have only mild involvement, but if there is a combination of S and C hemoglobin—double hemoglobinopathy—there is considerable skeletal involvement.

During early infancy, after only a few months, the bones of the hands and feet may show these changes. Such infants suffer from acute local pain, edema and swelling, together with slight fever. Within 10 days there are radiologically recognizable bone changes, mainly affecting the metacarpals or metatarsals. The bone seems widened with a prominent medullary space, and there are periosteal oppositions masking an underlying bony destruction (Fig. 9-3). These lesions, on the whole, do not show progression. Eventually metaphyseal growth may be disturbed. The metaphyses can show cupping and adjacent triangular or conical epiphyses, occasionally with premature local fusion. The fingers may be short, thick and plump.

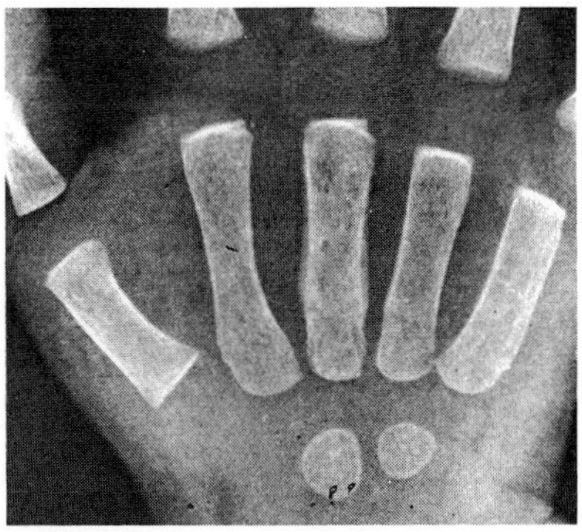

Fig. 9-3. Sickle cell disease in a 1-year-old boy. There is widening of the 3rd metacarpal and periosteal double contour. (Courtesy of J. Sauvegrain)

During later childhood the most characteristic

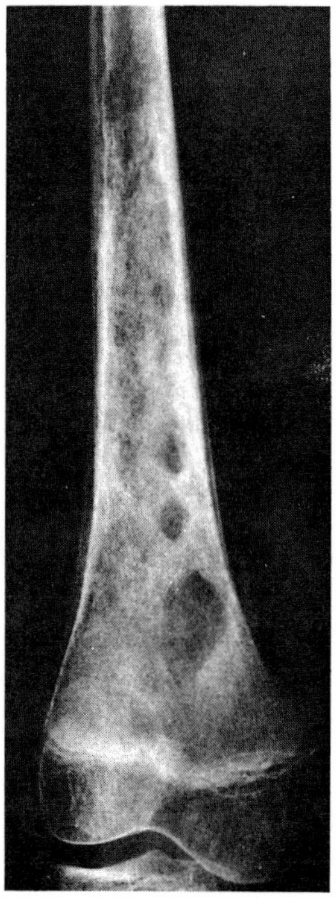

Fig. 9-4. Sickle cell disease in a 13-year-old boy. There is marked alteration of the bone structure, the cortex, and the periosteum of the femur. (Courtesy of P. Rigault)

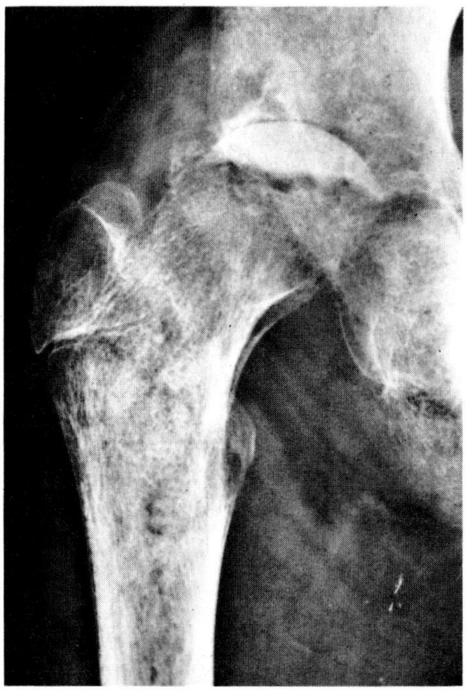

Fig. 9-5. Sickle cell disease in a 13-year-old boy. There is collapse and condensation—necrosis—of the femoral head. (Courtesy of P. Rigault)

changes are those of the long bones, especially of the humerus and femur, often in an asymmetrical arrangement. On the whole the joints are spared. Medullary hyperplasia will alter the form of the bones, as in thalassemia, and their structure will be osteoporotic. Flat bones, including the skull, are involved. Vertebrae can be abnormally shaped. Most frequently there is involvement of the lower thoracic region with biconcave vertebrae, loss of vertebral height and occasionally an increased transverse diameter. The aspect of severely involved vertebral bodies is sometimes referred to as fish vertebrae. Zones of ischemic necrosis, not always the result of vascular thrombosis, may be discovered during severe local pain, which is reminiscent of that experienced during osteomyelitis. Local areas surrounded by lytic lesions may soon be noted. Later there will be a sclerotic reaction surrounding these centers in a more or less regular fashion (Fig. 9-4). Eventually there may be generalized thickening of the trabeculae within this area. If there is superficial ischemia lamellar adjacent periosteal apposition can result in fusion with the cortex. A longitudinal radiolucent band may separate the two and lead to "bone in bone" appearance. Local swelling and severe pain are the clinical manifestations of such involvement of the more superficial parts of long and flat bones. In the older child ischemic necrosis will by preference involve the head of the femur and sometimes the head of the humerus in a ratio of about 6 to 1. The clinical appearance is that of Legg-Perthes-Calvé disease at a somewhat advanced stage, but the radiologic aspect differs, since the epiphyseal involvement is not uniform, but mono- or pluri-focal in the presence of a usually completely normal femoral neck. In the sub-chondral zone there may be very small lytic centers and marginal sclerosis. Deformity or even destruction of the femoral head can occur if weight bearing continues (Fig. 9-5).

Infection may occur in anyone of these ischemic zones, either periosteal, metaphyseal, or, as is most frequently the case, within the diaphysis. Most frequently situated distally in young infants, the location is quite variable later on. The causative microorganism is quite variable: staphylococcal or gram negative, or very often salmonella (other than Eberthella). Without antibiotic therapy there will be severe osteolysis and progressive periosteal reaction with ensuing sequestration and spontaneous fracture.

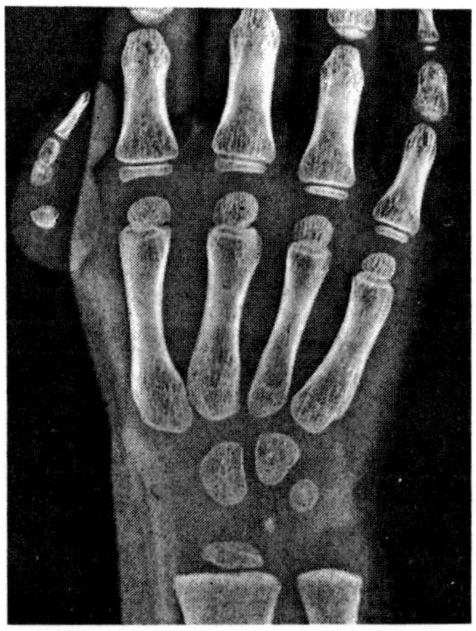

Fig. 9-6. Fanconi's anemia. Note the hypoplastic thumb. (Courtesy of M. Laval-Jeantet)

Spherocytosis of Minkowski-Chauffard

The erythrocytes assume a completely spherical appearance and have a markedly diminished resistance to hypotonic solutions. The most frequently involved regions of the skeleton are the skull and osteoporosis of long bones. Splenectomy leading to a very low subsequent rate of hemolysis without changing the basic hematologic criteria of this disorder also result in a marked reduction of the bony changes.

FANCONI'S ANEMIA

This is a severe type of hypoplastic anemia, which is refractory to therapy. Erythrocytes are involved only after granulocytes and megacaryocytes. This autosomal recessive disorder has an irregular manifestation electively in males.

Besides brownish pigmentation, patients have a growth deficit, microcephaly and anomalies of the bones of the hand or of the forearm. The latter are short, with valgus of the elbow and a laterally deviated hand. The thumb is hypoplastic or even absent. The little finger is short and curved. The involvement of the arm is quite variable and can be unilateral. In the most severe forms there is total absence of the radius and of the carpal ossification centers on the radial side. The ulna may be short and bowed, the phalanges of the thumb may be absent and the first metacarpal may be hypoplastic. The size of the second phalanx of the fifth finger may be small. Some patients have less skeletal involvement, such as hypoplasia of the phalanges of the thumb, the first metacarpals and of the distal radius (Fig. 9-6).

These malformations of the radius and fingers will allow recognition of this disorder in an involved family much before the hematologic problems become apparent, usually at the age of 5 to 7 years. The medullary hypoplasia may be recognized long before the peripheral cellular manifestations. Thrombocytopenia resulting from bone marrow failure and associated with malformations of the fingers and/or the radius also should support this diagnosis.

Other types of hypoplastic anemias such as the Blackfan-Diamond type usually are not associated with such bony anomalies. On the other hand, lack of formation of the radius has been described as part of the syndrome of amegacaryocytic thrombopenia, the syndrome of radius aplasia-thrombocytopenia.

OTHER ANEMIAS

Other anemias of long standing may also be accompanied by radiological signs. Thus, in fetomaternal incompatibility with fetal hemolysis the skeleton of an Rh positive baby born to a Rh negative previously sensitized mother can show transverse metaphyseal bands of increased radiolucency. These changes are bilateral and symmetrical and show up particularly well because of denser metaphyseal borders. Round bones and the epiphyses may show rings of increased density. These findings, however, are not specific for this disorder. They are simply the expression of a precocious interruption of ossification because of hemolytic interference. The density of the bones, where present, is entirely normal in relation to the age.

In babies suffering from nutritional hypochromic iron deficiency anemia, one can also see changes of the skull comparable to those already described. The face and long bones, however, are never involved. Possible associated findings because of coexisting rickets are entirely different.

Widening of the medullary cavity characteristically found in anemias does not occur, but can be recognized in another context. Singleton, for example, has described a syndrome showing this especially well in the area of metacarpals and phalanges in combination with aortic calcifications and abnormal dentition. An unusual facial appearance, hypotonia and anomalies of the skin—lentiginous lesions, psoriasis—seem to complete this syndrome (Brown et al.).

LEUCOSES AND RETICULOSES

The leucoses and Hodgkin's disease will be discussed, followed by histiocytosis and mastocytosis.

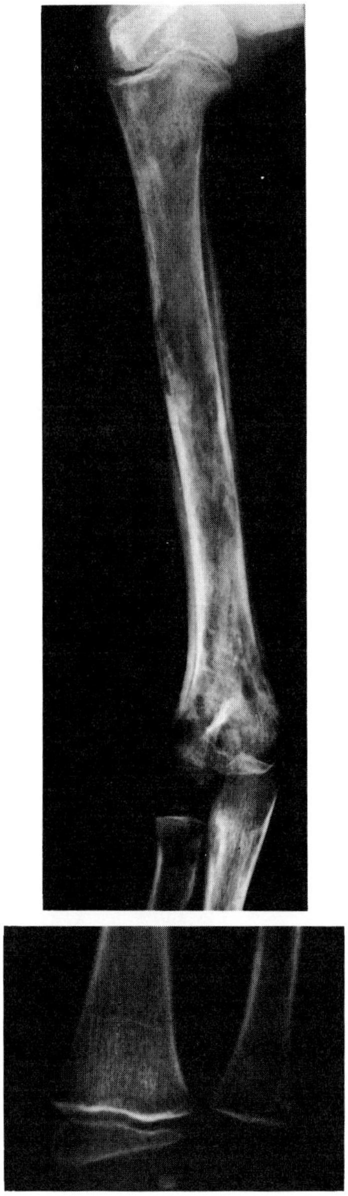

Fig. 9-7. Acute leukemia in a 5-year-old boy. Note the periosteal reaction *(top)* and the clear submetaphyseal band *(bottom)*.

THE LEUCOSES

Acute leukemia is the most frequently seen malignant disorder of the elements of the blood during childhood (95 per cent of all childhood leukemias), and its cellular characteristics are most often lymphoblastic. Bone marrow study, prior to the beginning of corticotherapy, is mandatory to fully establish this diagnosis. Invasion of the bone marrow by a significant number of young lymphoblastic or myeloblastic elements is adequate for the diagnosis, even though the peripheral blood may appear normal.

During the clinical course there are often bony and articular changes. Almost 25 per cent of all patients may initially present such changes.

Skeletal pain is mentioned in 60 per cent of all patients. The long bones are usually the seat of intensive pain, which may become even more severe with the progression of the disease. A decrease in pain is a good sign of effective therapy. The complete disappearance of these pains leads towards remission. If there is a recurrence it often happens in the exact same location. Such a recurrence may be strictly localized with intense local symptoms, so much so, that the diagnosis of an osteomyelitis or repeated strain is entertained. Clinical investigation will show palor, hepato- and splenomegaly, adenopathies and occasionally lesions of the buccal mucosa, strongly suggestive of the diagnosis. The severe local pain seems to be due to leukemic infiltration and cortico-subperiosteal involvement.

Arthralgias are seen somewhat less frequently than bone pain. One of several joints may be involved, often symmetrically. Rheumatoid arthritis can be simulated, especially since local inflammatory symptoms may be present and because of the usually febrile general condition.

Radiologic findings involving the skeleton are present in two out of three cases. They may be somewhat latent and only become manifest in the weeks and months after the clinical recognition of the disease. They affect zones of rapid growth. Four principal types of lesions can be distinguished: clean bands of increased lucency at the metaphyses, osteolytic foci, cortico-periosteal lesions and rarely osteosclerosis.

Clear radiolucent bands have the highest incidence and occur early, in about half of the cases. They are associated with other findings of bony involvement (Fig. 9-7). They reflect general metaphyseal involvement of the long bones and occur bilaterally and symmetrically. They are of variable thickness – 2 to 15 mm – and extend from one cortex to the other between the intact metaphyseal border and the zone of increased density on the diaphyseal side, where the spongiosa fades gradually. In flat bones, such as the ischium or the ilium, these clear bands extend alongside the cortex. They result from disturbed enchondral ossification, which produces a reduced number of abnormally fine trabeculations while the growth in length of the bone progresses actively. In addition, there is bony atrophy because of pressure from the prolifer-

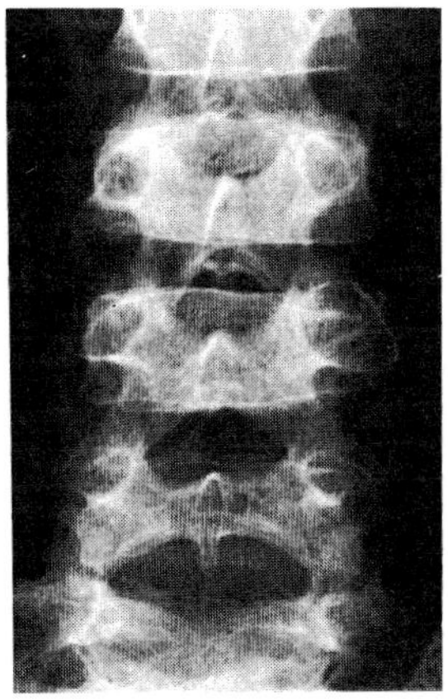

Fig. 9-8. Hodgkin's disease in a 7-year-old boy. There is marked widening of the left pedicle at L4. (Courtesy of M. Lamy)

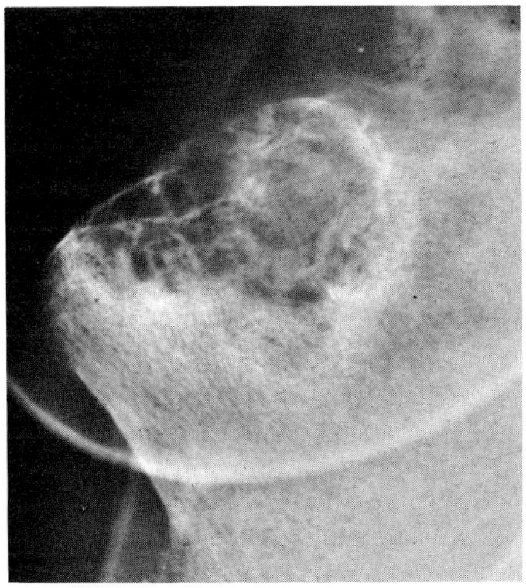

Fig. 9-9. Hodgkin's disease in a 7-year-old boy. Notice the lytic lesion with its wide involvement of the right iliac crest and wing. (Courtesy of M.Lamy)

ation of abnormal cells, and probably also in response to a nutritional factor. In spite of the fact that they are nonspecific, these findings in a child older than 2 years are highly suggestive. This is never seen in neuroblastoma, where metastases can radiologically mimic the signs of advanced leukemia.

Osteolytic foci are also seen relatively frequently (Fig. 9-7). They are exclusively seen within the spongiosa of long bones without specific localization. Their size is variable, most frequently they are only of pinhead size, but they can form larger zones of bony destruction which may alter the appearance of one or several regions of a bone. Occasionally there is even diffuse dimineralization, predominantly of the metaphyseal region, and the bony structure assumes a washed-out appearance. Fractures in these areas are only rarely noted, but wedging of vertebrae is occasionally present. This seems to result from a qualitative structural disturbance of the bone rather than from increased osteoclastic activity or a diffuse formation of osteoid. Lysis of trabeculae may also combine with local hemorrhage or medullary necrosis.

Cortico-periosteal lesions are somewhat unusual. They result from a localized cortical destruction or diaphyseal periosteal reaction along the long bones, especially of the legs, altering the bony contours (Fig. 9-7). Occasionally there is a newly ossified mass elevating the periosteum. Such a lesion is said to be the result of osteoblastic stimulation by the presence of abnormal cells located within the cortex and under the periosteum. *A limited osteosclerosis* can be seen in some rare patients. Most frequently this finding is associated with lytic lesions (Fig. 9-7). Bony infarcts can be noted, and sometimes a number of such lesions appear simultaneously. These findings must be carefully looked for in radiographs centered on the exact area involved: knee, wrist, the entire extent of both legs and the skull. If, indeed, radiolucent bands are mostly asymptomatic, one will usually find lytic or corticoperiosteal lesions in patients suffering from osteoarticular pain. They show remission or complete disappearance during clinical improvement, but have a tendency to recur in the same location, if a relapse sets in. If they are noted, they do not by themselves worsen the prognosis and have no significance in a prediction of the duration of the patient's survival. Several lines of growth arrest can help in the evaluation of the follow-up, focusing on the metaphyseal alterations during the course of leukemia. During therapy there is usually growth arrest resulting from the drugs given, especially during cortico-therapy.

Widening of the cranial sutures may be an indication of increased intracranial pressure resulting from CNS-leukemia.

HODGKIN'S DISEASE

The incidence of Hodgkin's disease is relatively low, since it barely represents 10 per cent of all malignant disorders during childhood. Besides superficial and deep involvement of lymph nodes of the liver and spleen, bony changes are only rarely noted. A high incidence, however, of positive bone marrow findings resulted from autopsy study in patients without any radiologic findings. Bone marrow studies or better bone marrow biopsy have resulted, in a number of cases, in the discovery of Sternberg cells within myelosclerotic foci, accompanied by intensive fibrosis.

Radiologically recognizable bony involvement is unusual and can only be found in 10 to 15 per cent of the patients. For the diagosis itself no significance can be attached to such findings. In an occasional patient, however, the first presenting symptom is severe localized bony pain, especially manifesting at night, sometimes even with local swelling in superficial bony involvement. Such a local lesion can be inflammatory, or simply due to edema of the soft tissue. These signs appear together with the radiologic findings. If there is involvement of the central or peripheral nervous system, radiographic findings usually are already clearcut.

Three pathogenetic modalities are possible to explain the bony lesions. Deep adenopathies immediately next to bone frequently have a direct eroding effect. Occasionally there is bony involvement by way of lymphatics around capillary vessels within the canals of Havers. The rarest possibility is that of hematogenous dissemination, resulting in an intraspongy granuloma, by preference localized at the metaphyseal zones. Some authors believe that such a finding is a de-novo appearance of a lesion within the reticular bony structure.

If the fact of proven bony involvement does in itself not aggravate the prognosis, it is still evidence of a markedly advanced or diffuse stage of the disease: stage IV. Often radiologic changes are only recognized considerably later than peripheral adenopathies, sometimes two to four years after the initial diagnosis. If they are recognized as an isolated finding, a carefully planned and directed search will discover deep lesions, normally inaccessible to clinical study. Radiologic lesions within the skeleton, even though they may be latent, are usually multifocal. They are usually lytic, but secondary osteosclerosis may set in, leading to a densification of the adjacent trabeculae and the surrounding zone. Local compensation, with an ivory appearance, can be seen. Any bone may be involved, even the skull. However, bones with a rich spongiosa, or those directly adjacent to ganglia are involved by preference. By decreasing frequency the principal sites involved are: the spine, the pelvis, the ribcage and the sternum.

Vertebral involvement occurs most frequently in the thoraco-lumbar area. The intervertebral disks are always spared. One or several vertebral bodies may be involved. The anterior surface of vertebral bodies may be eroded. This is suggestive of the presence of an adjacent mass lesion. This can be proven by lymphangiography. Vertebrae can be affected by osteolysis, resulting in a marked compression, which can be complete or wedge-shaped and which may deform a pedicle (Fig. 9-8). Often local reactive sclerosis leads to trabecular thickening, thus maintaining the normal vertebral contour. This mechanism can lead, within a number of months, to the classical ivory vertebra. In the case of thoracic involvement, there is often a palpable mass lesion in the neighboring area, and involvement of the posterior arch of the rib is often associated.

The ilium is frequently involved directly adjacent to the sacroiliac joint. The local lesions are of a mixed type with lytic areas, irregularly surrounded by condensed zones (Fig. 9-9). A lacunar and lacy appearance of the acetabulum can also be seen.

Within ribs there are lytic lesions with destruction of trabeculae and erosion of the inner cortical surface. The manubrium sterni can be similarly affected, and have a thickened and deformed appearance because of the underlying osteolysis. A mild degree of periosteal reaction is not rare. This radiologic image, together with the findings during local palpation of an infiltrating more or less edemateous mass lesion, may simulate a sarcoma.

Finally, there can be lesions electively involving the upper metaphyses of humerus or femur by multiple well delineated areas of lytic lesions within spongy bone, but with the tendency to erode and even elevate the cortex. Sometimes there is lamellar periosteal reaction around such lesions.

THE HISTIOCYTOSES

This is basically a review of histiocytosis X with comments on other reticuloses which occasionally involve the skeleton.

Radiographic Findings

A number of syndromes are grouped under the heading of histiocytosis X: isolated eosinophilic granuloma, Letterer-Siwe disease, and Hand-Schüller-Christian disease. They have similar histologic characteristics: marked cellular polymorphism, always with the proliferation of large histiocytic elements with an irregular nucleus, containing a nucleolus and a fine chromatin network. The cytoplasm is only mildly chromophile and contains numerous vacuoles and lipid inclusions as evidence of an intensive phagocytic activity. Zones of focal necrosis are surrounded by polymorphnuclear eosinophilic infiltrates. Lymphoplasmocytic elements may also be present. Electron

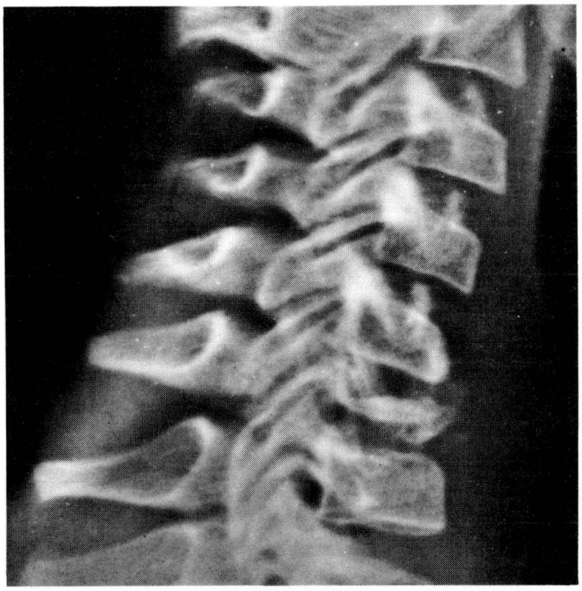

Fig. 9-10. Eosinophilic granuloma with vertebra plana in a 15-year-old boy.

microscopy has led to the finding of curious elongated filaments, of unknown significance, with a symmetrical ribbonlike structure and a transverse striation constructed around a simple axis. They are located only within the cytoplasm of cells of histiocytic characteristic, and seem to have a close relationship with the cytoplasmatic membrane and the vacuoles of the endoplasmatic reticulum.

In spite of this apparent histologic similarity there is great variation in the clinical expression of these syndromes. The disease of a given child may go from one expression to another. Skeletal localization is of considerable importance. The typical lesions are highly destructive and can be localized anywhere in the skeleton, either within membranes or within long bones. The skull is one of the main localizations.

Eosinophilic granuloma is an isolated bone tumor, most frequently manifesting painful local symptoms. A tumor, swelling, and only few other local findings may be present, if a superficial bone is involved. The most frequent location is within the vault of the skull, the ilium, or a vertebra.

In cranial involvement a lacunar defect often has a geographic contour, a clear border and no peripheral condensation. The internal, just as the external, table may have undergone lysis without any periosteal reaction (Fig. 9-11).

In the pelvis a slowly developing granuloma is typically located in the supra-acetabular area. Often a sclerotic border outlines its upper limit.

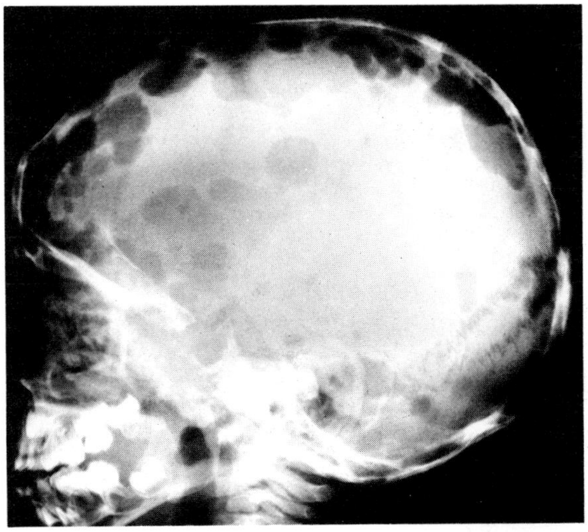

Fig. 9-11. Histiocytosis X in a 2-year-old boy with multiple defects throughout the skull. (Courtesy of R. LaPlane)

Vertebral involvement can lead to a reduction of the anterior portion of a vertebral body resulting in wedging, or in total collapse. The result is a vertebra plana. The pedicles are always spared (Fig. 9-10). Such a vertebral collapse may be clinically silent and is occasionally discovered as an incidental finding. Sometimes there are vague cervical or thoracolumbar pains. Involvement of a single vertebra with a perfectly normal appearance of the adjacent intervertebral disks will form a strong argument for this diagnosis. However, it is not unusual to have several adjacent vertebrae involved. Neurologic complications have been reported. Therapy will depend on the exact diagnosis and location. Biopsy and local curettage of a lacunar defect of the vault may be possible, but we do not advise this approach in patients with vertebral involvement. If there is a markedly progressive lesion present, radiotherapy can be beneficial.

In the *Hand-Schüller-Christian syndrome* diabetes insipidus may be the only presenting symptom for a long time. Multiple bony lacunae and the classical finding of exophthalmus may only appear after several years. Even though any bone may be involved, localization of lesions within the skull, ribs, the pelvis, the humerus or the femur are most frequently encountered. Localized bony expansion can be palpated above the involved area. Radiographic study will show more or less rounded, well delineated zones of increased radiolucency. Density will vary since these defects can superimpose on one another, or on healthy bone. The borders usually are not dense, but occasionally are bivalved, since the defect may extend quite

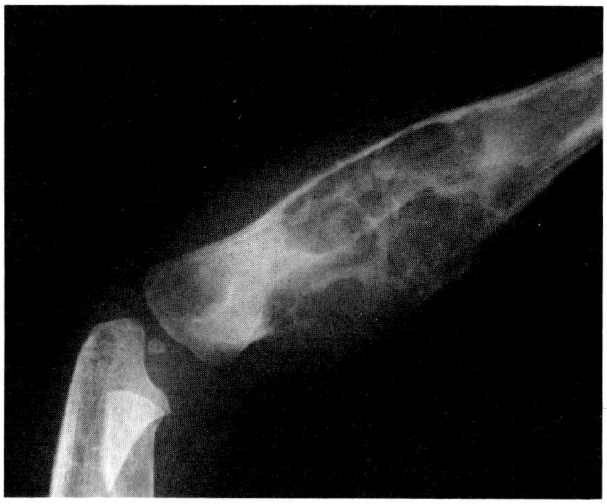

Fig. 9-12. Letterer-Siwe disease in a 2-year-old boy with multiple lytic defects involving the distal humerus. (Courtesy of R. LaPlane)

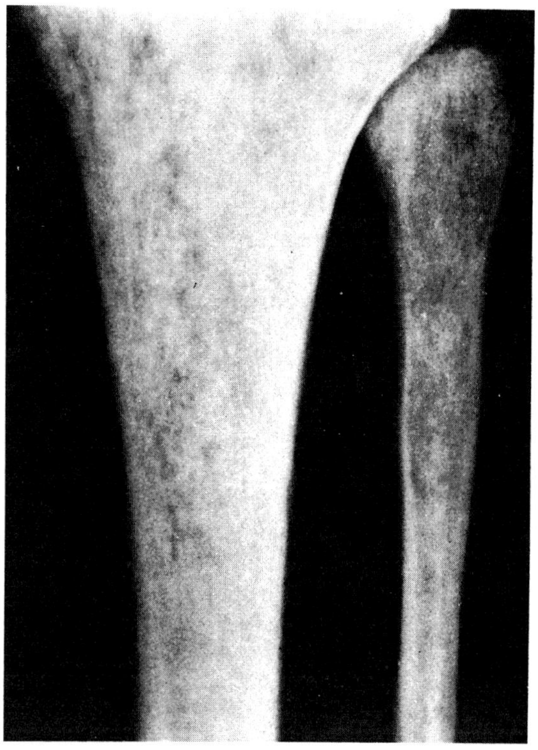

Fig. 9-13. Mastocytosis in an adult with nonspecific changes of the bones. (Courtesy of J. A. Lièvre)

deeply (Fig. 9-11). Occasionally periosteal reaction can be present, particularly in involvement of ribs. Faint peripheral sclerosis may be an indication of the repair of a lytic lesion with subsequent fading of the borders. This local healing is usually occurring at an early slow pace, and new lesions, sometimes in the same bone, may appear. Often these are more central or cortical in location.

Involvement of the base of the skull is frequently noted, especially in the petro-mastoid region, and simultaneously in the temporal bone. The body of the sphenoid is only rarely the site of lesions, in spite of the high incidence of diabetes insipidus. Orbital lesions are frequently seen, together with exophthalmus. In mandibular lesions there is often erosion of the lamina dura around the apex of teeth. In a more advanced stage these seem to float freely within the "empty" mandible. Corticotherapy, usually given to such a patient, will add osteoporosis to the multiple lytic defects.

In *Letterer-Siwe disease* there may be many lytic lesions. They are, however, not required for the diagnosis (Fig. 9-12). Chronic weeping skin lesions and involvement of the middle ear in early infancy together with hepato- and splenomegaly and lymphadenopathy, support this diagnosis. The course is somewhat chronic. Corticosteroid and velbe are presently the best therapeutic agents.

THE MASTOCYTOSES

The mastocytoses are rare disorders. In three out of four cases young infants are affected. Clinical findings are nodular, vesicular, or pigmented skin lesions. Localization within the bone or its medulla is possible. This finding, which will occur in 10 per cent of all cases, is somewhat rare in children. Hepatosplenomegaly and adenopathies are much less frequently present than bony lesions.

The latter are latent and could be overlooked if no skeletal survey were obtained, and bone marrow puncture were neglected. Bone marrow smears must be studied after toluidine blue staining for the presence of mastocytes. Bony lesions are, on the whole, circumscript without special localization. They appear as more or less clearly delineated lesions with an aspect of geodes, or simply as small areas of rarefaction. Small foci of condensation can also be present. Rarely, there is a diffuse nature of these lesions. There may be reticular osteoporosis, especially well marked in the pelvis, vertebrae and ribs (Fig. 9-13). Sometimes there is a somewhat denser aspect of the diaphysis or of the ends of the long bones as evidence of osteosclerosis. Frequently development is centripetal within the bone, and not always homogeneous in distribution.

Different stages of involvement can be seen in the same child. Bone biopsy may show the presence of mastocytic foci and, if decalcification of the specimen has been avoided, trabecular atrophy together with a fibroblastic lamellar apposition. The production of heparin or one of its precursors may explain this. These skeletal lesions, like the skin lesions, may disappear, but not necessarily in a parallel fashion. In the generalized forms of this disorder hepatosplenomegaly and adenopathies are present. It is recommended that one carefully and regularly follow these children, since leukemia has been noted with a high frequency.

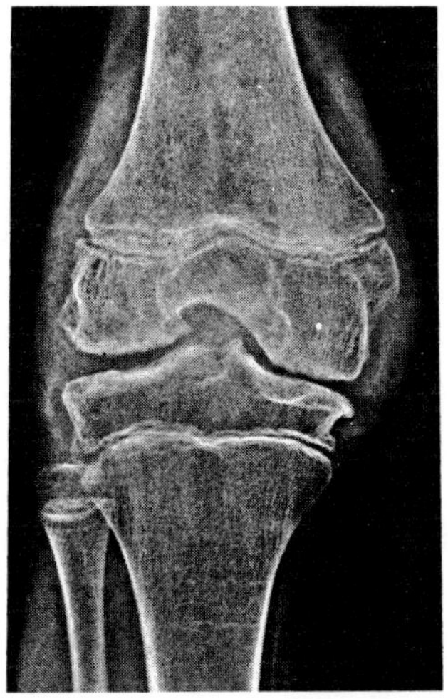

Fig. 9-14. Hemophilia in a 12-year-old boy. There is considerable alteration of the ends of the bones which form the knee joint exhibiting also an abnormal lucency. (Courtesy of M. Lamy)

BLEEDING DISORDERS

Hemophilia has multiple effects on joints.

HEMOPHILIA

The high risk of developing hemorrhages for a hemophiliac child is well known. Thanks to the possibility of therapy by plasma fractions and their derivatives, death can be prevented for most of these patients. Because of their possible effect on the skeleton, two forms of hemorrhage require our attention here: hemarthroses and bleeding within bone.

The Hemarthroses

From the moment a baby starts to actively move around, there is the risk of hemarthroses and in two out of three children with hemophilia this happens before 2 years of age. They are the presenting symptom in 15 per cent of all hemophiliacs. The severity of the effusion and the rapidity of the occurrence are the key factors in the clinical course.

Most frequently without any apparent reason or after only minimal, usually overlooked, trauma, such a child starts to complain about a painful extremity. Local pain results in limitation of motion and use. The affected joint is markedly swollen. Radiologic study reveals no fracture or deviation from the normal articular axis, rather it shows marked distension of the capsule and of the joint space by a hemarthros.

If the patient is already known to suffer from this disorder it is obviously easy to make the diagnosis. Immobilization in good functional position and corticotherapy will result in rapid healing and complete normalization of function. If this, however, is not the case, there should be a high index of suspicion in a boy with such a lesion and one should not easily accept the diagnosis of simple trauma, of early polyarthritis or suppurating arthritis. The latter suspicion would actually entail articular puncture and aspiration, which would be dangerous in a hemophiliac, since it could markedly aggravate the local condition. A careful family history should be reconstructed to establish if another boy or an uncle or maternal great uncle might be so affected. An immediate study of hemostasis should be requested—not simply a coagulation time—which should quickly result in the diagnosis of a deficit of anti-hemophilic factor A or B.

Even with all possible precautions and efforts to allow healing of the joint, there is a high risk of local recurrence. Normal activity of these children will expose them to new trauma. The simple act of walking represents repeated microtrauma to an already altered joint.

Involvement may be unilateral, but eventually will mostly be bilateral. The large joints are most frequently affected. This refers to the joints in decreasing order as follows: the knee, the elbow or tibial-talar joint, the shoulder, the wrist and also the hip. Every bleeding episode will result in immobilization of the child for 2 or 3 weeks. Muscular wasting occurs rapidly, further jeopardizing the joint. In this way there is progressive aggravation of the local pathology, resulting in synovial thickening, local hypertrophy, and cartilage erosion, which eventually will become fibrous. Sub-chondral small hemorrhages will result in irregularly arranged micro-osteolysis. Local increased hyperemia results in accelerated maturation and hypertrophy of some epiphyses.

This leads to the chronic arthropathy which incapacitates the hemophiliac child. The eventual outcome may not only be limitation of one or several joints, but ankylosis in poor position. Professional counseling of hemophiliac children concerning these risks is advised.

Radiologic follow-up allows a careful progressive evaluation of these lesions with a peak incidence around 8 to 10 years. The most characteristic appearance is that of the knee with dense bands of the synovial membrane. This can be recognized in the area of capsular insertion especially well, since muscles and soft tissues have undergone atrophy. Articular narrowing of uneven distribution is best seen on a lateral film, first in the femoro-patellar, then femoro-tibial region, predominating on the medial side. The joint space is irregular and the femoral condylar surface scalloped. Metaphyseo-epiphyseal demineralization is an expression of fibrillar osteoporosis. Axial deviation is frequently present, especially in valgus position. Identical events can be seen in other joints. It is not rare to note the development of tibio-tarsal equinovarus position or flexion deformity of the elbow. The concomitant muscular wasting can be appreciated on good radiographs.

After some months there are profound changes, such as abnormal axis of the joints with local deformity, unevenly distributed abnormal epiphyseal growth. This can explain the ensuing hypertrophy of the internal condyle, widening of the intercondylar groove and flattening of the medial tibial plateau. The articular surfaces are often scalloped. Sometimes there are osteophytes. Osteolytic foci can be recognized affecting the juxtaarticular demineralized bone containing geodes of variable size. These have a tendency to deform the ends of the bones (Fig. 9-14). Small subchondral cysts can be recognized on tomograms.

Orthopaedic treatment attempts to reestablish a somewhat normal articular axis. Cautious physiotherapy constantly attempts to counteract muscular wasting, especially by maintaining a good quadriceps. Therapeutic indications depend on a large number of factors, the most important ones being the severity of the bony and articular involvement, the degree of effective alteration of the bone—diffuse demineralization, and the number and size of juxta-articular geodes—skeletal maturation, the existing, and predictable further course of deformities (keeping in mind the eventual further growth and the remaining muscular power and capacity). There must be a careful and general therapeutic plan, well worked out individually and supervised by a team of pediatricians, orthopaedic surgeons and physiotherapists.

Intra-osseus Hematomas

The incidence of bleeding into the joint is definitely much higher than that of localized bleeding into bone. This complication must be recognized in spite of its somewhat rare occurrence, since an improper diagnosis may have disastrous results. Hematomas can occur into the spongiosa or epiphyses. Sub-periosteal bleeding is unusual.

Hematomas into spongy bone result in bones of resorption and the local formation of geodes surrounded by a lacy condensation or by local new bone formation. Some specific locations will result in surprising local bony deformity. The patella may assume a triangular shape or even become square. The calcaneus may blow up in size and appear to be filled with multiple cysts. Phalanges may seem to be totally "empty" or filled by "fat" resulting from a complete loss of trabeculation.

If there is hemorrhage into an epiphysis, the result is disappearance of the bony structure and a cystic image. If the involved epiphysis is part of a weight-bearing joint, such as the head of the femur, an aspect similar to an aseptic necrosis will result. Such a coxa plana will eventually be accompanied by narrowing of the joint space and alterations of the acetabular cortex. On rare occasions there may be slipping of the head and premature fusion of the cartilage. The resulting hypervascularity leads to accelerated maturation and an epiphysis which is too large and abnormally shaped.

Sub-periosteal hemorrhages have a low incidence and if present can lead to lamellar bony apposition. There is also the possibility of erosion of the underlying cortical bone and there may be scattered calcifications within the organizing hematoma with bony spicula formation perpendicular to the axis of the bone. This results in the impression of a malignant sarcomatous tumor. This finding can be especially misleading in the femur (see Fig. 14-24), of the cortex is elevated by the borders of the hematoma with its own border ossifying and partially surrounding the bone like a socket. Involvement of the iliac wing can be even more misleading, since it may assume the appearance of a tumor. There may be a large irregular lytic zone of considerable extent accompanied by rare areas of calcification within the soft tissues and periosteal new bone formation in places displaced by underlying bony fragments. A local mass lesion may be palpated. This lesion may be painless and well covered. A careful additional history may reveal some trauma several months previous or simply that the patient has noted a localized swelling. Obviously biopsy of such a lesion would be disastrous.

REFERENCES

General Works on Topic

CAFFEY (J.). Pediatric X-ray diagnosis. *5e édit., Chicago, 1967, Year Book med. publ., éd.*

MOSELEY (J. E.). Bone changes in hematologic disorders (Roentgen aspects). *New York, 1963, Grune and Stratton, éd.*

Anemias

BISMUTH (V.) et BÉNACERRAF (R.). Etude radiologique des manifestations osseuses des anémies hémolytiques héréditaires. *Ann. Radiol., 1967,* **10**, *559-574 et 723-736.*

BROWN (A. C.), PLAVTH (W. H.), GAY (B. B.), BLACKSTON (D. R.), GIANSANTI (J. S.) et MATTINA (P. J.). A distinct and anusual syndrome with characteristic facies, shorth stature, bony defects, aortic calcification with aortic valvular stenosis, abnormal dentition, hypotonia, lentiginosis and psoriasis. *Birth Defects, conference (abstract), Newporth Beach, 1974, 106.*

DIGGS (L. W.). Bone and joint lesions in sickle-cell disease. *Clin. Orthop., 1967,* **52**, *119-145.*

HALL (J. G.) et LEVIN (J.). Congenital amegakaryocytic thrombopenia with bilateral absence of the radius : radius-platelet hypoplasia or RPH. *Birth Defects, Original Article Series, 1969, V n° 3, 190-195.*

HALL (J. G.), LEVIN (J.), KUHN (P. P.), OTTENHEIMER (E. J.), VAN BERKUM (K. P.) et MCKUSICK (V. A.). Thrombocytopenia with absent radius (TAR). *Medicine, 1969,* **48**, *411-439.*

JUHL (J. H.), WESENBERG (R. L.) et GWIN (J. L.). Roentgenographic findings in Fanconi's anemia. *Radiology, 1967,* **89**, *646-653.*

JUIF (J. G.), STOLL (C.) et KORN (R.). Thrombopénie hypoplastique congénitale avec aplasie du radius. *Arch. franç. Pédiat., 1972,* **29**, *513-526.*

MASSON (A.), CRONMULLER (G.), ROUSSELOT (P.), LUTZ (D.), BERGER (J.) et SCHNEEGANS (E.). La thrombocytopénie hypoplastique congénitale avec aplasie radiale. Description d'un cas. *Ann. Pédiat., 1971,* **18**, *777-788.*

MCDONALD (R.) et GOLDSCHMIDT (B.). Pancytopenia with congenital defects (F. A.). *Arch. Dis. Childh., 1960,* **35**, *367-372.*

MINAGI (H.) et STEINBACH (H. L.). Roentgen appearence of anomalies associated with hypoplasic anemias kof childhooe : Fanconi's anemia and congenital hypoplastic anemia (erythrogenesis imperfecta). *Amer. J. Roentgenol., 1966,* **97**, *100-109.*

NILSSON (L. R.). Chronic pancytopenia with multiple congenital abnormalities (Fanconi's anemia). *Acta paediat., 1960,* **49**, *518-529.*

O'HARA (A. E.). Roentgenographic osseous manifestations of the anemias and the leukemias. *Clin. Orthop., 1967,* **52**, *63-83.*

ORSINI (A.), RAYBAUD (Cl.), SAGNET (H.) et PERQUIS (P.). Manifestations osseuses de la drépanocytose chez l'enfant. *Pédiatrie, 1966,* **21**, *255-271.*

POCHEDLY (C.) et ENTE (G.). Effects of sickle cell disease on the skeletal system of children. *Clin. Med., 1969,* **76**, *16-23.*

RIGGS (W.) et ROCKETT (J. F.). Roentgen chest findings in childhood sickle-cell anemia. A new vertebral body finding. *Amer. J. Roentgenol., 1968,* **104**, *838-845.*

SCHONENBERG (H.) et SCHEIDHAUER (E.). Beidseitige radiale Hemimelie mit Megakariocytopenie. Ein neues Missbildungs syndrom. *Z. Kinderheilk., 1966,* **97**, *240-263.*

SINGLETON (E. P.) et MARTEN (D. F.). An anusual syndrome of widened medullary cavities of metacarpals and phalanges, aortic calcification and abnormal dentition. *Pediat. Radiol., 1973,* **1**, *2-7.*

Malignant Dyscrasias

BEACHLEY (M. C.), PECK LAU (B.) et RICHARD KING (E.). Bone involvement in Hodgkin's disease. *Amer. J. Roentgenol., 1972,* **114**, *559-563.*

FISHER (A. M. H.), KENDALL (B.) et VAN LEUVEN (B. D.). Hodgkin's disease : a radiological survey. *Clin. Radiol., 1962,* **13**, *115-127.*

FUCILLA (I. S.) et HAMANN (A.). Hodgkin's disease in bone. *Radiology, 1961,* **77**, *53-60.*

GROSSMAN (H.), WINCHESTER (P. H.), BRAGG (D. G.), TAN (Ch.) et MURPHY (M. L.). Roentgenographic changes in childhood Hodgkin's disease. *Amer. J. Roentgenol., 1970,* **108**, *354-364.*

O'HARA (A. E.). Roentgenographic osseous manifestations of the anemias and the leukemias. *Clin. Orthop., 1967,* **52**, *63-83.*

HORAN (F. T.). Bone involvement in Hodgkin's disease. A survey of 201 cases. *Brit. J. Surg., 1969,* **56**, *277-281.*

PAPILLON (J.), CROIZAT (P.), REVOL (L.), CHASSARD (J. L.), BOTHIER (F.) et COSTE (J.). Les localisations osseuses de la lymphogranulomatose maligne. *J. Radiol. Electrol., 1964,* **45**, *109-116.*

ROUSSEL (J.), SCHUMACHER (P.), PERNOT (M.), CANDELA (A.), METZ (R.) et KESSLER (Y.). Considérations sur les localisations osseuses de la maladie de Hodgkin. *J. Radiol. Electrol., 1966,* **47**, *482-485.*

TEILLET (F.) et SCHWEISGUTH (O.). La maladie de Hodgkin chez l'enfant. Etude de 72 observations personnelles. *Arch. franç. Pédiat., 1968,* **25**, *313-330.*

THOMAS (L. B.), FORKNER (C. E.), FREI (E.), BESSE (B. E.) et STABENAU (J. R.). The skeletal lesions of acute leukemia. *Cancer, 1961,* **14**, *608-621.*

WILLSON (J. K. V.). The bone lesions of childhood leukemia. A survey of 140 cases. *Radiology, 1959,* **72**, *672-681.*

Reticuloses

AVERY (M. E.), MCAFEE (J. G.) et GUILD (H. G.). The course and prognosis of reticulo-endotheliosis (eosinophilic granuloma, Schüller-Christian disease and Letterer-Siwe disease). A study of forty cases. *Amer. J. Med., 1957,* **22**, *636-652.*

COLE (A. R.). Mastocytosis. Report of a case in a 15 1/2 -week-old infant with cutaneous and generalized skeletal changes. *Arch. Dis. Childh., 1965,* **40**, *677-683.*

DESHAYES (P.), ARINAL (C.), DREYFUS (P.), DRYLL (A.), HUBAULT (A.), MATRAJT (H.) et SÈZE (S. DE). Les localisations osseuses de la mastocytose. *Sem. Hôp. Paris, 1969,* **45**, *524-530.*

GRIFFITHS (D. L.). Orthopaedic aspects of myelomatosis. *J. Bone Jt Surg., 1966,* **48-B**, *703-728.*

LEFEBVRE (J.) et CHAUMONT (P.). Le devenir du granulome éosinophile cnez l'enfant. *J. Radiol. Electrol., 1958,* **39**, *705-712.*

LIÈVRE (J. A.), CAMUS (J. P.), MAY (Mme V.), BÉNICHOU (M. C.), PRIER (Mme A.) et LIÈVRE (Mme J. A.). Sur sept observations de mastocytose osseuse. *Bull. Acad. nat. méd., 1973,* **157**, *521-524.*

MAGAI (K.), SUGIYAMA (Y.), ISONO (Y.) et YOSHIDA (K.). An autopsy case of primary osteomyelosclerosis in a 6-years old girl. *Acta path. jap., 1969,* **19**, *81-93.*

MALLET (R.), RIBIERRE (M.), LABRUNE (B.), REYROLE (L.), NEZELOF (C.) et BASSET (F.). Deux observations d'histiocytose X du jeune enfant. Présence dans les lésions osseuses de filaments intracytoplasmiques d'apparence virale. *Bull. et Mém. Soc. méd. Hôp. Paris, 1966,* **117**, *385-391.*

NEZELOF (CH.). L'histiocytose X. *Rev. franç. Etud. clin. biol., 1966,* **11**, *22-39.*

VAILLAUD (J. C.), MANASSERO (J.), VISSIAN (L.), VAILLANT (J. M.) et MAISSA (S.). Les mastocytoses de l'enfant et du nourrisson. Aspects cliniques et considérations nosologiques à propos de 4 cas. *Pédiatrie, 1968,* **23**, *763-777.*

WOLFSON (J. J.), KANE (W. J.), LAXDAL (S. D.), GOOD (R. A.) et QUIE (P. G.). Bone findings in chronic granulomatous disease of childhood. *J. Bone Jt Surg., 1969,* **51-A**, *1573-1583.*

Coagulopathies

ALAGILLE (D.), QUÉNEAU (P.) et HANTRAYE (M.). Les aspects radiologiques des arthropathies hémophiliques. *Ann. Radiol., 1961,* **4**, *749-758.*

BOLDERO (J. L.) et KEMP (H. S.). The early bone and joint changes in haemophilia and similar blood dyscrasias. *Brit. J. Radiol., 1966,* **39**, *172-180.*

BOURDON (R.), BERNARD (J.), CAEN (J.), BARD (M.) et PATRUX (Cl.). Données évolutives des lésions ostéo-articulaires radiologiques de l'hémophilie. *Sem. Hôp. Paris, 1963,* **39**, *2818-2824.*

FAURÉ (Cl.). Manifestations ostéo-articulaires et musculaires de l'hémophilie. *Encyclopédie méd.-chir. Radiol., 1968, 31375 A10.*

LAYANI (F.), MAY (V.), PAQUET (J.) et PELISSON (J.). Les ostéo-arthropathies hémophiliques. A propos de 6 cas. *Sem. Hôp. Paris, 1959,* **35**, *3435-3448.*

10 Neurologic Diseases

C. Fessard

This chapter is devoted to a study of alterations of the skull and the spine, and the remote effects of neuromuscular disorders. It concludes with a discussion of the phacomatoses.

THE SKULL AND NEUROLOGIC PATHOLOGY

In a large number of disorders with central nervous system involvement a careful analysis of well centered and properly exposed skull films can reveal information of great value. We will successively discuss brain tumors, abnormal increase of one side of the skull, cerebral atrophy and finally certain malformations.

BRAIN TUMORS

Many expanding intra-cranial lesions lead to radiologic manifestations. These may be changes in the structure and form of certain bones of the vault or of the base of the skull. More frequently, however, signs of increased intracranial pressure will result. The absence of findings in no way rules out the possibility of such a lesion.

Direct Findings

Skeletal changes directly due to a tumor can occasionally be seen if the malignancy is located within the *posterior fossa*. The possibility of diagnostic significance might be attached to the prominence of the cerebellar fossa, if the squama is locally thinned out, protruding, or has an abnormal posterior concavity in the area of the basi-occipital bone on a well centered, strictly lateral film (Fig. 10-1). In an unusual patient, where local palpation reveals in this region the presence of a small nonexpansile mass during crying (midline), one should search by tangential views of varying penetration for a notch within the external table or a small lacunar lesion of a dermoid cyst. This structure is always located in the midline, slightly lobulated or rounded and surrounded by a fine dense line. After having developed within the diploe, this lesion may extend into the epidural space.

Supra-tentorial tumors usually have no such radiologic expression. Those with superficial hemispheric development could lead to local thinning, or even a localized prominence of the vault (Fig. 10-2). Tumors with a slow development, such as astrocytomas, can lead to a protrusion of the parietal and especially the temporal region. Meningeal masses, however rare in children, are well known for their local hypervascular effect in certain patients. These lead also to localized hyperostosis. The unusual size of vascular grooves for the branches of the middle meningeal artery and for the diploic veins assumes definite value if this is a bilateral finding and if accompanied by an abnormal branching in an atypical zone. The entire thickness of a portion of the vault may show up as local hyperostosis, sometimes with local perpendicular spicules of the external table between the bone and the galea (Fig. 10-3).

Certain paramedian anterior tumors can, on lateral

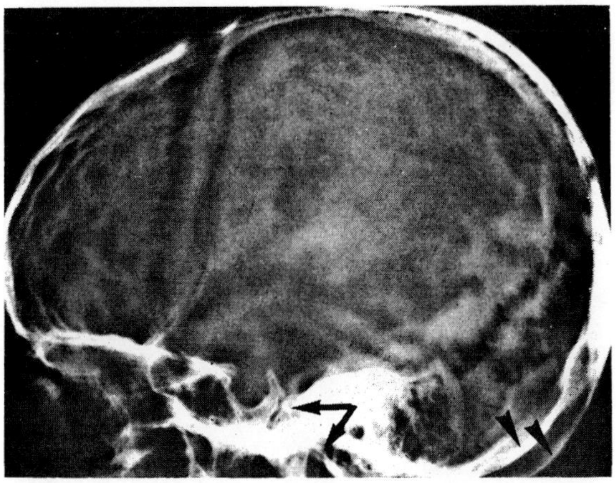

Fig. 10-1. Tumor of the posterior fossa in a 10-year-old girl. In addition to thinning of the cerebellar fossa, there are other classic symptoms of increased intracranial pressure. These are widening of the sutures, changes in the sella, and a concave clivus. (Courtesy of M. Hassan)

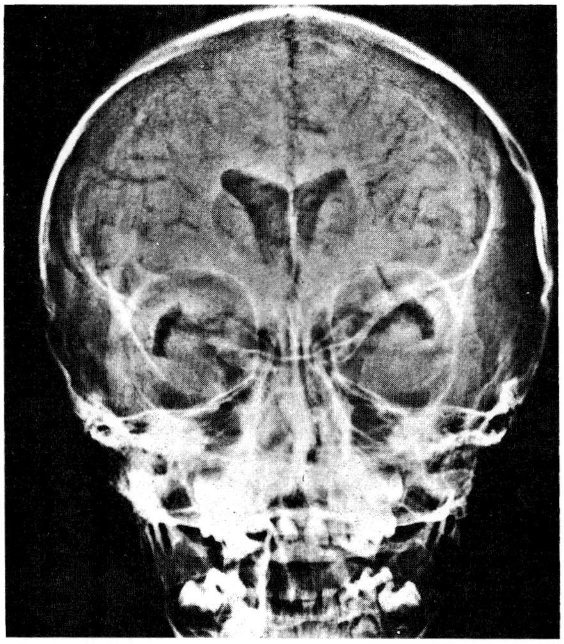

Fig. 10-2. Arachnoid cyst of the Sylvian fossa in a 3½-year-old boy. Note the prominence of the left temporal fossa and the disappearance of the innominate line of the greater sphenoid wing. (Courtesy of M. Hassan)

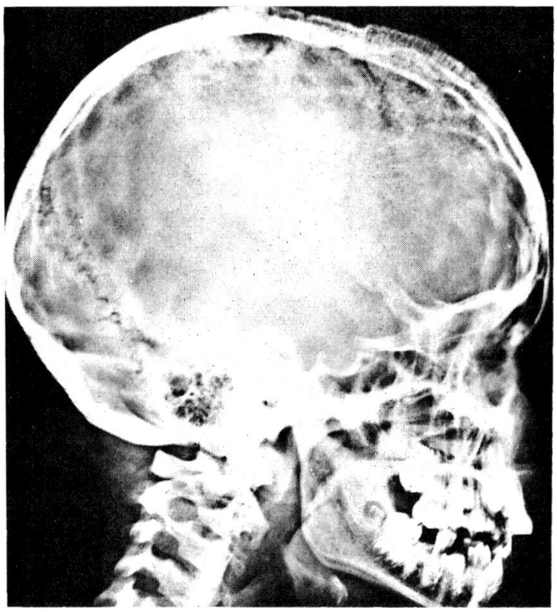

Fig. 10-3. Meningioma of the convexity in a 11-year-old girl: hyperostosis of the cranial vault with spicule formation. (Courtesy of J. Aicardi)

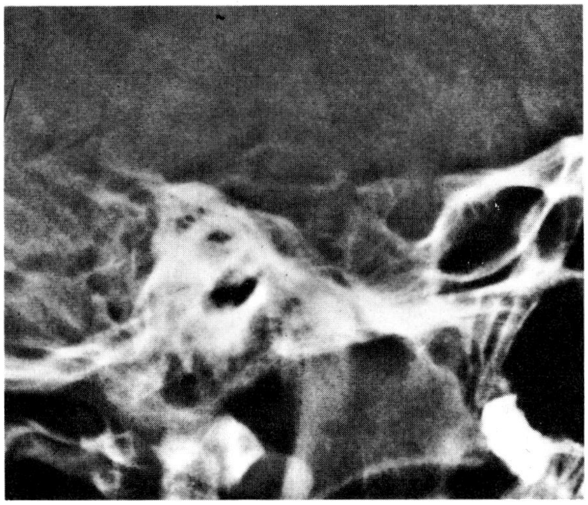

Fig. 10-4. Chordoma in a 7½-year-old boy. Note the local destruction of the clivus. (Courtesy of M. Hassan)

films, push the tips of the greater wing of the sphenoid, which surmounts the sphenoidal plane, forward, and result in a projection separate from that of the other side.

Tumors of the *base of the skull* lead to a number of signs. Partial lytic lesions (sometimes of moderate extent) of the floor of the cerebral fossa should result in a suspicion of bony invasion by a sarcoma or a metastasis of a hematogeneous or neurogenous tumor. A mixed local lesion in the region of the clivus with destructive signs and those of bony condensation should raise the suspicion of the presence of a chordoma, which often extends laterally towards the tip of the petrous bone and the sphenoid (Fig. 10-4). The combination of such findings with intra-cerebral calcification or sequestrated bony fragments visible on tomographic cuts form a strong argument for such a diagnosis.

Changes in the area of the *sella turcica* will help with the diagnosis of a tumor with intra- or suprasellar development. In children this will be either an optico-chiasmatic glioma, or a cranio-pharyngioma, which have a clearly differing radiologic expression. The glioma of the chiasma frequently leads to a deformity of the anterior portion of the sella (Fig. 10-5). Depending on whether there is only a depression of the sub-chiasmatic region or also of the tuberculum of the sella, this results in a ω or a W. Sometimes this impression is more elongated and pear-shaped. The dorsum of the sella is often eroded and the posterior clinoid processes may be demineralized and thin. Correctly centered views of the optic foramen will permit

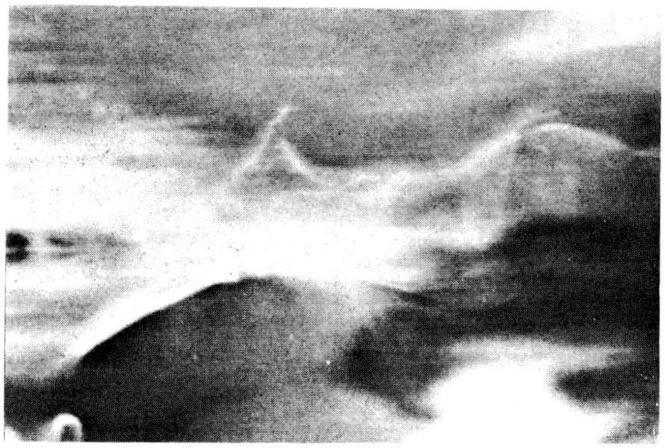

Fig. 10-5. Glioma of the optic chiasma. The elongated appearance of the sella turcica is well demonstrated by tomography. (Courtesy of M. Hassan)

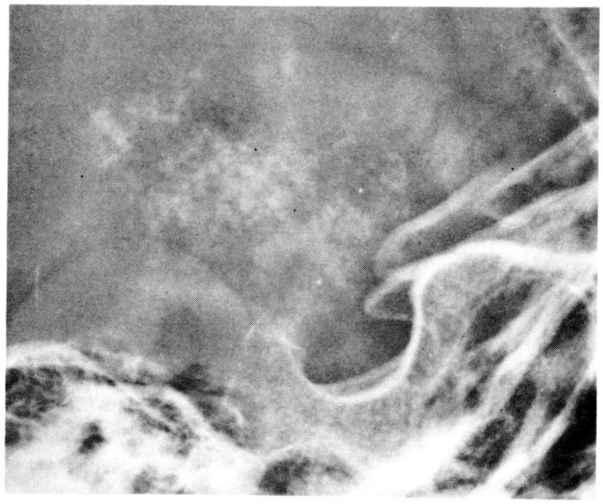

Fig. 10-6. Craniopharyngioma. There are numerous calcifications above the sella turcica.

judgment of unilateral or bilateral enlargement. Such involvement is somewhat unusual, since it is not accompanied by any local erosion or bony alteration of the surrounding structures. The form of the optic canal remains the same or simply becomes somewhat oval. During normal growth the definitive size is reached towards the third year and the largest diameter is about 6.5 mm. An asymmetrical appearance, together with a difference greater than 2 mm or clearcut enlargement of one or both sides, always have pathologic significance. Sellar changes associated with those of one or both optic foramina will give diagnostic confirmation. Cranio-pharyngiomas always spare the optic canal. They usually are accompanied by calcifications, either within or just above the sella turcica, which is itself abnormal in more than two-thirds of all patients (Fig. 10-6). Tomographic study in the AP and lateral directions will further verify the local findings. Most frequently the sella is enlarged, either only in the AP diameter or in all directions by direct ballooning of the intrasellar masslesion. If the enlargement is uneven and predominates toward one side, the sella seems to have a double contour. An abnormal outline is usually associated with possible shortening of the back of the sella as if it were amputated at its base. Sometimes it is also elongated to the point where one can no longer recognize its superior delineation other than by a small ridge. Erosion can occur in all directions, and this may result in a doubled aspect like a "flute's mouthpiece." The floor is often disappearing either in a uniform or uneven fashion, but is rarely completely destroyed by the threatened invasion of the sphenoid sinus. On the AP view there is frequently widening and deepening of the median concavity, and its walls then are clearly visible and angulated. The chiasmatic groove may be especially well delineated. Erosion of the inferior portion of the anterior clinoids results in their clearcut appearance. The lesser wing of the sphenoid sometimes seems to press on them, since the structure may assume a more vertical position and will project in its entire width on a lateral view. Therefore, if a tumor is pre-chiasmatic in location the sella is distended and mainly ballooned; if the location is retrochiasmatic, there is an elongation of the sella. If its dimensions appear normal, there is usually an amputated and flat dorsum. There is a direct relationship between the density of the sellar contours and the speed of tumor growth. If there is a slow development there may be adequate time for the cortical bone to repair itself.

These direct signs of the presence of a tumor must be carefully analyzed, since they are not always readily noted. This also applies to calcifications and their possible intra- or peritumoral location. Calcification of the pineal region is always abnormal prior to 6 years of age and must be considered suspicious before 10 years of age. Contrary to the general opinion, craniopharyngiomas do not always spare the optic canals. This finding can therefore occasionally be noted in such a tumor developing an anterior extension.

Indirect Findings

Less frequent and nonspecific for the presence of a tumor are findings of *elevated intracranial pressure.*

Before the second year of life the skull can be easily distended by widening of the sutures and thinning of the vault. In the older child these changes differ somewhat with the patient's age and the speed of the clinical

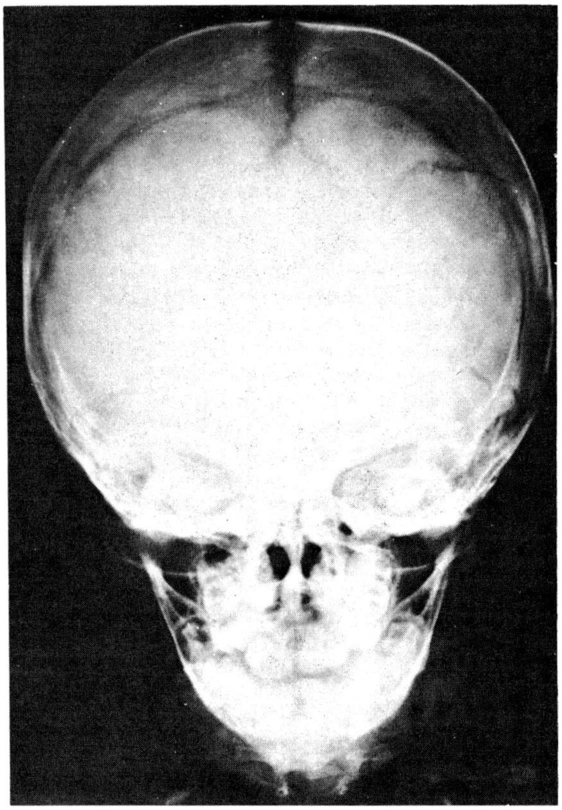

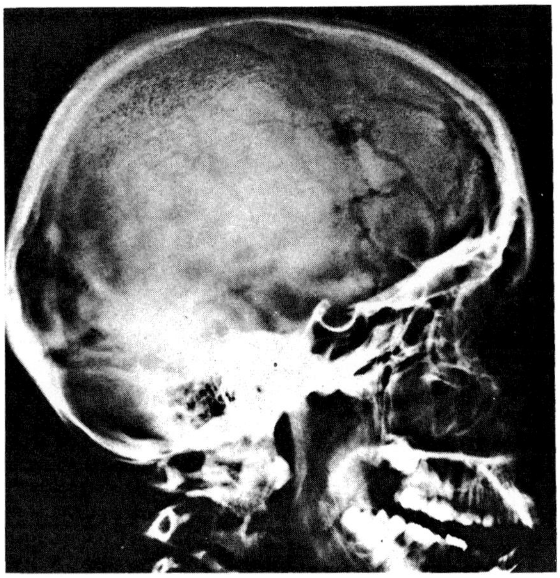

Fig. 10-7. Normal variants in the appearance of the skull. *(Top)* A supernumerary suture line in an infant. (Courtesy of J. Lefebvre) *(Bottom)* Vascular imprinting in a 14½-year-old girl. (Courtesy of C. Fauré).

progression. The key findings are separation of sutures, digital impressions of the vault and sellar changes (Fig. 10-1).

Split sutures are those with widening above 2mm. Splitting can extend over the entire skull and affect all sutures or it can be limited to the coronal and lambda sutures. If there is chronic development, the interdigitation of the external table will be stretched apart. This is best seen near the coronal sutures.

Digital impressions are a normal finding during childhood. They may be noted from the first few months in the frontoparietal upper region, towards the sixth month. They may also be present in the occipital region, and after the eighth month more posteriorly than the fronto-temporal region. Their prominence may actually increase up to 4 years of age, but towards 8 to 10 years they will practically disappear. These local effects, reducing slightly the thickness of the inner table, do not exactly reflect the anatomic relationship of the directly underlying cerebal convolutions. This imprinting will only have a clinical significance if it is extensive and deep, and especially if there is associated splitting of sutures.

In an advanced degree of increased intracranial pressure and after the sutures of the skull have already fused, marked dilatation of the canals of emissary veins may become evident, but changes of the sella are the most dramatic expression. The sella will assume a generally increased and dilated form with the shape of a "bucket." Its cortex will be thin and the dorsum more or less demineralized and shortened (Fig. 10-1).

THE LARGE SKULL

A large skull due to an increase of intracranial volume can result from many different etiologies. Increased intracranial pressure resulting from an expanding lesion is only present in about 20 per cent of such patients and most frequently results from a posterior fossa tumor.

Subdural effusions are seen somewhat more frequently. An enlarging skull with prominent bossing of the parietal region is frequently noted. Its exact etiology in a baby is not completely clear. Trauma, sometimes overlooked, can help to explain this finding. Careful attention should be directed to possibly finding a fine fracture of the skull. Confusion with an accessory suture line should be avoided, particularly in small babies with the possibility of the presence of the metopic, mendosal or interparietal suture or wormian bones (Fig. 10-7, *Top*). Deep venous grooves can add to the confusion. These are usually carved within the diploe of the parietal or of the frontal bones with

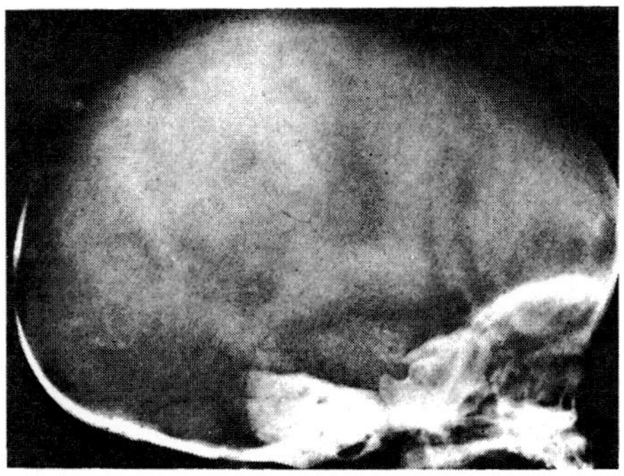

Fig. 10-8. Aqueductal stenosis in a newborn. There is increased volume in the occipital region with poor ossification of the cranial vault. (courtesy of M. Hassan)

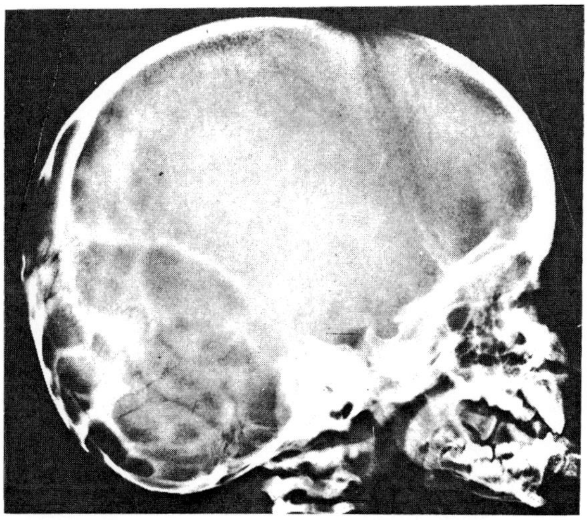

Fig. 10-9. Dandy-Walker syndrome in a 1-year-old infant. Note the lacunar appearance of the posterior fossa. (Courtesy of M. Hassan)

slightly dense borders, and, usually, a winding course leading towards a venous lake having a deep, rounded impression within the internal table (Fig. 10-7, *Bottom*).

If unilateral, such an aspect may lead to errors. Subdural effusions are usually bilateral, but if they are unilateral and chronic there may be changes affecting the middle cerebral fossa with local widening and elongation. The adjacent bones may be eroded and the lesser wing of the sphenoid may be projected more anteriorly than that of the other side.

Hydrocephalus is the most frequent cause of a large skull in babies. The bony changes usually confirm the clinical findings. There will be a craniofacial dysproportion, widening of the sutures, many wormian bones, an unusually thin aspect of the vault and only occasionally a flat sella. In three particular conditions special significance can be attached to radiologic findings. In the presence of congenital aqueductal stenosis the posterior fossa appears to be very small and flat, since the dilatation is limited to the supra-tentorial ventricles (Fig. 10-8). Contrary to this, a Dandy-Walker cyst with its huge distention, usually limited to the 4th ventricle, results in an enormous occipital protuberance which is in a very high position at the level of or above the lambda suture (Fig. 10-9). The lateral sinuses originating at this point show up as an impression obliquely extending towards the area of the mastoids. All these findings can be well seen once the baby is a year old. Sometimes there is dolichocephaly, and widening of the bitemporal diameter may be lacking, but a marked posterior bulge can be prominently present. All this can be accompanied by a bulge which begins behind the parieto-occipital region, and the posterior fontanelle can be huge. The possible importance of the findings on radiographs of the cervical spine and of the atlanto-occipital region in the diagnosis of *Arnold-Chiari's malformation* has already been emphasized. A base view will help in an evaluation of the possibly enlarged foramen magnum and a curvilinear depression of the postero-medial surface of the petrous bone. Deprivation dwarfism described by Silver and Finkelstein can also lead to widening of sutures. In this disorder babies are small, have an excessive appetite and delayed bone maturation. Widening of the suture is sometimes only noted during the healing phase, but may be noted earlier (Afshani et al.). It is quite difficult to understand this phenomenon. The rapid growth of the brain, offered as a cause, does not seem to explain the early appearance of this finding. This condition should not be confused with other reasons for elevated intracranial pressure.

A fenestrated skull or "congenital lacunar skull," more frequently present with spina bifida with meningocele, does not always appear to be an expression of increased fetal intracranial pressure (see p. 310).

CEREBRAL ATROPHY

While working up a child for epilepsy, mental retardation or hemiplegia, careful analysis of well-centered skull films — AP, lateral, half axial Waters view or axial base view — will sometimes reveal findings indicative of underlying cerebral atrophy (Fig. 10-10). Adequate growth of the brain is the underlying force for normal growth of the skull. Local findings will be more pronounced if there is an asymmetric atrophy, of the

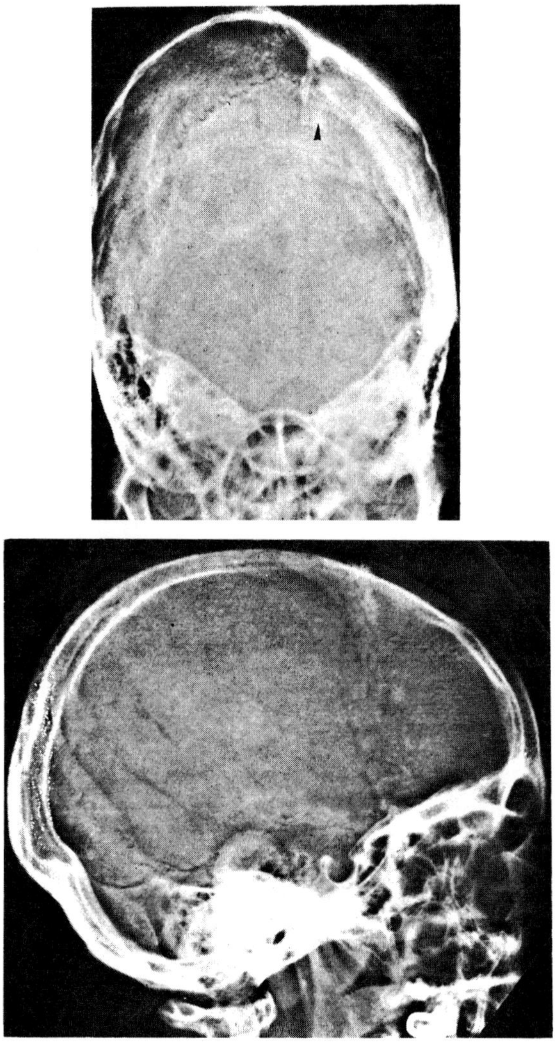

Fig. 10-10. Unilateral cerebral atrophy on the left in a 12-year-old girl. (Courtesy of M. Hassan)

brain, especially in unilateral involvement of one entire hemisphere. Findings depend largely on how, and how massively, the cerebral parenchyma has been damaged, and also on the degree of associated ventricular dilatation.

The radiologic findings are those mainly involving the cranial vault, but can also extend to the base of the skull. One half of the skull is underdeveloped with a flat parieto-temporal curve, thickening of the diploe, which may appear denser and show a smooth inner table. Digital impressions may be widely spaced or lacking.

The anterior fontanelle and the groove of the longitudinal sinus may be slightly displaced towards the involved side. The temporo-sphenoidal fossa is shrunken, since the petrous bone is higher in position. The same applies to the lesser wing of the sphenoid, which may become enlarged. The crista galli may lean towards the atrophic side. The sinuses may appear prematurely, with exaggerated development. This refers to the ethmoid cells, the supra-orbital recess and the pneumatization of the sphenoidal and frontal sinuses, which are frequently asymmetrical. Taken together these findings are clearly different from those associated with an asymmetrical expansion of the skull resulting from a unilateral and chronic subdural hematoma. A further development in older patients or adolescents with cerebral atrophy, seen with a relatively high incidence, is internal frontal hyperostosis. In massive cerebral atrophy the markedly dilated lateral ventricle will almost touch the skull. The total volume of the skull will be increased and the cranial vault will be thin. If there is a uniform total reduction of the cerebral parenchyma, microcephaly resulting from bilateral atrophy has an entirely different radiological appearance than total craniosynostosis (Fig. 10-11).

CEREBRAL MALFORMATIONS

A number of bone findings can be noted in the presence of cerebral malformations. Thus absence of ossification of the vault will be found in anencephaly. Micro-encephaly is associated with a severe degree of neonatal microcephaly with a markedly small cranial size, which will not grow and may develop premature closure of its sutures. A large midline defect in the occipital or frontal region is frequently a sign of an abnormal development of the underlying nervous structures. A meningocele of varying size is usually present with this finding and is referred to as *cranium bifidum*.

A lacunar skull is also almost exclusively present in newborns with meningomyelocele, meningocele or an encephalocele. The typical findings are lacunae of the cranial vault clearly outlined by denser bone (Fig. 10-12). This finding is especially well seen close to the sagittal, coronal or lambdoid sutures. It results from the disappearance of the internal table and of the diploe. Often the external table will also disappear. This condition is referred to as cranio-fenestria. This aspect is transitory and will disappear very rapidly, within one or two months. It takes a longer time to repair a cranium bifidum.

A small midline defect may be the expression of the presence of a congenital dermal sinus. Such a round, sometimes very small defect can be due to a dermoid cyst, especially within the occipital region. Occasionally this can also be found in the frontonasal region. Every patient with a history of repeated attacks of purulent meningitis must be carefully investigated for the presence of such a finding, but also for the possible presence of a defect of the tegmen tympani of the petrous bone or of the cribriform plate of the ethmoid resulting from trauma.

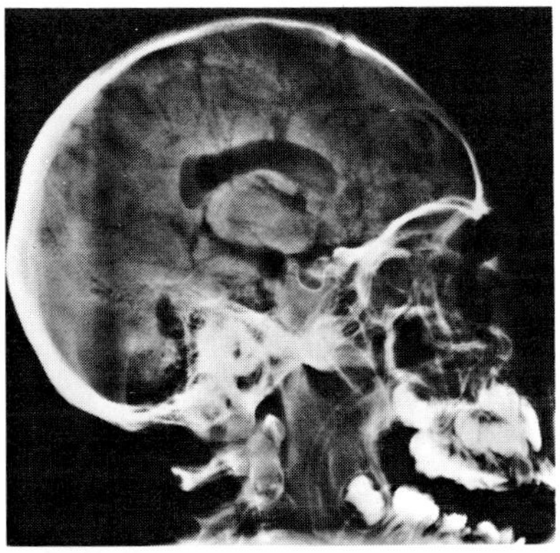

Fig. 10-11. Air study of autosomal recessive microcephaly. Girl aged 6½ years.

THE SPINE AND NEUROLOGIC PATHOLOGY

We have concluded that within the framework of this book, a discussion of the spine in its relation to neurologic disorders is necessary. Actually, the presenting signs and symptoms in this respect can be quite misleading, and a careful study of the skeleton can yield valuable clinical information. This refers, in particular, to the presence of tumors, which we will discuss before dealing with local malformations.

TUMORS

Motor or sensory disturbances of sphincters can be an expression of the presence of spinal pathology; this may also be the case in an occasional patient presenting with arthralgias, torticollis and lumbar pain. Spinal deformity of recent onset, even if asymptomatic, may be the only implication, for a number of months, of the presence of a medullary tumor. The index of suspicion should be particularly high if there is only localized spinal involvement and marked pain. In such patients a detailed radiologic study is mandatory. The entire spine should be carefully investigated, since the lesions are often located at a higher level than the local findings or pain. Study should consist of AP and lateral films of the spine, oblique views, and, when necessary, tomographic cuts. The documents obtained must allow careful analysis of the morphology, structure and topographic relationship of each vertebral body and its arch. The normal anatomy and its variants must be well known.

It is possible, but rather unusual, to discover structural findings suggestive of a *bone tumor* in a larger child (see 5th part). Thus, a reticulosarcoma will result in a homogeneous density of a vertebral body or its irregular destruction. If this is noted, and there are neurologic findings, an epidural extension of the tumor is suspected. An aneurysmal bone cyst can lead to vertebral collapse, but the local involvement may be limited to a pedicle, giving a "one eyed appearance" to a vertebral body on the AP view. Localized osteolysis of the sacro-coccygeal region, accompanied by clearly defined calcifications on a tomogram, will support the diagnosis of a chordoma.

An hourglass extradural tumor results in the marked widening of one or more foramina (Fig. 10-13). This is a reliable finding. Local enlargement can be best appreciated by simply comparing both sides. Both adjacent pedicles may be eroded, but more frequently only the one below the tumor is. Erosion may extend to the articular apophyses and to the posterolateral vertebral surface. If the process has been of long standing there may be changes of the bony structure. A local condensation may be noted besides the widening of the foramen by a neurofibroma. Occasionally we note an increase of the interpedicular distance involving a single vertebra. This finding has diagnostic value only if the borders of both pedicles are clearly visible, if there is no abnormal position or rotation of the spine, and if a normal distance for the intervertebral disk is maintained. In the presence of a tumor located in the thoracic region, and with an extra-spinal extension of sufficient size, local extension may involve the posterior aspect of ribs and lead to local widening of the intercostal space (Fig. 10-13). A careful search for the presence of tumoral calcification is recommended. This finding supports the suspicion of a neurogenic tumor, most frequently a sympathoblastoma.

Purely medullary tumors are rare, and have only late bony manifestations. The expanding mass must have sufficient size and consistency. Its growth in the transverse and mainly sagittal direction has important consequence for the diagnosis (Fig. 10-14). The search for such a lesion is often neglected or poorly conducted. In babies the growth of the tumor may even delay the midline fusion of the posterior arches or result in an abnormal posterior bulge of one or two spinous pro-

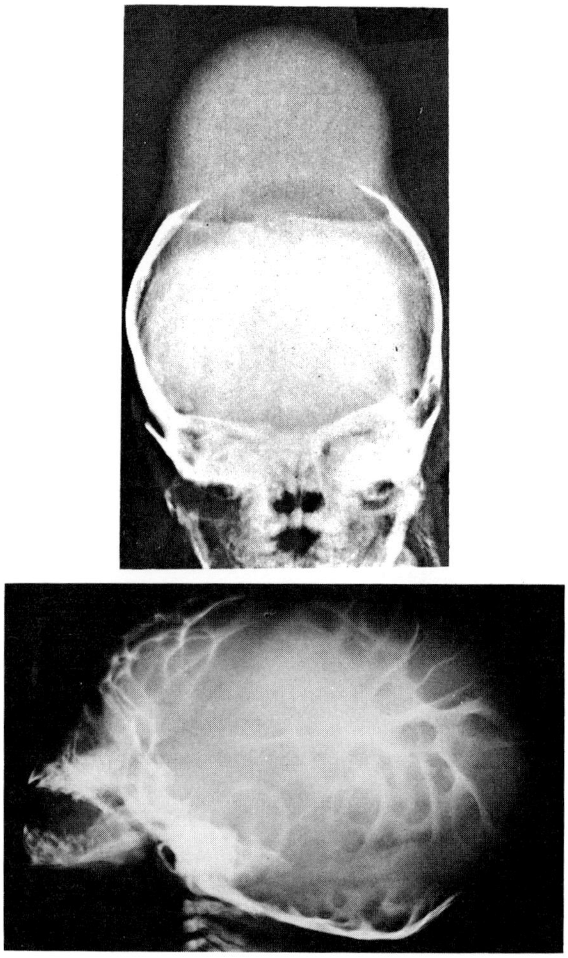

Fig. 10-12. Cranial anomalies associated with malformations of the central nervous system in the newborn. *(Top)* Cranium bifidum with encephalocoele. (Courtesy of J F. Hirsch) *(Bottom)* Lacunar skull associated with spina bifida. (Courtesy of R. LaPlane)

cesses. Sometimes there is scalloping of the posterior border of vertebral bodies and the pedicles may assume an unusually elongated and narrow form. The interpediculate distance can be increased in a single or in several vertebrae. In the latter situation widening may be fusiform. Without the presence of bony lysis, the altered appearance of the internal surface of one or both pedicles may be thin, laminated or abnormally concave. These findings are only rarely all present in a given patient, and widening of the spinal canal may go unnoticed if one is not meticulous in the analysis of each individual vertebra, comparing them with one another.

Several authors have attempted to measure, in normal infants and children throughout growth, the sagittal diameter of the spinal canal and the interpedicular distance at the different levels of the spine. This requires sufficient vertebral ossification, especially to determine the sagittal diameter. The numbers are only significant after 3 years of age. Such an objective evaluation will help significantly not to consider a physiologic finding as abnormal. The spinal canal is somewhat wider in its cervical and lumbar area and has its narrowest region in the midthoracic portion. On AP films pedicles will have a rounded or oval shape, but below the 7th thoracic vertebra their aspect is either transversely flattened or even slightly concave. The foramina usually are larger at the level of the 2nd and 3rd cervical vertebrae. Two levels below they are somewhat smaller, but still of greater size than those of the thoracic region. Great caution should be exercised before making a statement on an abnormal widening of the spinal canal. Careful measurements must be available, and one should only designate clearcut findings as abnormal. Such findings, however, do have considerable significance, if limited to one or two vertebrae which vary strikingly from the immediately adjacent bodies. By the same token, it must always be kept in mind that a total absence of spinal findings does not exlude the possibility of a tumor. Local findings may be limited to a slightly abnormal curve over a short spinal segment, a mild kyphotic or kyphoscoliotic posture.

A progressive scoliosis in a big child or an adolescent may, for several years, be the only clinical expression of syringomyelia. Neurologic and bony findings, such as widening of the medullary canal may appear much later.

MALFORMATIONS

A number of congenital malformations of the nervous system can be accompanied by spinal changes.

Radiographic investigation of meningocele or myelomeningocele reveals the presence of a spina bifida, a large defect of the posterior vertebral arches extending over a variable distance (Fig. 10-15). Sometimes there are only some minor remnants of these arches, but the interpedicular distance is always enlarged. These local defects also have a remote effect. Besides hydrocephalus, many newborns may also have a congenital lacunar skull.

Other spinal anomalies, such as anomalies of vertebral bodies and partial agenesis of the sacrum, may be present with a spina bifida. Intra-dural tumors are frequently associated, and they may erode the poste-

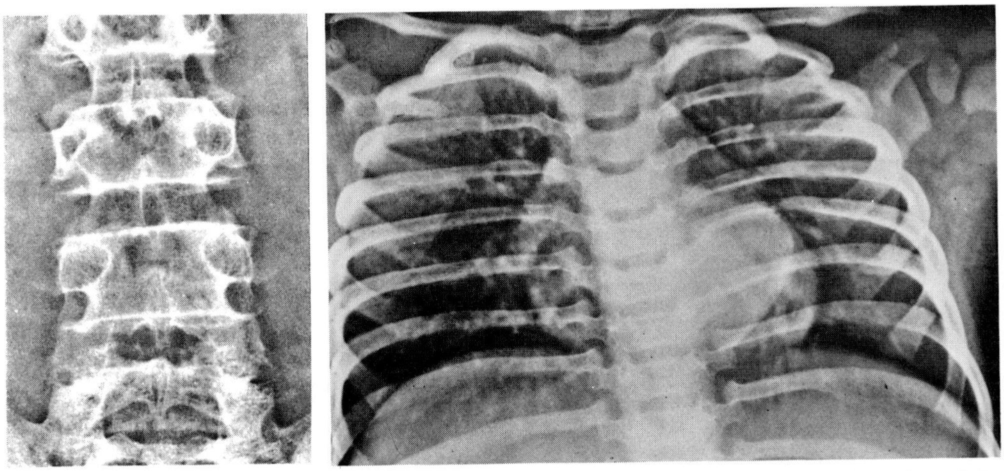

Fig. 10-13. Extradural tumor with spinal manifestation. *(Left)* Neurinoma with partial erosion of the right pedicle at the 3rd lumbar vertebra in a 15-year-old boy. *(Right)* Neuroblastoma which led to marked widening of the 6th left intercostal space in this 11-year-old girl. (Courtesy of J. Sauvegrain)

rior surface of the vertebral bodies and reduce the size of the pedicles.

Diastematomyelia should be mentioned as a separate entity. Besides a defect of segmentation and fusion of vertebral bodies, there is often an osteo-dural or dural spur extending across the spinal canal from either a posterior arch or the posterior surface of a vertebral body. This spur cuts across the spinal cord dividing it into two separate lateral parts. This cleavage becomes accentuated during growth, since the development of the spine is more rapid than that of the spinal cord. Localized hypertrichosis is often present, overlying the malformation, and can help by leading to an investigation for the presence of this lesion.

Radiologically, diastematomyelia can show a complex spinal block with abnormal fusion, especially posteriorly. There may be an aspect of spina bifida. Furthermore, there is widening of the spinal canal with its maximum usually corresponding to the location of the spur. On AP films, and even better on tomograms, this spur can be recognized as a dense, sometimes bony opacity (Fig. 10-16). If, however, this structure is only formed by dura it may not be visible. In such patients myelography will reveal an opaque defect located in the middle of the spinal canal and within the contrast agent.

A midline dimple in the sacral region should never be overlooked. Such a finding should always lead to radiologic study of the spine. Such a dermal sinus may be blind and simply continue in the subcutaneous tissues as a fibrous tract, but it may form a communication with the spinal canal and with the meninges, where it can even be connected to a dermoid or an epidermoid cyst. Normal growth and migration of the nervous tissues are frequently disturbed in such patients. Radiographic study will show the frequent association

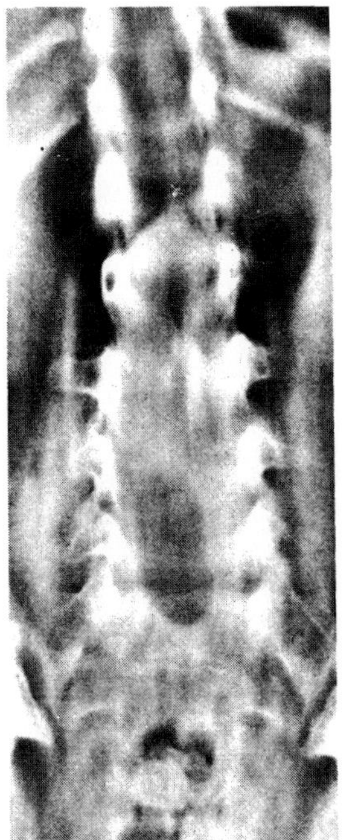

Fig. 10-14. Intraspinal dysembryoma with widening of the spinal canal. (Courtesy of J. Sauvegrain)

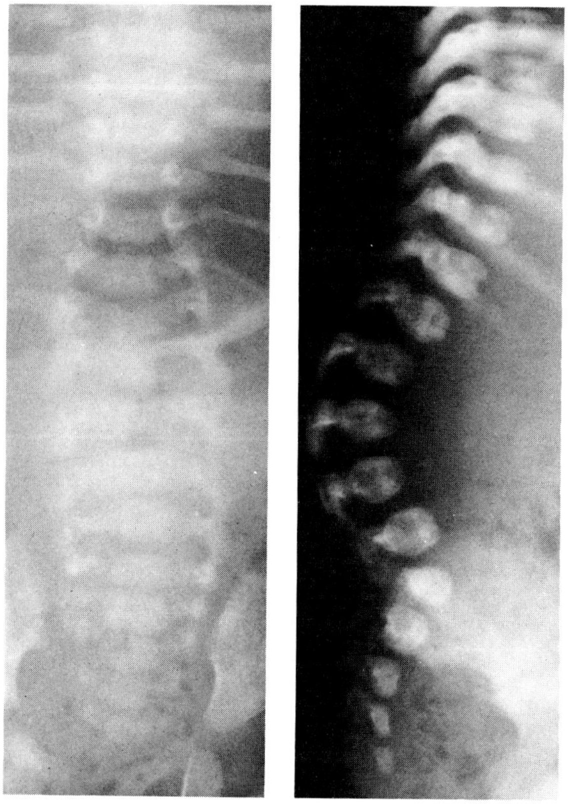

Fig. 10-15. Spina bifida in a newborn. (Courtesy of R. Laplane)

of localized spiny bifida and tumor with local imprints on the spine by erosion. Myeloradicular symptoms are usually present, and repeated bacterial meningitis with ectodermal spinal dysraphism has been reported in such patients.

If a patient has an abnormal gait combined with uneven growth of the legs, deformity of one foot or an unexplained limp, and especially if there is monoparesis, the possibility of a medullary malformation must be considered. The index of suspicion will be particularly high if there is some local vertebral finding or a superficial dermal anomaly in the lumbo-sacral region. Radiographic study may show an extensive spina bifida, widening of the spinal canal and sometimes a transfixing spur, the direct evidence of diastematomyelia.

Having been discussed with the respective dysostoses (p. 160), anomalies of the atlanto-occipital region will only be briefly mentioned here. They may remain asymptomatic for a long time. Discovery may result from trauma, painful torticollis or medullary compression. Symptoms are frequently misleading. Well centered and good quality radiographs, with the head held in flexion and extension, must be obtained.

Arnold-Chiari's malformation, frequently associated with basilar impression, can be the cause of such neurologic symptoms. An abnormally short neck, a low insertion of the hairline and torticollis should lead to a full radiologic investigation. Measurements of the sagittal diameter of the cervical canal may reveal an unusual widening of its upper region and narrowing of C_6-C_7 in patients with an ectopic location of the bulbocerebral structures, always part of an Arnold-Chiari malformation.

BONE LESIONS SECONDARY TO NEUROMUSCULAR DISORDERS

Neurologic disorders can have an effect on a part of, or the entire, locomotor system. Such changes are in no way limited to the bony structure around the central nervous system (skull and spine). The different anomalies secondary to cerebral, medullary and peripheral nervous disorders will be discussed and followed by pathology of the muscles and ligaments.

CEREBRAL INVOLVEMENT

We will successively deal with various encephalopathies and cerebral motor defects.

Encephalopathies

Many encephalopathies result in poor growth. Affected small patients have delayed bony maturation, but no abnormal epiphyseal development. Proven abnormal epiphyseal development should always lead to a careful search for hypothyroidism. In rare instances, gigantism has been reported. Delayed awakening is of variable intensity, but not progressive. Greater than normal height is a constant feature from birth; the subsequent growth rate, however, is regular during the first years. Once these children reach adolescence they will not be giants. The prediction of their definitive height is a function of the degree of the advancement of bone maturation over the chronologic age of the child. Craniofacial dysproportion has been noted in such patients. There is a large, prominent forehead and deep seated eyes, within prominent orbits (see p. 277).

Patients with severe retardation are chronically bedridden, muscular cripples. They show an excess of tubulation, a coxa valga, and an increased vertebral height. Prolonged immobilization, frequently combined with poor food intake, can lead to severe skeletal demineralization. In such a situation the bones are markedly radiolucent with very thin diaphyseal cortex, an occasionally lamellar appearance, and a poorly defined metaphyseal bony structure with markedly washed out trabeculae. Osteoporosis is severe, and in some patients there is a severe calcium loss, actually a form of osteomalacic, late onset of rickets. Diaphyseal bowing, sometimes also involving the metaphyses, especially of the legs, is frequently present. Minimal passive motion can lead to fractures. These are sometimes very difficult to recognize on radiographs. If the bony structure remains almost normal, and if patients have fractures, a careful investigation is indicated whether such unhappy children have not been the victims of unrecognized, concealed, active or accidental trauma. Sometimes there appears to be bony fragility with a high degree of osteoporosis subsequent to the cerebral pathology. This syndrome is the condition Neimann et al. have described as associating mental retardation, amyotrophia and degenerative lesions of the central nervous system.

Certain encephalopathies are part of more complex syndromes which have a possible effect on the skeleton. Lissencephaly, for instance, leads to the disappearance of cerebral convolutions with microcephaly and mental retardation, and is often associated with anomalies of the fingers—polydactyly, camptodactyly. The facial appearance of these patients is quite characteristic. There is a high forehead, a protruding occiput, marked eyebrows, a wide bridge of the nose, abnormalities of the ear position and helix formation, and micrognathism. Corneal opacities in a peripheral location have been noted. Hirsutism is also on record. The transmission is probably as an autosomal recessive disorder.

In the chapter on dysostoses, mention was given to the association of anomalies of the hands and feet with different types of mental retardation (see p. 170).

Homocystinuria

This disease results from a metabolic block because of a defect in cystathionine-synthetase. Most frequently it is noted because of mental retardation. Morphologic findings rarely lead to its recognition.

The appearance of patients may be similar to Marfan's disease, since they often are very tall with very slender extremities. This is especially true of the acra. This is, however, not a constant feature. Usually there is also genu valgum, thoracic deformity, either in the form of a funnel chest or pectus carinatum, and kyphoscoliosis. Patients often have a disturbed gait. Dislocation of the lens may also be a key feature. Arterial and venous thromboses occur relatively frequently.

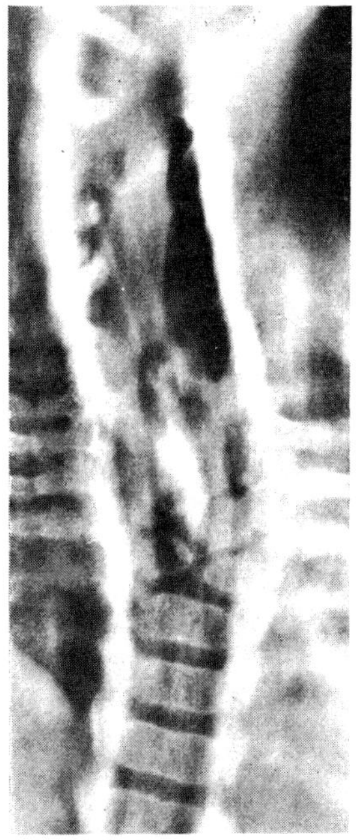

Fig. 10-16. Diastematomyelia. Note the widening of the spinal canal and the demonstration of the medial comma-like spur revealed by tomography in this 7-month-old infant. (Courtesy of J. Sauvegrain)

Radiographically, this disorder is characterized by the association of osteoporosis and epiphyseo-metaphyseal changes (Fig. 10-17). Osteoporosis of a moderate degree is present in more than half of all cases. An occasional patient may develop spontaneous fractures. This form of osteoporosis is generalized, but for some reason more pronounced in the spine. The epiphyses are fragmented, flattened and deformed. Their structure is frequently uneven in the area of the metacarpals, the distal ulnar and the femoral head. The metaphyseal border is often irregularly outlined and slightly dense. Sometimes this area has a concave border into which the markedly concave epiphysis inserts. Frequently there is local widening with lateral prolongation in a spur. Bony maturation is unusual, since it is not uniformly retarded, but anarchic. This refers especially to the carpal bones, which have an unusually disturbed pattern of individual appearance and development. The diaphysis appears to be somewhat long, but this is not a constant feature.

Platyspondyly, with transverse widening of the vertebral body, and biconcave vertebral shape are sometimes present. Abnormal spinal curvature can be seen. A study of the skull may reveal microcephaly, thickening of the vault, and sometimes hyperostosis frontalis interna. It is possible that some of these findings result from disturbed metabolism, since similar findings have been noted in the metaphyses of phenylketonuric children fed a phenylalanine-free diet. Others, however, may result from ischemic vascular disturbances, such as defects of the vertebral endplates or metaphyseal borders, and epiphyseal pathology.

Unlike Marfan's disease, which is a dominant disorder, homocystinuria follows an autosomal recessive mode of transmission. This diagnosis must always be considered in a patient with arachnodactyly and mental retardation.

Aspartylglycosaminuria

This is a recently described metabolic disorder (Autio et al.), characterized by an abnormal urinary excretion of aspartylglucosamin.

Affected patients have signs of mental retardation and an unusual facial appearance. Their coarse features are somewhat reminiscent of mucopolysaccharidoses, especially in somewhat older patients. Their height is slightly below the mean. Patients often have a dorsal kyphosis and a heart murmur. Their lymphocytes are vacuolated.

Radiographic study reveals that the cortex of the long bones is thin, as is that of the bones of the hands and feet. The ulna is slightly shorter than the radius. The vertebral endplates are irregular, and wedging of vertebral bodies attributed to local fracture has been reported. The cranial vault may be thick. Transmission is as an autosomal recessive.

Phenylketonuria

Phenylketonuria does not lead to similarly characteristic bony changes as do the two preceding diseases. Still, there are some findings at the distal end of radius and ulna which are seen quite regularly. These are widening of the metaphyseal line with slight demineralization, and the presence of spicules across the growth cartilage. These are seemingly a direct continuation of small bands of condensation within the metaphysis, and are arranged parallel to the axis of the bone.

This condition is clearly related to a regimen poor in phenylalanine. It is much more prevalent during restricted intake, and seems to have a direct relationship with the lowering of alkaline phosphatases. Because of this finding, careful supervision of the skeleton during dietetic therapy of phenylketonuria has been recommended (Murdoch and Holman).

Wilson's Disease

This autosomal recessive disorder leads to severe cerebral degenerative changes and cirrhosis of the liver. It is the result of an abnormal copper metabolism. The symptoms have their onset frequently during childhood or adolescence. Bone and joint involvement is in the background during the course of this feared disease. Still, there may be pain and swelling of joints with a moderate degree of limitation of motion and crepitation during passive mobilization. These findings may mimic rheumatoid arthritis. These findings are present in patients of advanced age, and only unusually before adolescence or adulthood. During childhood radiographs will not show more than a mild degree of osteoporosis with a thin cortical aspect and prominent trabeculation. Occasionally, osteochondritis dissecans, especially of the knee, has been noted. Fragmentation of epiphyses or of a vertebral body occurs late. There may be loose bodies within joints and sometimes a small dense line is suggestive of chondrocalcinosis, which can be seen in addition to the degenerative changes (Fig. 10-18). In some instances multilocular cysts have been described within the metaphyses. Such findings are more readily noted and present in the neighborhood of the wrist and the tibio-tarsal joint. Osteomalacia, or renal rickets, can occur with marked involvement of the metaphyses, Looser-Milkman zones, and even fractures (Mindelzun). The sella turcica can be small (Askoy et al.).

It is difficult to explain the mechanism leading to these skeletal manifestations, since experimental copper intoxication has not led to joint involvement. The changes of osteomalacia, however, seem to be secondary to renal involvement, which is frequently seen in Wilson's disease.

Menkes' syndrome, with its severe degree of mental retardation, spasticity, and convulsive crises, would also seem to be due to abnormal copper metabolism—affected intestinal absorption. It is transmitted as a sex-linked recessive disorder. The hair is abnormal—pili torti—which has led to the descriptive term of "kinky hair syndrome." Towards 2 or 3 months babies with this disorder will show the radiologic findings of osteoporosis, and somewhat later cortical hyperostosis of long bones accompanied by mild metaphyseal widening, occasionally of irregular type.

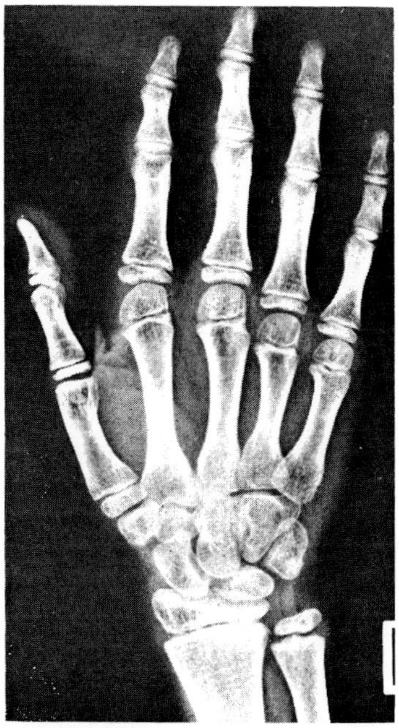

Fig. 10-17. Homocystinuria in a 13-year-old boy along with osteoporosis and some changes in the epiphyses. (Courtesy of J. C. Dayras)

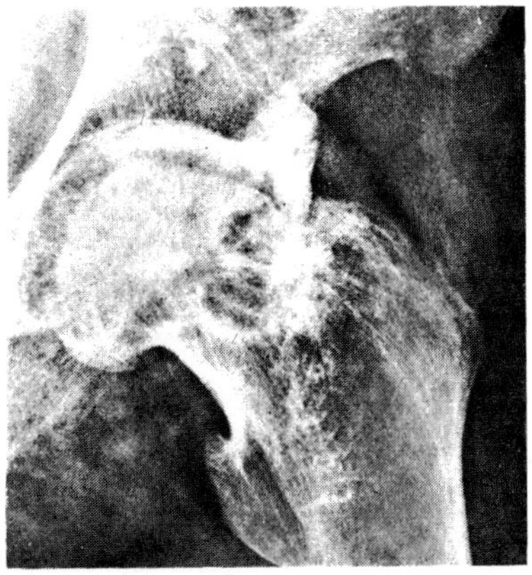

Fig. 10-18. Wilson's disease in a young adult. Note the severe deformity of the femoral head and neck. (Courtesy of B. Pépin)

The clavicle and the scapula may be involved and the anterior ends of the ribs may be widened. Such changes have some similarity with the sub-periosteal hematomas of the battered child syndrome or infantile cortical hyperostosis (see p. 343 and see p. 345). Occasionally, there are some wormian bones present, and microcephaly has also been reported. After 1 year of age it seems that the cortical changes disappear (Wesenberg et al.).

Cerebral Motor Dysfunction

Children suffering from hemiplegia often show asymmetry of the length of their extremities. The shortening of a leg is often noted, usually distally. If the condition progresses, shortening happens especially within the first years of life. It is never of great significance, but seems to be more clearcut in patients with severe motor deficit who also have disturbed sensitivity. It is possible to also have delayed bony maturation of the affected side, since the ossification centers, mainly of the carpal region, are of smaller size, not delayed in their appearance.

The hips of babies with spastic disorders must be carefully watched. There is a high incidence of uneven muscular tonus resulting in a local disequilibrium, which may lead to progressive dislocation. Weakness of the glutaeus medius and the predominance of the adductors of the thigh play an important role. Two local situations can favor this development: bilateral and symmetrical coxa valga, and markedly weakened gluteal muscles with a marked disturbance of gait. There is a vicious circle resulting in flexion and especially adduction of one thigh, which leads to obliquity of the pelvis. The tilting of the thigh results in altered weight bearing, anteversion of the femoral head, fixation of the diaphysis in abduction and internal rotation while in the upright position and during attempts to walk. In such cases the hip is no longer properly centered and there will be changes of the acetabular roof, and loss of the lateral lip. A normal acetabular roof in this area must always be carefully investigated (Fig. 10-19). If there is asymmetrical weight bearing there may soon be dystrophy of the femoral head with loss of structure and deformity, sometimes with considerable alteration of the shape and marked local pain. Affected children have a great handicap. The obliquity of the pelvis accompanying the dislocation of the hip constantly alters the alignment of the spine. Sometimes it may also be a marked lumbar scoliosis resulting in pelvic tilt. The hip will thus eventually undergo dislocation. In many patients these factors augment one another.

Cerebral motor invalidity does not only lead to malposition of the hip and spine. The foot can assume marked valgus or varus deformity and even the knee may be locked in a flexed position.

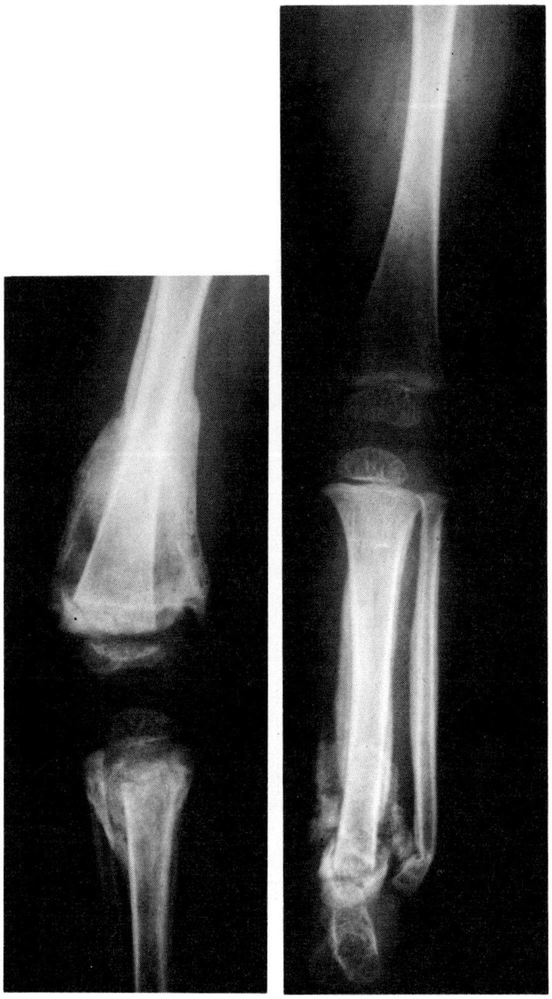

Fig. 10-19. Paraplegic infant 21 months of age. There are multiple fractures at different stages of healing combined with the dislocation of the distal femora and proximal tibial epiphyses on the right.

SPINAL CORD AND PERIPHERAL NERVOUS DISORDERS

Some lesions of the spinal cord may lead to considerable bone or joint pathology. Peripheral neuropathy caused by anterior horn lesions of the cord as a result of poliomyelitis is one example. Retraction and muscular imbalance can lead to severe deformity of the extremities and the spine. Abnormal growth of skeletal elements in regions with severe paralysis will result in uneven longitudinal growth. Similar involvement of vertebrae and of the pelvis is even more serious. The excessive slenderness of the bones and local osteoporosis, together with the wasting of the musculature, are in marked contrast with the frequent thickening of the subcutaneous tissue. Because of abnormal local fragility, minimal trauma may result in fractures. Similar local changes can be seen during the course of Werdnig-Hoffmann's disease, a hereditary disorder transmitted as an autosomal recessive.

Patients suffering from chronic paraplegia of whatever etiology may develop similarly severe bony demineralization. A specific complication of paraplegics secondary to myelitis or trauma is the development of para-osteo-arthropathies with abnormal calcification within some bursae, especially that of the gluteus medius above the trochanter and that of the adductors medial to the femoral neck. These lesions have an ankylosing effect. They should be left alone, because surgical attempts to remove them inevitably are followed by local recurrence. Para-articular calcifications can be seen following coma or encephalitis.

These serious troubles with walking may be associated with pes cavus. On radiographs there is a small angle resulting from the abnormal growth location of the two pillars of the plantar arch, the anterior metatarsals and the posterior calcaneal pillars. If this finding is present a careful study should be directed to determine if there are signs of a heredo-degenerative spinocerebellar lesion or a cervico-occipital spinal malformation. There are also other disorders, such as Charcot-Marie's disease and poliomyelitis, which can result in this deformity.

If there is a major disorder of the sensory system, such as loss of pain sensation or of the deep sensitivity, unusual and surprising osteoarticular changes can occur (Fig. 10-20). The lack of pain after fractures will result in severe hypertrophic callus formation with totally irregular proliferation. True osteoarthropathy can occur. Some joints show signs of rapid swelling. This swelling appears to be inflammatory, but is painless and will be only present for a number of hours. After a while the joint space can no longer be recognized, because of marked local deformity. Sometimes there is also dislocation. Besides local atrophy and lysis of the most distal bony elements, there may also be a proliferative juxta articular reaction, recognizable by the presence of anarchic calcifications and exuberant hyperostosis with flaky and sometimes ill-defined contours. The bony architecture is completely altered and the joint space may no longer be visible. The pathogenetic mechanism of these neurotrophic disturbances is not generally agreed upon. However, many authors believe that the degree of vasomotor disturbance present seems to offer a logical explanation for these findings.

The distribution and localization, together with the eventually recognized neurologic defects, usually will

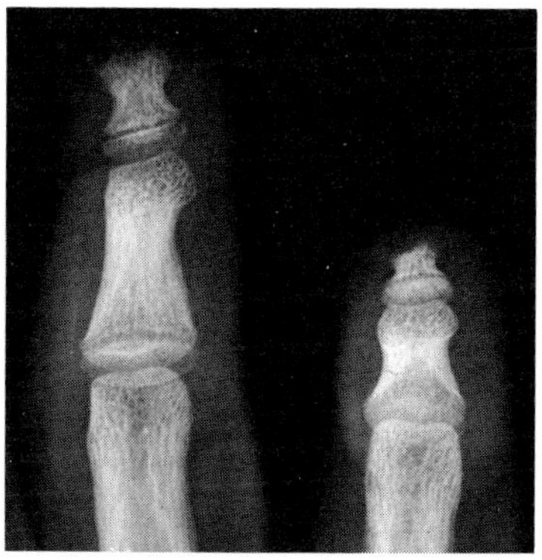

Fig. 10-20. Congenital insensitivity to pain. There is a lytic effect on the end of the terminal phalanx which involves the middle and index finger.

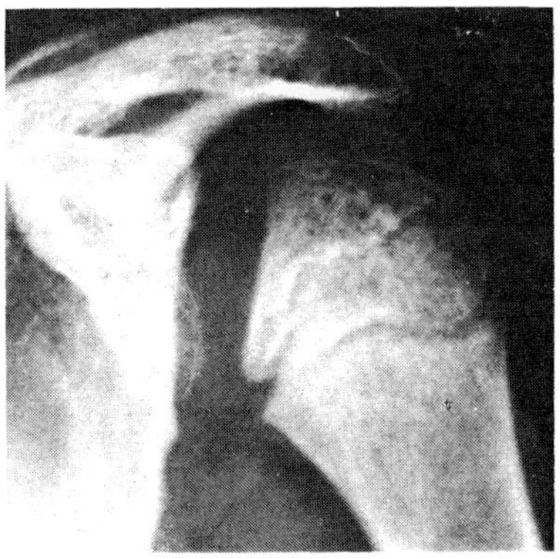

Fig. 10-21. Neglected obstetrical paralysis of the brachial plexus in an 11-year-old girl. Significant alterations involve the humeral head and joint. (Courtesy of P. Rigault)

help in recognizing an etiology. Thus, syringomyelia will frequently result in neurogenic arthropathies of only the arms, since thermo-algesic dissociation follows a special topographic distribution resulting from the location of the spinal anomaly limited to the cervico-thoracic area. In patients with congenital indifference or insensitivity to pain, just as in those with familial dysautonomia, the main joints are most frequently involved, even though initially this involvement may be limited to crepitation or simply a restriction of movements. Joint mobility is usually maintained because of a lack of pain. This makes more understandable the frequently associated bone destruction and the presence of multiple scars from injuries and burns and also from deep bites into the tongue. These patients usually also have some mutilation of their fingers or toes. Patients with spina bifida or paraplegia with transsection of the cord may also develop bony lesions because of secondary insensitivity to pain (Fig. 10-19). These lesions can be similar to those of the battered child syndrome (see p. 345). In acrodystrophic neuropathy, or the Thévenard's syndrome, with lesions of the roots and posterior spinal ganglia, skeletal involvement is usually limited to the lower legs. There is articular lysis of the toes with local bony resorption, and geode formation of the distal phalanges. Certain types of progressive hereditary acro-osteolysis are somewhat similar, but differ in that there is always marked involvement of the hands. There may also be pyramidal tract signs (see p. 179).

Neglected obstetrical brachial plexus paralysis with secondary deformity of the bones of the shoulder manifest clinically in a marked internal rotation and elevation of the humero-scapular joint. Posterior subluxation of the head of the humerus is not unusual. Its posterior portion is flattened, while its anterior portion becomes ovoid (Fig. 10-21). Such lesions are the result of retraction of the internal rotator muscles of the shoulder and those of the anterior articular capsule.

MUSCULAR AND LIGAMENTOUS INVOLVEMENT

Children suffering from advanced *myopathies* have a high risk of developing changes in their hips and spine. Reduced height of the vertebral bodies can be quite prominent. Some authors have observed slenderness of the diaphysis of long bones of the extremities, in spite of a normal bony structure. There is a rather striking widening of the fibula on lateral views (Fig. 10-22; Kaufmann). The most striking radiologic finding, resulting from a fatty infiltration of the hypertrophic gastrocnemius, can be recognized as fine feathery striations within the muscle, of either normal or increased size.

We shall review the following separate conditions: myositis ossificans, osteochondromuscular dystrophy or the syndrome of Catel-Schwartz and Jampel, and arthrogryposis.

Myositis Ossificans

Myositis, or progressive ossifying fibrodysplasia, is characterized by the formation of lamellar bone within connective tissue and muscle.

The leading symptom is limitation of movement of one or several joints, together with the appearance of subcutaneous nodules. This can occur with a febrile

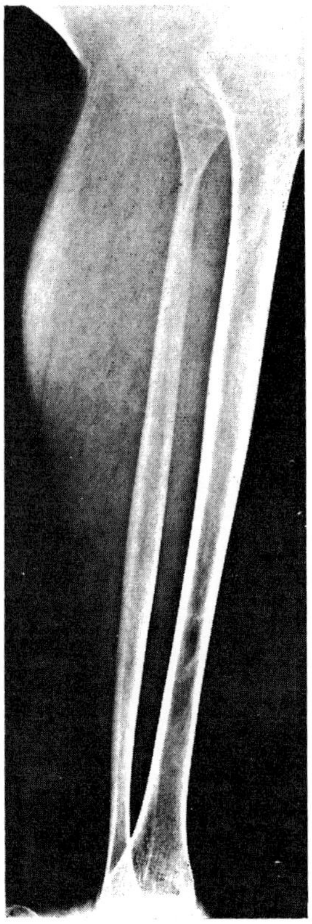

Fig. 10-22. A 15½-year-old boy with muscular dystrophy. Besides muscular involvement the tibia is thin in appearance and there is marked widening in the AP diameter of the diaphysis of the fibula. (Courtesy of C. Fauré)

episode. Locally there may be limitation of specific movements only, and examination may reveal muscular induration or a fluctuating, sometimes painful mass. Preferred areas for involvement are para-vertebral, cervical, shoulder, proximal tibial, and the region of the arms. A frequent finding is shortening and deviation of the thumb, the big toe, and the phalanges, and occasionally incurving of the 5th finger. The evolution of myositis ossificans is slowly progressive by relapses. It eventually leads to very extensive involvement, the so-called "petrified man," and eventual death.

Radiologically, early signs are small dense bands within muscle, or ossification in the area of muscular insertions mimicking exostoses. Subsequently larger areas of ossification will form ridges between different skeletal parts (Fig. 10-23, *Top, left*).

Abnormal findings of the hands and feet are of particular interest, since such congenital anomalies are frequently present and can offer reliable diagnostic information, even before abnormal ossification can be recognized. The most characteristic findings are those of the first metatarsal and the phalanges of the big toe (Fig. 10-23, *Top, right*). The metatarsal is short and plump, especially its distal portion, and it appears shrunken and is medially deviated. Occasionally this portion may form a separate bony piece. The first phalanx is usually very short, triangular or trapezoid, with an oblique base. This bony element, if present, is often fused with the second phalanx. The latter is deviated laterally and is sometimes too short. The most constant abnormality of the hand is that of the 1st metacarpal bone (Fig. 10-23, *Bottom*). The phalanges of the thumb may be hypoplastic, and sometimes there is also an abnormal and deformed epiphysis of the 1st phalanx. This bony structure may be triangualr with an oblique metaphyseal line. The 2nd phalanx is often short and narrow at its tip. The most distal phalanx of other fingers may be similarly affected. An additional finding may be hypoplasia of the middle phalanx of the fifth finger.

Even though the majority of observed cases are isolated, there is evidence that this disorder is transmitted as a dominant trait. The manifestation of the gene is most likely irregular, since in one family there are patients with the full disorder while other members only show the presence of skeletal anomalies.

The basis for the induction of such an abnormal bony development is unknown. Treatment of the disorder is rather disappointing. Corticosteroids have only a limited effect during active phases of the disease. The diphosphonates seem to have a somewhat better effect, but great care must be exercised in their use.

Besides this generalized form of progressive myositis ossificans there are also localized types of traumatic origin. Myositis ossificans should not be confused with multiple cartilaginous exostoses (see p. 88), osteoma cutis, with its more superficial lesions, or the other types of subcutaneous calcifications.

Osteochondromuscular Dystrophy

This syndrome, also known as the Schwartz-Jampel syndrome, has been mentioned by Catel as enchondral dysostosis type Catel-Hempel. It refers to the combination of myotonia and an abnormal development of skeletal growth, similar to spondylo-epiphyseal dysplasias.

Besides manifesting dwarfism, affected children have a peculiar appearance, a pinched face with a small mouth and narrow palpabral fissures. Ocular anomalies are regularly present—micro-cornea, myopia and juvenile cataract. The neck and trunk are short, with sternal protrusion and thoracic kyphosis. The joints of the extremities are somewhat prominent and limited in their movements.

Radiographic studies show a reduced vertebral height with irregular endplates. There is marked deformity of the epiphyses of the long bones, especially of the femoral head, also of the carpal and tarsal bones. The metaphyseal border is irregular in outline. Coxa vara is frequently present. Local involvement of the base of the skull has been reported—platybasia, basilar impression, and excessive development of the posterior clinoid processes.

Anatomic study reveals the coexistence of abnormal development of growth cartilage and muscle. Recessive autosomal inheritance has been proven. Therapy with procainamid seems sometimes beneficial (Huttenlocher et al.).

This disease should not be confused with myotonia dystrophica of Steinert, with its dominant inheritance and clinical expression reminiscent of Marfan's disease, including craniosynostosis, micrognathia, kyphoscoliosis and clubfoot.

The Arthrogryposes

Multiple congenital arthrogryposis is a well known disorder leading to multiple stiff joints. The large joints are mainly involved. Usually they are frozen in flexion, as are the hands and feet. Limited movements are possible, and seem to indicate that the articular surface is intact.

At birth radiographic examination will not reveal significant skeletal findings. There may be an unusual slenderness of the bones and a relatively high incidence of neonatal fractures and dislocation of the hips. Later, and especially if such babies are not properly treated, there will be abnormally formed epiphyses in the areas of local deviation, or abnormal articulation. The diaphyses of long bones remain slender and seem to be poorly modeled (Fig. 10-24). The tarsal bones and those of the carpus often have an abnormal appearance. It is not unusual for these patients to also have coxa vara, absent patella and scoliosis. The bony structure is abnormally loose and osteoporotic. Sometimes a craniofacial dysproportion can be recognized—plagiocephaly or unusual bossing of the forehead. Underexposed films of the extremities can show the marked degree of muscular atrophy.

There is an occasional association of skeletal malformations with arthrogryposis: polydactyly, syndactyly, hypertelorism and mandibular hypoplasia.

Serial bone biopsies have demonstrated that the local changes are of a reactive nature, since in early life normal bone is present. The same is true of the articular structures. After a number of years there is progressive bony atrophy and a disturbed ossification of cartilage with widely spaced bony trabeculae and unossified cartilaginous islands (Jacobson).

Arthrogryposis really is a heterogeneous group of clinically somewhat similar disorders. Besides the most frequently observed classical form, there are also familial types with recessive transmission. For instance, this is the type seen among the Alaskan eskimos (Wright) and in a Palestinian family described by Lebenthal.

Muscular rigidity is already extreme at birth and early physiotherapy is indicated. In order to improve the condition of such infants, orthopaedic therapy must be systematic, energetic and unrelenting.

Besides arthrogryposis, there are other syndromes showing a limitation of joint movements, for instance, the two brothers studied by Laplane et al., with articular ankylosis having its onset after the second year in combination with marked dwarfism. Skeletal involvement was mild—excessive radiolucency of the epiphyses, and irregular development of the acetabulum and of the proximal end of the femoral neck. In the patient of Moore and Federman onset was somewhat later and there were also ocular lesions—cataract, glaucoma, hyperopia and uveitis—and dominant transmission. A somewhat plump appearance of the hands led these authors to discuss a possible relationship with pleonosteosis of Léri, which is, however, quite different.

THE PHACOMATOSES

Bony involvement of the phacomatoses has a varying incidence and aspect depending on the type studied. In neuro-angiomatosis of Sturge-Weber discussed at the end of this chapter, there is no direct skeletal involvement.

Contrary to this, however, there is a high incidence of skeletal changes in Bourneville's tuberous sclerosis and in Von Recklinghausen's neurofibromatosis. These disorders frequently go unrecognized for a prolonged period of time and may become clinically evident only during childhood. During adolescence they may become very marked. Such changes may be a leading symptom of the presence of these diseases and will help to establish the diagnosis in latent involvement, for instance in a family with variable manifestation of the respective phacomatosis.

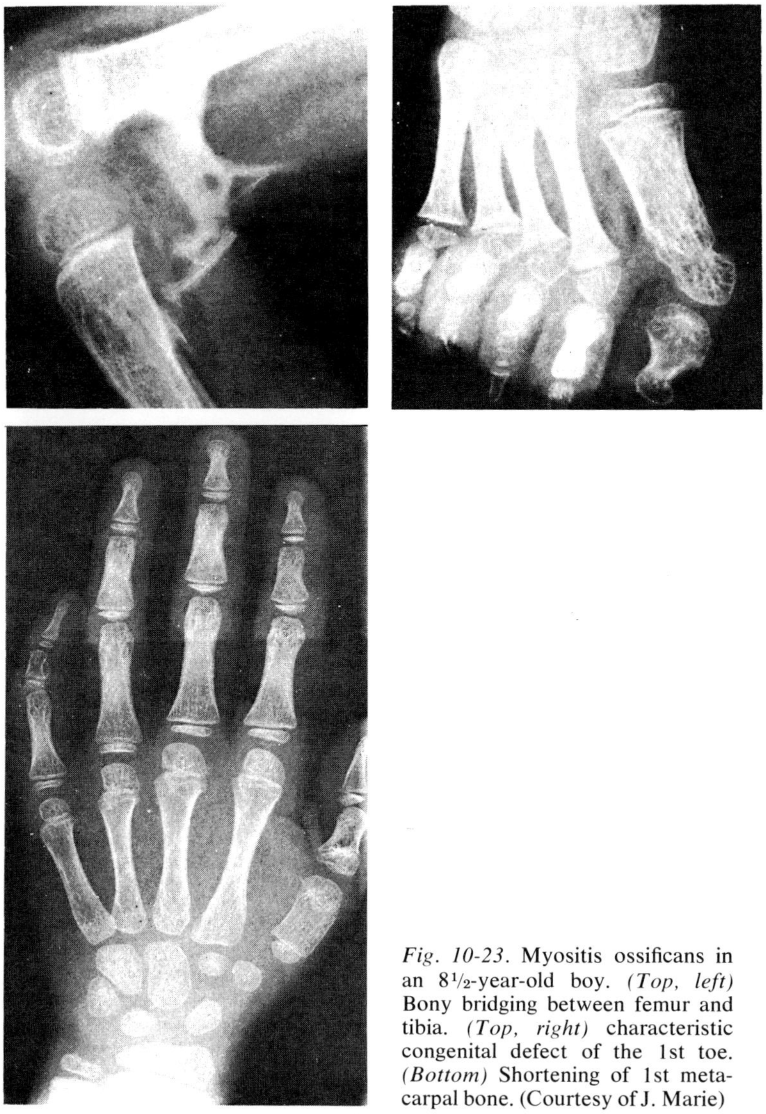

Fig. 10-23. Myositis ossificans in an 8½-year-old boy. *(Top, left)* Bony bridging between femur and tibia. *(Top, right)* characteristic congenital defect of the 1st toe. *(Bottom)* Shortening of 1st metacarpal bone. (Courtesy of J. Marie)

BOURNEVILLE'S TUBEROUS SCLEROSIS

In this disorder patients suffer from the association of epilepsy, mental retardation and adenoma sebaceum of the face. The skeletal involvement does not lead to clinical symptoms. Affected patients show the first symptoms, convulsive seizures, as babies. If there is known familial involvement the presence of unpigmented spots or of "café au lait" spots of the skin or possibly retinal phacomas will help to establish the proper diagnosis. Bony lesions will hardly ever be noted before the patient is 5 years old. They are present in big children towards adolescence with a 60 per cent incidence. Favoured areas are the skull, the bones of the extremities, the pelvis and the spine.

Skull films may show the presence of more or less rounded osteosclerotic foci within the diploic space. These can be floccular, of variable size and may be confluent. A local reaction within the internal table can be recognized immediately adjacent to superficial tuberous nodules (Fig. 10-25). There may also be deepseated paraventricular rounded calcifications.

The lesions of the small bones of the extremities are quite different in nature. They involve mainly the metaphyseo-epiphyseal region. They are round and pseudocystic (Fig. 10-25). They increase in number and size with advancing age. Their contours are usually ill-defined by nonspecific fibrous zones, replacing the normal trabeculation. Periosteal ossification sometimes overlies some of these, especially when metacarpals or metatarsals are involved. This finding may also be noted as an isolated irregular manifestation without subperiosteal resorption. Fine fracture lines lacking displacement in apparently normal bone may be recognized. Such findings together with pulmonary fibrosis have led in some patients to the confusion of this disorder with sarcoidosis, a disease only rarely seen in children (see p. 341).

Osteoblastic or sclerotic changes involving the pelvis and the spine are frequently present. Within the central portion of the iliac bones there may be irregular flamelike densities with a poorly defined border. These lesions, however, are not reticulated and do not destroy bone. Within vertebral bodies these opaque lesions are somewhat less marked. Careful search may reveal their presence within the vertebral bodies as well as the posterior arches. Others bones, such as ribs, may also be affected, with lesions of a mixed character. Long bones have a somewhat higher tendency towards irregular periosteal lesions of the diaphyses or simply zones with increased trabeculations.

NEUROFIBROMATOSIS (VON RECKLINGHAUSEN'S DISEASE)

One-third of all affected patients will have skeletal involvement. In some patients these may be unrecognized. Their presence in others will lead to the discovery of the underlying disorder, particularly in the presence of vertebral malalignment and uneven length of extremities. Some radiographic appearances may offer problems for the differential diagnosis in patients with only mild or minimal skin lesions and in the absence of a positive family history. Vertebral anomalies with a high incidence of spinal deformity are frequently encountered and represent the most important skeletal changes.

Patients with spinal involvement frequently have a scoliosis. About 50 per cent of them will have thoracic involvement with convexity towards the left. The scoliosis affects only a small number of vertebral bodies.

There is a high incidence of vertebral wedging. The bodies may assume a diabolo shape resulting from concavity of the anterior and posterior surface. There may also be loss of substance of the posterior arches involving the pedicles, the laminae and the articular and spinous processes (Fig. 10-26). One of the consequences is a marked enlargement of the intervertebral foramina and of the spinal canal in the transverse as well as the AP diameter. This aspect can be suggestive of the presence of a spinal cord tumor or of a neurofibroma. Myelography will, however, reveal, in the majority of cases, the presence of a simple hygroma without a nervous tissue tumor.

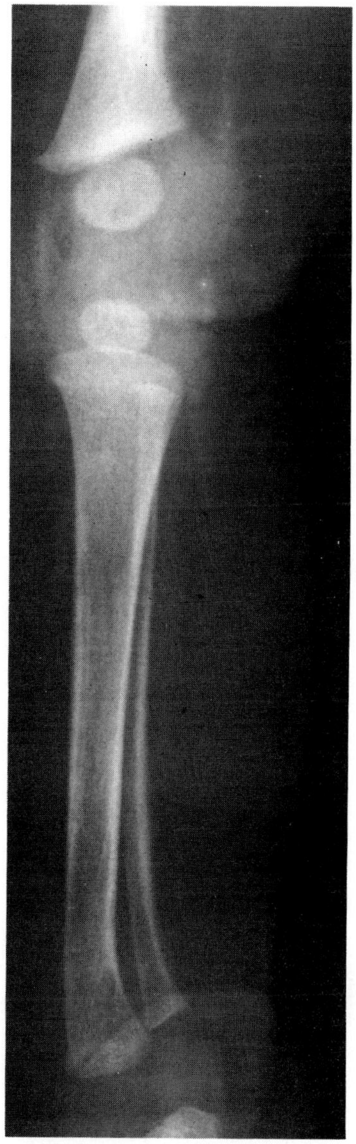

Fig. 10-24. Arthrogryposis involving a 5-month-old baby. Note the changes which involve the ends of the long bones. (Courtesy of J. Lefebvre)

The prognosis for the scoliosis is serious, since there is progression towards rotational dislocation of the spine including a true vertebral dislocation. This is a

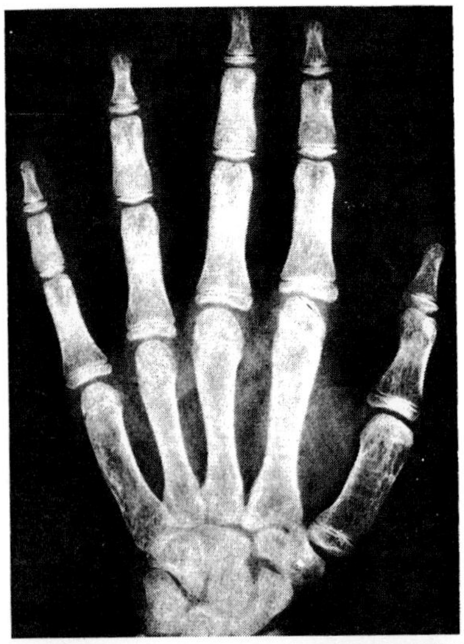

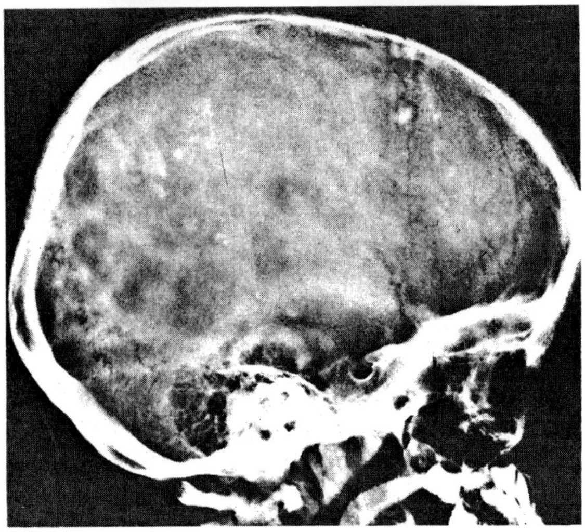

Fig. 10-25. Bourneville's tuberous sclerosis. *(Top)* 14-year-old boy with an abnormal bone structure of the metacarpals, particularly the 1st and 5th. *(Bottom)* 3-year-old boy with intracerebral calcifications. (Courtesy of R. Dailly)

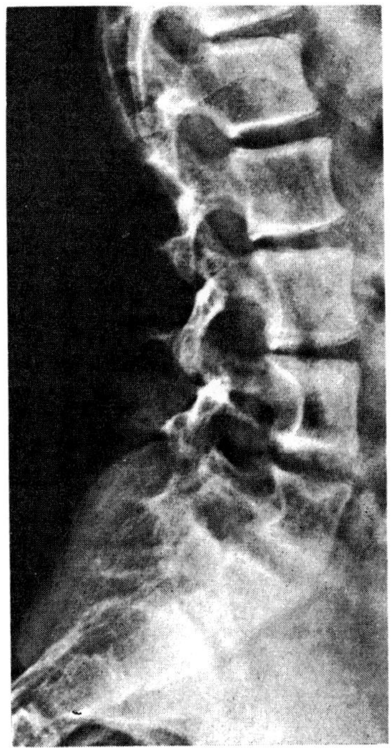

Fig. 10-26. Von Recklinghausen's disease in a 14-year-old boy. There is considerable widening of the spinal canal with concave deformity of the posterior borders of the lower lumbar vertebrae. (Courtesy of M. Lamy)

secondary phenomenon, which follows the destruction of the posterior articular process. In spite of the severe deformity, paraplegia is only rarely seen in the adult. If present, this is the result of the growth of a tumor.

The pathogenesis of these kyphoscolioses is still under discussion. An extending spinal cord lesion is an exceptional finding. The presence of a neural tumor developing from the nerve sheath in the presence of marked widening of the foramina, resulting in changes of the alignment of the spine could be suspected. This has hardly ever been observed. Some authors favor the theory of neurofibromatous infiltration of bone or of a regional mesodermal dysplasia.

If a patient with neurofibromatosis is suffering from scoliosis a very careful and sustained follow-up, together with active therapeutic measures, is mandatory. Often this requires posterior or anterior arthrodesis at an early moment.

Cranial involvement is relatively less frequent. Only one in six patients will be affected. Macrocranium, seen in more than one third of all patients (Weichert et al.), may be a latent finding, occasionally clinically evident by unilateral exophthalmus.

Radiographic findings may be those of local loss of thickness, an ovoid lacunar defect in the parietal or lower lambdoidal region (Fig. 10-27), and a somewhat larger, almost midline defect of the posterior region of the vault. This may look like a cranium bifidum. Sometimes there is a large defect of the entire posterior and superior border of one of the orbits, leading, in these patients, to congenital exophthalmus. Such a lytic process may involve both wings of the sphenoid and part of the frontal bone. In addition, the orbit and the sphenoidal groove, as well as the middle cerebral fossa, can be involved. The clinoids may be absent or deformed. This aspect of hypoplasia or osteolysis occasionally results in errors of interpretation leading to surgery or radiotherapy. Such interventions are not only unnecessary, but outright dangerous.

Similar to the findings mentioned for the spine, there may be a number of widened openings in the base of the skull. Similar etiologic theories have been proposed. Here again the possibility of the presence of intercranial expansile lesions or a neurinoma of one or several cranial nerves must be entertained. During infancy an optic glioma must be considered. Local calcifications and a supra-sellar expansion may mimic the symptoms of a craniopharyngioma. There may be a marked local uptake of isotopes in the region of osteolytic foci in the absence of brain tumors.

The involvement of the extremities can be strikingly variable. Bowing, sometimes congenital, may involve the leg and the forearm (see p. 168). In these patients there is always an anterior convexity. The presence of this finding should immediately alert one to the danger of pseudarthrosis, which may suddenly appear. Localized gigantism of the hands or feet with very thick subcutaneous and soft tissue structures may look like elephantiasis. Radiographic findings can lead to the diagnosis of the underlying disease.

Bowing mainly affects the lower or midportion of the tibia with anterior angulation. The bony structure may be abnormally clear. Histologic study of this region will demonstrate the presence of fibrous tissue, and occasionally that of a neurofibroma. Some patients have a congenital pseudarthrosis with a long distance between the remaining bony elements. Their facing ends may be blunt or rounded and sometimes pointed towards one another. There may be segmental bony hypoplasia. Sometimes there is a total absence of the fibula.

With local gigantism there is an unusual extent of the bone, a wavy appearance, and occasional thickening of the periosteum, but the width may be reduced. All these changes have been interpreted as trophic changes of neural origin, or as resulting from regional hypervascularity.

Occasionally a routine radiograph study will detect asymptomatic findings involving the long bones. The most characteristic sign is that of a small erosion of an adjacent neurofibroma resulting in an abnormal contour of the bone with localized thickening, or an uneven appearance of the cortex (Fig. 10-28). Occasionally periosteal elevation, leading to a bony edge outlining a local lesion, appears to have had its onset within the bone. This, however, is a false impression. In some cases clear centers can be recognized within the bone. These simulate a cortical defect or a nonossifying fibroma. Such erosive lesions are seen involving ribs with a relatively high incidence, where they sometimes mimic the appearance of coarctation of the aorta.

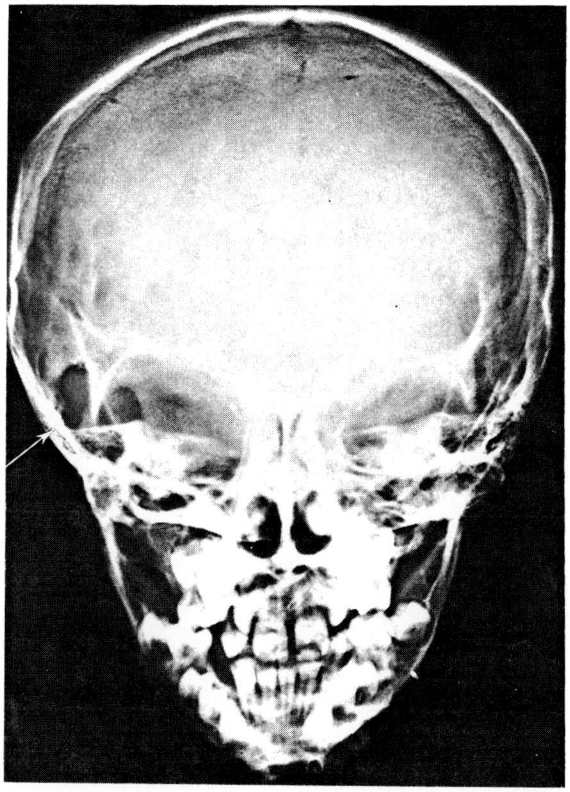

Fig. 10-27. Von Recklinghausen's disease in a 7½-year-old girl. Note the parieto-occipital defect on the right, and the plexiform neurinoma of the right orbit. There is an elevation of the orbital roof and an effacing of the sphenoidal ridge. (Courtesy of M. Hassan)

Careful radiographic investigation and follow-up, particularly of the spine, is therefore important in the care of patients with neurofibromatosis. Radiographic studies may help to properly establish the diagnosis in those patients who only have minimal cutaneous involvement.

STURGE-WEBER'S NEROANGIOMATOSIS

The classical finding is that of double contour "gyriform" patterns of intra-cranial subcortical calcifications primarily in the parietal and the occipital region (Fig. 10-29). They can be present after the patients are 2 or 3 years old. They result from calcifications lo-

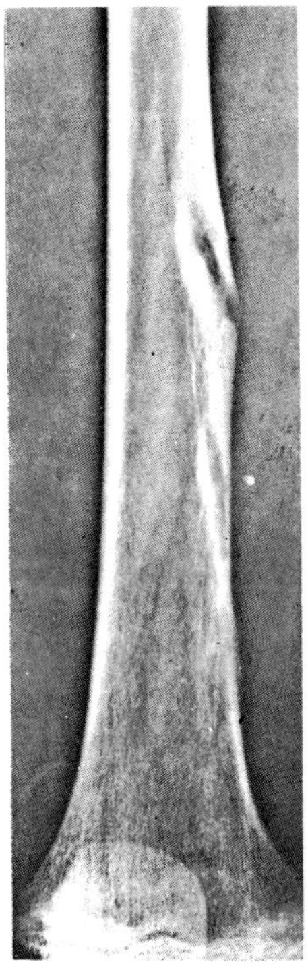

Fig. 10-28. Von Recklinghausen's disease in an 8-year-old girl. Notice the neurofibroma by its local erosion of the femur.

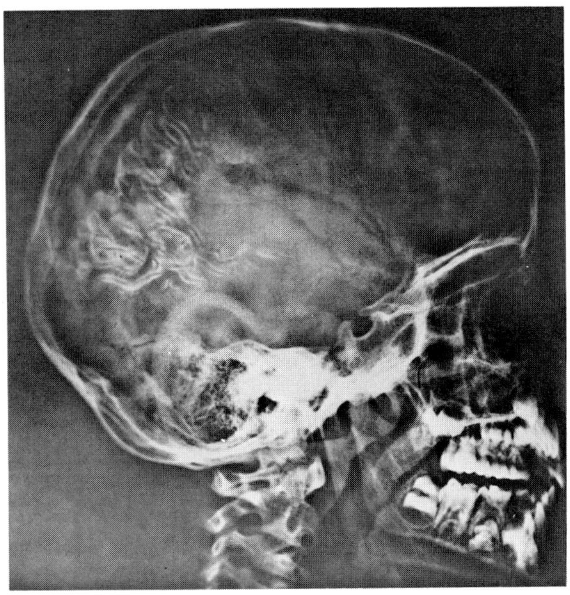

Fig. 10-29. Sturge-Weber neuroangiomatosis with its characteristic "double track" appearance. (Courtesy of J. Sauvegrain)

cated within the deep cellular layers of the cerebral cortex. At a somewhat earlier moment it is possible to recognize cerebral atrophy. Such signs may be readily recognized if one of the hemispheres is completely involved, but may be much less evident and only limited to local thinning or thickening of the vault if the atrophy is localized. In the area underlying the angioma of the face local hypertrophy of the facial structures and of the sinuses has also been reported. These changes may be localized to the trigeminal region on the same side as the meningo-encephalic anomalies with predominance in the frontal supra-orbital region.

REFERENCES

Basic Books and Works on Radiographic Approaches

CAFFEY (J.). Pediatric X-ray diagnosis. 5e édit. *Chicago, 1967, Year Book med. publ., éd.*

EPSTEIN (B. S.). The spine. A radiological text and atlas. *Philadelphia, 1969, Lea and Febiger, éd.*

HAWORTH (J. B.) et KEILLOR (G. W.). Use of transparencies in evaluating the width of the spinal canal in infants, children, and adults. *Radiology, 1962,* **79**, *109-114.*

HINCK (V. C.), HOPKINS (C. E.) et SAVARA (B. S.). Sagittal diameter of the cervical spinal canal in children. *Radiology, 1962,* **79**, *97-108.*

HINCK (V. C.), CLARK (W. M.) et HOPKINS (C. E.). Normal interpediculate distances (minimum and maximum) in children and adults. *Amer. J. Roentgenol., 1966,* **97**, *141-153.*

LEFEBVRE (J.), ERRERA (A.) et CHAUREY (M.). Note préliminaire sur la mesure des distances interpédiculaires vertébrales chez l'enfant. *J. Radiol., 1958,* **39**, *229-231.*

LUSTED (L. B.) et KEATS (T. E.). Atlas of roentgenographic measurement. *Chicago, 1959, Year Book med. publ. éd.*

NAIK (D. R.) et EMERY (J. L.). Diagnosis of Cleland-Arnold-Chiari deformity on plain radiographs of the spine. *Develop. Med. Child. Neurol. 1969, suppl. 20, 78-81.*

NORDQVIST (N. L.). The sagittal diameter of the spinal cord and the subarachnoïd space in different ages groups. A roentgenographic post mortem study. *Acta radiol., 1964, suppl. 227.*

SCHWARZ (G. S.). The width of the spinal canal in the growing vertebra with special reference to the sacrum. Maximum interpediculate distances in adults and children. *Amer. J. Roentgenol., 1956,* **76**, *476-481.*

SILVERMAN (F. N.). Roentgen standards of size of the pituitary fossa from infancy through adolescence. *Amer. J. Roentgenol., 1957,* **78**, *451-460.*

SIMRIL (W. A.) et THURSTON (D.). The normal interpediculate space in the spines of infants and children. *Radiology, 1955,* **64**, *340-347.*

TAVERAS (J. M.) et WOOD (E. H.). Diagnostic neuroradiology. *Baltimore, 1964, William Wilkins, éd.*

The Skull and Neurology

AFSHANI (E.), OSMAN (M.) et GIRDANY (B. R.). Widening of cranial sutures in children with deprivation dwarfism. *Radiology, 1973,* **109**, *141-144.*

DEBRUN (G.) et LE GAL (J.). Tumeurs supra-tentorielles de l'enfant. *Encyclopédie méd.-chir. : Radiol., 1964, 31626 K10 et M10.*

EPSTEIN (J. A.) et EPSTEIN (B. S.). Deformities of the skull surfaces in infancy and childhood. *J. Pediat., 1967,* **70**, *636-647.*

FAURÉ (CL.) et GRUSON (B.). L'exploration radiologique des cranio-pharyngiomes de l'enfant (à propos de 17 observations). *Ann. Radiol., 1959,* **11**, *197-228.*

FAURÉ (CL.) et DEBRUN (G.). Apport de la radiographie simple du crâne à l'examen d'un sujet porteur d'une tumeur cérébrale évoluant sous le masque d'une épilepsie chronique d'apparence primitive. *Cah. Epilepsie, 1971,* **1**, *55-66.*

FESSARD (CL.). Cerebral tumors in infancy. 66 clinico-anatomical case studies. *Amer. J. Dis. Child., 1968,* **115**, *302-308.*

GUTHKELCH (A. N.). Occipital cranium bifidum. *Arch. Dis. Childh., 1970,* **45**, *104-109.*

LAVAL-JEANTET (M.), OLIGO (N.) et JUSTER (M.). Les impressions digitales crâniennes chez le nouveau-né. *Bull. Ass. Anat., 1966, 51e réunion, 571-579.*

LEFEBVRE (J.), GUY (E.) et METZGER (J.). Evolution des signes radiographiques des atrophies cérébrales unilatérales. *Acta radiol., 1953,* **40**, *314-324.*

LEFEBVRE (J.), FAURÉ (CL.), DEBRUN (G.), LABRUNE (M.) et LE GAL (J.). Les tumeurs du cervelet et du quatrième ventricule. Sémiologie radiologique. *XXIe Congrès Ass. Pédiat. Lang. franç., Paris, 1967, Expansion Scient. franç., éd., t. I, 106-132.*

LIEBESKIND (A.), JACOBSON (R.) et SCHECHTER (M. M.). Craniolacunia diagnosed prenatally. *Neuroradiology, 1971,* **3**, *109-112.*

MCRAE (D. L.). Observations on craniolacunia. *Acta radiol., 1966,* **5**, *55-64.*

MIRIBEL (J.) et MARINIER (R.). Apport de la radiographie simple du crâne à l'examen d'un épileptique. *Rev. Neuropsychiat. infant., 1968,* **16**, *847-861.*

SHOPFNER (C. E.), JABBOUR (J. T.) et VALLION (R. M.). Craniolacunia. *Amer. J. Roentgenol., 1965,* **93**, *343-349.*

SILVER (H. K.) et FINKELSTEIN (M.). Deprivation dwarfism. *J. Pediat., 1967,* **70**, *317-324.*

SOMOGYI (Zs.). Craniofenestria, craniolacunaria. *Fortschr. Röntgenstr., 1962,* **96**, *502-507.*

VOUTILAINEN (A.). A case of lacunar skull of the newborn. *Ann. Paediat. Fenn., 1964,* **10**, *57-63.*

The Spine and Neurology

FISCHGOLD (H.) et WACKENHEIM (A.). La radiographie des formations intrarachidiennes. *Paris, 1965, Masson, éd.*

GODLEWSKI (S.) et DRY (J.). Les anomalies congénitales de la charnière cervico-occipitale. *Paris, 1964, Expansion scient. franç., éd.*

LEFEBVRE (J.), KLEIN (M. R.), LEPINTRE (J.) et FAURÉ (CL.). Etude radiologique des tumeurs médullaires chez l'enfant. *Acta radiol., 1956,* **46**, *48-53.*

MOYSON (FR.) et WITTEK (FR.). La diastématomyélie. *Acta orthop. belg., 1968,* **34**, *419-432.*

RIGAULT (P.), POULIQUEN (J.-C.), GUYONVARCH (G.) et DURAND (Y.). Quatre cas de diastématomyélie. *Rev. Chir. orthop., 1972,* **58**, *33-50.*

RIGAULT (P.), POULIQUEN (J.-C.), LEPINTRE (E.) et HOUTTEVILLE (J.-P.). Malformations médullaires chez les enfants atteints de malformations vertébrales congénitales (en dehors des myélo-méningocèles). *Ann. Pédiat., 1972,* **19**, *775-783.*

Distant Effects on the Skeleton

AUTIO (S.), VISAKORPI (J. K.) et JARVINEN (H.). Aspartylglycosaminuria (AGU). Further aspects on its clinical picture, mode of inheritance and epidemiology based on a serie of 57 patients. *Ann. clin. Res., 1973,* **5**, *149-155.*

AKSOY (M.), CAMLI (N.), DINCOL (K.), ERDEM (S.) et AKGÜN (T.). Osseous changes in Wilson's disease. A radiologic study of nine patients. *Radiology, 1972,* **102**, *505-509.*

BECKER (P. E.) et KNORRE (G. V.). Myositis ossificans progressiva. *Ergebn. inn. Med. Kinderheilk., 1968,* **27**, *1-31.*

BONA (C.), STANESCU (V.), DUMITRESCU (M. S.) et IONESCU (V.). Histochemical and cytoenzymological studies in myositis ossificans. *Acta histochem., 1967,* **27**, *207-224.*

BUCKNALL (W. E.), HASLAM (R. H. A.) et HOLTZMAN (N. A.). Kinky hair syndrome : response to copper therapy. *Pediatrics, 1973,* **52**, *653-657.*

CATEL (W.). Differential-Diagnostische Symptomatologie von Krankheiten des Kindesalters. *Stuttgart, 1951, G. Thieme, éd., p. 48-53.*

CUSWORTH (D. C.) et DENT (C. E.). Homocystinuria. *Brit. med. Bull., 1969,* **25**, *42-47.*

EDWARDS (M. J.). The experimental production of arthrogryposis multiplex congenita in guinea-pigs by maternal hyperthermia during gestation. *J. Path., 1971,* **104**, *221-229.*

FEINBERG (S. B.) et FISH (R. O.). Roentgen findings in growing long bones in phenylketonuria. *Radiology, 1962,* **78**, *394-398.*

FELLER (E. R.) et SCHUMACHER (H. R.). Osteoarticular changes in Wilson's disease. *Arthr. and Rheum., 1972,* **15**, *259-266.*

FISCH (R. O.), GRAVEM (H. J.) et FEINBERG (S. B.). Growth and bone characteristics of phenylketonurics children. *Amer. J. Dis. Child., 1966,* **112**, *3-10,*

FRIEDLANDER (H. L.), WESTING (G. W.) et WOOD (W. L.). Arthrogryposis multiplex congenita. *J. Bone Jt Surg., 1968,* **50-A**, *89-112.*

GAUDIER (B.), RÉMY (J.), NUYTS (J.-P.), CARON-POITREAU (CH.), BOMBART (E.) et FOISSSAC-GÉGOUX (M.-CH.). Etude radiologique des signes osseux de l'homocystinurie (à propos de six observations). *Arch. franç. Pédiat., 1969,* **26**, *963-975.*

GIBSON (D. A.) et URS (N. D. K.). Arthrogryposis multiplex congenita. *J. Bone Jt Surg., 1970,* **52-B**, *483-493.*

HOOSHMAND (H.), MARTINEZ (A. J.) et ROSENBLUM (W. I.). Arthrogryposis multiplex congenita. Simultaneous involvement of peripheral nerve and skeletal muscle. *Arch. Neurol., 1971,* **24**, *561-571.*

HUTTENLOCHER (P. R.), LANDWIRTH (J.), HANSON (V.), GALLACHER (B. B.) et BENSCH (K.). Osteochondromuscular dystrophy, a disorder manifested by multiple skeletal deformities myotonia and dystrophic changes in muscles. *Pediatrics, 1969,* **44**, *945-958.*

JACOBSON (H. C.), HERBERT (E. A.) et POPPEL (M. H.). Arthrogryposis multiplex congenita. *Radiology, 1955,* **65**, *8-17.*

KAPLAN (M.), NAHUM (H.), GRUMBACH (R.), DRAPEAU (P.), GOROUBEN (J. C.) et ANIZAN (B.). A propos d'un cas de myosite ossifiante progressive. *Ann. Pédiat., 1963,* **39**, *1776-1785.*

LAMY (M.), JAMMET (M. L.) et AJJAN (N.). Arthrogrypose ou syndrome arthrogryposique ? A propos de dix observations. *Sem. Hôp. Paris, 1965,* **41**, *2419-2430.*

LAPLANE (R.), FONTAINE (J.-L.), LAGARDÈRE (B.) et SAMBUCY (F.). Nanisme syndesmodysplasique familial. Une entité morbide nouvelle. *Arch. franç. Pédiat., 1972,* **29**, *831-838.*

LEBENTHAL (E.), SHOCHET (S. B.), ADAM (A.), SEELENFREUND (M.), FRIED (A.), NAJENSON (T.), SANDBANK (U.) et MATOTH (Y.). Arthrogryposis multiplex congenita : Twenty-three cases in an arab kindred. *Pediatrics, 1970,* **46**, *891-899.*

LEFEBVRE (J.), GUY (E.), LERIQUE (J.) et CHAUMONT (P.). Les données des explorations physiques des myopathies. *Excerpta Med. Internat. Congress series, 1964, n° 107, 648-650.*

LLOYD ROBERTS (G. C.) et LETTIN (A. W. F.). Arthrogryposis multiplex congenita. *J. Bone Jt Surg., 1970,* **52-B**, *494-508.*

MCEWEN (G. D.) et FLOYD (G. S.). Congenital insensitivity to pain and its orthopedic implications. *Clin. Orthop., 1970,* **68**, *100-107.*

MAROTEAUX (P.). La myosite ossifiante. *Rev. Rhum., 1965,* **32**, *512-513.*

MASSÉ (P.), BARON (P.), CAHUZAC (M.), LACHERETZ (M.), MARTIN (CH.), QUÉNEAU (P.) et ROULET (J.). La chirurgie de l'infirmité motrice cérébrale chez l'enfant. *Rev. Chir. orthop., 1967,* **53**, *729-793.*

MINDELZUN (R.), ELKIN (M.), SCHEINBERG (I. H.) et STERNLIEB (I.). Skeletal changes in Wilson's disease. A radiological study. *Radiology, 1970,* **94**, *127-132.*

MOORE (W. T.) et FEDERMAN (D. D.). Familial dwarfism and « stiff joints ». Report of a kindred. *Arch. intern. Med., 1965,* **115**, *398-404.*

MURDOCH (M. M.) et HOLMAN (G. H.). Roentgenologic bone changes in phenylketonuria. *Amer. J. Dis. Child., 1964,* **107**, *523-532.*

NEIMANN (N.), VIDAILHET (M.), MARTIN (J. J.), ANDRÉ (Mme M.), FLOQUET (J.) et GRIGNON (J.). Fragilité osseuse, amyotrophie, arriération et lésions dégénératives du système nerveux central. *Arch. franç. pédiat., 1973,* **30**, *899-913.*

POUYANNE (L.), VERGER (P.), GUILLARD (J.-M.), MORTUREUX (Y.), SANDLER (B.), GUINARD (F.) et DANDELOT (G.). Myosite ossifiante progressive (maladie de Munchmeyer) chez un enfant de treize mois. *Bordeaux méd., 1968, 1345-1350.*

SCHWARTZ (O.) et JAMPEL (R. S.). Congenital blepharophimosis associated with a unique generalized myopathy. *Arch. Ophthal., 1962,* **68**, *52-57.*

SIEGELMAN (S. S.), HEIMANN (W. G.) et MANIN (M. C.). Congenital indifference to pain. *Amer. J. Roentgenol., 1966,* **97**, *242-247.*

SILVERMAN (F. N.) et GILDEN (J. J.). Congenital insensitivity to pain : a neurological syndrome with bizarre skeletal lesions. *Radiology, 1959,* **72**, *176-190.*

SMITH (D. M.), ZEMAN (W.), JOHNSTON (C. C., Jr.) et DEISS (W. P., Jr.). Myositis ossificans progressiva. Case report with metabolic and histochemical studies *Metabolism, 1966,* **15**, *521-528.*

SMITH (S. W.). Roentgen findings in homocystinuria. *Amer. J. Roentgenol., 1967,* **100**, *147-154.*

TURPIN (R.), CRUVEILLER (J.), LAFOURCADE (J.), BOCQUET (L.), CAILLE (B.), GORIN (R.) et VIALETTES (M.-L.). L'arthrogrypose multiple congénitale : maladie ou syndrome (étude de 9 observations). *Ann. Pédiat., 1966,* **42**, *1-18.*

WESENBERG (R. L.), GWINN (J. L.) et BARNES (G. R.). Radiological findings in the kinky hair syndrome. *Radiology, 1969,* **92**, *500-506.*

WRIGHT (G.) et AASE (J.). Kuskokwim syndrome : an inherited form of arthrogryposis in the Alaskan Eskimo. *Birth Defects, Original Article Series, 1969, V n° 3, 91-95.*

Phacomatoses

« Les phacomatoses ». *18e Congrès Ass. Pédiat. Langue franç., Bâle, 1961, vol. II.*

COSTE (F.), GUIDET (M.), LABROUSSE (C.), ROYER (J.) et LAUGIER (P.). Le rachis dans la sclérose tubéreuse de Bourneville. *Rev. Rhum., 1966,* **33**, *17-22.*

DAVIDSON (K. C.). Cranial and intracranial lesions in neurofibromatosis. *Amer. J. Roentgenol., 1966,* **98**, *550-556.*

DEBAENE (A.), ACQUAVIVA (P.), DUFOUR (M.) et LEGRÉ (J.). Hyperconcavité (scalloping) vertébrale lombaire au cours de la maladie de Recklinghausen. *J. Radiol. Electrol., 1973,* **54**, *149-151.*

DELAITRE (R.), PASQUIER (CH.) et GROSIEUX (M.-F.). La maladie de Recklinghausen chez l'enfant. *Rev. Pédiat., 1967,* **3**, *237-244.*

DICKERSON (W. W.). Nature of certain osseous lesions in tuberous sclerosis. *Arch. Neurol. Psychiat. (Chic.), 1955,* **73**, *525-529.*

FOURNIER (A. M.), PADOVANI (J.) et DENIZET (D.). La neuro-fibromatose de Recklinghausen, son polymorphisme radio-clinique. *J. Radiol. Electrol., 1963,* **44**, *513-522.*

GRIFFITH (B. H.), MCKINNEY (P.), MONROE (C. W.) et HOWELL (A.). Von Recklinghausen's disease in children. *Plast. reconstr. Surg., 1972,* **49**, *647-653.*

GUILLEMINET (M.), CREYSSEL (J.), MOURGUES (G. DE) et FISCHER (L.). Neurofibromatose de von Recklinghausen. Hypertrophie congénitale d'un membre inférieur dans l'enfance et luxation spontanée de la hanche homolatérale à l'âge adulte. *Presse méd., 1970,* **78**, *1269-1271.*

HUNT (J. C.) et PUGH (D. G.). Skeletal lesions in neurofibromatosis. *Radiology, 1961,* **76**, *1-19.*

LABRUNE (B.), REYROLE (L.), ELCHARDUS (J. C.), LEBEAU (J. C.), RIBIERRE (M.) et MALLET (R.). Localisations rénales et osseuses au cours de la sclérose tubéreuse de Bourneville. *Ann. Pédiat., 1970,* **46**, *774-782.*

MESZAROS (W. T.), GUZZO (F.) et SCHORSCH (H.). Neurofibromatosis. *Amer. J. Roentgenol., 1966,* **98**, *557-569.*

PITT (M. J.), MOSHER (J. F.) et EDEIKEN (J.). Abnormal periosteum and bone in neurofibromatosis. *Radiology, 1972,* **103**, *143-146.*

SALERNO (N. R.) et EDEIKEN (J.). Vertebral scalloping in neurofibromatosis. *Radiology, 1970,* **97**, *509-510.*

SMITH (T. K.), GREGERSEN (G. G.) et SAMILSON (R. L.). Orthopaedic problems associated with tuberous sclerosis. *J. Bone Jt Surg., 1969,* **51-A**, *97-102.*

ZEIGLER (R. L.), HARLE (T. S.) et FRED (H. L.). Roentgenographic features of tuberous sclerosis. *Amer. Fam. Physcn., 1970,* **i**, *88-91.*

Part Five:

Acquired Bone Diseases

In this part we shall first study infectious disorders such as osteomyelitis, tuberculosis of bone, mycoses, congenital syphilis, congenital rubella and sacroidosis. Two disorders of uncertain etiology are also included: pulmonary hypertrophic osteoarthropathy and infantile cortical hyperostosis.

Within the context of trauma, a limited discussion will be devoted to the battered child syndrome. Fractures cannot be dealt with here, since they are well covered in most surgical or orthopaedic books. Some comments are included on practical orthopaedic problems.

Chronic atrophic polychondritis will not be covered, since its manifestations are limited to cartilage. Bony lesions are not part of this disorder. A number of bibliographic references are appended with respect to this disease.

11 Infectious and Traumatic Disorders

P. Rigault

OSTEOMYELITIS

During the last 20 years a complete change of all the aspects of acute osteomyelitis has taken place. Historically this was a very serious, frequently fatal, disease requiring surgery and eventually leading to chronic persistent suppuration or much feared deformity.

Better health care for infants and children, early and effective therapy for acute infections with antibiotics, and altered epidemiologic factors, possibly related to improved hygiene and general health, are all part of the significant progress achieved in the therapy of osteomyelitis and the dramatic reduction of its serious nature. The incidence, however, has been the same for the last several dozens of years. Hospital statistics reveal that even though the age of the patients is now even lower, since more and more babies and newborns are affected, the total number of cases with osteomyelitis remains about the same. Involvement in acute osteomyelitis during infancy up to adolescence, if recognized early and properly treated, has today an entirely different prognosis. Practically always complete, often rapid and permanent, healing will result without any complications. Unhappily, however, there is still too high a number of patients in whom the nature of the disorder is initially unrecognized, and for whom therapy is inadequate. Often a number of unfavorable factors play a significant role, such as in the newborn period or early infancy. Unfavorable or sometimes disastrous familial conditions may further contribute to a poor prognosis, and the disease may progress as in the pre-antibiotic days. The diagnosis of osteomyelitis has a number of extremely complex aspects. We will successively discuss acute, subacute and chronic osteomyelitis.

ACUTE OSTEOMYELITIS

It is important to handle patients suspected of suffering from acute osteomyelitis from the start as a *true emergency*. The condition must be quickly recognized. If suspected, all measures directed to its recognition must be rapidly taken and therapy immediately instituted.

Out of full well-being a child or adolescent will suddenly complain of excruciating pain at one of the ends of a long bone of a limb. This sudden pain may be progressive and is usually accompanied by a febrile infectious symptomatology. Prominent clinical findings are marked swelling of the metaphyseal region of the involved bone with local pain and pain to palpation. Such findings are sufficient for clinical suspicion. The immediate next steps are: casting of the involved limb, administration of antibiotics (after having taken a throat and blood culture), and the drawing of blood for sedimentation rate and white count. A careful clinical search is required for the possibility of staphylococcal rhinopharyngitis, otitis or other infections. Radiographic study completes the initial work-up. It may be entirely normal (Fig. 11-1). In spite of the fact that this aspect of osteomyelitis should be generally known there are unhappily too many situations where this is not recognized. There are several reasons for this. Because of local trauma this may be considered simply as a contusion or a minimal fracture in spite of a negative roentgenfinding. Because of the high fever and local inflammation cellulitis with lymphangitis may be suspected. An adjacent joint may be held in flexion, but could actually be moved and diagnosis of acute rheumatoid arthritis is sometimes suspected, sometimes with the disastrous consequence of the prescription of corticosteroid therapy. Because of the immobility of the limb poliomyelitis has also been suspected.

All these errors are highly detrimental to the patient, since they result in the delay of proper treatment. Only the earliest possible diagnosis and the imediate beginning of therapy will fully control or abort an osteomyelitis. All errors are avoidable, if the clinical rules known for many years are not overlooked, particularly that: acute bone pain in children accompanied by infection and fever must be considered to be early osteomyelitis.

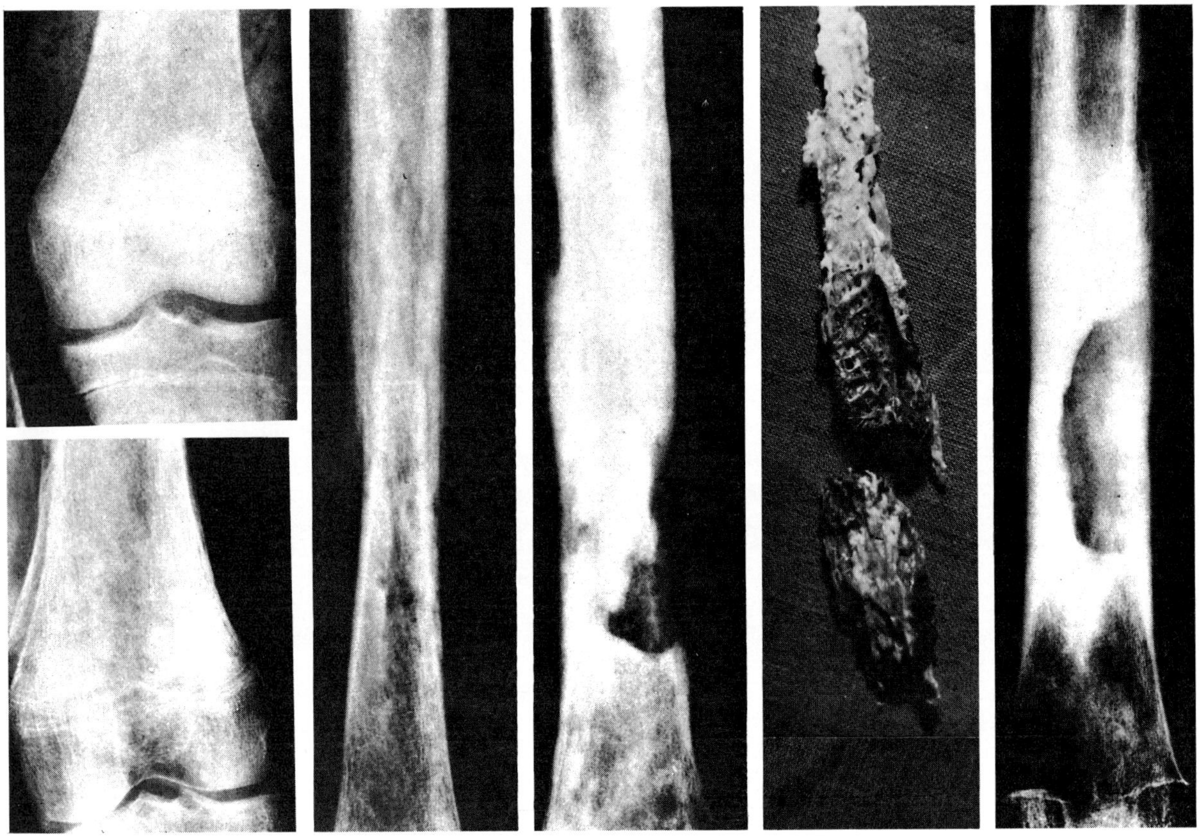

Fig. 11-1. (*Far left, top*) Acute osteomyelitis of the lower end of the femur in a 13-year-old girl. The onset was sudden with acute knee pain and fever up to 40°C. Therapeutic measures consisting of casting and antibiotics by infusion were withheld for several days. Ten days later the radiographic appearance is still normal. This is not unusual. (*Far left, bottom*) During the 3rd week a sudden periosteal abscess was opened and drained. (*Second from left*) As therapy was delayed the course is that of prolonged osteomyelitis. After 3 months there is a complete destruction of the femoral diaphysis. (*Third from right*) Sequestration of the large diaphyseal fragment can be recognized with the appearance of a fistula along an earlier incision and drainage of the abscess. (*Second from right*) Surgically removed sequestrum. (*Far right*) Definitive healing was possible 7 years after the onset of osteomyelitis. Several surgical interventions included an incision for abscess formation, the removal of sequestra, curettage, along with other procedures were required. Several large bony defects remain and there is a considerable loss of cortex. This is a typical course of prolonged osteomyelitis.

It is a grave mistake to wait for several days in order to follow the infectious symptoms. There will be formation of an abscess palpable in its subperiosteal location, sometimes quite expansive in location and extending completely around the bony shaft requiring surgical drainage. Radiographic study can show this in the image of a cortical double contour combined with early bony symptoms, such as local motteling and irregularity of the compact bone and metaphyseal geodes (Fig. 11-1, *Far left, bottom*).

If there is no therapy or if the early phases have been overlooked and if the patient does not develop further complications, the usual sequence of events is abscess formation with a fistula tract to skin. There will be chronic discharge of pus as long as the osteomyelitic process continues. Patients with a prolonged course eventually suffer from chronic secondary osteomyelitis.

Clinical Types

The clinical aspect of osteomyelitis is so varied that it is almost impossible to enumerate all the possible symptoms. The *onset* can also be quite variable in its intensity and presentation.

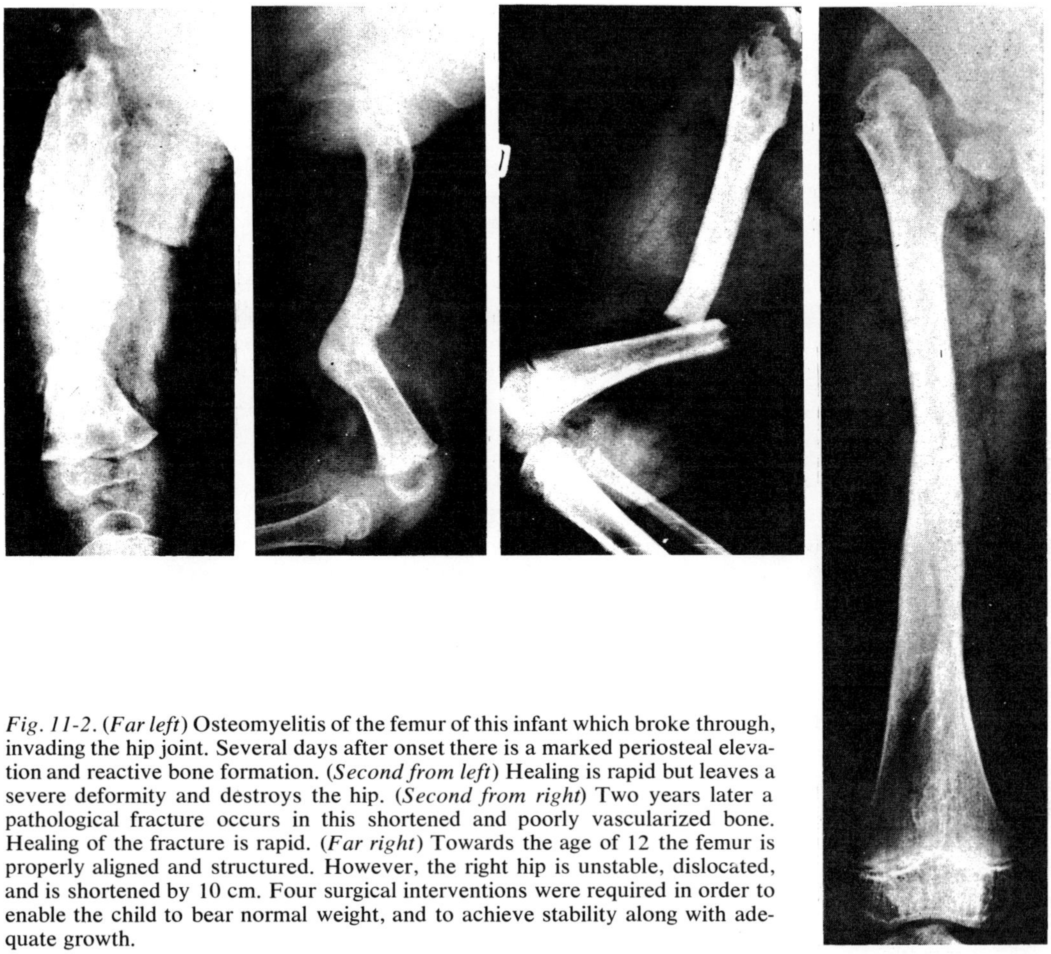

Fig. 11-2. (*Far left*) Osteomyelitis of the femur of this infant which broke through, invading the hip joint. Several days after onset there is a marked periosteal elevation and reactive bone formation. (*Second from left*) Healing is rapid but leaves a severe deformity and destroys the hip. (*Second from right*) Two years later a pathological fracture occurs in this shortened and poorly vascularized bone. Healing of the fracture is rapid. (*Far right*) Towards the age of 12 the femur is properly aligned and structured. However, the right hip is unstable, dislocated, and is shortened by 10 cm. Four surgical interventions were required in order to enable the child to bear normal weight, and to achieve stability along with adequate growth.

Sometimes there are only findings of minimal intensity and only mild spontaneous pain. This is sub-acute osteomyelitis. There will always be acute pain from pressure to the bone, which will support this diagnosis.

Sometimes, however, bony localization occurs during a severe acute clinical infection by staphylococcal intoxication or more frequently during septicemia or staphylococcal sepsis from a variety of primary local lesions. In such clinical circumstances a careful systematic examination, almost segment by segment for the presence of bone pain or early abscess formation, is indicated.

The condition of the host is a key factor and two special aspects should be distinguished.

Neglected acute osteomyelitis in transplant recipients, and patients in poor nutritional states or severely neglected hygienic conditions today have the highest incidence of severe involvement. In these cases multiple localization with severe destruction of extensive bony segments, even entire diaphyses, joint involvement and a general tendency towards chronic fistula formation can occur. Affected patients have a high risk of damage to the growth cartilage with serious consequences.

Acute osteomyelitis in the infant has its own special characteristics (Fig. 11-2). Frequently occurring in newborns or prematures, the initial location may often be within epiphyses, and is therefore clinically hard to recognize. It may be recognized only after the formation of an abscess. This may lead to the radiologic discovery of the extensive bony and articular involvement. In this patient group early joint involvement is the rule. There may even be septic arthritis. The usual port of entry is the skin, sometimes the umbilicus, the airway (rhino-pharynx, lungs), or the digestive tract (diarrhea with toxicosis). Infectious hospitalism is today a serious problem. A special sub-group is that of patients developing this complication from contaminations after infusions. Fever may be absent or mild, but the general condition and a lack of weight gain may be the key symptoms. Laboratory findings may not be dramatic. The systematic search for localized pain is not a foolproof method of identification.

A number of other symptoms must be carefully investigated to help in recognizing the basic disorder. A careful search of all movements of the baby in the crib and while being held up by the shoulders should be made. The baby should be placed face down. During this investigation one should cause the baby to cry and move in order to see if part of the body or a segment of a limb is held in a fixed position. Local edema, especially of the shoulders and groin and of the para-articular region may be an important finding, together with some crying during passive cautious mobilization of the limbs and their segments, studied successively. Such a systematic examination is correct approach to early detection of localized osteomyelitis in the baby who may be suffering from infection, or who is already under treatment. Radiographs may be helpful during an early phase. Good films will reveal the presence of edema of the soft tissues. Changes and destruction of bones may be visible after a few days.

It may be surprising how rapidly these changes develop. Clinical or radiologic study may uncover large abscess formation requiring drainage, extensive periosteal elevation and local calcification, epiphyseolysis with a very poor prognosis, and abnormal positioning and dislocation of the neighboring joints.

The course of acute osteomyelitis of the baby may be in two markedly different directions. On the one hand bony destruction, joint involvement and destruction of the growth zone, can occur so rapidly, and be so extensive, that serious functional defects result—severe shortening, dislocation, bowing, etc. (Fig. 11-2). On the other hand, an excellent prognosis can be given if it is possible to rapidly effect evacuation of the pus from the deep abscess or necrosis. This evacuation may be spontaneous, or surgically induced by puncture and aspiration. If these measures are successfully performed, there is excellent healing without chronicity or relapse. The ground rule in the handling of osteomyelitis of the newborn, premature or baby is its earliest possible diagnosis and therapy, since this is the key element for the prognosis.

The location of osteomyelitis may have considerable importance for the course of the disorder. Long bones or extremities and especially the lower end of the femur and the proximal region of the tibia are areas of frequent involvement. Still, any bone can be affected. The proximal end of the femur is a particularly feared location, especially in babies, because of frequent local involvement of the hip. Early diagnosis may prevent difficulties. Painful mobilization of the hip and regional edema extending into the pubic and perineal region, combined with edema of the soft tissues and abnormal centering within the joint on radiographic study are some of the most telling local findings. Fibular involvement is not unusual, with, on the whole, a good prognosis since the bone can be resected in its major extent without ill effect. Involvement of the humerus is seen frequently and may be extensive and serious extending to the shoulder with resulting functional disturbances. Osteomyelitis of both bones of the forearm, as pandiaphysitis, frequently has a serious prognosis, since even if there is healing there will be persisting disturbances of pronation and supination. Osteomyelitis of the clavicula may appear first as a local infiltration resulting from the superficial location of the bone. There is an inherent risk of early fistula formation.

Short bones are often the site of osteomyelitis. It should be suspected if there is pain localized in a foot or a hand coexisting with fever. Calcaneal localization is not unusual and local abscess formation with a relatively superficial location is a frequent consequence. Chronic prolonged local involvement is, however, rare.

Vertebral involvement is frequent. It almost always involves the intervertebral disk, and occurs together with arthritis. The differential diagnosis may be somewhat difficult, since there are similarities with Pott's disease and even meningitis. A para-vertebral abscess may develop. Such a lesion is seen with increasing frequency; it usually has a good prognosis. Involvement of the maxilla is now rare in babies. If present, there are early ocular findings together with subsequent bony destruction and severe dental sequelae. Somewhat more unusual localizations are those involving ribs, the skull, the sternum and the scapula.

Staphylococci are the responsible *pathogens* in nine out of ten patients. Streptococcal osteomyelitis has become quite rare. Salmonella osteomyelitis is occasionally seen and may take a subacute or chronic course. Its preferred localization is in the tibia, ribs or the spine.

CHRONIC OSTEOMYELITIS

A chronic course may be the result of a prolonged initially acute osteomyelitis or a special type of "directly chronic" osteomyelitis.

CHRONIC OSTEOMYELITIS AFTER ACUTE OSTEOMYELITIS

This is simply a prolonged course of the basic disease. The diagnosis should not offer any problem, since the early phase should have led to the proper recognition of the disorder. The prognosis is serious and relapses must be feared. This course of osteomyelitis is seen from childhood on and results usually from a delayed onset or insufficient therapy of the disorder.

The anamnestic information is practically always the same. There is an acute osteomyelitis which has not healed completely. Its inflammatory signs persist. They may slowly disappear, only to recur. An incised abscess sometimes does not fully dry up, and there may be renewed fistula formation with repeated bouts of suppuration.

Radiologically, marked thickening of the cortex and unusual density of the bone will develop frequently together with a number of cavities. There is necrotic sequestrum formation of irregular and varying sizes, which may be spontaneously evacuated. Bowing of long bones with superficial destruction of joints and of the growth cartilage may also be present if arthritis complicates the picture or if there is indirect extension of the process into the neighbouring joints. If a particularly large bony segment has thus disappeared, the danger of the formation of a pseudarthrosis is real.

Such a prolonged course of osteomyelitis, which may assume any aspect of the whole spectrum of possible changes from a localized defect of one bony end to the total involvement of the entire extent of a long bone, is very difficult to successfully treat. The number of needed surgical interventions may be considerable and relapse may even occur many years later.

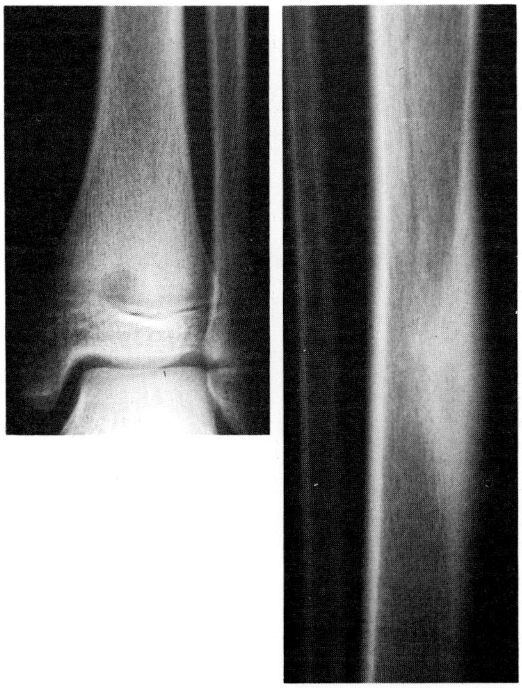

Fig. 11-3. Chronic osteomyelitis. (*Left*) Typical appearance of a central bony abscess in a 14-year-old boy who has been suffering from this disorder for several months. Local symptoms are increasingly painful, especially at night. The local lesion, when surgically approached, was found to be filled with pus. Culture revealed staphylococcus aureus. (*Right*) Another type of chronic osteomyelitis is localized periostosis. Surgery revealed that the causative microorganism was a staphylococcus. The intervention resulted in a complete relief of painful symptoms which this adolescent girl has been experiencing for several months.

PRIMARY CHRONIC OSTEOMYELITIS

This is a somewhat rare type of osteomyelitis. Proper recognition may be difficult and slow, since the aspect may mimic that of a number of other bony lesions—tumors, local dystrophy or infection.

Often local biopsy and a direct bacteriologic examination will lead to the correct diagnosis, especially if there is a central bony abscess—a Brodie abscess (Fig. 11-3). Such patients complain of chronic persisting pain, especially unpleasant at night, of a progressive nature. Otherwise there is no sign of a generalized disorder, and only radiographs will lead to the recognition of a metaphyseal centrally located small bony defect within a dense zone. The degree of subjective complaint and the local findings are markedly variable. Radiographic appearance may be that of a cyst of multiple dense central foci, or simple loss of local bone structure with variable localization. These lesions may be diaphyseal or diaphyseometaphyseal, sometimes with periosteal thickening.

A surgical approach is always justified, since besides confirming the diagnosis it will lead to eventual local healing.

Necrosing osteomyelitis with hyperostosis is an unusual type (Fig. 11-3) characterized by an extensive painful bony tumefaction involving the entire diaphysis or a diaphyseo-metaphyseal segment. Radiographs show an increased volume of the involved bone with a local irregular spotty densification of zones of geodes or sequestra.

Inflammatory signs are only moderate, localized and generalized, and occasionally only local biopsy and direct culture will lead to the proper diagnosis and the exclusion of a possibly suspected sarcoma or reticulosarcoma.

Periostitis albuminosa of Ollier and Poncet is seen only exceptionally in children. It is characterized by a collection of abscesses, often sterile, located directly next to bone and with only the most minimal bony lesion recognizable. The latter has to be considered as the result of a minor degree of acute osteomyelitis having healed spontaneously with some necrotic debris remaining as the causative agent for the local symptomatology. Surgical evacuation will result in complete cure.

Pathology and Pathogenesis

In the great majority of patients the causative agent is a staphylococcus.

The local infection, most frequently metaphyseal during childhood and epiphyseal in the baby, leads to local pus formation. This results from the necrotizing effect of staphylococcal toxins leading to local thrombophlebitis of potentially extensive nature. This process can involve the entire diaphysis and result in the formation of extensive sequestra.

Once suppuration has set in, even when this process forms a fistula opening onto the skin, it cannot evacuate the abnormal material like an abscess of the soft tissues can because it has no capacity to simply contract and fuse its walls. This is not possible because of the rigidity of the bony bed, where pus formation occurs. This fact explains why surgical evacuation of an osteomyelitic abscess is required and why simple spontaneous evacuation of sequestra will lead to the unhappy and discouraging chronicity of the lesions once established (Fig. 11-1 *C* to *F*).

Treatment

Therapy varies with the type of osteomyelitis.

Acute osteomyelitis requires emergency therapy, which must include: first, immobilization of the involved segment by casting and immobilizing both neighboring joints, and second, intensive high dosage intravenous therapy by infusion for 8 to 10 days.

Since one rarely knows the exact characteristics of the causative microorganism and its sensitivity to antibiotics, one must systematically use a bacteriolytic antibiotic—penicillin or a semi-synthetic penicillin Y in combination with a synergistic antistaphylococcic antibiotic drug. The dosage must be high: 10 to 20 million U of penicillin or even more, or 100 to 150 mg/kg of semi-synthetic penicillin per day. This dosage must be maintained for ten days under careful supervision of the general condition, the temperature, the sedimentation rate, and the numbers and counts of the white and of the red cells. After this period the cast is removed and radiographs are obtained.

If there are no more findings, which is quite frequently the case, it can be assumed that the osteomyelitis has, in fact, been aborted. The cure is often so dramatic that the original diagnosis may even be questioned. This is, however, of no importance! The antibiotic treatment should be continued by mouth for at least 2 months.

If there are still local inflammatory findings or general symptoms, but no clinical or radiologic signs for abscess formation, a new cast is applied and the antibiotic therapy renewed for another ten days, either intravenously or by mouth, depending on the severity of the clinical and laboratory findings. A new assessment is required after this second ten day period.

If there is abscess formation, recognized either by clinical or radiologic investigation, surgical intervention is the next step. A wide incision will lead to adequate evacuation of the accumulated pus after trepanation of the cortex in search of deep suppuration. All necrotic debris are excised and multiple suction tubes are placed before closure and renewed immobilization by casting. Culture should lead to the recognition of the responsible microorganism and its antibiogram. On this basis it is possible to offer a rational antibiotic treatment by infusion.

If there is a good response there will be only minimal radiologic findings visible after 2 to 4 weeks. In any case, immobilization should be continued until all clinical and laboratory findings have normalized and there is no further recognizable local inflammatory finding. Simple bed rest is indicated if one of the legs is involved until the sedimentation rate is markedly improved. Antibiotic therapy by mouth should be continued for at least 4 months after the end of casting. This is the only reliable way to avoid a possible relapse. Normal activity can be allowed when all the findings locally as well as the laboratory tests have returned to normal. It is obvious that such strict measures and careful supervision practically always require hospitalization of the child at least during the initial period.

Peracute osteomyelitis or its occurrence during sepsis will require in addition to these above outlines even higher doses and general supportive measures, such as intravenous alimentation, blood transfusion, etc. Prolonged hospitalization may be needed.

Only sub-acute forms or markedly localized types of osteomyelitis can be treated simply by oral antibiotics and without immobilization.

Inadequate application of these rules and delayed diagnosis are the key causes for therapeutic failures resulting in chronic osteomyelitis.

The care of *chronic osteomyelitis* requires indefinite follow-up. Medical therapy with antibiotics and immobilization must be maintained until all signs of inflammation have completely disappeared. This requires many weeks, months and sometimes several years with an occasional remission.

There are several possible indications for a surgical intervention for the evacuation of an abscess, removal of affected soft tissues and necrotic pieces of bone, for the curettage and for removal of sequestra. Such interventions will always try to carefully respect the bony continuity in order to avoid further complications such as a local fracture or the formation of pseudarthrosis. Still, the entire infected and dead extent of the bone, wherever possible, must be removed with closure of the remaining spaces and removal of fistula tracts. The local healing obtained in this way is usually, but not always permanent.

During this stage of the disease it is surgery alone which may bring about complete healing. Antibiotic therapy only has a supportive role to play, since by itself it is incapable of bringing about healing.

True chronic osteomyelitis is also a surgical disorder. Again, removal of a sometimes deep seated abscess or of a sequestrum should improve conditions, but may leave the problem of how to fill cavities within bones. Transplants or partial muscle insertion can be beneficial.

We will close this chapter on a pessimistic tone by commenting on the therapy of the sequelae of osteomyelitis. Some of these serious complications, such as uneven and abnormal growth, shortening or atrophy of part of a limb, bowing or pseudarthrosis, stiff joints sometimes in very poor position, and permanent or recidivating suppuration, all offer serious challenges. Surgical treatment of any one of these sequelae is long, difficult and not always rewarding. It should be added that in some of the worst situations, rare as they are, amputation will be the only reasonable approach after many years of repeated efforts or where the chronic local suppuration threatens the life of the patient, or finally where the functional disturbance of a leg is such that replacement by a prosthesis will be an improvement for the patient.

In the final analysis it is important to be fully aware that the total incidence of osteomyelitis has not changed. Even so it actually has practically no mortality. It remains, in those cases, however rare, where healing does not promptly occur, a much feared disorder resulting in chronic invalidity of childhood and persisting for life.

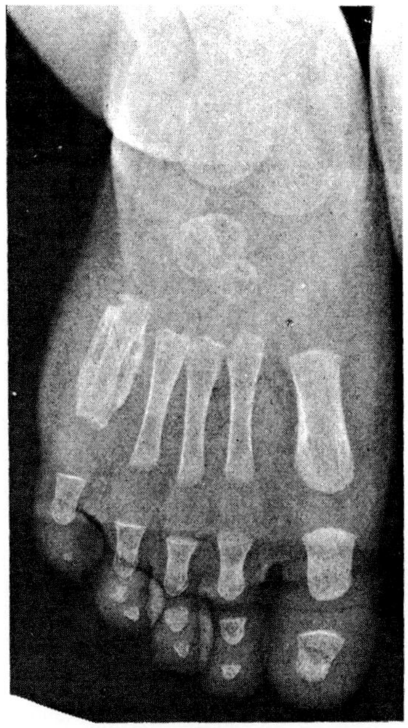

Fig. 11-4. Tuberculosis of the bone in a 1-year-old infant. Note the typical appearance of the spina ventosa involving the 5th metatarsal. (Courtesy of R. Mallet)

TUBERCULOSIS OF BONE

We shall consider here tuberculosis in multiple locations, since osteoarticular tuberculosis results from involvement of the joints.

Skeletal tuberculosis occurs in young children, but not exclusively. It is an unusual disorder, seen with a higher incidence in black children. It is a localized manifestation during the second phase of the disease, but it can occur simultaneously with primo-infection.

Most frequently involved patients will show up with a swollen finger, or, more rarely, a swelling of the cranial vault. Sometimes this disorder is recognized during a routine examination or because of some other complications.

Clinically, there is an increase in size of the finger. The swelling is hard, painful and there is slight local inflammation. Sometimes swelling of a limb or marked tumor of the orbit may be noted. The later stages of the natural course of the disease, with infiltration of the soft tissues and fistulae, are no longer seen because of the modern specific therapy.

The most characteristic radiographic finding is the presence of a spina-ventosa. Its early aspect is that of local swelling, widening and double contour of the cortex. The bone assumes a fusiform shape. This is followed by local bony destruction with a mottled or geodic appearance (Fig. 11-4). The radiographic findings may well be less characteristic and the phalangeal invovement may simply manifest as an increase in size with multiple small geodes and adjacent condensation. Within long bones one may recognize pseudo-cysts with marked periosteal reaction. These changes occur mainly in the diaphysis. Multi-geodic images, however, can be noted within the femoral metaphysis (Cremin et al.). In the cranial vault lacunar images may be present with ill defined borders, and surrounded by a large zone of condensation.

In a given patient there are quite often several areas of involvement. Besides a typical spina ventosa of a phalanx, simple widening of the cortex may be noted in other phalanges, in a metacarpal or a long bone. We emphasize that these typical round lytic lesions—*multiple geodes*—characteristically seen in sarcoidosis are not part of this disease.

Considering the rarity of skeletal tuberculosis its main risk is in being overlooked. In the presence, therefore, of the phalangeal lesions with a marked periosteal reaction or in the presence of multiple small lytic lesions the diagnosis of tuberculosis should be entertained. Every effort to rule out the possibility of contamination, the presence of other visceral lesions, especially within the chest, must be undertaken, and a tuberculin test is mandatory. Therapy should start soon combining several antibiotics. The duration of therapy is 12 to 18 months. This should result in rapid and complete cure without the addition of corticoids (Mallet et al.).

The appearance of this disorder should not be confused with that of sarcoidosis, which is a rare disorder in the baby or young child (see p. 341). The aspect of the lesions in syphilis is entirely different and careful analysis should lead to full differentiation. However, there are patients with chronic osteomyelitis with a remarkable periosteal reaction and the radiographic diagnosis may be extremely difficult to establish in the presence of localized spina ventosa.

Besides this type, mainly affecting the baby, there is tuberculous osteitis, which may be seen in bigger children. This form will involve the skull and the metaphysis of long bones. Occasionally, if there is articular tuberculosis, an epiphysis may be involved. It results in a markedly geodic appearance, sometimes containing a sequestrum. Usually there is no condensation and no periosteal reaction. Actually, however, the latter may be present, and there is considerable difficulty in distinguishing this lesion from chronic osteomyelitis.

As a consequence of BCG vaccination some rare patients develop bony lesions 6 to 12 months later. The aspect is quite similar to tuberculosis of the skeleton. There may be a metaphyseal lytic lacuna with a clear center and a surrounding periosteal reaction with a good prognosis.

THE MYCOSES OF BONE

These lesions are unusual and will be discussed only shortly.

Histoplasmosis must be mentioned especially, since this disorder can be seen regularly in babies. It is discovered because of the presence of a reduced general condition. A large liver and spleen are usually found, sometimes lymphadenopathies are found.

Radiographic findings are multiple: small radiolucencies within the skull, the diaphyses of long bones, the scapula, the pelvis and the clavicles. These geodes have a variable size and a round or oval form. The long bones frequently have a periosteal reaction seen as a double contour, sometimes with a slight elevation. Osteoporosis is frequently also present.

Cryptococcosis, coccidiomycosis and actinomycosis can also lead to limited clearly defined lytic lesions. Cryptococcosis has only a minimal periosteal reaction, whereas such a finding can be seen much more impressively in coccidiomycosis. In both these disorders dissemination occurs by hematogenous spread, and the lesions may be located in the metaphyses of long bones, the skull, the spine, the pelvis or the scapulae. Cryptococcosis is often combined with sarcoidosis or with one of the reticuloendothelioses. In actinomycosis bony lesions may occur secondarily to involvement of soft tissues. The most frequent locations are ribs or the spine, especially the cervical area. Often there is also a pleural reaction and opacification of the apex of both lungs.

The bony lesions due to the different mycoses often have an aspect very close to that of osteomyelitis or local tuberculosis. This leads to the comment that their radiologic diagnostic recognition may offer real difficulties, especially when no information is available on skin tests or serologic studies.

CONGENITAL SYPHILIS

This disorder has become exceedingly rare. We shall simply mention the precocious form and refer briefly to the late bony manifestations.

Clinical Findings

Congenital syphilis in its precocious form presents the following clinical findings: cutaneous and mucosal changes—palmo-plantar pemphigus, macular or papular syphilides, coryza, perionyxis—and by visceral involvement mostly hepatitis with an icterus. We shall focus exclusively on the bony manifestations.

These may be latent or present with mild edema or bony swelling discovered by palpation. Sometimes such patients already suffer from a pseudo-paralysis of Parrot. Clinically, this can lead to the loss of the function of one or several limbs, usually the arms. An involved extremity is limp, hanging passively with the hand held in pronation. Sensibility and reflexes are normal and there is no true paralysis. If a leg is involved, it is always held in flexion. A warm, painful local swelling may be noted in the metaphyseal region of long bones.

The course of the disorder, if properly treated is always favorable. During the first few weeks of treatment there may be an apparent aggravation in lacunar images and thickening of the periosteum. Subsequently the lesions will diminish and disappear, usually more slowly than the clinical signs.

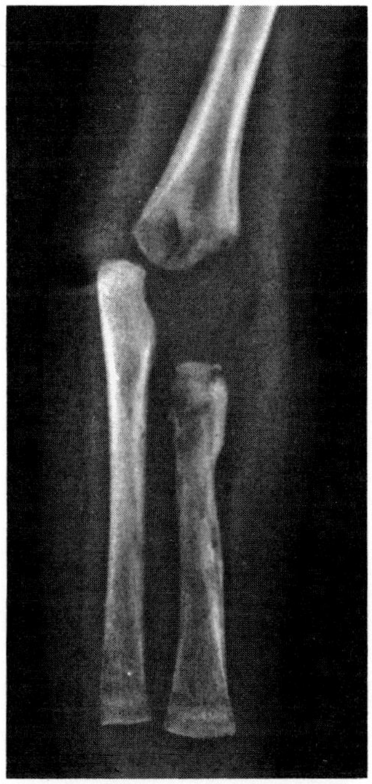

Fig. 11-5. Congenital syphilis in a 2½-year-old girl. There are radiolucent submetaphyseal lines, double contours of the cortex, and small lytic defects of the proximal region of the radius. (Courtesy of M. Lamy)

Radiographic Findings

The appearance of the disease is quite variable. Sometimes it is simply limited to slightly dense metaphyseal zones with an immediately adjacent band of increased radiolucency. This may be the only finding. Other patients, however, have a severely disturbed metaphyseal region with alternating clear and dense bands of irregular character. Occasionally a pathologic metaphyseal fracture may be noted, leading to exuberant callus formation.

Sometimes there are additional lytic findings also located within the metaphyses (Fig. 11-5). They have a variable aspect, most frequently they appear as small islands, sometimes almost in a columnar arrangement. If it is extensive, it can result in the so called celery stalk appearance which is characteristic of rubella (Cremin and Fisher). Sometimes these images may result in a peripheral ossification defect, most frequently involving the medial border of the tibia—Wimberger's sign. The entire bone may have a mottled appearance.

Along with these changes there may also be considerable periosteal reaction. This is the most constant radiologic finding, which may appear as a duplicated cortex. This duplication may be by two parallel fine lines, with local thickening in between the lines, or by multiple layers. Long bones are quite frequently involved, often together with phalanges, metacarpals, ribs and even the long bones of the cranial vault. A biopsy of cartilage shows marked disorganization of the columnar cartilage and the presence of fibrous tissue. This aspect should not be confused with that of other congenital disorders, such as rubella, hypoparathyroidism, hemoglobinipathies and especially not with the battered child syndrome (see p. 345).

LATE CONGENITAL SYPHILIS

Early involvement is seen much less and it does not have the same characteristic appearance. The most frequent involvement is that of the tibia, skull, nose and the phalanges.

The predominating lesion is the gumma. This leads to a number of clinical findings, such as deformity of the tibia by anterior convexity, sometimes with marked local pain, the destruction of the root of the nose and swelling of a finger. Such a finding is sometimes noted during a general clinical examination with findings of joint effusion, keratitis and dental anomalies. The latter can be present in two ways: Hutchinson's teeth, involving the upper incisors, and Parrot's atrophy of the cusps of the first molars.

The radiographic appearance is that of hyperostosis with lytic lesions (Fig. 11-6). Hyperostosis of the tibia

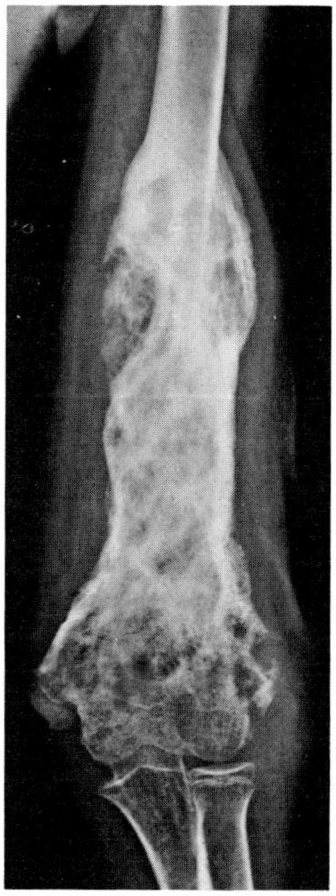

Fig. 11-6. Congenital syphilis tarda in this 13-year-old girl. Its appearance here can hardly be distinguished from a chronic bacterial osteomyelitis. (Courtesy of R. Mallet)

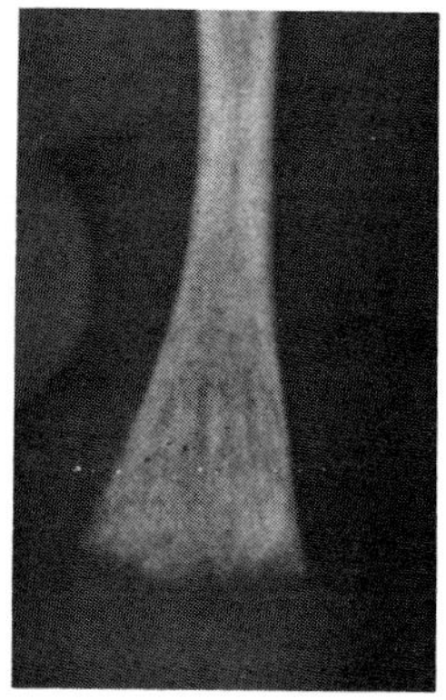

Fig. 11-7. Congenital rubella in a 2-month-old boy. Note the striated metaphyses with a "celery stalk" appearance. (Courtesy of C. Fauré)

is most prominent as thickening of the cortex, which in places assumes a layered appearance. The lytic or geodic lesions are mostly localized at the metaphyses of long bones, phalanges or flat bones. They can be present in large numbers or as a single lesion. If grouped, there are usually fine, dense separating bands. The involvement of fingers is reminiscent of tuberculous spina ventosa. Cranial involvement may present a specific local aspect.

It is quite difficult to distinguish these different lesions from other types of osteitis, especially those of bacterial etiology, since their incidence is much higher. Because of this they must always be considered first.

In spite of its rare occurrence congenital syphilis should never be overlooked. The association of periosteal reactions and metaphyseal lytic lesions should lead to serologic study, which will readily confirm the suspicion of the presence of this disease.

CONGENITAL RUBELLA

No exhaustive discussion of congenital rubella is attempted. Affected newborns have clinical findings of purpura, hepatomegaly and central nervous system involvement, a tense fontanelle, and electroencephalographic findings.

The skeletal signs are quite characteristic and may support this diagnosis strongly. These findings are transitory and recognizable during the first 1 to 3 months. Besides the disturbed growth of these babies, the findings are mainly recognized on radiographs.

The bony lesions involve only the metaphyses of the long bones, especially the lower femur and the proximal tibial metaphyses. They spare the diaphyses. There is abnormal metaphyseal trabeculation with fine parallel clear lines oriented in the axis of the bone, the so-called "celery stalk" appearance (Fig. 11-7). These changes are localized at some distance from the growth cartilage, separated by an irregularly dense zone or a radiolucent band. If seen alone this clear band does not have any meaning, since it is seen with a high incidence in babies suffering from many different disorders resulting in intrauterine growth disturbance.

Examination of the skull may reveal the presence of an excessively large, anterior fontanelle extending between the frontal bones into the metopic suture area. Prominence of the soft tissue structures may be associated. Sometimes intracranial calcifications are also recognizable.

The development of the lesions is rapidly regressive. Abnormally dense metaphyses, together with mild irregularity of the growth zone, may persist for a considerable length of time. They may appear widened and form a small lateral spur.

Anatomic study of a growth cartilage has shown the constant presence of local irregularity, inadequate formation of osteoid tissue, which calcifies poorly, and persisting small irregularly outlined cartilaginous islands. In some patients arrangement of the cartilaginous islands and the penetration by capillaries may be somewhat irregular. Usually there is a marked osteoblastic activity. It is entirely possible that these lesions result from a local metabolic disturbance secondary to the process rather than to bony infection by the virus.

OTHER VIRAL INFECTIONS

A similar appearance can be found in cytomegalic inclusion disease (Graham et al., Brandner). We have also noticed such changes in a patient with neonatal hepatitis with icterus.

Besides congenital viral infection, there have been rare cases of skeletal involvement after an initial smallpox vaccination. Local findings were hyperostosis and periosteal reaction. Occasionally there appears to have been a slightly abnormal bony structure in the involved area. These lesions usually disappear without sequelae.

SARCOIDOSIS

Bony involvement is a frequent finding in sarcoidosis. It has an incidence of about one in five patients. This lesion, however, is hardly ever seen prior to 10 years of age. The local skeletal lesions are also known under the name Perthes-Jüngling's diseases.

Clinical Findings

The lesions may be recognized because of an abnormal appearance of fingers or in a systematic radiologic search in patients with a disease in other locations.

If fingers are involved, there may be local swelling of the clubbed fingers with local redness or bluish discoloration. These usually painless changes can be responsible for a limitation of movements. The interphalangeal joints, however, remain normal. Usually there are several fingers involved, without any repetitive pattern.

The lesions have a tendency to stabilize. Sometimes, however, they are progressive and may lead to considerable local functional disturbances. A number of clinical manifestations of this disorder—thirst, polyuria and nausea—may result from hypercalcemia, which occurs in about one-third of these patients. This finding does not have any direct bearing on the skeletal involvement and may be present without the latter. Hypercalciuria is seen even more frequently and it appears that these patients behave like persons with an abnormal sensitivity to vitamin D.

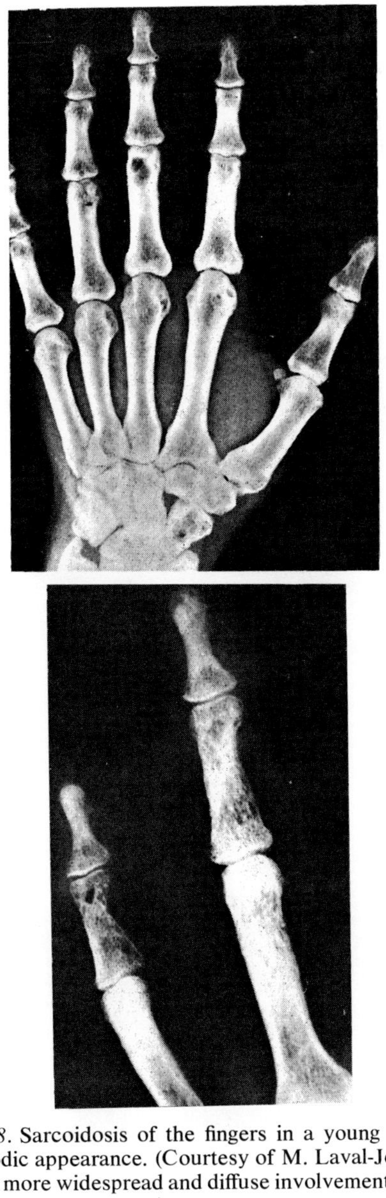

Fig. 11-8. Sarcoidosis of the fingers in a young adult. *(A)* Multigeodic appearance. (Courtesy of M. Laval-Jeantet) *(B)* Here is a more widespread and diffuse involvement of phalanges. (Courtesy of J. A. Lèvre)

Radiographic Findings

Lesions of variable size are localized within fingers and bones (Fig. 11-8). There may sometimes be several small geodes riddling the phalanges. In other instances there are small lacunar or pseudocystic changes of a somewhat larger size inflating the diaphysis and resulting in a locally thin cortex. The phalanx may be even more involved by a diffuse process resulting in a mottled appearance (Fig. 11-8). There are

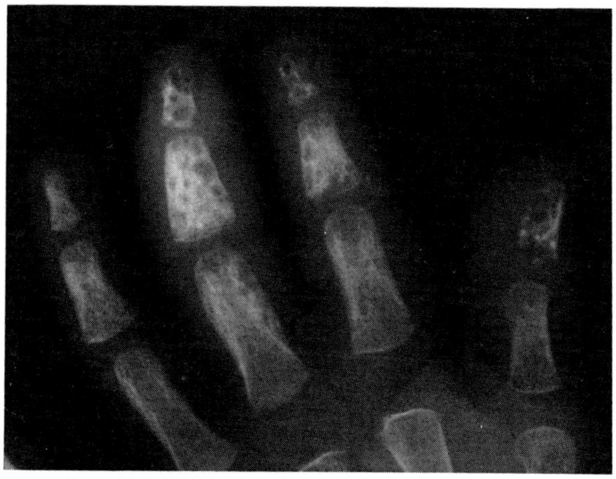

Fig. 11-9. Microgeodic involvement of several phalanges in a 22-month-old male infant. (Courtesy of M. Aussanaire)

many transitional changes possible between these different types of lesion.

Long bones are rarely affected. The forearm and the fibula may be involved. Lesions of the spine and of the pelvis are even more unusual. There are rare instances of cranial involvement usually underlying skin lesions. Small islands of increased density within the pelvis, the femur, ribs or the skull are on record. They are unusual and it would appear that they have locally been described in adults, where they may simulate metastatic lesions.

The microgeodic appearance of phalanges is a characteristic finding in another disorder in babies we have described. This "disease" of unknown etiology is discovered during the second year of life because of local swelling and redness of fingers. Spontaneous healing has been observed within several months.

Radiographic changes involve the middle or distal phalanges of fingers as slight local enlargement and a marked change of structure because of local formation of numerous small geodes. The middle and index fingers are most frequently affected, but other fingers may also be involved. The rest of the skeleton is normal (Fig. 11-9).

During the course of an oro-digito-facial syndrome small phalangeal lacunar defects may also be noted. This syndrome, however, should be easily diagnosed, because of its oral manifestations (see p. 177).

PULMONARY HYPERTROPHIC OSTEOARTHROPATHY

This disorder is seen in older children. The bony lesions appear as a secondary manifestation subsequent to a chronic disorder, most frequently involving the lungs (infection or tumor).

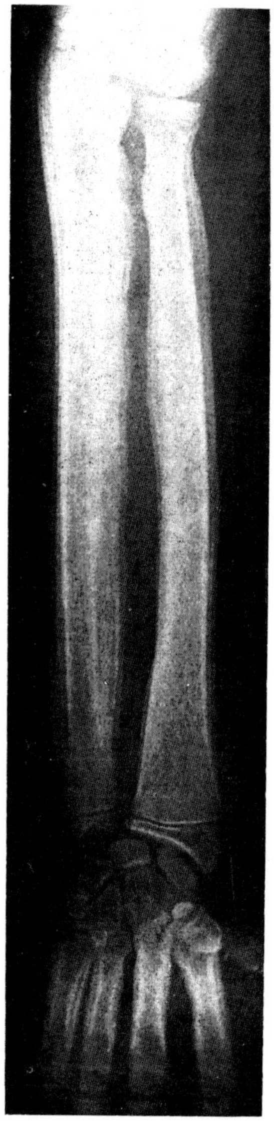

Fig. 11-10. Hypertrophic osteoarthropathy in a 13-year-old boy suffering from a mediastinal thymoma. (Courtesy of D. Nusslé)

The clinical findings of swollen fingers and clubbing are associated in about one-third of the patients with flexed joints, stiffness and pain. Vasomotor disturbances and paresthesias may also be present.

The radiographic findings are marked periosteal apposition, which mainly affect the bones of the hands and feet, but also the long bones (Fig. 11-10). The newly formed cortex is often wavy in its contour and may be separated from the original cortex by a more or less radiolucent zone. The joints do not seem to be involved.

The course of these lesions is variable and reflects the basic disorder. If the underlying disease can be fully treated, complete disappearance of these findings is possible. There have been patients in whom the bony changes preceded the clinical manifestation of a pulmonary disorder and actually led to its discovery.

Mention should be given to *pachydermoperiostosis,* which has a higher incidence in men with its onset usually during adolescence. This disorder is not usually seen during childhood. Clinical findings are limited to thickening of the skin of the face and a massive appearance of the extremities. The radiologic manifestations are very similar to those of pulmonary hypertrophic osteoarthropathy. This disorder is genetically determined and is transmitted as a dominant in some families.

Observations are reported of patients with idiopathic arthropathy without skin lesions, but with a very similar symptomatology.

We should separately consider the patients described by Currarino et al. and by Chamberlain et al. Onset of the disorder has been towards the second year of life, with local painful swelling of fingers and toes combined frequently with generalized eczema and widening of the cranial sutures and of the anterior fontanelle. After 2 years of age there may be painful crises with marked swelling of the large joints—knees and tibiotarsal joints. Periosteal apposition occurs along the diaphyses of all the long bones and the clavicles. There may be numerous wormian bones within abnormally wide cranial sutures. The disorder seems to have a spontaneously regressive tendency, so that around 6 years of age there may be a practically normal appearance of the long bones. The etiology of this disease is unknown, but a familial tendency—after observing two sisters—is reported by Currarino.

Other reports also mention cortical hyperostosis during childhood appearing in the course of a chronic respiratory infection accompanied by fever and an increase of gamma globulins, especially IgG. The development is towards spontaneous disappearance (Goldbloom et al.).

INFANTILE CORTICAL HYPEROSTOSIS (CAFFEY'S DISEASE)

In spite of earlier descriptions, this disease has been clearly defined in the publications by Caffey and Silverman. Its etiology is still unknown.

Clinical Findings

The disease is recognized during the first three months of life, usually during the second or third month. Sometimes it is present at birth, or even in utero from the 31st week on (Bennett and Nelson). Individual patients may show severe involvement, and an occasional baby was born dead. It is unusual to recognize the beginning of this disorder later than the fifth month.

Affected babies are highly irritable, constantly crying and agitated. They sleep poorly. A pale general aspect may be noted and a marked loss of appetite can accompany the abnormal behavior. Slight fever is usually reported, occasionally up to 39° or 40° C.

During the initial phase of the disorder there may be marked swelling of soft tissues, which may be the first finding. The cheeks and mandibular region are the most frequently involved sites. There is an occasional involvement of the extremities, especially the shins. In the presence of local swelling and redness skin temperature may be elevated. Local palpation shows a certain firmness, or, at the onset of the disorder, the skin will be soft. In a rare patient there may be abnormal posture of one of the limbs simulating pseudo-paralysis (Brooksaler).

Hematologic study may show slight anemia with moderate leucocytosis. Sedimentation rate may be high in 20 per cent of the cases, and alkaline phosphatases may be slightly elevated.

The disorder proceeds by successive exacerbations during the initial months of life. Healing usually occurs during the second year of life. There are numerous babies with a markedly longer, chronic course with recurrences during early childhood, sometimes even into adult age. There are no effects on skeletal growth, but diaphyseal bowing has been reported.

Radiographic Findings

The radiologic signs can occur very early, even in utero. There is predominant involvement of the diaphyses of the long bones by excessive cortical thickening. The border of the cortical widening is often uneven and of a wavy contour. The original cortex is well seen and the density of the hyperostosis seems to correspond to normal bone at least at the beginning of a new exacerbation (Fig. 11-11).

The lesions can assume many different aspects. Occasionally there is simply local fusiform widening of a part of a diaphysis. This may be unilateral. Sometimes two such local changes may be present, each at one end of a diaphysis. There are patients with extensive cortical thickening, extending along the entire diaphysis giving the appearance of the ends of the bone being connected by the string of a bow. In extreme cases hyperostosis can result in irregular widening of the bone to three or four times its normal diameter with the loss of its original shape.

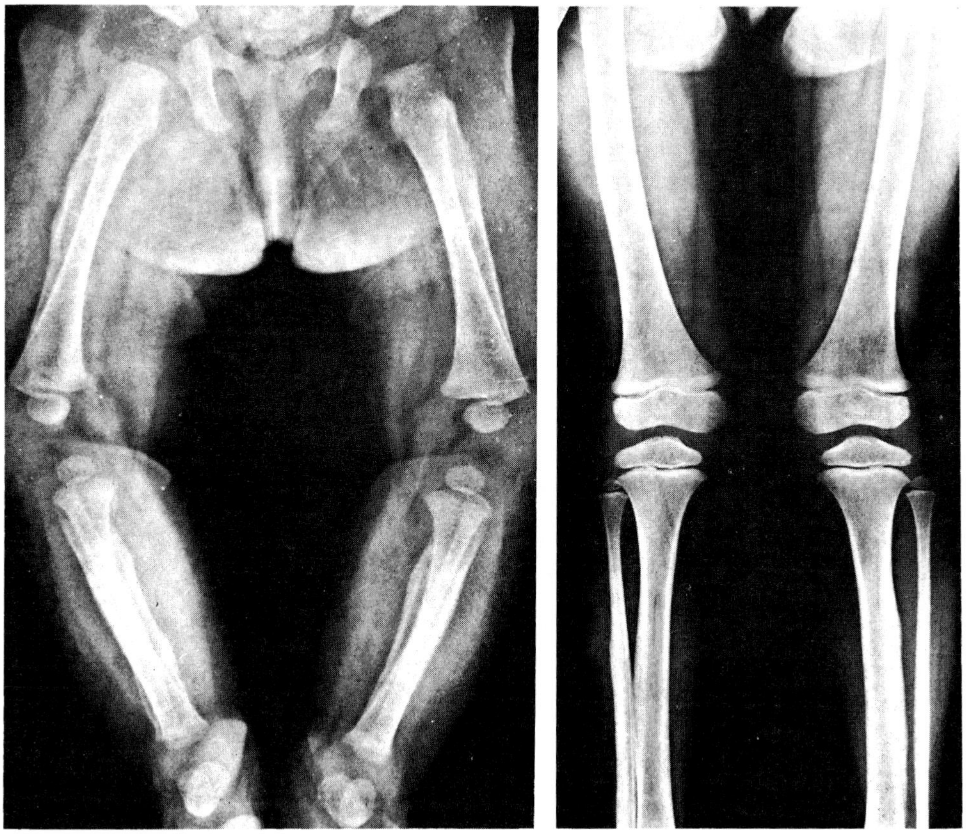

Fig. 11-11. Infantile cortical hyperostosis. (*Left*) In an infant $2\frac{1}{2}$ months old. (*Right*) Relapse at the age of 3 years. This patient had several relapses up until he was 8 years old.

The further course of events results in a reduction of hyperostosis, local increased density and eventually more or less persisting cortical thickening. If there are relapses, some previously unaffected bones may be involved and others already healing may show the recurrence of hyperostosis.

The most frequently seen localizations are the mandible, clavicle, scapula, iliac bones, ribs, metacarpals and metatarsals. Only rarely will there be involvement of frontal, parietal or nasal bones. Local small geodes can be noted within the skull. The vertebral bodies are never affected.

Anatomy and Pathogenesis

Histologic study (Eversole) at the beginning of the disorder reveals a richly cellular tissue with many polymorphonuclear cells and vessels replacing almost the entire periosteum. This process extends into the neighboring soft tissues with marked edema. Eventually there is periosteal reorganization. Between its new surface and the earlier cortex there is fibrous and osteoblastic proliferation. The deposition of calcium within the new osteoid tissue corresponds to the radiologically recognizable bony apposition. During the last stage incorporation of this hyperostotic zone into the original healthy portion of the bone takes place. The bony tissue, initially rich in osteoblasts, loses those cells. Sherman and Hellyer emphasize the proliferation of the intima within arterioles immediately below the inflammatory zone. The question is raised whether secondary hypoxia could play a role in the development of hyperostosis.

The etiology of this disorder remains unclear. There are a number of familial observations which include radiographic findings in parents. This would suggest the possibility of a dominant transmission. It would, however, be impossible to explain all the cases of this disease on the basis of genetic factors alone. No proof has been so far presented to support the possibility of an infection or an immunologic or allergic etiology.

Treatment

Corticosteroids seem to have an excellent effect on the clinical manifestation of this disease. It would seem advisable to use them for a relatively short time only in patients with severe pain, irritability and insomnia. Such treatment will not influence the development of the radiologic lesions and cannot prevent recurrences. Some authors have advised prolonged therapy, but the drawbacks and dangers of such therapy do not seem to be justified considering the usually benign course.

Infantile cortical hyperostosis should not be confused with hyperostoses of traumatic origin and especially with the battered child syndrome. Traumatic hyperostoses are seen with a significantly higher incidence and have frequently led to confusion.

It should not be overlooked that many prematures will develop a double contour of the cortex of long bones as a normal finding. During chronic, severe hypoparathyroidism with tetany, this same aspect, sometimes even with a layered cortex, can be noted (see p. 207).

THE "BATTERED CHILD" SYNDROME (SYNDROME OF SILVERMAN OR AMBROISE TARDIEU)

This disorder, often with severe skeletal lesions, is seen with an infinitely higher incidence than the diseases with which it is frequently confused, such as Caffey's disease, syphilis or scurvy. If the true nature of the disorder is not recognized, it will expose these babies to severe danger and may result in their death. This is why special emphasis is given to its diagnostic features.

According to Silverman the initial description of abuse of infants and their consequence goes back to Ambroise Tardieu. Actually the significance of the clinical and radiologic changes was only made clear in the publications by Silverman and by Caffey.

Clinical Findings

The circumstances leading to the recognition of an affected patient can be quite variable. Often babies are hospitalized because of a painful inability to use a limb accompanied by local swelling. Sometimes skin lesions are the main symptom—ecchymoses, local swelling, ulcers, burns. In other instances general neglect, weakness, malnutrition and even convulsive seizures may lead to an investigation.

Skeletal changes can be more or less prominent. Occasionally they are incidental discoveries during a workup, because of a wrist or elbow deformity resulting in local stiffness and flexion. Most frequently localized swelling of a limb and the inability of the patient to properly use it will lead to a local study. Active or passive mobilization will be painful and a slight increase of the local temperature may be noted. Swelling is usually superficial and may also involve an abnormal angulation of part of a limb with an obvious underlying fracture. There may be fever leading to the erroneous impression of a possible bony or osteo-articular infection.

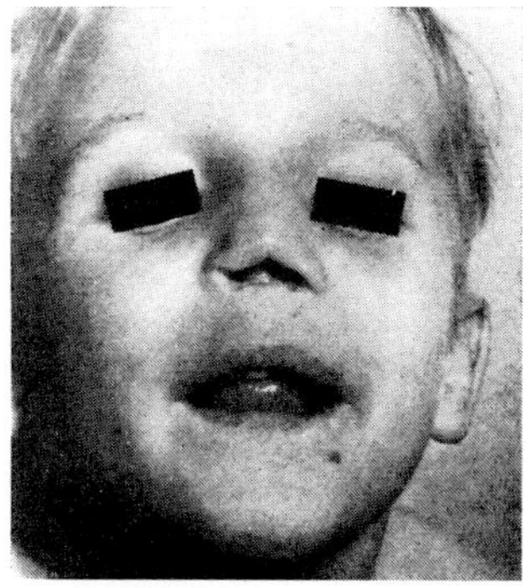

Fig. 11-12. The battered child syndrome. Note the marked defect of the nasal septum.

The nose may be markedly abnormal with a pugilistic aspect or evidence of the disappearance of the septum between the nostrils (Fig. 11-12). The significant involvement of the skin should never be overlooked. There may be ecchymoses or white scars, possibly the result of burns. Lesions within the mouth, ulcerations of the palate, fractured teeth may be present. Vomiting, abnormal crying and convulsive episodes can all result from subdural effusion.

Radiographic Findings

One or several long bones may be involved with a rather typical pattern. There is a combination of cortical diaphyseal and metaphyseal changes.

Sometimes there is a true fracture of a diaphysis, and occasionally a marked displacement and shortening or deformity of the affected limb. Most frequently, however, there is only a "green stick fracture." Exuberant callus formation may be noted at the elbow or knee resulting from a lack of immobilization and repeated local trauma. Later, this callus will be resorbed and only a modeling defect or slight angulation will remain.

Double contour of the cortex and periosteal ossification appear rapidly outlining the periphery and later filling in the large hematoma, which may

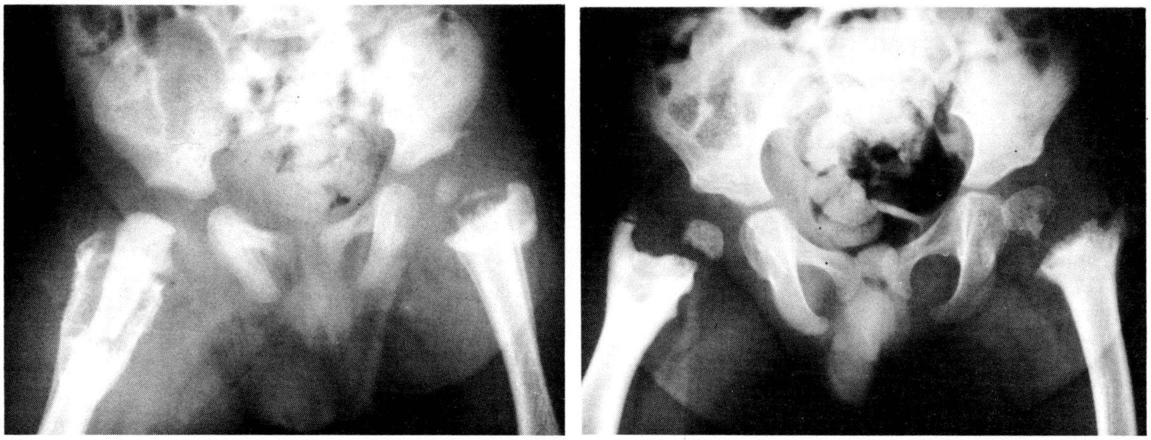

Fig. 11-13. Battered child syndrome with serious hip involvement after severe trauma which occurred at the age of 5 months. (*Left*) Patient at 6 months. (*Right*) Patient at 2 years. (Courtesy of R. Mallet)

envelop the entire extent of the diaphysis and metaphysis (Fig. 11-13). Occasionally there is only thickening of the diaphysis with a square, massive, almost rectangular, local aspect. Periosteal appositions are more or less considerable in extent and can narrow the space of the medullary canal. Such changes may be quite irregular and result in a cottony aspect or they can be arranged as fine individual lamellae resulting in a relatively uniform thickening of the diaphysis (Fig. 11-14, *Left*).

In some instances early pictures will simply show thickening of the soft tissues. A repeat examination 9 to 12 days subsequent to the appearance of local swelling or painful limitation of motion will then give evidence of the underlying bony changes.

Metaphyseal lesions are not only frequently present, but in babies they have a very special aspect, somewhat comparable to certain obstetrical fractures. The metaphysis itself may be clearly fractured and fragmented. One of the fragments may be displaced laterally, forming the corner sign. A fine radiolucent band seems to separate the metaphyseal border from the rest of the bone. This linear discontinuity may be complete or only partial and results in a lateral aspect like "a cut fingernail." Often there is only an irregularity of the metaphyseal end, which appears wavy and ill-defined (Fig. 11-14). Such metaphyseal lesions can be accompanied in some rare instances by a displacement of the epiphysis together with subluxation of the shoulder or of the hip. Anomalies of the small bone of the hand can also be present. Metacarpals and the 1st phalanges of some fingers are mainly involved with an irregularly outlined head or base and periosteal thickening.

Fractured ribs are often noted. Often affected is the internal portion of the posterior arch of the middle ribs, occasionally a whole series and with marked callus formation. The spine may show a bulge of the anterior and superior region of a vertebral body.

The cranial sutures may be unusually wide, even without intracranial fluid accumulation. A linear parietal or temporo-occipital fracture may be present.

Finally, bony maturation is clearly retarded in many patients and growth may also be affected. Many children have lesions of varying duration, which should immediately alert one that there has been repeated trauma. Such findings will help to rule out the possibility of a single serious accident, due possibly to negligence, and which, because an adult feels guilty, is simply denied.

Course, Etiology, and Diagnosis

The course is quite variable leading sometimes to death or severe permanent mental or neurologic defects from skull injury.

The prognosis for skeletal lesions is usually good, but it is absolutely essential to remove the children in danger from their normal surroundings. Exposure to abuse may have serious consequences, such as shortening of a limb, ankylosis of an elbow, kyphosis, rigidity of fingers, coxa vara and sometimes even severe dysplasia of the hip. The lesions resulting from a defect of the nasal septum are esthetically disturbing.

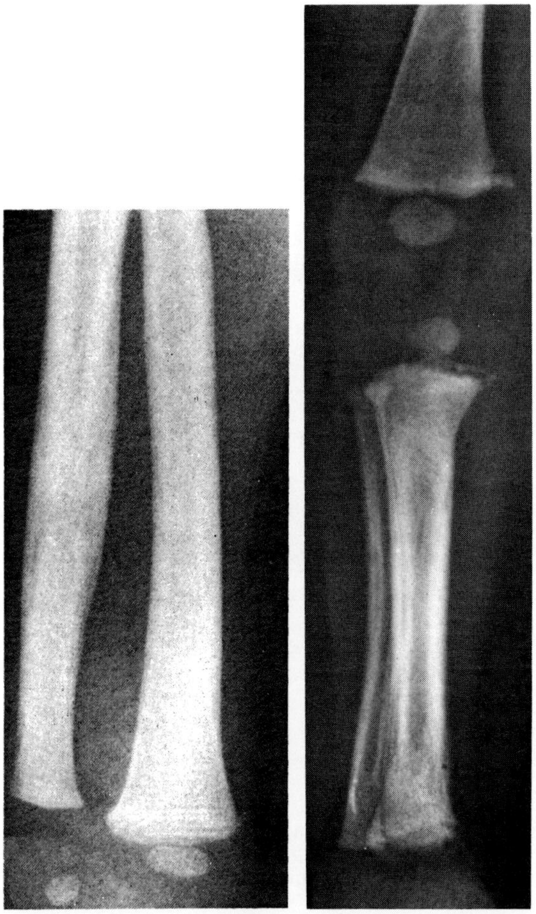

Fig. 11-14. Fractures overlooked during early infancy. (*Left*) 2-year-old boy with marked consolidated periosteal reaction. (*Right*) 9-month-old baby with irregular metaphyseal outline and double cortical contours.

Aron emphasizes the serious implication of lesions of the eyeground—greyish atrophic foci located at the very periphery of the temporal sector of the visual field—which suggests that they may not be noticed during a rapid examination.

This syndrome is not always the result of active and willful manipulation, but sometimes of simple, somewhat rough, but still normal handling of babies, who may have predisposing factors. Caffey has insisted on the fragility of the insertion of the periosteum in the baby together with a rich vascularity of this zone.

The differential diagnosis may offer an occasional problem, because of similarities of some of the findings with poliomyelitis, an osteomyelitis, Pott's disease and even tumors of the bone. A full initial study with repeated investigation of the patient and of the entire skeleton will soon clarify the situation. Caffey's disease never has changes of the metaphyseal border. It should thus be properly differentiated from the battered child syndrome, just as other disorders of abnormal bony density. Defects of the nasal septum may suggest the possibility of congenital syphilis, but the metaphyseal changes are again different and the serologic findings will help to differentiate the conditions in a questionable case. Many lesions are reminiscent of scurvy, but this condition has become so extremely rare that it will hardly ever cause real confusion. Furthermore, it should be remembered that in the battered child syndrome there is normal trabeculation of the bones and particularly of the epiphyses and no widening of the metaphysis itself.

It may be somewhat more difficult to differentiate the disorder from congenital indifference to pain (see p. 318), but here the babies have a normal sensitivity, and the age distribution is a helpful argument.

REFERENCES

Osteomyelitis. Chronic Polychondritis

Aractingi (Th. R.). Etude de 32 cas d'ostéomyélite du nouveau-né. *Rev. Chir. orthop., 1961,* **47**, *50-63.*

Capitanio (M. A.) et Kirkpatrick (J. A.). Early roentgen observations in acute osteomyelitis. *Amer. J. Roentgenol., 1970,* **108**, *488-496.*

Feinbloom (R. I.) et Halaby (F. A.). Acute pyogenic spondylitis in infancy. *Clin. Pediat., 1966,* **5**, *683-684.*

Ferguson (A. B.). Osteomyelitis in children. *Clin. Orthop., 1973,* **96**, *51-56.*

Giedion (A.). Weichteilveranderungen und radiologische Frühdiagnose der akuten Ostomyelitis im Kinderalter. *Fortschr. Röntgenstr., 1960,* **93**, *455-466.*

Gledhill (R. B.). Subacute osteomyelitis in children. *Clin. Orthop., 1973,* **96**, *57-69.*

Johner (C. H.) et Szanto (P. A.). Polychondritis in a newborn presenting as tracheomalacia. *Ann. Otol. Rhinol. Laryng. (St. Louis), 1970,* **79**, *1114-1117.*

Judet (R.) et coll. Ostéite et ostéomyélite chronique. *Gaz. méd. Fr., 1964,* **71**, *1017-1021.*

Lamy (M.), Jammet (M.-L.), Nezelof (C.), Laugier (J.) et Ajjan (N.). La polychondrite chronique atrophiante évolutive. *Arch. franç. Pédiat., 1967,* **24**, *633-650.*

Laplane (R.), Fontaine (J.-L.), Lagardère (S.), Paquelin (F.) et Navarro (J.). La polychondrite chronique atrophiante de l'enfant. *Nouv. Presse méd., 1973,* **2**, *1045-1048.*

Laurence (G.). Ostéomyélite du nouveau-né et du nourrisson. *Rev. Prat., 1963,* **13**, *883-897.*

Laurence (G.). Caractères généraux de l'infection à staphylocoques chez les nouveau-nés et les nourrissons. *Rev. Prat., 1968,* **18**, *19-30.*

Laurence (G.). Les localisations ostéo-articulaires et leur traitement. *Rev. Prat., 1968,* **18**, *65-75.*

Laurence (G.). Antibiothérapie de l'ostéomyélite aiguë. *Rev. Prat., 1968,* **18**, *suppl., 4825-4826.*

Rabuzzi (D. D.). Relapsing polychondritis. *Arch. Otolaryng., 1970,* **91**, *188-194.*

RIGAULT (P.) et PINAUD (J. B.). Les arthrites purulentes aiguës de la hanche chez le nourrisson. *Ann. Chir. infant., 1968,* **9**, *245-256.*

RIGAULT (P.) et BLANCHARD (J. P.). Spondylodiscites à germes banaux chez l'enfant. *Rev. Chir. orthop., 1970,* **56**, *367-382.*

STOPPA (R.) et DJILALI (G.). Aspects mal connus de l'ostéomyélite chronique. *Presse méd., 1968,* **76**, *suppl. Atlas n° 46.*

WICHTL (O.). Frühe Röntgenzeichen der akuten Osteomyelitis im Kindesalter. *Wien. klin. Wschr., 1968,* **80**, *552-554.*

Tuberculosis. Mycoses of the Skeleton

ALLEN (J. H.). Bone involvment with dessiminated histoplasmose. *Amer. J. Roentgenol., 1959,* **82**, *250-254.*

COWEN (N. J.). Cryptococcosis of bone. Case report and review of the literature. *Clin. Orthop., 1969,* **66**, *174-187.*

CREMIN (B. J.), FISHER (R. M.) et LEVINSOHN (M. W.). Multiple bone tuberculosis in the young. *Brit. J. Radiol., 1970,* **43**, *638-645.*

ENG (J.) et AANELAND (T.). BCG osteitis in a child. A bacteriological investigation. *Scand. J. Resp. Dis., 1966,* **47**, *182-186.*

GEHWEILER (J. A.), CAPP (M. P.) et CHICK (E. W.). Observations on the roentgen patterns in blastomycosis of bone. A review of cases from the blastomycosis, cooperative study of the Veterans administration and Duke University Medical Center. *Amer. J. Roentgenol., 1970,* **108**, *497-510.*

MALLET (R.), RIBIERRE (M.), LABRUNE (B.) et BRÉTI (C.). Tuberculose osseuse diffuse du nourrisson (Spina ventosa généralisées). *Ann. Pédiat., 1968,* **15**, *554-559.*

MARTINI (M.), BOUDJEMAA (A.) et BOULAHBAL (F.). Les ostéites tuberculeuses. *Rev. Chir. orthop., 1972,* **58**, *595-608.*

SINIOS (A. W.), SWOBODA (W.), MEISSNER (G.) et STUR (D.). Osteomyelitis als Folger der BCG Impfung. *Mschr. Kinderheilk., 1965,* **113**, *605-609.*

Syphilis of the Skeleton

CAFFEY (J.). Syphilis of the skeleton in early infancy, the non-specificity of many of the roentgenographic changes. *Amer. J. Roentgenol., 1939,* **42**, *637-655.*

CREMIN (B. J.) et FISHER (R. M.). The lesions of congenital syphilis. Part I. The early or perinatal lesions. *Brit. J. Radiol., 1970,* **43**, *333-341.*

LEVIN (E. J.). Healing in congenital osseous syphilis. *Amer. J. Roentgenol., 1970,* **110**, *591-597.*

McDONALD (R.). Congenital syphilis has many faces. *Clin. Pediat., 1970,* **9**, *110-114.*

MAGGI (G. C.) et GRASSI (E.). Aspetti radiologici delle localizzazioni scheletriche dell'eredolue precoce. *Minerva pediat., 1963,* **15**, *938-946.*

TOURAINE (R.). Syphilis congénitale (syphilis prénatale). *Rev. Pédiat., 1970,* **6**, *357-369.*

Congenital Rubella and Other Viral Infections

BAGGIO (P.). L'osteopatia nella sindrome neonatale da infezione rubeolica intrauterina. *Acta paediat. lat. (Reggio Emilia), 1967,* **20**, *42-67.*

BRANDNER (M.). Die Bedeutung der metaphysären Ossifikationsstörungen im Säuglingsalter mit besonderer Berücksichtigung der infektiösen Fetopathien. *Fortschr. Röntgenstr., 1973,* **118**, *531-537.*

GRAHAM (C. B.), THAL (A.) et WASSUM (C. S.). Rubella-like bone changes in congenital cytomegalic inclusion disease. *Radiology, 1970,* **94**, *39-43.*

MERTEN (D. F.) et GOODING (C. A.). Skeletal manifestations of congenital cytomegalic inclusion disease. *Radiology, 1970,* **95**, *333-334.*

MICHAELS (R. H.) et KENNY (F. M.). Postnatal growth retardation in congenital rubella. *Pediatrics, 1969,* **43**, *251-259.*

RUDOLPH (A. J.), SINGLETON (E. B.), ROSENBERG (H. S.), SINGER (D. B.) et PHILLIPS (C. A.). Osseous manifestations of the congenital rubella syndrome. *Amer. J. Dis. Child., 1965,* **110**, *428-433.*

SACREZ (R.), FRUHLING (L.), KORN (R.), JUIF (J. G.), FRANCFORT (C.) et GEIGER (R.). Three cases of cytomegalic inclusion disease. *Arch. franç. Pédiat., 1960,* **17**, *129-140.*

SAIDI (M.) et CHAGNON (J.). Les manifestations osseuses de la rubéole congénitale. *Un. méd. Can., 1971,* **100**, *1771-1774,*

SINGLETON (E. B.), RUDOLPH (A. J.), ROSENBERG (H. S.) et SINGER (D. B.). The roentgenographic manifestations of the rubella syndrome in newborn infants. *Amer. J. Roentgenol., 1966,* **97**, *82-91.*

WILLIAMS (H. J.) et CAREY (L. S.). Rubella embryopathy. Roentgenologic features. *Amer. J. Roentgenol., 1966,* **97**, *92-99.*

Sarcoidosis

BEAUDOING (A.), ROST (M.), COULOMB (M.) et PONT (J.). Affection microgéodique des phalanges d'étiologie inconnue chez l'enfant. A propos de deux nouvelles observations. *Pédiatrie, 1972,* **26**, *803-813.*

BERK (R. N.) et BROWER (T. D.). Vertebral sarcoidosis. *Radiology, 1964,* **82**, *660-663.*

BONAKDARPOUR (A.), LEVY (W.) et AEGERTER (E. E.). Osteosclerotic changes in sarcoidosis. *Amer. J. Roentgenol., 1971,* **113**, *646-649.*

CHAOUAT (Y.) et BENICHOU (Ch.). La maladie de Perthes-Jungling. *Gaz. méd. Fr., 1964,* **71**, *1120-1130.*

FITZGERALD (P.) et MEENAN (O. C.). Sarcoidosis of hands. *J. Bone Jt Surg., 1958,* **40-B**, *256-261.*

HOLT (J. F.) et OWENS (W. I.). Osseous lesions of sarcoidosis. *Radiology, 1949,* **53**, *11-30.*

LIN (S.-R.), LEVY (W.), GO (E. B.), LEE (I.) et WONG (W. K.). Unusual osteosclerotic changes in sarcoidosis, simulating osteoblastic metastases. *Radiology, 1973,* **106**, *311-312.*

MAROTEAUX (P.). Cinq observations d'une affection microgéodique des phalanges du nourrisson d'étiologie inconnue. *Ann. Radiol., 1970,* **13**, *229-236.*

SCHWEIZER (A. Th.) et KANAAR (P.). Sarcoidosis with polyarthritis in a child. *Arch. Dis. Child., 1967,* **42**, *671-674.*

TOOMEY (F.) et BAUTISTA. Rare manifestation of sarcoidosis in children. *Radiology, 1970,* **94**, *569-573.*

TURNER (O. A.) et WEISS (R.). Sarcoidose of the skull. *Amer. J. Roentgenol., 1969,* **105**, *322-325.*

YOUNG (D. A.) et LAMAN (M. L.). Radiodense skeletal lesions in Boeck's sarcoid. *Amer. J. Roentgenol., 1972,* **114**, *553-558.*

Idiopathic Osteoarthropathy. Pachydermoperiostosis

CAVANAUGH (J. J. A.) et HOLMAN (G. H.). Hypertrophic osteoarthropathy in childhood. *J. Pediat., 1965,* **66**, *27-40.*

CHAMBERLAIN (D. S.), WHITAKER (J. A.) et SILVERMAN (F. N.). Idiopathic osteoarthropathy and cranial defects in children (familial idiopathic osteoarthropathy). *Amer. J. Roentgenol., 1965,* **93**, *408-415.*

CURRARINO (G.), TIERNEY (R. C.), GIESEL (R. G.) et WEIHL (C.). Familial idiopathic osteoarthropathy. *Amer. J. Roentgenol., 1961,* **85**, *633-644.*

DUMONT (L. E.) et DIEU (Y.). L'ostéo-arthrite hypertrophiante. *Rev. méd. Liège, 1962,* **17**, *378-380.*

GOLDBLOOM (R. B.), STEIN (P. B.), EISEN (A.), MCSHEFFREY (J. B.), ST. JOHN BROWN (B.) et WIGLESWORTH (F. W.). Idiopathic periosteal hyperostosis with dysproteinemia. A new clinical entity. *New Engl. J. Med., 1966,* **274**, *873-878.*

RIMOIN (D. L.). Pachydermoperiostosis (idiopathic clubbing and periostosis). Genetic and physiologic considerations. *New Engl. J. Med., 1965,* **272**, *923-931.*

URSING (B.). Pachydermoperiostosis. *Acta Med. scand., 1970,* **188**, *157-160.*

Infantile Cortical Hyperostosis

ALBERTI (G. P.), GIANNASI (F.) et PANZETTI (G.). La sindrome di de Toni-Caffey-Silverman nel quadro delle periosteopatie dell'eta infantile. *Ann. Radiol. diagn. (Bologna), 1962,* **35**, *443-469.*

BENNETT (H. S.) et NELSON (T. R.). Prenatal cortical hyperostosis; case reports. *Brit. J. Radiol., 1953,* **26**, *47-49.*

BROOKSALER (F.). Infantile kortikale Hyperostose. *Kinderärtzl. Prax., 1957,* **25**, *459-462.*

BUSKIRK (F. W. van), TAMPAS (J. P.) et PETERSON (O. S., Jr.). Infantile cortical hyperostosis : inquiry into its familial aspects. *Amer. J. Roentgenol., 1961,* **85**, *613-632.*

CAFFEY (J.) et SILVERMAN (W. A.). Infantile cortical hyperostoses : preliminary report on new syndrome. *Amer. J. Roentgenol., 1945,* **54**, *1-16.*

EVERSOLE (S. L., Jr.), HOLMAN (G. H.) et ROBINSON (R. A.). Hitherto undescribed characteristics of the pathology of infantile cortical hyperostosis (Caffey's disease). *Bull. Johns-Hopk. Hosp., 1957,* **101**, *80-99.*

FAURÉ (CL.). Diagnostic radiologique des hyperostoses cortico-périostées du tout jeune nourrisson. *Concours méd., 1969,* **91**, *3799-3810.*

MARQUIS (J. R.). Infantile cortical hyperostosis. A report of an unusual case. *Radiology, 1967,* **89**, *282-284.*

NEUHAUSER (E. B. D.). Infantile cortical hyperostosis and skull defects. *Radiology, 1970,* **48**, *57-59.*

PAJEWSKI (M.) et VURE (E.). Late manifestations of infantile cortical hyperostosis (Caffey's disease). *Brit. J. Radiol., 1967,* **40**, *90-95.*

SHERMAN (M. S.) et HELLYER (D. T.). Infantile cortical hyperostosis; review of literature and report of five cases. *Amer. J. Roentgenol., 1950,* **63**, *212-222.*

SWERDLOFF (B. A.), OZONOFF (M. B.) et GYEPES (M. T.). Late recurrence of infantile cortical hyperostosis (Caffev's disease). *Amer. J. Roentgenol., 1970,* **108**, *461-467.*

VIALATTE (J.) et NODOT (A.). Hyperostose corticale infantile ou maladie de Caffey. *Ann. Pédiat., 1967,* **14**, *699-701.*

The Battered Child Syndrome

ARON (J. J.), MARX (P.), BLANCK (M. F.), DUVAL (R.). et LUCE (R.). Signes oculaires observés dans le syndrome de Silverman (syndrome des enfants mal traités). *Ann. Oculist. (Paris), 1970,* **203**, *533-546.*

CAFFEY (J.). Multiple fractures in the long bones of infants suffering from chronic subdural hematoma. *Amer. J. Roentgenol., 1946,* **56**, *163-173.*

FESSARD (C.), MAROTEAUX (P.) et LAMY (M.). Le syndrome de Silverman. « Fractures multiples du nourrisson » (étude de seize observations). *Arch. franç. Pédiat., 1967,* **24**, *651-665.*

GNEHM (H. P. E.). Le syndrome de l'enfant battu. *Helv. paediat. Acta, 1973, suppl. 31.*

GREINACHER (I.). Röntgenbefunde beim sogenannten Battered-Child-Syndrom. *Fortschr. Röntgenstr., 1970,* **113**, *704-710.*

HILLER (H. G.). Battered or not-a reappraisal of metaphyseal fragility. *Amer. J. Roentgenol., 1972,* **114**, *241-246.*

MAROTEAUX (P.), FESSARD (C.), ARON (J. J.) et LAMY (M.). Les séquelles du syndrome de Silverman (fractures multiples du nourrisson, syndrome dit des « enfants battus »). Etude de seize observations. *Presse méd., 1967,* **75**, *711-716.*

SILVERMAN (F. N.). The roentgen manifestations of unrecognized skeletal trauma in infants. *Amer. J. Roentgenol., 1953,* **69**, *413-426.*

SILVERMAN (F. N.). Unrecognized trauma in infants, the battered child syndrome, and the syndrome of Ambroise Tardieu. Rigler lecture. *Radiology, 1972,* **104**, *337-353.*

12 Some General Problems of Orthopaedic Surgery

P. Rigault

This discussion attempts to provide a sound basis for the handling of the numerous babies brought by parents to the consulting pediatrician or orthopaedic surgeon. Generally they have been alarmed by a deformity or anomaly of a leg, the spine, the trunk, or a disturbed gait. Experience has taught us that most of the cases are of a benign nature.

In the vast majority of cases the worries of the parents are, fortunately, unjustified. We are either faced with a basically normal condition that will disappear with growth, or it may simply be a "special condition," a mild variant which is still within normal development. This may prove to be familial, and simple measures may be the only required therapy.

It is our responsibility, however, to reassure the family and to define the normal and the borderline. To be able to properly distinguish these, one must not only know the stages of physiologic development of the legs and the trunk, not only collect adequate past histories of both the patient and his family, not only carefully study, segment by segment, the entire locomotor system, but have available a complete and adequate radiographic skeletal survey wherever necessary, as well as other diagnostic information. Many skeletal disorders which result in severe functional problems in the adult may be present during childhood as minor findings and are without any functional symptoms. Sometimes, a more serious generalized disorder is recognized during a careful investigation for a minor, seemingly benign local problem.

Parental worries, even though they are frequently unjustified, may lead to uncovering a serious problem. In this sense, then, there are no minor orthopaedic problems. When responding to questions that the family has voiced, we must be well aware of the ill-defined limits between the normal and the abnormal and exercise caution. It is sometimes necessary to postpone definitive judgment. We may want to follow the patient for some time before reaching a conclusion. We must also be aware of the limits of our knowledge. It may be important to emphasize the somewhat questionable character of certain decisions.

We shall successively discuss: anomalies of the feet, bowing and deviation of the legs, disturbed gait related to rotation anomalies of the skeleton of the lower extremities, limping, and spinal curvatures.

ANOMALIES OF THE FEET

Maternal preoccupation with these problems is as excessive as the number of unjustified prescriptions for corrective devices. In an attempt to clarify this, we will study distinct problems at different ages.

IN THE NEWBORN AND INFANT

We will not involve ourselves here with such serious types of local deformity as congenital club feet, equinovarus deformity, the congenital convex foot, the fixed talus or valgus of the foot, or metatarsus varus congenitus of any etiology. All these severe defects are usually recognized early and are promptly brought to the attention of a specialist. There are a number of minor anomalies which we would like to emphasize. The study of the newborn or infant must include a study of the morphology of the foot and its mobility. Active and passive function must be checked by inciting movements, for instance by local pinching or irritation with a toothbrush. Any local rigidity or slightly spastic posture must immediately raise one's suspicion. This will frequently just be the result of the intrauterine position of the foot in relation to the leg during the last weeks of pregnancy. This may give it the appearance of either a talus or varus in abduction. This condition has an entirely benign character as reduction is easily accomplished. The simple form of a pes talus is clinically manifested in an excessive spontaneous dorsal flexion and a limitation of passive plantar flexion. There is also sometimes valgus deformity. Three special points of interest are noted here.

One should first suspect the possible presence of a congenital dysplastic hip. All tests for this lesion must be carefully conducted. The approach must include radiographs of the hip (Fig. 12-1).

If only present on one side, there is often an associated, contralateral clubfoot of varying degrees. Both feet are affected, but inversely, the one in equino varus, the other in a valgus position. These are "mirror feet" resulting, most likely, from a malposition in utero, where both feet were in opposition planta to planta. This condition usually has a good prognosis.

The possibility of a paralytic nerve lesion within the posterior compartment of the lower leg may lead to pes talus in the infant who is affected by spina bifida or early poliomyelitis which can be clarified by careful neurologic investigation. Pes talus is frequently a benign, bilateral condition, often present in infants born by breech delivery. The prognosis is generally good. Corrective manipulation and maintenance by a splint and bandages will usually be adequate. If not, casting may be required for several weeks. The most benign types will actually correct themselves spontaneously when the musculature of the newborn starts to develop and mobility increases. However, it should be recognized that certain types of pes talus do not sufficiently correct themselves. It must be accepted that a number of patients with flat feet that are recognized at a later time are, without a doubt, the result of the lack of correction of an early, mild form of pes talus. This is also true of some high arched valgus deformities seen in the large child.

Two defects which are relatively unknown conditions that present at birth deserve our attention, especially since they may be confused with pes talus and might often be neglected. These are *congenital convexity of the foot* and the *true congenital flat foot.* They are rare and difficult to recognize. The presence of a certain local rigidity and a valgus of the calcaneus are suspicious findings. Any slightly abnormal foot, especially one which has lost its usual flexibility, should be brought to the attention of the orthopaedic surgeon, who should order radiographs and then follow it up. One should be able to recognize early an isolated metatarsus varus—pes adductus—a minor variant of clubbed feet. It requires early therapy as it usually has a refractory tendency.

IN EARLY INFANCY

From the time that the child begins to walk to the age of three or four years flat feet or similar lesions will become apparent. A considerable number of infants with these problems, such as true flat feet, a cavovarus deformity or congenital synostoses of tarsal bones

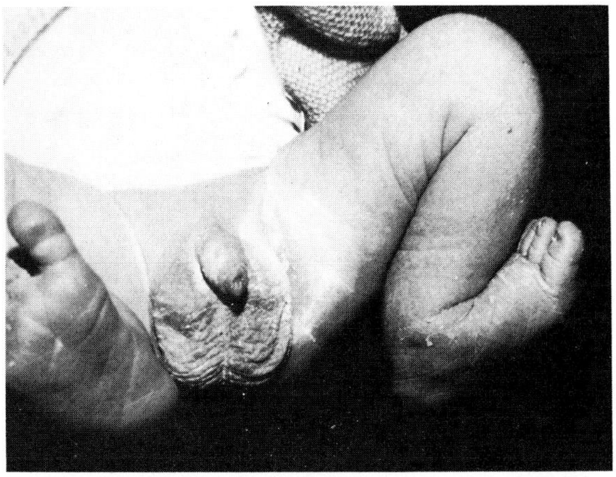

Fig. 12-1. Bilateral pes calcaneus in a newborn. This local finding of itself entirely benign, however, a careful clinical and radiographic examination of the hip should always be done in order to rule out the possibility of a congenitally dislocated hip.

may be suspected, if not proven, by a careful clinical examination even at this early age. A number of congenital malformations, such as pes convexus, can only be recognized at the time when the patient begins to walk. It is virtually a fact that the great majority of infants brought for consultation can be considered normal. On the other hand, if true malformations are brought to our attention too late, effective therapy is exceedingly difficult.

It is understandable that mothers of small children may be anxious when they note that their child touches the ground with the entire sole of his foot, which does not yet reveal an arch (Fig. 12-2). Good advice is all that is needed in such a situation. In the older child it can frequently be proven that the feet are indeed normal. This is done after studying the local condition under weight bearing, without weight bearing, and by studying footprints. It is very important to reassure the mother (Fig. 12-3). We are generally dealing with what is known as a "pseudo" flat foot, that is, one which, in addition to genu valgum, rests with its medial border upon the floor. This condition may also be due to the valgus position of the hind foot caused by hyperlaxity. This can easily be recognized from its posterior appearance. Observation of the foot while bearing weight on one leg only, or on the tips of the toes, will show that the arch will reveal itself perfectly. In such a situation the prescription of a small wedge with a slight posterior supination may be justified even though it may be questionable whether such

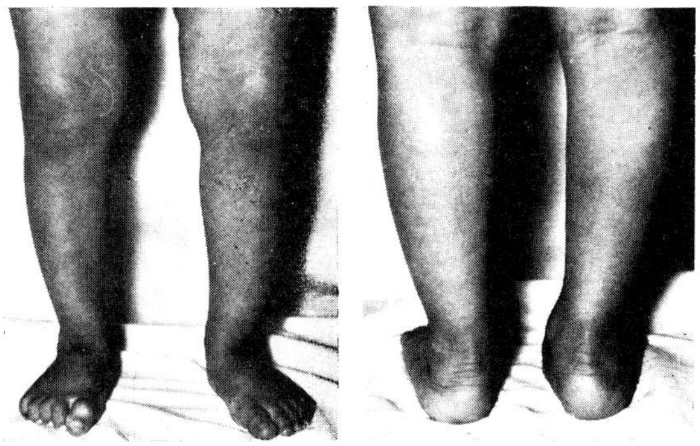

Fig. 12-2. "Pseudo-flat feet" in a 2-year-old. The pudgy appearance along with the apparent lack of a plantar arch is entirely normal at this age.

a measure actually helps in the correction of a congenital local anomaly.

It is important to be very discriminating in the prescription of arch support in this age group. One should suggest to the mother that she purchase shoes of moderate support, make good use of the visit by examining carefully the entire patient, especially with respect to the legs and posture, and recommend annual follow-up examinations.

Gymnastics and other forms of exercise are, on the whole, over prescribed. In the absence of an anomaly they are not heeded and if the anomaly is present, it is unlikely that they will be sufficient to be effective. They are rarely put to good use.

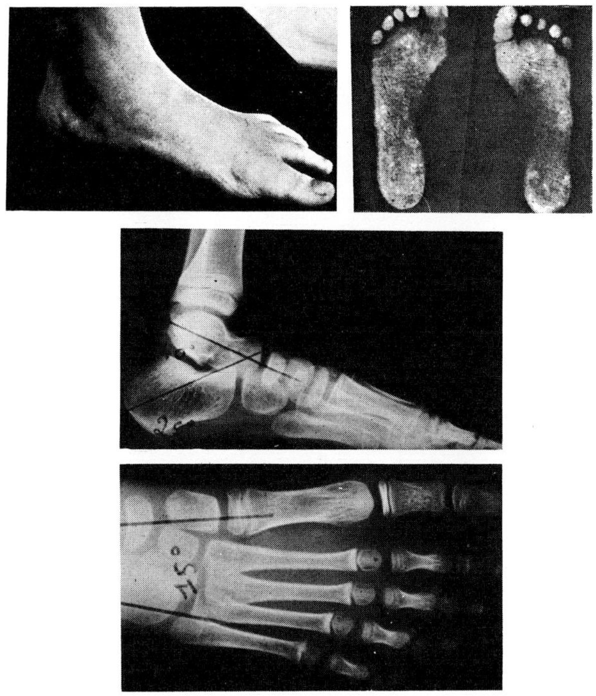

Fig. 12-3. The characteristics of a normal foot are: *(Top, left)* The arch remains hollow, even while bearing weight. *(Top, right)* Normal plantar imprint. *(Center, bottom)* There is a normal degree of talocalcaneal diversion on weightbearing radiographs. All these findings should be properly verified and evaluated during an examination if there is any question of a foot anomaly (see Fig. 12-4).

DURING LATER INFANCY AND ADOLESCENCE

Here the problems are much more clearly defined. If there is a true deformity of the foot, the examination, especially with a foot print will result in clear findings. It is important to ascertain the actual cause of the deformity and to offer rational treatment.

A true flat foot in valgus presents a classic appearance. The foot print is without a notch, and the talocalcaneal angle is increased on both the AP and lateral views during weight bearing. The etiology for this can be paralytic, congenital synostosis or idiopathic. If there are important functional difficulties, orthopaedic or surgical management will be required (Fig. 12-4).

Cavovarus deformity frequently results from a variety of neurologic disorders or from a painful underlying disorder, such as corns, claw foot, instability of the hind foot, or from pain on weight bearing or while wearing shoes. Foot prints and radiographs are very helpful and will assist in a painstaking follow-up under orthopaedic conservation or surgical management if there is progression of the underlying disorder.

Simple pes valgus frequently is an expression, in the older child, of abnormal laxity. This can be treated with arch support, as has been described for children in the younger group.

Cavovarus deformity, which is frequently confused with either a flat foot or a pes cavus, is often brought to the attention of the orthopaedic surgeon because of an abnormal protrusion of the internal malleolus, the head of the talus, or the base of the fifth metatarsal, is, in the majority of cases, the result of an abnormal rotation of the leg or femur. The aspect is that of a posterior pes valgus with a flat anterior portion and a markedly high plantar arch. This can be seen on a foot print. An arch support with a posterior supinator wedge and an anterior pronator wedge will rarely lead to the improvement of this anomaly, as it usually results from pathology located at the knee or the hip.

It will not often be possible to locate the underlying etiology. If there is familial occurrence of minor findings, one can reassure the mother of the probably benign character of the child's condition. However, it is wise to prescribed periodic follow-up during the active growth period. Only in this manner will it be possible not to overlook lesions that will manifest themselves at a later time.

Additional anomalies are those of the toes which result from a deviation or from a wide range of local deformities. Therapy is conservative, or may utilize surgery, depending on the characteristics of the lesion. Hallux valgus in young girls is seen quite frequently and presents a somewhat special problem. After puberty this lesion can be quite disturbing and there may be local pain and irritation of the head of the first metatarsal while wearing shoes. The leg may be long and slender or short and square. Usually spreading of the forefoot can be found. Local complaints may be self limited and normalization may result after a few months, while high heeled narrow shoes are worn. In this age group it is unusual that surgery is required.

One more common anomaly should be mentioned. In the older girl there is often an extra bony element, an os tibiale externum, located on the medial side of the tarsal scaphoid. This causes local pain while wearing shoes. This finding can be best recognized on AP films of the foot. If several local injections of corticosteroids do not result in complete healing of the reactive symptoms which are the result of local pressure, it may become necessary to resect this small extra bony structure. During surgery this may be located like a sesamoid within the most distal tendon of the musculus tibialis posterior (see Fig. 4-37, p. 171).

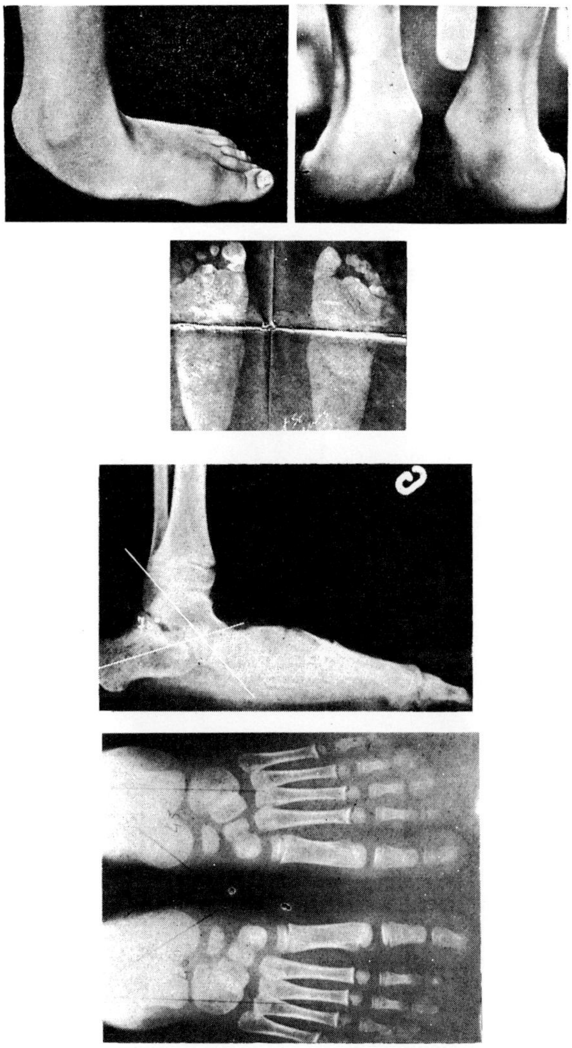

Fig. 12-4. The characteristics of a flat foot are: *(Top, right and left)* disappearance of the plantar arch with a marked prominence at the head of the talus and at the valgus position of the heal. *(Second from top)* Changes in the plantar imprint. *(Second from bottom, bottom)* An exaggerated talocalcaneal eversion while bearing weight is shown on this radiograph. These characteristic findings must be fully documented before the diagnosis of flat feet can be made.

BOWING AND DEVIATIONS OF THE LEGS

This is another area where preoccupied and worrying parents frequently require help from their pediatrician.

BOWING OF THE LEGS

In the Newborn and Baby

Physiologic bowing of both legs is regular or "comma" shaped in its uppermost portion, sometimes at different levels, and is accompanied by internal rotation of the foot and of the leg. This simply corresponds to the intrauterine position, where one leg was overlying the other and both were pressed against the trunk. This position can easily be assumed during the first few months of life and represents the physiologic pos-

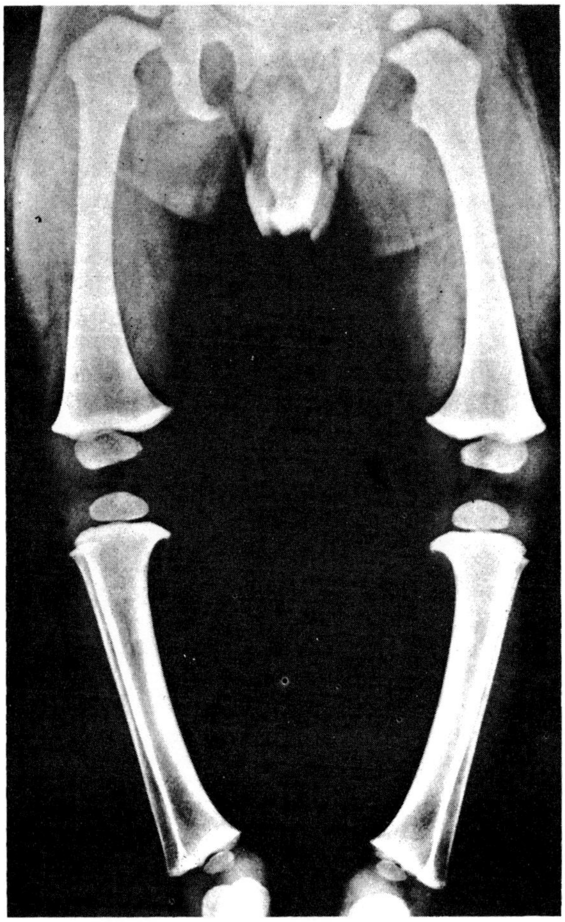

Fig. 12-5. Bilateral bowing of the lower portion of both legs in an 18-month-old infant during the early stages of walking.

ture. It will spontaneously correct itself after a few months.

Mothers will often be disturbed that their baby at several months of age is normal in appearance with prominent calfs. Radiographic study, if there is any doubt, can confirm the normal alignment of the skeleton.

During Infancy

There is sometimes generalized curving of the tibia, which may be more prominent in the upper-third or two-thirds. Besides medial concavity which give the legs a bowed or cowboy appearance. There will also be radiographic evidence of the actual incurving of the tibia (Fig. 12-5). In the majority of cases this will erroneously be called Blount's disease, since this type of bowing is definitely a simple continuation of the previously described posture. This is confirmed by the tendency to spontaneously disappear. Proper radiographs will confirm a normal skeleton and show, occasionally, a mild degree of high bowing of the tibia.

This finding should not be confused with bowing seen in rickets, which is low and with anterior convexity. It is good policy to completely examine the infant and to obtain radiographs of both legs in their entirety. There are cases where a careful study for bowing of the legs will reveal the presence of Blount's disease (Fig. 12-6) or of some other constitutional disorder of the skeleton (see p. 77).

In the Larger Child

Frequently there is an unsightly proximal bowing of the tibia which is limited to its upper-third. This finding is almost always accompanied by marked anomalies of the rotation of the femur and of the entire leg. No conservative orthopaedic measure will help in this situation and a surgical approach utilizing either an osteotomy or lateral epiphyseal fusion, depending on the patient's age, can be recommended. It should never be overlooked that this generally isolated local lesion can sometimes be the expression of a generalized disorder.

GENU VALGUM

During growth many infants will have a mild degree of physiological genu valgum. Many mothers will require help and encouragement during this phase. Between the mothers' fears and the frequent indecision of the physician, the right decision must be reached. If there is marked deformity, it is easily recognized, there are, however, possible causes for error.

Error by default. It is not unusual for young infants to be sent to the orthopaedic surgeon because of flat feet, when they actually suffer from genu valgum. The somewhat changed axis of the leg results in a foot pressed to the ground at its medial border since the infant cannot correct its posture in the subtalar joint. The child cannot place its foot on the ground in a normal manner. By observing the child in the AP view, it should be easy to recognize the abnormal angulation of the knees. Weight bearing on one leg brings out the condition even more clearly by revealing a pronounced deviation of the knee while the position of the foot becomes normalized.

Errors by excess: A large proportion of infants have genu valgum resulting from an excessive intermalleolar distance, which can result from a marked degree of obesity of the thighs, particularly in girls who cannot get their knees close to one another. This may also result from a condition known as "large knees," which can be seen in a number of adolescents during active growth, when the marked protrusion of the external condyles prevents a proper approximation of the medial malleoli. Careful clinical investigation in these conditions will verify that there is no deviation from the normal axis of the leg. This can be fully confirmed, if needed, by radiographic study.

Once the presence of genu valgum has been recognized, careful measurement is needed to fully appreciate its significance and to follow its development. The classical method utilized to measure the intermalleolar distance, while in the upright or prone position, is highly unreliable, since it is difficult to fix the actual front where the condylar region enters into direct contact. The simplest measurement is that of the axis which is formed by the thigh and the lower leg. This measurement, although coarse, is convenient. It can be obtained either lying down or standing upright, and standing on both or only one leg. This method is quite helpful in following developments. The most reliable measurement is the radiograph. This allows one to fully appreciate the angle formed between the axis of the femur and the tibia. It is not often obtained and requires strictly AP film exposure of either supine or upright positioning. This form of evaluation should be used at least once, in order to properly appraise the skeletal parts. Clinical evaluation in the follow-up may be adequate as the problem of such patients is commonly esthetic.

The so-called "spontaneous disappearance" of genu valgum is based on the entirely false assumption that there is a laxity in the ligaments of the knee. This is almost never true. In early infancy, growth of the genu valgum is accompanied by a slight recurvation which is responsible for the easy fatigability of these infants, whose knees are only stable in hyperextension. The "reductibility" results from the fact that during examination of the completely straight knee in the supine infant, the lateral ligaments relax, since the genu recurvatum is slightly flexed. Genu valgum of the growing infant seems to be the result of asymmetric growth between the internal and external halves of the distal long bones of the knee, especially of the femur. It is also possible that this is the reason for the occasional motheaten appearance which is frequently seen affecting the medial condyle during infancy (see Fig. 2-9, p. 20). The approach taken to a true genu valgum, with an angle of more than 10°, or to very unsightly characteristics is dependent upon the patient's age.

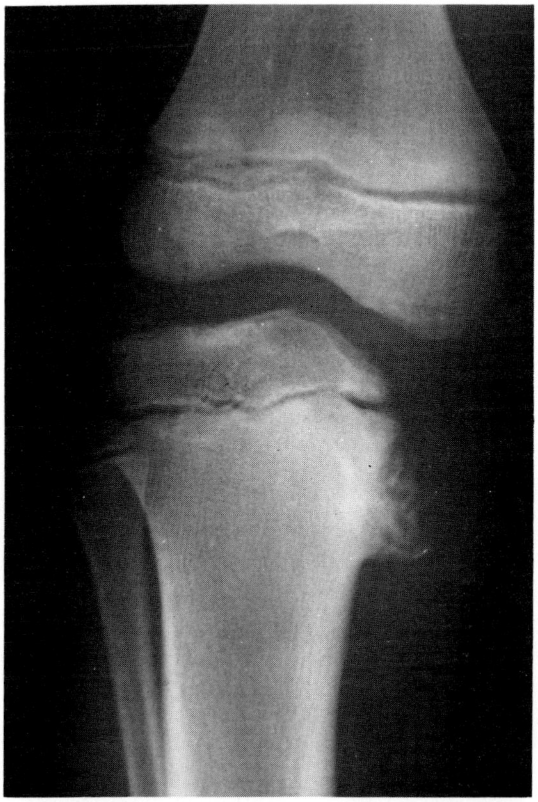

Fig. 12-6. Blount's disease in a 7-year-old boy. Note the severe changes in the medial portion of the tibial metaphysis along with the partial destruction of the corresponding plateau. (Courtesy of J. Lefebvre)

From the beginning of walking to four or five years, a mild degree of genu valgum is almost physiologic. After the initial phase, in which the condition might progress for six months to one year, it will become stable for six months, whereupon spontaneous improvement will follow. In the great majority of cases this will happen within another six months to one year. This improvement may occur during the following spurts of growth or may be noted after holidays. A reassuring attitude and a conservative approach is important.

There are, however, patients with a more severe degree of involvement with 15°, 20°, or an even greater deviation with progressive local involvement, ensuing pathology of the feet and back, and in whom surgical correction may become necessary. If there is unilateral or predominantly one-sided genu valgum, an abnormal tilt of the pelvis and a scoliotic attitude may result.

The use of supports is, on the whole, an illusory cure. The underlying idea is to correct the pressure axis at the medial portion of the knee. Such an effect is most unlikely, and a genu valgum, which will disappear after the application of supports, in all likelihood would have undergone spontaneous correction. The same might be said for other forms of treatment, and one must be extremely cautious in attempts to evaluate effectiveness.

On the other hand, a correcting cast should be considered effective. In order to achieve positive results, it is necessary to use long casts with a forced varus position. These must be changed approximately every four weeks. Therapy is usually rapidly successful within three or four months. The casts are very demanding as one should leave the casts on permanently, and this severely affects the daily lives of these infants.

Ideally, one should use night splints in the attempt to progressively bring the malleoli closer together. This form of therapy is reliable, nontraumatic and tolerable. In patients with uncooperative parents, this approach will not work. However, the majority of infants and parents will accept this form of therapy. During the day the infant is free of any interference, the only inconvenience being the fact that the correction is slow, requiring 8 to 12 months of constant attention. Splints or cases have a therapeutic effect for up to six or eight years. Later, other forms of more aggressive therapy must be used. Between the ages of 6 and 12 problems of genu valgum are rarely seen.

Later, however, genu valgum is frequently noted during adolescence and puberty. At this time overweight boys are primarily affected. At this age it may become necessary, depending on the bone age and the local radiographic findings, to perform epiphyseal fusion or an osteotomy. The exact decision must be left to the orthopaedic surgeon, who should be able to achieve an ideal correction of the condition. Corrective management is indicated if there is marked deviation of the knee, as this condition leads to arthroses in adulthood.

DISTURBED GAIT RESULTING FROM ABNORMAL ROTATION OF THE SKELETON OF THE LEG

We are dealing here with a very real, frequently encountered, and well known problem of some controversy. The orthopaedic surgeons are very familiar with this condition which is, however, poorly known and understood by pediatricians and family physicians. The latter will often attribute the local abnormal findings of the feet or knee to local pathology, whereas the underlying disease process is almost always situated much higher in the hips.

The most typical patient is a child, usually female, between 6 and 12 years of age, who while walking or at rest, shows internal rotation of the knees, so that the patellae face medially. In addition they have bowing of the upper tibia with a medial concavity and high recurvation together with the cavovalgus deformity, which is often misinterpreted as a flat foot and confirmed by a foot print (Fig. 12-7). Careful history will reveal that the child has slept for a long time on the abdomen or on all four extremities, especially with flexed legs. Also, when playing on the ground, such children frequently sit with their knees pressed together and feet pushed outwards. They are incapable of sitting cross-legged, can hardly run or jump, and develop pain in their groin after prolonged walking. Often one will find out that these children walked with the knees facing medially. As this posture slowly was corrected the feet were positioned normally, whereas the tibia developed bowing while the knees remained in internal rotation.

Examination reveals that there is external rotation of the skeleton of the leg, so that the axis of the foot forms an angle with the plane of flexion of the knee at 20° to 40° or greater. This may be the case in an advanced case with marked tibial bowing and pes cavovalgus. On the other hand, there may be excessive internal rotation of the hip of 60° or as high as 90°, while external rotation is limited to 10° or less. Extreme flexion may also be markedly limited. Radiographic study may confirm that there is excessive anteversion of the femoral necks up to 50° or more. Sometimes there is only an abnormal orientation of the acetabular roof, but this may be difficult to prove.

The combining feature here seems to be an abnormal rotation of the femoral axis. We may be dealing here with an isolated anteversion, which instead of progressively disappearing, not only persists, but affects the compensating external rotation of the skeleton of the leg and thus is responsible for the changes of the knee and foot. The local disturbance may be located only in the hip, also affecting the acetabulum or it may affect the entire femur. There is a certain analogy with excessive anteversion seen leading to the identical symptoms in congenital dislocation of the hip. Family history is sometimes very revealing.

How should one deal with these problems? The answer is not simple. In dealing with a very young infant without femoral pathology, a careful clinical and radiographic study of the pelvis and both legs, including measurements for the anteversion with annual follow-up is recommended. If there is a tendency towards improvement, conservative management is recommended along with plans to follow the patient to the

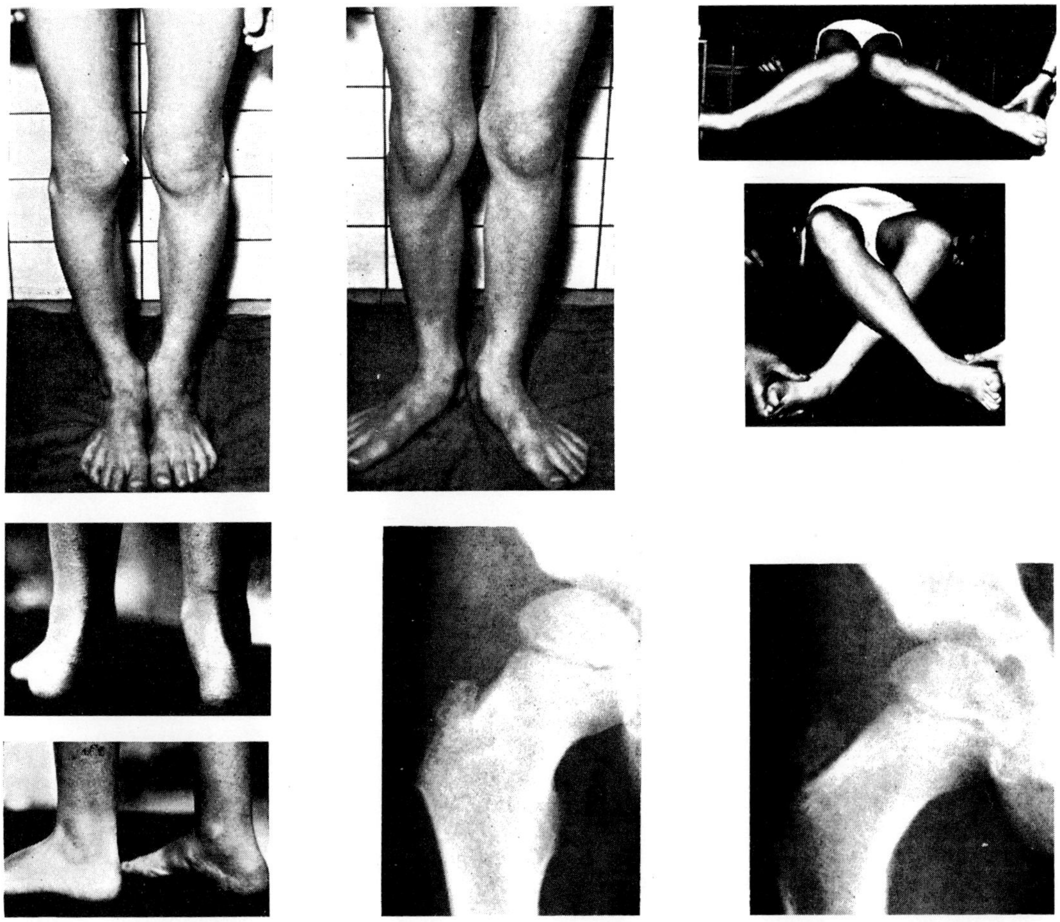

Fig. 12-7. Abnormal rotation of the skeletal element of the leg. *(Top, left and second from left)* The knees rotate inward during walking revealing a high tibial arch. If the knees face anteriorly, the tips of the feet will have a tendency to diverge too much, resulting in an increased external rotation of the bones of the leg. *(Top, right)* There is an exaggerated internal rotation of the hips with equal limitation in their external rotation. *(Bottom, left)* Often there is an associated pes valgus excavatus. *(Bottom, right and second from right)* The exaggerated anteversion of the femoral necks is the base of this syndrome and can be corrected by a derotation-osteotomy.

end of the growth period. However, if the patient walks with internal rotation and there is no improvement of the femoral anteversion after one or more years, an intervention with femoral derotation may be the only means of reestablishing a normal physiological orientation of the legs. This intervention should not be recommended too early. One must wait until all possibilities of spontaneous correction are exhausted. However, one should not wait until external rotation of the leg occurs spontaneously as a compensatory mechanism. This would require a double osteotomy of the femur and tibia, which is a much more complicated intervention. An age limit cannot be set of, for instance, six to eight years, but one should rather rely on the length of observation available in an individual patient.

In the older child it is practically no longer possible – if only for reasons of schooling – to offer a double osteotomy. One is then forced to approach the esthetically most disturbing lesion, which is the bowing of the upper portion of the tibia. This approach leaves the total skeletal rotation out of consideration. The operation will depend on the age of the patient. Fusion of the epiphyses of the fubula and external tibia or an osteotomy can be recommended.

It is much more desirable to operate on the younger

child for a minor anomaly as opposed to attempting a symptomatic and incomplete surgical correction during adolescence. Pediatricians and family physicians should, therefore, devote their attention to these alterations of skeletal rotation of the legs and refer such problems to the orthopaedic surgeon as early as possible.

THE LIMPING CHILD

This is a frequent finding. We cannot discuss here the entire orthopaedic pathology affecting the legs and hips, however, we would like to stress the following points.

It is a ground rule to always carefully and completely investigate the entire lower extremity along with the pelvis and the trunk, when investigating a patient for a limp. Studies must include the patient's walk, articular mobility throughout the body, measurements for all segments, radiographic study, and neurologic status. In many instances investigation for a limp results in the recognition of inequalities in leg lengths, or a neurologic disorder, such as unrecognized paralysis or contracture.

Radiographic study of the hips must be obtained. This study should not only consist of the frontal view of the pelvis, but should include the lateral views of both hips. Whenever a patient is investigated for painful knees, a radiograph of the hip is mandatory. It is very disturbing to see patients repeatedly in whom a congenital dislocation of the hip was recognized too late, or in whom osteochondritis of the hip, epiphysiolysis of the femoral head, coxa vara congenita, or other local pathology is present because, at an earlier time, detailed study of an infant or a young child with a limp was neglected. If the local findings are normal, radiographic studies should be repeated 45 to 60 days later, even if the initial presenting symptoms have disappeared. This is the only reliable way to recognize local pathology.

During childhood and adolescence a limping child with sudden local pain, limitation of motion, and fever may present without any local radiographic findings. Under therapy with traction the condition disappears after a few days and follow-up radiographs will again show no bony involvement. There may however be local edema of the soft tissues around the hip. The term "observation hip" has been applied to this condition which has an unknown, possibly viral etiology.

One should never overlook the possible infectious or inflammatory joint involvement of the hip, the knee, the foot, the spine, or of the sacroiliac joints. There are also subacute types of osteomyelitis. Nothing is lost if a patient is unnecessarily put in a cast and treated with antibiotics. This sometimes happens with a misdiagnosed patient with acute rheumatoid arthritis. On the other hand, administration of corticosteroids in osteitis or for a painful hip is not without danger.

There are many minor reasons we should not overlook a limp. These include a number of local soft tissue lesions, osteochondritis, fatigue fractures and other conditions that are not always considered.

A limp must eventually be considered to represent a psychosomatic problem in young girls, if all clinical etiologies have been carefully ruled out. It may be helpful to guide such a young lady with the necessary firm and clear approach. If this does not help, the psychiatrist may have to take over.

SPINAL INVOLVEMENT

We only consider minor anomalies of form of the spinal curvature so frequently seen in the daily pediatric practice and would like to exclude the marked local anomalies.

The acquisition of the final, normal static appearance of the spine evolves over a rather lengthy period of an individual's life. The baby has a spine in total kyphosis from the occiput to the sacrum, which is easily appreciated at the time when the child starts to sit. There is no harmonious curvature present as in the adult, that is, a lumbar lordosis, thoracic kyphosis and cervical lordosis. These will only establish themselves progressively starting from the moment when the individual begins to walk. Frequently growing children have "bad posture", especially a round back, and lumbar hyperlordosis. All the rules for a careful examination of the spine during infancy must be properly applied in order to distinguish between abnormal posture and true pathology:

a) The child must be examined in the nude, in order to recognize even mild imbalance. Besides the general physical development the genital status and development can be appreciated.

b) During the investigation, the following landmarks should be identified: Interspinous line, tips of the scapulae, spinae iliacae posteriores and the iliac crests.

c) The child must be examined upright viewing it from the back, the front and in the side view by evaluating the spinal curvatures using a lead line. In the frontal view the line must pass from the spinous process of C7 through the fold between both buttocks

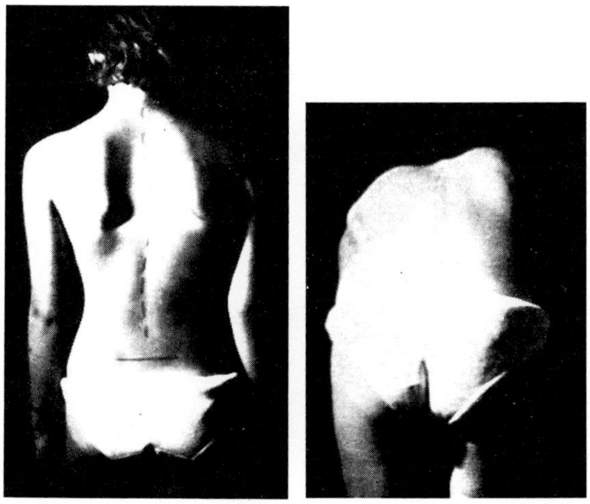

Fig. 12-8. The clinical search for the presence of a gibbus is fundamental as part of spinal examinations. If present it implies the existence of an abnormal underlying structure.

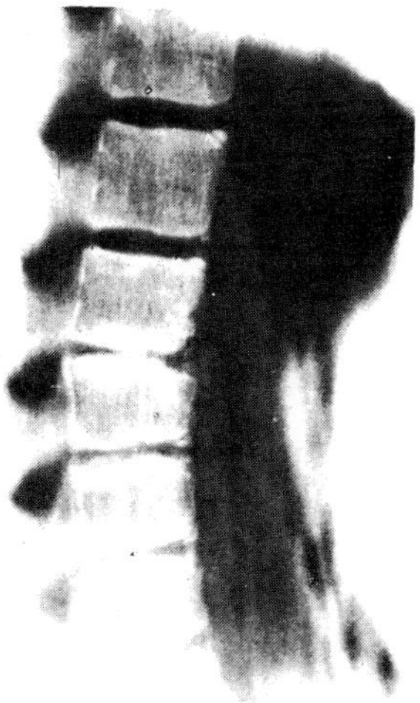

Fig. 12-9. Vertebral osteochondritis was discovered in this child, who did not present with any subjective symptoms but simply had a fixed dorsal kyphosis.

and in the lateral view from the external auditory canal to the trochanter major. A clear deviation is the expression of a usually fixed spinal malalignment.

d) A most important phase is the investigation of the flexed spine with the child touching with the tips of the fingers, the toes and then coming up slowly forming a completely round back. During this maneuver the examiner must stand directly behind the patient. In this way it should be easy to recognize even the slightest degree of gibbus resulting from vertebral rotation and from a real structural scoliosis (Fig. 12-8).

e) By checking the patient and his mobility in the horizontal and sitting positions and flexing anteriorly, posteriorly and to the sides, it is possible to recognize local rigidity or fixation of a segment. Such findings would be the expression of a true lesion, whatever its course involving the spine, and would not simply reflect on the posture.

f) The legs must be carefully measured, just as must be the position of the pelvis. Careful attention should be given to the way a child walks.

g) A general work-up, including history, reflexes, weight, height, muscular status, physical activities and involvements in sports is necessary.

h) If there is the slightest doubt, after the completion of the physical examination, radiographic study of the spine, including at least an AP view of the entire spine from the base of the skull to the upper portion of the pelvis in the upright position must follow.

Only after such an examination and after having eliminated all the possible inflammatory, traumatic, tumoral, structural and other spinal lesions, can we possibly conclude that there is simply a poor spinal posture.

Poor posture is a problem frequently encountered during school physical examinations. It results in maternal anxiety. During adolescence this may be an almost physiologic problem, since correction is possible by having the child retract its belly, hold its shoulders, and particularly the head, straight, thereby assuming a proper curvature of a normal spine.

Hypotonic and overweight children and also particularly tall, prepubertal girls, are in need of some activities in gymnastics or sports and a lot of patience rather than orthopaedic measures. Still, it is important to carefully supervise such patients from time to time, because of the danger of a fixed abnormal attitude. Careful study, especially by radiographs may reveal some underlying pathology, especially Scheuermann's disease (Fig. 12-9).

One final word should be added here on the so-called scoliosis of the baby. This always refers to one complete curvature of the spine, usually towards the left, which can be practically straightened out without rotation. The condition usually is corrected within some weeks after hyperreduction with a plaster shell. This is, in all likelihood, a persistent intrauterine posture, often accompanied by torticollis. Radiographic study is always required, in order not to overlook congenital anomalies. The same goes for the patient in whom this type of a scoliosis persists or becomes worse. In such a situation we would have to deal with the very unusual, but serious problem of infantile scoliosis with precocious onset.

Part Six:

Bone Tumors

Clément Fauré

13 Bone Tumors: The Interpretation of Radiographs and the Technical Radiographic Approach

Tumors of the skeleton, whether primary or secondary, represent an important part of pathology of the bones occurring during childhood. Radiology plays an important role in their discovery, in the proper diagnostic recognition of a lesion and especially in the decision whether an existing lesion is benign or malignant. The importance that is attached to it in the following description is therefore not surprising. This approach is only one of the many necessary for the establishment of a dignosis. It is unusual that radiology alone reliably solves a clinical problem. Generally it is necessary to correlate the results of a careful and detailed radiologic study with the result of a pathologist's expert interpretation of properly obtained biopsy material in order to arrive at a reliable diagnosis.

THE DIAGNOSTIC APPROACH IN RADIOLOGY

Most frequently primary bone tumors are present as a solitary lesion of a bone, recognized because of variable underlying clinical findings. Secondary tumors most frequently start out with multiple and disseminated skeletal involvement, but may occasionally be solitary. A solitary bony lesion recognized on a radiograph may be congenital or acquired. If acquired, the five following categories must be considered:

For many radiologists it is almost too risky to venture a diagnosis in the presence of a solitary bone lesion and they will simply enumerate a number of diagnostic possibilities without selecting a specific diagnosis. A careful and systematic radiologic approach to bony lesions and the involvement of the adjacent soft tissue structures will permit a markedly reduced number of possible diagnoses. All hypothetical etiologies must be considered in each of the five categories mentioned below. If one also includes such considerations as the age and the sex of the patient, the presenting clinical findings and the duration of local findings, one can eliminate a number of possibilities and arrive at a very small number of, and occasionally only one, diagnosis.

THE REACTION OF BONE TO A LESION

Bones have only two ways of reacting to a local aggressive process, whatever its nature. Either bone becomes destroyed secondary to osteoclastic stimulation by the local lesion, eventually recognized as osteolytic zones, or there may be condensation by new bone formation resulting from a stimulation of normal osteoblasts present within bone or under the periosteum. Condensation may also be present as calcification of the matrix, the product of certain types of tumor cells, such as osteoblasts and chondroblasts. The reaction of the bone can be purely osteolytic or purely condensing, or both, which is the rule. This bony reaction is not specific. Sometimes there may be a particularly striking appearance, especially in osteolytic and mixed types.

The Different Types of Osteolytic Reaction

Osteolysis, even in its extensive form, may not be radiographically visible if it occurs in a very loose spongy tissue, such as markedly osteoporotic bone. Osteolytic lesions will only become recognizable radiographically, if they involve either the compact bone of a diaphysis, the metaphyseo-epiphyseal cortex, or that of a flat or short bone. According to Lodwick we can define different types of involvement depending on the extent, the limitation and aspect of osteolysis.

Geographic type (Figs. 13-1, 14-5 to 14-9, and 14-19): Defects with clearly defined borders of the bony defect, sometimes with a polycyclic outline and with a clearly recognizable appearance between osteolysis and the neighboring bone. The cortex is either completely destroyed, eroded or thinned, but still present. This type of osteolysis can be seen in a number of primary bone tumors, benign or malignant, in certain metastatic tumors and also during infectious disorders and in the course of histiocytosis X.

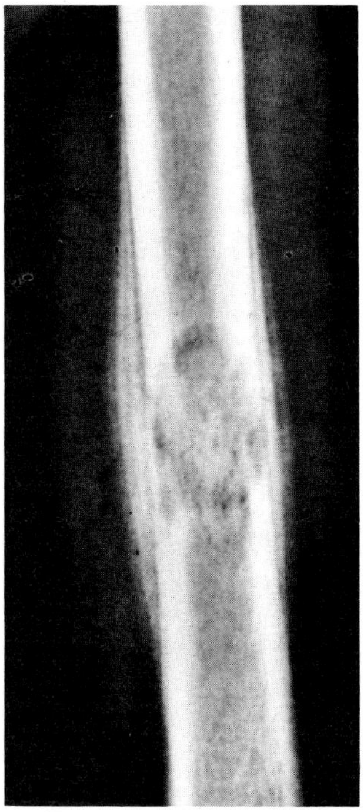

Fig. 13-1. Geographic osteolysis. Corticoperiosteal ossification which occurred in parallel layers during the course of osteomyelitis in the humerus of an 8-year-old child.

Motheaten type (Figs. 15-4, 15-7 and 15-17 *B*): The osteolysis can be seen in the form of many small confluent defects destroying the cortex, leading in some places to local fractures. This type of osteolysis is often noted in the presenee of primary malignant tumors, at an early stage and in metastatic involvement.

Permeated type (Figs. 15-10 *A* and 15-17 *A*): The osteolysis assumes the aspect of tiny holes within the cortex. When such lesions are seen strictly in the AP view they may be completely overlooked. They are better recognized if recorded tangentially. In this situation the cortex will simply appear to have lost some of its density without being destroyed or eroded. Its normal preserved area and the affected part are not divided by a clear border. This type of osteolysis is frequently combined with marked periosteal reaction. Usually it occurs during a primary or secondary tumor-lesion with a rapidly progressive and extensive character.

Mixed type (Figs. 15-5, 15-8, 15-14, 15-15, 15-18, and 15-19): This type is seen frequently. In most patients there is a combination of central geographic osteolysis and a permeated appearance at the periphery. In this combination of signs the osteolysis is evidence of a rapidly progressive tumor with extensive involvement.

Purely isolated condensating reactions (Fig. 15-22) are rarely present, if differentiation from condensation resulting from calcification of the tumor stroma is attempted. This will be discussed later.

The Different Types of Mixed Reaction

Geographic osteolysis, clearly delineated by a sclerosing zone of variable extent, frequently of rather thin appearance (Figs. 14-1 and 14-2, 14-4, 14-10, 14-13, 14-20 and 14-21), is highly characteristic for a slowly growing and therefore benign underlaying process. Such findings can be seen among others during the course of enchondramas, bone cysts, nonossifying fibroma (Figs. 14-1 and 14-2), monostotic fibrous dysplasia and epidermoid cysts (Figs. 14-20 and 14-21). This appearance can also be seen during certain infectious processes, especially those involving the cranial vault.

Another type of mixed reaction is due to a rounded or oval osteolysis of limited extent—several millimeters to a centimeter in diameter—surrounded by a uniformly thick zone of sclerotic bone with its own periphery loosing itself gradually within the normal neighboring bone (Figs. 14-11 and 14-12). This involvement is also suggestive of a benign process, primarily an osteoid osteoma. Chronic condensating osteomyelitis of Garré may lead to a similar appearance, but such a lesion occurs only rarely.

Mixed reactions with condensating and lytic characteristics may have a more complicated appearance, or they can alternate without any recognizable order between osteolysis and condensation (Figs. 13-2, 15-1 and 15-3). Such involvement is seen especially in flat bones and should alert one to the possibility of metastatic tumor involvement or primary malignant lesions such as Ewing's sarcoma, osteosarcoma, the local involvement during Hodgkin's disease, and even to the remote possibility of a benign lesion, such as a hemangioma or an enchondroma.

REACTIVE PERIOSTEAL OSTEOGENESIS

All local involvement of the periosteum by an abnormal process usually originating from the underlying bone, but occasionally also from the adjacent soft tissues, will result in an osteogenetic reaction by the subperiosteal osteoblasts. Usually it takes just about 15 days for the radiologic manifestation of this osteogenesis. This periosteal reaction can assume different aspects depending on the duration of the local irritation and especially on the rapidity of the underlying process.

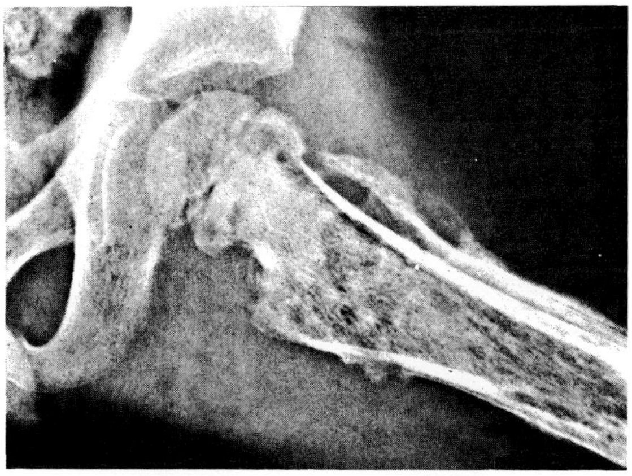

Fig. 13-2. Osteolysis and associated bone condensation. Dense masses and even periosteal reaction occurs during severe osteomyelitis.

Spiculation

Any lesion invading the cortex from the medullary cavity, whether infectious or neoplastic, will usually elevate the periosteum and detach it from its contact with the cortex. Within this space there are a number of perpendicular structures with respect to the cortex and the periosteum—Sharpey's fibers and vessels—radiologically not recognizable, but capable of eventually forming a sort of scaffolding and support for osteoblastic activity after bony tissue is formed along these structures. They are visible radiologically as fine spicules perpendicular to the cortex. This type of periosteal reaction is seen usually in rapidly progressive tumors. Most frequently this would refer to primary, but sometimes also secondary, local lesions. There is practically no bony definition under the periosteum and the location of the periosteum itself corresponds to the line going through the most distal points of all these spicules. This type of spiculation can occasionally occur in periosteal reaction after local infection. As an explanation, the theory has been put forth that a destruction of Sharpey's fibers and of vessels by proteolytic enzymes are its cause, since this usually occurs in the course of such infections (Nelson).

Lodwick distinguishes five types of spiculation: a) "Hair-on-end"-appearance (Fig. 15-2). Ewing's sarcoma invading a diaphysis has a high association with this finding. b) "Sunburst" appearance (Fig. 15-8 and 15-12). A high incidence of this finding is noted in sarcomas with local development, especially osteosarcoma. c) "Velvety" appearance with fine spicula formation of uneven size and often obliquely arranged with an ill-defined lateral border. This finding is said to occur with relatively high incidence in chondrosarcoma, but can be seen exceptionally during infections. d) A regular type with thicker, occasionally confluent spiculation showing a clear peripheral delineation (Fig. 15-4) seen in slowly progressive tumors or in non-tumor processes, such as hypertrophic callus formation during osteogenesis imperfecta (Fig. 14-22). e) Unclassifiable type. This type corresponds to a series of different aspects of spiculation, which cannot be classified in anyone of the preceding four groups (Figs. 14-24 and 15-16). Usually there is an underlying malignant process, but we should emphasize that we have seen an occasional patient with periosteal hematoma, especially the pseudo-tumoral types, during hemophilia (Fig. 14-24).

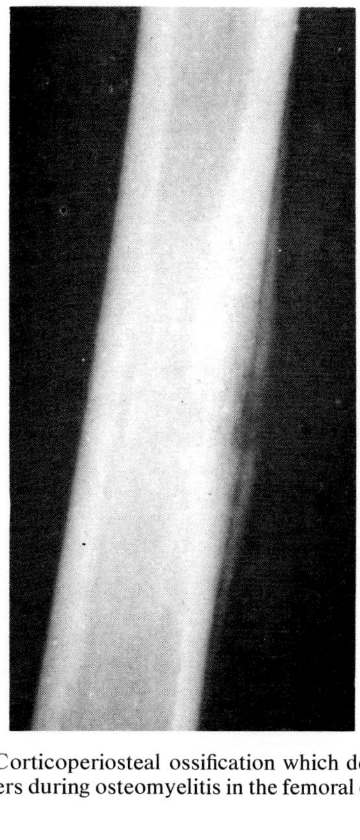

Fig. 13-3. Corticoperiosteal ossification which developed in parallel layers during osteomyelitis in the femoral diaphysis.

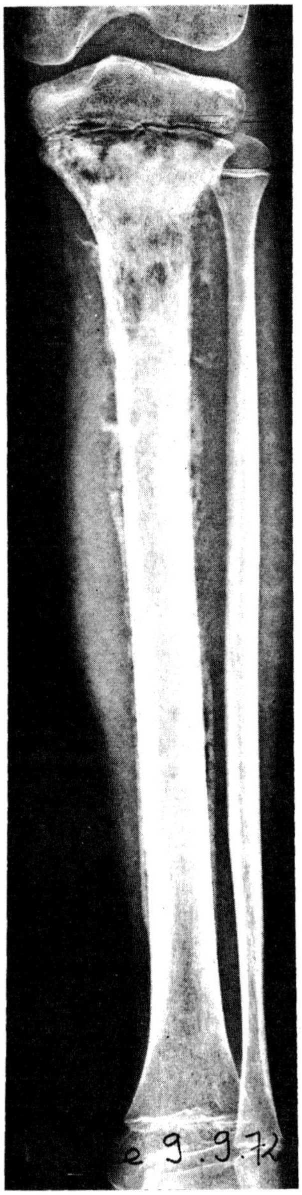

Fig. 13-4. This later stage of osteomyelitis has the appearance of a pseudo-tumor. Fully developed periosteal reaction of homogeneous characteristics at the region of the middle and upper-third of the tibia.

Subperiosteal Ossification in Parallel Layers

Here periosteal stimulation results in the construction of bony lamellae, but there is not sufficient time for full assimilation into the cortex or complete fusion before a new abnormal process outside of this layer of bony tissue occurs moving the periosteum yet further distally. The result is a succession of bony layers resulting in the onion peel aspect (Figs. 13-1, 13-3, 13-7, 15-11 and 15-12). This appearance is not specific for a tumor. It simply results from a rapidly progressive local lesion. This finding can be present during an infectious process, histiocytosis X, periosteal hematoma, and malignant tumors of primary or secondary nature. If the underlying lesion is rapidly progressive and its development is faster than that of subperiosteal osteogenesis there will be, in addition to the layered reaction, either local spiculation or simply direct invasion of the neighboring soft tissue structures across the periosteum in the form of a local mass with its matrix possibly showing local calcification. In such a situation there will be a periosteal reaction forming a local spur at the periphery of such a tumoral effraction—Codman's triangle.

Solid Homogeneous Periosteal Reaction

Osteogenesis occurs in one single homogeneous sub-periosteal bony layer of 1 mm thickness or more. It has uniform density and may be confused with the external surface of the cortex appearing as a more or less extensive hyperostosis on the surface of the bone. This aspect may persist unchanged for many weeks or even months. This is the reflection of a very slowly progressive underlying lesion, usually of a benign type. It may assume a number of different aspects: thin and regular—eosinophilic granuloma, osteoid osteoma, sub-periosteal hematoma, sub-periosteal fracture, hypertrophic pulmonary osteoarthropathy and osteomyelitis, thin and wavy—hypertrophic pulmonary osteoarthropathy, thick and wavy—vascular disturbances and varicose veins, thick, dense, elliptic and regular in outline—osteoid osteoma (Fig. 14-12), Ewing's sarcoma treated by irradiation, possibly malignant tumors with markedly slow progression, or thick with a smooth surface or an interrupted surface, directly adjacent or somewhat separated from the cortex—osteomyelitis (Figs. 13-2 and 13-4), storage disorders, especially Gaucher's disease.

Cortical Expansion (Periosteal Remodeling)

Certain slowly progressive lesions originating from the medulla or the deeper layers of the cortex may occasionally become large enough to lead to a progressive cortical destruction of endosteal bone. The cortex will become thin and at the same time there will be a stimulation of the periosteum, which will form new bone in order to maintain the stability of the affected skeletal part. With the progression of the deeper part of the lesion, this bone will become hollow from within, whereas the newly deposited layers of the periosteum will envelope it. The result is an expansion of the bone. By radiograph there will be a convex external protrusion with a cortical ridge projecting outwardly and a second cortical ridge forming a somewhat thinner arch at the tip of the convexity (Figs. 14-5 and 14-15 to 14-17). If the expansile lesion is not uniform and growth occurs in different directions, there will be zones of bony erosion separated by other zones, where the bone is more or less destroyed. Seen at its inner surface, the lesion contains a number of defects separated by active bone-bridges. On radiographs these appear as remodeled trabeculae which are not stretched out totally, as this has been assumed, across the cavity.

This type of bony expansion with conservation of the cortex, even though it may be thinner, is the hallmark of a slowly progressive lesion and usually evidence of benign involvement. This finding has also been recorded in certain types of secondary tumors—hypernephroma and cancer of the thyroid—but in such instances it will be very unusual not to have a destruction and brake within the cortex, at least in some areas of the zone of the bony expansion.

The Periosteal Spur or Codman's Triangle

When a local lesion displaces the periosteum so much that the fixation of the periosteum is broken, there will be at the transition between the remaining normal periosteum and the adjacent elevation a formation of a triangular homogeneous spur or apposition of bone. The tip of this spur with a triangular form points to the still normal cortex and the external tip to the displaced periosteal portion (Figs. 15-6 *A*, 15-8 and 15-15). This sub-periosteal triangle simply indicates that there has been periosteal elevation and not, as was assumed for a long time, a malignant lesion. This finding can be seen during osteomyelitis, in the course of several benign and slowly developing tumors, in aneurysmal bone cysts, in periosteal hematomas and in histiocytosis X (Fig. 13-5).

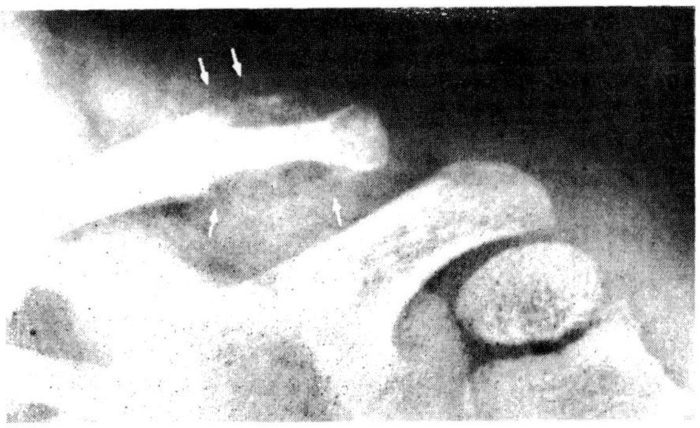

Fig. 13-5. Periosteal spurs which are the result of trabecular localization of histiocytosis X.

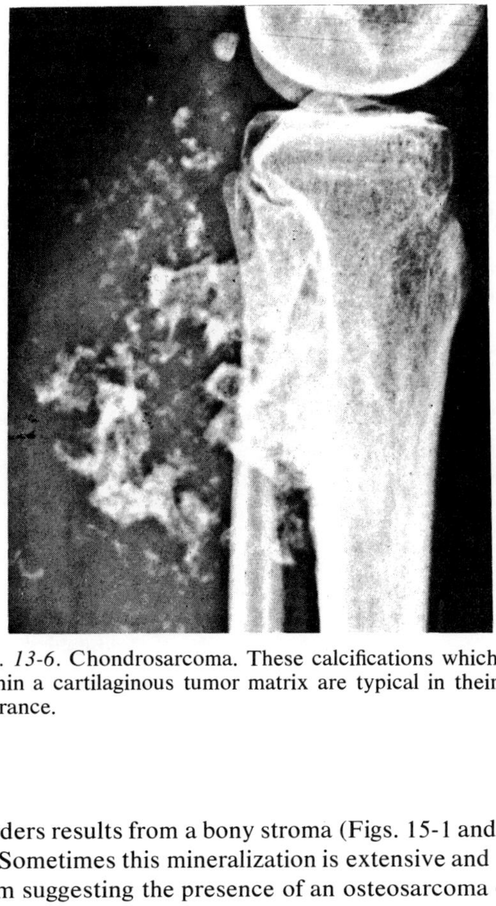

Fig. 13-6. Chondrosarcoma. These calcifications which are within a cartilaginous tumor matrix are typical in their appearance.

TUMORAL MATRIX CALCIFICATION

The matrix formed by tumor as it invades the soft tissues in the extra-cortical region or within the medullary cavity can take up calcium. The aspect of such calcium deposits will vary according to the type of cells. Flocular calcifications of the "popcorn" type or sometimes even more punctate are suggestive of a benign or malignant cartilaginous matrix (Figs. 13-6 and 14-7). Calcification in a homogeneous layer with ill-defined borders results from a bony stroma (Figs. 15-1 and 15-3). Sometimes this mineralization is extensive and uniform suggesting the presence of an osteosarcoma or a periosteal sarcoma, but it may also be less uniform, or grossly lumpy—as seen in osteosarcoma.

OTHER DIAGNOSTIC CONSIDERATIONS

If there is only a single skeletal lesion, the following further points deserve careful consideration.

The Extent of Bony Involvement

A neoplastic process initially will be localized and limited to the involved bone, usually its metaphyseal region, whereas an infection will have the tendency to involve a large segment of the bone, since it expands rapidly throughout the medullary cavity. Therefore, if a lesion involves a large portion of the diaphysis of a long bone one should first think of the possibility of this being an infection (Fig. 13-4); only Ewing's sarcoma, amongst tumors of bone, may show this tendency to diaphyseal extension.

Localization of Lesions

Certain abnormal processes have a predilection for flat bones, some for short bones and yet other ones for long bones.

Several tumors have a tendency to involve certain regions and locations within the skeleton with a relatively high frequency. The vast majority of primary benign tumors will develop in metaphyses of long bones. Seventy-five to eighty per cent of all osteogenic sarcomas are localized in the neighborhood of the knee, either within the distal femoral or the proximal tibial metaphysis. Chordomas, by perference, are localized within the sacrum, the cervical spine and the base of the skull. Benign osteoblastomas have a high incidence of involvement of the posterior arch of vertebrae. If the pathological lesion is within a long bone its precise location is equally important. The epiphysis, for example is the favored location for benign chondroblastomas and giant cell tumors. The metaphysis, as we have seen, is frequently the site for the onset of many different types of malignant or primary tumors. The diaphysis can be involved either by an infectious or tumoral process. If there is involvement by tumor, this is most frequently a metastatic secondary lesion. If primary, the most frequent type of involvement is by Ewing's sarcoma rather than an osteogenic sarcoma.

Relation of Tumor to the Growth Plate

A local infectious lesion will almost always sooner or later invade the growth cartilage. After completely crossing this structure the infection will reach the epiphysis and also the joint. The articular cartilage itself may be rapidly destroyed resulting in a reduced joint space.

Tuberculosis and other bony infections by non-pyogenic micro-organisms can also develop on either side of the growth cartilage, but this after a much longer period of time—several months instead of several weeks. Similarly, if the joint is involved the process of articular cartilage destruction is much slower and it takes much longer to result in a narrow joint space.

Primary or secondary tumors, whether malignant or benign, behave differently with respect to growth cartilage, which represents a sudden and total barrier (Figs. 15-3, 15-7 and 15-15). This, therefore, is a very important radiologic criterium for the differentiation between infectious and tumoral lesions. If a lesion abruptly ends at the limit of the growth cartilage, its nature is most likely tumor and only rarely infectious. If, however, it crosses the cartilage, it is most likely an infectious lesion. Bony involvement of Hodgkin's disease with a rapidly progressive course and also osteogenic sarcoma in the older child can both cross the growth plate.

Speed of Progression and Duration of Course

If, in a given case. there are earlier radiographs showing that the lesion under discussion has remained unchanged during months and even years, chances are that this is a benign lesion. If no earlier films are available, a number of points may help in an evaluation of the speed of progression of the disorder. Punctate or moth-eaten osteolysis are evidence of a rapidly progressive underlying process, whereas a geographic type of defect gives evidence of a somewhat less rapidly progressive course. A sclerotic rim around the osteolytic centers will also be evidence of a relatively slow evolution, and if in addition there is an arched cortical elevation together with local thinning it can be concluded that the lesion grows very slowly. Remote changes of the skeleton are also of interest. A regional osteoporosis usually takes several months to develop. The exception is a patient after an initial trauma with an osteoporosis of Sudeck. The same goes for a bone that had sufficient time to undergo changes of form and size. If there has been bowing without loss of continuity by stimulation of growth one can conclude that the lesion is old with an evolution of many months, if not years (Fig. 13-7).

Incidence, Age, and Sex Distribution

On the basis of large statistical material on bone tumors, such as Dahlin's, who reviewed 1,025 benign and 2,962 malignant tumors, we must first of all consider the general incidence of each type of tumor. Bony adamantinomas are most unusual, whereas Ewing's sarcoma or osteosarcoma occur frequently.

Table 13-1. Age Distribution of Benign and Malignant Bone Tumors

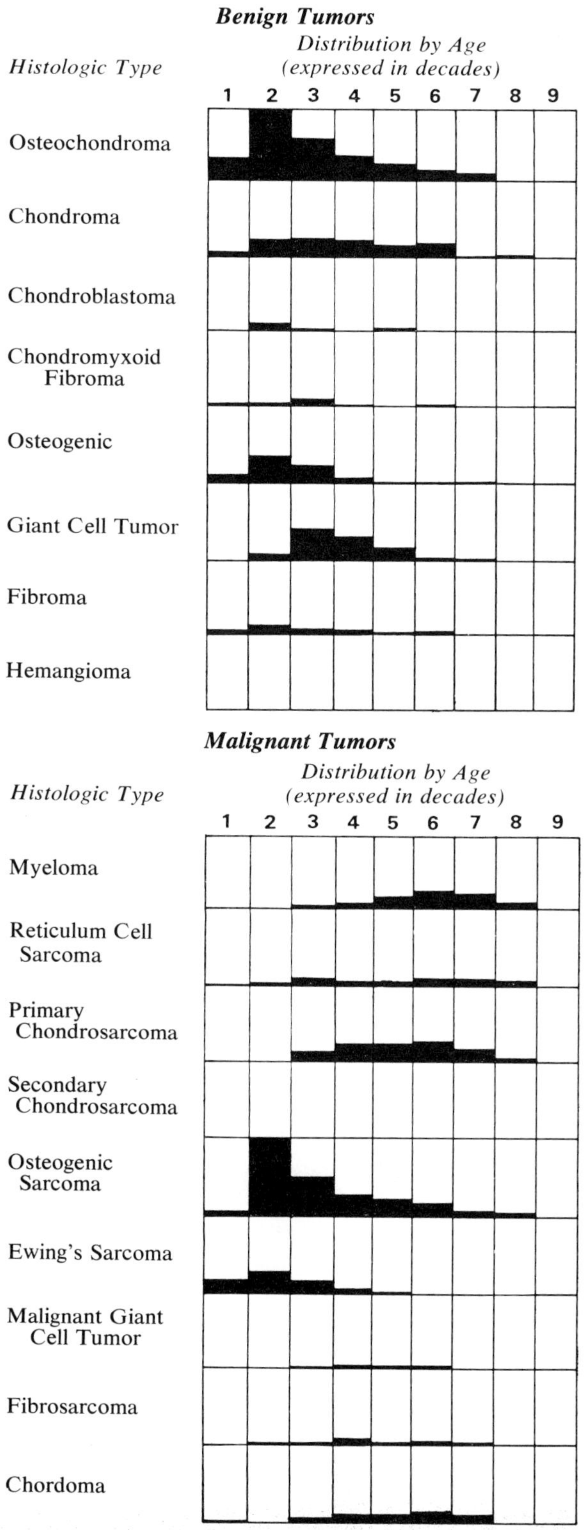

(from Nelson)

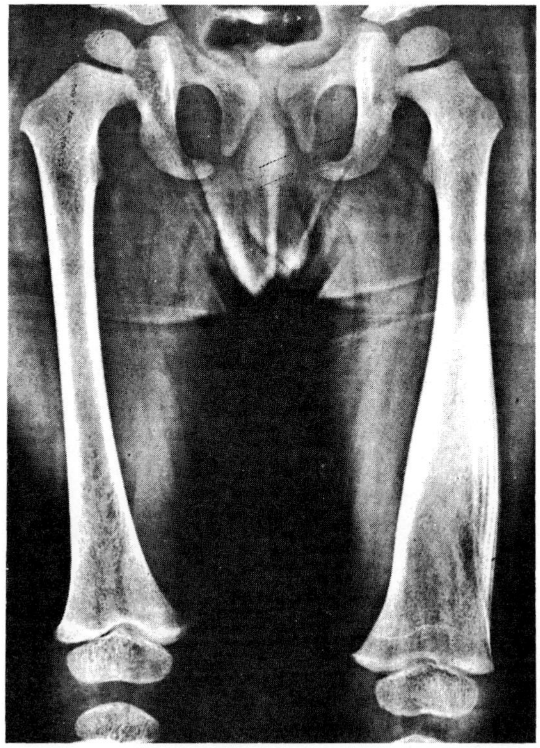

Fig. 13-7. Corticoperiosteal ossification in lamellar and parallel layers involving the left femur as a result of subperiosteal hemorrhages. The left femur is also lengthened signifying a long-standing and slowly progressive local involvement.

The incidence of any given type of tumor is also an expression of the age of the patient, which may be of great significance. Giant cell tumors are practically never seen before the disappearance of the growth plate and fusion of the epiphyses with the metaphyses. Chondrosarcomas, myelomas and metastatic bone tumors have a high frequency starting with the fourth decade and thereafter. Table 13-1, from Nelson, illustrates the incidence as a function of the patient's age. One comment, however, must be made: it appears very logical and easy to make an exact statement on the age at the onset of a rapidly progressive tumor such as an osteosarcoma or Ewing's sarcoma, but such a judgment may be entirely deceptive and very difficult in the presence of a slowly progressive benign type of a lesion. One is not at all sure if these have been present for only a few months or maybe for many years. An enchondroma or a monostotic lesion in fibrous dysplasia would fall into this category.

This age-related incidence does not only apply to neoblastic involvement. Other pseudo-tumoral lesions

Table 13-2. Differentiating Radiographic Features Between Infections and Tumors of Bones

I. Radiologic Findings
Suggestive of an Infectious Lesion of Bones

Localization in the long segment of the bone, especially within the diaphysis

Presence of a sequestrum. Formation of a sequestrum is unusual in neoplasia with the exception of metastases to the cranial vault.

Full massive periosteal reaction, sometimes completely enveloping involucrum

No visible spiculation

Destruction of cartilage immediately next to the lesion. Rapid local destruction supports the presence of a local infection, whereas a slow destruction supports nonpyogenic microorganism, especially tuberculosis.

II. Differential Findings Supporting a Benign or Malignant Tumor

Findings	*Benign Lesions*	*Malignant Lesions*
Borders	Regular, sometimes wavy, clear, distinct, sometimes with a slight, sclerotic border	None, ill-defined, sometimes bordered by zones of punctated osteolysis
Extent	Limited, located either in the medullary cavity or within the cortex, which is simply eroded, but not destroyed	Originating from the medullary space with extension along the medullary cavity and across the cortex, which is destroyed. Presence of an ill-defined and poorly limited mass within the soft tissue
Shape	Large diameter usually below 6 cm	Large diameter usually above 6 cm.
Internal texture	Homogeneous sometimes with trabeculations	Irregular, inhomogeneous, motheaten punctate or mixed lesions, some condensing and some lytic
Periosteal reaction	Rare. If present, it is solid, filled in and homogeneous.	Frequently present, but may be totally lacking. Irregular, interrupted, onion peel, multilayered, or with spiculation.
Duration of lesion	Evidently chronic with little modification from a preceding film: peri-tumoral sclerosis; cortical expansion; remodelling and deformity of the bone	Punctate osteolysis around the lesion
Localization	Tumors located within epiphyses or short bones are more frequently benign.	

also do have a varying incidence depending on the patient's age. Thus, a bone cyst, an aneurysmal bone cyst or fibrous dysplasia are all seen with a high incidence in young individuals during the first two decades of life. Histiocytosis X has a peak in patients under 10 years of age, and brown tumors of primary hyperparathyroidism are seen only in the adult. Secondary hyperparathyroidism can also be found during childhood, but only exceptionally with brown tumors or osteoclastomas.

The sex of the patient has only minimal importance, since there are only a few tumors with a predominant incidence in boys or girls.

We have reviewed the different criteria for the analysis of diagnostic findings, which may guide the radiologist in his evaluation of a solitary bone lesion which may be due to tumor. We shall now follow this outline in our discussion of the different variants of bone tumors. Before doing this, however, we would encourage a review of the tables and of the different considerations for the differential diagnosis supporting certain types of lesions (see Table 13-2).

RADIOGRAPHIC INVESTIGATIVE TECHNIQUES

The radiographic investigation of bone tumors requires films of high quality with fine-detail screens and the use of a small focal spot. Two views at right angles generously covering the areas involved are absolutely necessary, and often additional views must be taken with varying degrees of rotation of the extremity so that the borders of the lesion can be fully appreciated. This is especially true of the cortical and periosteal region. It is a good policy to obtain several films of the exact same view with differing penetration in order to have a good basis for evaluating the lesions within the soft tissues as well as within the denser cortico-periosteal region.

Tomograms (Norman) are sometimes helpful, especially in order to get a better appreciation of the loss of tissue in the center of a condensing lesion—osteoid-osteoma, in order to demonstrate the presence of calcifications within the tumor stroma, and to better document osteolysis of spongy bone, which is not clearly apparent on plain films.

Direct radiographic magnification is occasionally helpful for the better appreciation of local structures in the presence of a small osteolytic lesion or localized periosteal reaction.

A complete skeletal survey is necessary if it is unknown whether the patient is suffering from a primary localized or a secondary tumor.

Angiography has been favored by a number of authors. The information derived from this procedure can be of variable interest and depends largely on the type of tumor (Halpern et al., Lagergren et al., 1958, 1962; Lindbom et al., Kittredge et al.).

As a rule, the majority of benign tumors have only poor vascularization. This is the case in osteomas, osteochondromas, enchondromas and bone cysts. If these tumors invade the neighboring soft tissues they simply push the vessels aside. There are however some benign tumors with a high degree of vascularity, such as osteoid osteomas, aneurysmal bone cysts, osteogenic fibromas, giant cell tumors and angiomas.

Malignant tumors are usually hypervascular and to a certain degree will have a tumor type vascularity with neoformed vessels of irregular caliber, a curved angulated course and arterio-venous shunts. This is the case in osteosarcoma (Fig. 15-6 *B*), and in chondro-sarcoma. There are some malignant tumors with poor vascularization, for instance, periosteal fibrosarcomas.

Angiography cannot offer reliable criteria, since we have noted that even some benign tumors are hypervascular. Furthermore, there are patients with local inflammatory lesions resulting in pseudotumoral hypervascularity, such as a chronic abscess, myositis ossificans and villo-nodular synovitis. Angiography does not help one to arrive at a final decision between benign and malignant characteristics of a given lesson. This is contrary to the statement in 1951 by Columella and Mucchi, who claimed that arteriography could obviate the need for biopsy. Still, arteriography will help in selecting a good region for the biopsy, since it is capable of revealing necrotic avascular regions.

Arteriography is also helpful in the evaluation of the extent of a tumor and can influence the decision where exactly to limit the surgical excision, or the choice of the field of irradiation, if radiotherapy is required.

Radiographic study of a surgically removed specimen – either as is or cut in sections – should always be obtained, since this may help the pathologist in his correlation of macroscopic and microscopic histologic findings.

Isotope studies (Charkes, Charkes et al., Guerin) with ^{85}Strontium have been performed in adults in the search for metastases, where the primary lesion was known. According to Guerin, repeated scintigraphies, together with differential concentration curves, can be helpful in distinguishing a malignant tumor from subacute osteitis.

Scintigraphy would show the extent of the tumor better than the radiograph and would thus be helpful in determining the site for biopsy. This method, however, will result in a certain delay in establishing the diagnosis. The long – 65 days – half life of this radioactive substance results in too much irradiation, so that it is contraindicated in childhood. Some authors actually would not utilize this substance in patients other than those suffering from proven cancer. During childhood different isotopes with a shorter half-life have been used (^{47}Ca, ^{67}Ga, ^{87}Sr, ^{18}F) but anyone of these substances is either too difficult to obtain, too costly or too difficult to handle without possible errors, so that they are not generally used (Charkes et al.).

The more recent substances available, pyrophosphate or polyphosphate of technetium – ^{99m}Tc – have fundamentally changed this situation. It is now possible to perform skeletal uptake studies during infancy and childhood. Since the price is reasonable and the substance is readily available, this short-lived radioactive substance is now widely used. It also results in excellent images (Rain et al., Subramanian et al.).

Isotope studies have the great advantage of revealing metastatic lesions at a time when conventional radiography cannot detect them (Helson et al.).

Thermography can bring the same results in studies for metastases (Gershon-Cohen) not yet visible on films. Thermography is a diagnostic approach devoid of any danger, since this method simply registers the skin temperature. This method is not yet widely used, since not many hospitals have thermographic equipment available. The method is in no way specific, since fractures, sprains, osteomyelitis, arthritis and a slipped disk may all result in infrared emission from an "abnormal" local lesion. However, in a patient known to be suffering from metastatic bone disease and who complains of painful areas without local x-ray involvement, the discovery of a hot lesion by thermography will allow us, with a high degree of reliability, to recognize such a metastases. Some authors are so sure of this positive correlation, that they use this finding as a guide for radio-therapy (Gershon-Cohen). If radiotherapy is effective there will be a return to a normal local skin temperature.

REFERENCES

AEGERTER (E.) et KIRKPATRICK (J. A.). Orthopedic diseases. Physiology, pathology, radiology. *Toronto, 1968, Saunders, éd.*

AEGERTER (E.). Diagnostic radiology and the pathology of bone. *Radiol. Clin. N. Amer., 1970,* **8**, *215-226.*

CAFFEY (J.). Pediatric X-ray diagnosis. *5e édit., Chicago, 1967, Year Book, éd.*

CALLE (R.) et CHAVANNE (G.). Tumeurs osseuses. *In* R. Trial, Traité de radiodiagnostic, vol. 10 : Os, Pathologie générale. *Paris, 1969, Masson et Cie, éd.*

CHARKES (N. D.). Bone scanning : principles, technique and interpretation. *Radiol. Clin. N. Amer., 1970.* **8**, *259-270.*

CHARKES (N. D.) et SKLAROFF (D. M.). The radioactive strontium photoscan as a diagnostic aid in primary and metastatic cancer in bone. *Radiol. Clin. N. Amer., 1965,* **3**, *499-509.*

COLUMELLA (F.) et MUCCHI (L.). L'arteriografia nei tumore ossei. *Atti de XVI Congresso Naz. Radiol. Med., 1950, 93.*

DAHLIN (D. C.). Bone tumors. *2e édit., Springfield, Ill., 1967, Ch. C. Thomas, éd.*

DARGEON (H. W.). Tumors in childhood. A clinical treatise. *New York, 1960, Paul B. Hoeber, éd.*

EDEIKEN (J.) et HODES (Ph. J.). Roentgen diagnosis of diseases of bone. *Baltimore, 1967, Williams et Wilkins, éd.*

FERGUSON (A. B.). Benign tumors of bone in childhood. *Pediat. Clin. N. Amer., 1967,* **14**, *683-704.*

FEVRE (M.). Aspects tumoraux ou pseudo-tumoraux des affections « inflammatoires » des os, infectieuses, mycosiques, parasitaires et d'origine inconnue. *Rev. Prat., Paris, 1969,* **19**, *2069-2091.*

GERSHON-COHEN (J.). Thermography and panography in diagnosis of bone disease. *Radiol. Clin. N. Amer., 1970,* **8**, *241-249.*

GESCHISTER (Ch. F.) et COPELAND (M. M.). Tumors of bone. *Philadelphie, 1949, Lippincott J. B. and Co., éd.*

GUERIN (R. A.). La scintigraphie dans l'ostéosarcome. *Chirurgie, 1970,* **96**, *50-52.*

HALPERN (M.) et FREIBERGER (R. H.). Arteriography as a diagnostic procedure in bone disease. *Radiol. Clin. N. Amer., 1970,* **8**, *277-288.*

HELSON (L.), WATSON (R. C.), BENUA (R. S.) et MURPHY (M. L.). 18 F Radioisotope scanning of metastatic bone lesions in children with neuroblastoma. *Amer. J. Roentgenol., 1972,* **115**, *191-199.*

HOPE (J. N.) et BORNS (P. F.). Radiologic diagnosis of primary and metastatic cancer in infants and children. *Radiol. Clin. N. Amer., 1965,* **3**, *353-374.*

JACOBSON (H. G.) et SIEGELMAN (S. S.). Some miscellaneous solitary bone lesions. *Seminars Roentgenol., 1966,* **1**, *314-331.*

JAFFÉ (H. L.). Tumors and tumorous conditions of bones and joints. *Philadelphie, 1958, Lea and Febiger, éd.*

KITTREDGE (R. D.). Arteriography in Ewing's tumor. *Radiology, 1970,* **97**, *609-610.*

KIRKPATRICK (J. A.). Tumors of bone. *Pediat. Clin. N. Amer., 1959,* **6**, *557-571.*

KOZLOWSKI (K.), GORSKA (M.), DEPOWSKI (M.) et SIKORSKA (B.). Tumeurs osseuses rares, primitives ou secondaires, de l'enfant. A propos de neuf observations. *Ann. Radiol., 1970,* **13**, *219-228.*

LAGERGREN (C.) et LINDBOM (Å.). Angiography of peripheral tumors. *Radiology, 1962,* **79**, *371-377.*

LAGERGREN (C.), LINDBOM (Å.) et SÖDERBERG (G.). Hypervascularization in chronic inflammation demonstrated by angiography. *Acta radiol., 1958,* **49**, *441-452.*

LAGERGREN (C.), LINDBOM (Å.) et SÖDERBERG (G.). Vascularization of fibromatous and fibrosarcomatous tumors : histopathologic, microradiographic and angiographic studies. *Acta radiol., 1960,* **53**, *1-15.*

LAGERGREN (C.), LINDBOM (Å.) et SÖDERBERG (G.). Blood vessels of osteogenic sarcomas : histologic, angiographic and microradiographic studies. *Acta Radiol., 1961,* **55**, *161-176.*

LAGERSEN (C.), LINDBOM (Å) et SÖDERBERG (G.). The blood vessels of chondrosarcoma. *Acta radiol., 1961,* **55**, *321-328.*

LEMERLE (J.) et SCHWEIGUTH (O.). Carcinologie infantile. *Concours méd., Paris, févr. 1970, suppl. au no 7-14.*

LICHTENSTEIN (L.). Bone tumors. *3e éd., Saint-Louis, 1965, The C. V. Mosby Co., éd.*

LODWICK (G. S.). Reactive response to local injury in bone. *Radiol. Clin. N. Amer., 1964,* **2**, *209-219.*

LODWICK (G. S.). A probabilistic approach of the diagnosis of bone tumors. *Radiol. Clin. N. Amer., 1965,* **3**, *487-497.*

LODWICK (G. S.). Solitary malignant tumors of bone. The application of redictor variables in diagnosis. *Seminars Roentgenol., 1966,* **1**, *293-313.*

LODWICK (G. S.). The bones and joints. *Chicago, 1971, Year Book, éd.*

MAROTEAUX (P.). Aspects tumoraux des maladies constitutionnelles du squelette. *Rev. Prat., Paris, 1969,* **19**, *2093-2104.*

MURRAY (R. O.) et JACOBBSON (H. G.). The radiology of skeletal disorders. Exercises in diagnosis. *Edimbourg et Londres, 1971, Churchill Livingstone, éd.*

NELSON (S. W.). Some fundamentals in the radiologic differential diagnosis of solitary bone lesions. *Seminars Roentgenol., 1966,* **1**, *244-267.*

NEZELOF (Ch.). Communication personnelle.

NORMAN (A.). The value of tomography in the diagnosis of skeletal disorders. *Radiol. Clin. N. Amer., 1970,* **8**, *251-258.*

PICARD (J. D.) et SCHWEISGUTH (O.). Le diagnostic radiologique des tumeurs osseuses primitives malignes de l'enfant. *Médecine infant. (Paris), 1960,* **67**, *31-44.*

RAIN (J. D.), KUNTZ (D.) et NAJEAN (Y.). Importants progrès en scintigraphie osseuse grâce à l'emploi de pyrophosphate de technetium (^{99m}Tc). *Nouv. Presse méd., 1973,* **2**, *3-186.*

SCHWEISGUTH (O.). Les tumeurs malignes primitives des os longs chez l'enfant. *In* Journées Parisiennes de Pédiatrie. *Paris, 1967, Flammarion, éd., p. 201-212.*

STEWART (J. R.), DAHLIN (D. C.) et PUGH (D. G.). The pathology and radiology of solitary benign tumors. *Seminars Roentgenol., 1966,* **1**, *268-292.*

SUBRAMANIAN (G.), MCAFEE (J. G.), BELL (E. G.), BLAIR (R. J.), O'MARA (R. E.) et RALSTON (P. H.). ^{99m}Tc-labeled polyphosphate as a skeletal imaging agent. *Radiology, 1972,* **102**, *701-704.*

TAYBI (H.). Solitary bone lesions in children. *Seminars Roentgenol., 1966,* **1**, *392-406.*

TEILLET (F.), BISMUTH (V.), BOURDON (R.) et BERNARD (J.). Aspects tumoraux osseux au cours des leucémies, des lympho et réticulosarcomes ganglionnaires et de la maladie de Hodgkin. *Rev. Prat., Paris, 1969,* **19**, *2441-2458.*

TRIFAUD (A.), BUREAU (H.) et PAYAN (H.). Tumeurs bénignes des os. *Paris, 1959, Masson et Cie, éd.*

VENOUIL (J.) et RAY (A.). Diagnostic des tumeurs osseuses primitives de l'enfant. *Maroc. méd., 1970,* **50**, *631-645.*

14 Benign Tumors and Pseudotumors

In an attempt to describe the different types of benign lesions we could follow the classification of Lichtenstein (Table 14-1) as others have done and then move on to a chapter devoted to pseudotumoral lesions. However, we prefer, along with Stewart, Dahlin and Pugh, a different approach which combines the problems of tumors and pseudotumoral lesions, as their histologic substrate is of the same cellular type. We shall, therefore, discuss the following successively: fibrogenic tumors or pseudotumoral lesions: cortical defects and residual fibrous islands, nonossifying fibroma, monostotic fibrous dysplasia and desmoplastic fibromas;

Chondrogenic tumors or pseudo-tumoral lesions: osteochondromas, enchondromas, chondromas, benign chondroblastomas and chondromyxoid fibromas;

Osteogenic tumors or pseudotumoral process lesions: osteomas, ostoid osteomas and benign osteoblastomas;

Tumors or pseudotumoral lesions of differing origin: angiomas, lymphangiomas or osteolysis of vascular origin (vanishing bone) lipomas and neurilemmomas;

Tumors or pseudotumoral lesions of differing origin: giant cell tumors, aneurysmal bone cysts and simple bone cysts;

Other benign pseudotumoral lesions: epidermoid cysts, pigmented villonodular synovitis, hypertrophic callus formations, periosteal hematomas and myositis ossificans.

FIBROGENIC BENIGN TUMORS

Fibrogenic tumors are the centers of nonspecific fibrous tissue which are located either entirely, or predominantly, within the cortex of the bone. This is probably not a true neoplasm. It is more likely simply the result of errors in osteogenesis. The tumors in this group differ only in their manner of development and radiographic appearance.

METAPHYSEAL CORTICAL DEFECTS

These defects have a high incidence, according to Sontag and Pyle and Caffey, 30 to 40 per cent of infants followed for a period of time are affected at one time or another. At any given time during their development 2 per cent of all children have a metaphyseal defect.

There is no sex predilection for this lesion. Age, however, is of considerable interest, since cortical defects are seen from infancy to adolescence with maximum incidence rates between 6 and 11 years.

There is virtually no clinical symptomatology. Frequently the finding is noted during a radiographic investigation for trauma or another reason. If there is local pain, the best rule to follow is not to correlate the two directly. Control radiographs which are taken of the other side because of local pain reveal the presence of cortical defects with just about the same incidence.

Skeletal localization is of importance. These defects are located within the metaphyses of long bones close to the growth cartilage. The most frequently seen location is at the posteromedial distal femoral metaphysis. Other localizations, in order of decreasing incidence, are the proximal ends of the tibia, the proximal region of the fibula, the distal region of the tibia, and the proximal end of the humerus. There may be multiple lesions within the same bone or in several different ones. In such a situation they may either have a parallel course or they may follow one another.

Their radiographic appearance is relatively consistent. There is a localized osteolytic defect with well defined borders, sometimes surrounded by a dense edge, of rounded or oval form, oriented within the longitudinal axis of the bone, and usually of relatively small size, between 2 and 3 cm. If viewed tangentially, the lesion is located within the cortex, which is slightly altered having an "hourglass" appearance. Its external border is frequently very thin, but is never destroyed. There is no periosteal reaction and the adjacent soft tissues are unremarkable. During the course of further development this defect will progres-

Table 14-1. Classification of Lichtenstein

Origin		*Benign Tumors of Bone*	*Malignant Counterpart (If Any)*	*Malignant Tumors of Bone (Arising Through Malignant Change or Independently)*
Of cartilage-cell or cartilage-forming connective-tissue derivation	Peripheral	Osteocartilagenous exostosis (multiple exostosis)	Peripheral chondrosarcoma	Chondrosarcoma
	Central	Enchondroma (skeletal enchondromatosis)	Central chondrosarcoma	Chondrosarcoma
		Benign chondroblastoma		
		Chondromyxoid fibroma	(Not known)	
		Other chondroid tumors	(Not known)	
Of osteoblastic derivation		Osteoma	(Not known)	Osteogenic sarcoma
		Osteoid-osteoma	(Not known)	
		Benign osteoblastoma	(Osteogenic sarcoma)	
Of nonosteoblastic connective-tissue derivation		Nonosteogenic fibroma	(Not known)	Fibrosarcoma
		Least-aggressive giant-cell tumors →	More aggressive & malignant giant-cell tumors →	Frankly malignant giant-cell tumors
Of mesenchymal connective-tissue origin		———		Ewing's sarcoma
Of hematopoietic origin		———		Multiple myeloma; Chronic myeloid leukemia; Acute leukemias; Malignant lymphoma (Reticulum-cell sarcoma, "Lymphosarcoma, Hodgkin's disease)
Of nerve origin		Neurofibroma; Neurilemoma	(Malignant schwannoma)	
Of vascular origin		Hemangioma; Hemangiopericytoma-(glomus)	(Hemangioendothelioma)	Hemangioendothelioma
Of fat-cell origin		Lipoma		Liposarcoma
Of notochordal derivation		———		Chordoma
Of adamantine or possibly basal-cell derivation		———		So-called adamantinoma

sively move away from the growth cartilage as the patient grows. Metaphyseal ossification is never affected. This is a very important negative finding. The natural course takes about two to three years and always results in the complete disappearance of the local finding after the area has gone through a phase of local densification.

The diagnosis must be based on the age of the patient, the metaphyseal localization, and radiographic appearances. There is no need for verification by biopsy.

The prognosis is excellent and, the great majority of cortical defects will eventually disappear without any form of therapy. However, there are cases when this lesion is the starting point for a nonossifying fibroma, which will grow in size and depth.

NONOSSIFYING FIBROMA

Included under this heading are nonosteogenic fibromas, fibro-xanthomas, and osseus xanthomas.

As defined by Jaffe and Lichtenstein, this is a lesion close to the cortical defect, but occurring much less frequently. If in Dahlin's statistics this lesion represents less than 5 per cent of all benign tumors, its exact incidence is very elusive, since many cases remain asymptomatic and often are not detected. Those lesions which are recognized by radiographic study may never reach the surgeon or come to the attention of the pathologist.

Again there is no sex predilection. The patient's age is, however, of significance, since nonossifying fibromas are only seen in the older child, during adoles-

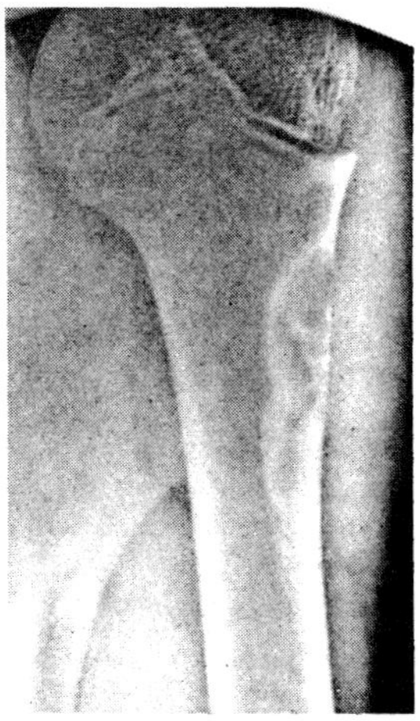

Fig. 14-1. Nonossifying fibroma of the proximal humeral metaphysis.

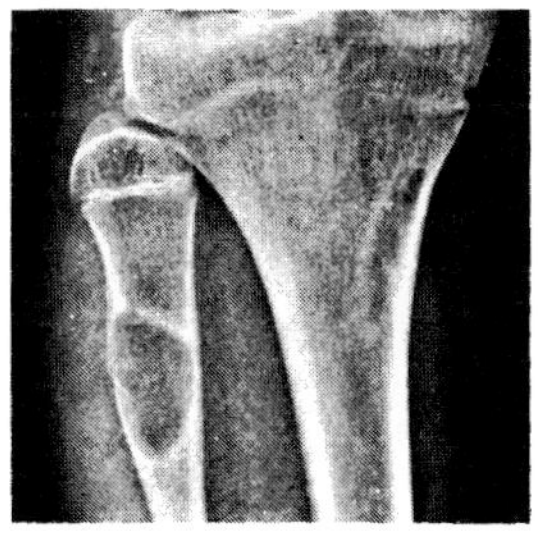

Fig. 14-2. Nonossifying fibromata involving the proximal ends of the tibia and fibula.

cence, and in young adults. This lesion occurs then in a group of patients slightly older than those affected by cortical defects. The oldest patient in Dahlin's statistics was 25 years of age.

The clinical manifestations are either nonexistent or mild. This is frequently an incidental radiographic finding at the time of study, performed because of trauma or pain, and is unrelated with the actual lesion. Still, if extensive, a nonossifying fibroma can result in a local fracture or may be the cause for a pathological fracture. This is particularly true, if the distal tibia is affected (Rigault and Klisowski).

The localization within certain parts of the skeleton is quite characteristic. Generally, the metaphyses of long bones are the site of these lesions, usually at some distance from the growth cartilage. This differentiates them from the cortical defects. It is the distal metaphyses of long bones that are most frequently involved and in order of their decreasing incidence we find involvement of the distal end of the femur in one-third of all patients, the distal end of the tibia seen in slightly less than one-third of all patients, and rarely the proximal end of the tibia, the proximal or distal ends of the fibula, the proximal end of the humerus, the distal end of the radius, and the proximal end of the femur.

The radiographic appearance is very typical (Figs. 14-1 and 14-2). There is a localized rounded or oval defect, somewhat similar to a cortical defect, but more extensive in height and width, often extending onto a larger part of the bony circumference, usually in a somewhat eccentric manner. The contours are often rounded, polycyclic, and bordered by an edge or a narrow line of dense sclerotic bone. If seen on an AP film this defect often contains very dense lines representing sclerotic cristae which separate the individual lobules of the fibrous lesions. Seen tangentially, which may require several views, it can be noted that the lesion is located within the cortex which may be elevated in an "hourglass" fashion, and, although thin, it is not destroyed. There is no periosteal reaction and the neighboring soft tissues are perfectly normal. The defect may extend deeply towards the spongiosa with a dense, sometimes thick border. In some patients it is possible, in certain views, to view the impression of a central bony defect, which may mimic the lesion of monostotic fibrous dysplasia. Some fibromas do not have dense borders at their periphery. In slender bones such as the fibula they may soon involve the entire width of the bone (Fig. 14-2). At the distal end of the tibia it is not unusual for a pathologic factor to extend through the area of a fibroma.

The prognosis for this lesion is excellent. Within a few months or years there will generally be displacement towards the diaphysis of the nonossifying fibroma. The lesion will become circumscribed and will progressively fill in and then eventually disappear. This whole development takes somewhat longer however than the course of a metaphyseal cortical defect. Therefore, it is the rule not to recommend surgical intervention with the exception of the localization at the distal end of the tibia. A number of authors suggest curettage followed by the insertion of bone chips. Occasionally a patient will develop a local recurrence, even after surgical correction. For such a lesion to develop into a malignancy is very unusual and is actually doubted by Skrede.

The differential diagnosis usually does not offer any problems, because of the typical radiographic appearance. There is an occasional patient where it may be necessary to think of the possibility of a chondromyxoid fibroma or an aneurysmal bone cyst. Verification by biopsy may be necessary in such an exceptional situation.

Microscopic study will reveal a tumor of fibrous tissue arranged in homogenous whirls containing neither bony trabeculae, necrosis, nor signs of infection, but which in rare places will contain multinucleated cells. The presence of such multinucleated cells have resulted in occasional confusion with giant cell tumors, chondromyxoid fibromas and aneurysmal bone cysts, since they also can contain this type of cells. In a few areas one may fund vascular spaces and hemorrhagic pools. These findings, along with the frequent combination with osteochondrotic lesions by an ischemic necrosis involving different skeletal regions—osteochondritis dissecans of the knee, osteochondritis of the femoral head and anterior tibial apophysitis—have led to the theory of a common vascular factor, leading also to metaphyseal cortical defects and nonossifying fibromas (Lefebvre et al.). Some nonossifying fibromas can also contain masses of cholesterol or lipophages which may lead them to become classified within the group of bone xanthomas or fibroxanthomas. According to Dahlin, however, such inclusions of cholesterol and lipophages are not seen exclusively in nonossifying fibromas, since they can also be present during the course of the spontaneously regressive evolution of other benign lesions such as simple bone cysts, giant cell tumors, monostotic fibrous dysplasias, aneurysmal bone cysts, and even in the osteoclastomas of hyperthyroidism.

MONOSTOTIC FIBROUS DYSPLASIA

Fibrous dysplasia, after having been confused for a long time with the bony manifestations of hyperparathyroidism because of its polyostotic types, was recognized as a distinct entity by Lichtenstein in 1938 (see p. 97). The monostotic form of this disorder was recognized by Jaffe and Lichtenstein in 1942. Patients with this localized type are frequently suspected of suffering from a bone tumor. The incidence of such lesions should not be overlooked since Pritchard in 1951 was able to collect 256 patient cases published in the literature. Firat and Stutzman in 1968 maintained that they represent 2.5 per cent of all bone tumors or 7 per cent of all benign bone tumors.

This disorder is, in all likelihood, congenital without familial or hereditary characteristics. It is evenly distributed between the two sexes. At the time of discovery more than half of the patients are adolescents, with the other half being evenly distributed over the ensuing decades.

Clinical manifestations are primarily those of pain, especially if the local lesion is in a weight-bearing bone. Sometimes a pathologic fracture leads to the recognition of the lesion. More rarely a local bowing or other deformity in a portion of a limb may lead to the discovery. It is not unusual, however, to recognize the disorder as an incidental finding during radiographic investigation for trauma or other reasons. The presence of "café au lait" spots may be of diagnostic help.

The primary skeletal localizations are maxillofacial, skull, rib, femoral and tibial bones.

The radiographic appearance is not consistent. Generally, there are osteolytic, geodic images of a larger size than those seen in other fibrous lesions. Contrary to the other lesions these are most frequently located within the medulla rather than the cortex. The cortex itself can be somewhat thin, and although eroded from within, it is never destroyed. The peripheral limitation is often marked by a clear border with a sclerotic zone. In some places this sclerosis may be more marked by denser islands. The bone is often widened and even deformed. If the lesion is localized in a long bone, it most frequently involves the diaphysis. This is in contrast to the other fibrous lesions which have an affinity for the metaphysis, or at least the diaphyseo-metaphyseal region. The epiphysis is never involved (Louyot et al.).

If there is involvement of flat bones such as the ribs, the skull or facial structures, the local lesions may assume an expansile characteristic and appear mixed with considerable, clearly delineated condensation. All of these findings give the lesion a strictly benign appearance. Involvement of the base of the skull may be by expansile lesions with marked condensation.

The prognosis is good, although some complications can occur. For example, complications observed have included spontaneous fractures, compression of nerves at the base of the skull, disturbing deformities of the face, and leontiasis ossea. Only patients with this type of complication will require some form of therapy according to their exact type of involvement. Radiotherapy is contraindicated. Dahlin states that six cases of malignant degeneration have been seen after radiotherapy, five of which were within the maxilla.

The radiographic diagnosis is not always easy to make and other benign osteolytic tumors which widen the affected bone and are surrounded by a narrow sclerotic border must be considered. These are, for example, fibrous lesions, chondromyxoid fibromas, aneurysmal bone cysts, and if the mandible is involved, in particular bilaterally, cherubism should be considered. In a number of the mentioned localizations, biopsy and histologic studies will be required in order to find out if the bone lesion is composed of dense collagen tissue and if osteoid trabecular islands are within. In the presence of many such islands, and if they are confluent the radiographic appearance of such a lesion may be rather dense mimicking an osteoma. If such a lesion is located in the facial, and especially in the cranial structures, the radiographic appearance of a meningioma may be closely simulated.

DESMOPLASTIC BONE FIBROMA

This lesion is extremely rare, with only three cases noted in Dahlin's material. It is similar in appearance to other desmoid fibrous tumors, and originates from soft tissues, especially of the abdominal wall. Its highest incidence is during the second decade without any sex predilection. Long bones are involved as well as flat bones.

The radiographic appearance is characterized by a central defect of a metaphysis or diaphysis (Ferguson), frequently with marked trabeculation. The cortex is thin, occasionally irregular in structure, suggesting the possibility of a malignant process. In flat bones the most frequent shape is polycyclic and often surrounded by a sclerotic border.

The diagnosis can only be fully established after histologic study of biopsied material. The lesion is composed of bundles of collagen tissue with interspersed cells with small pisiform nuclei. The lack of abnormal findings within the nuclei separates this type of tumor from a fibrosarcoma. There are occasional types which may be very difficult to diagnose. According to Nilsonne this type of tumor may be considerably less rare than is generally thought. Included in this category would also be a number of differentiated fibrosarcomas, especially in surviving patients.

BENIGN CHONDROGENIC TUMORS

OSTEOCHONDROMA

An osteochondroma or osteocartilaginous exostosis is a skeletal protrusion with a base remaining in continuity with the adjacent cortex and the underlying bone from where it originates. Its tip is formed by cartilage which assures its growth. This growth is parallel to that of the affected individual and as a rule the tumor will terminate its growth at the same time the growth plate disappears, and the fusion of the epiphyses to the metaphyses is concluded. Because of this fact, some authors (Levy et al.) would prefer to call this lesion enchondral osteoma, since there seems to be a bony structure with an enchondral origin as opposed to osteomas, which usually result from intramembranous ossifications. The question must be raised to determine if this is not rather a congenital malformation and not a benign tumor. It is logical, however, to group this type of a lesion within the bone tumors because of the clinical findings, and the possibility, although rare, of malignant degeneration.

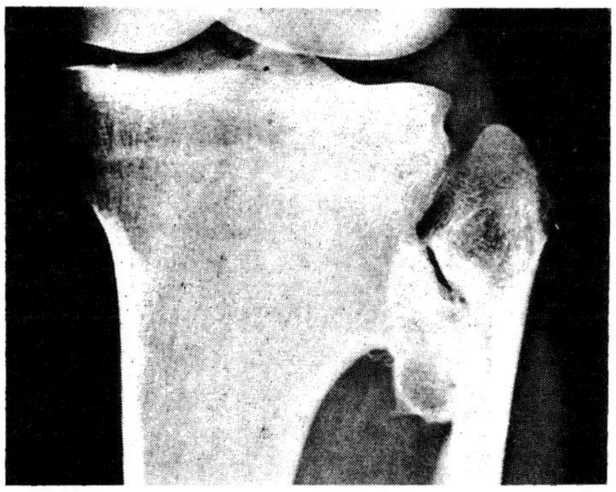

Fig. 14-3. Enchondral exostosis of the tibia resulting in the displacement of the fibula laterally in addition to eroding its proximal end.

The incidence of this type of tumor is high. In the statistical data of Dahlin it represents 12 per cent of all bone tumors and 45 per cent of all the benign lesions. Both sexes are equally affected.

These lesions are usually discovered during the most active enchondral growth of the patient. Therefore, 50 per cent of all cases are less than 20 years old at discovery with a peak incidence during the second decade.

Clinical symptoms are local swelling which may be discovered accidentally by the patient, or during an unrelated physical examination, occasionally there is local pain following repeated trauma or friction of the exostosis and a nerve. Vascular compression at times may occur. The lesion is rarely discovered because of acute local pain which results from trauma.

Preferred localizations are the metaphyses of long bones with a frequent involvement of the distal femoral metaphysis and the proximal humerus. These two localizations together represent almost 50 per cent of all cases. Other localizations listed by decreasing frequency are the proximal tibial metaphyses, the proximal femur, the pelvis, the proximal fibular metaphyses, the distal tibia, the hands, and the ribs. All other skeletal areas can also be affected, but they occur less frequently. The base of the skull is rarely affected.

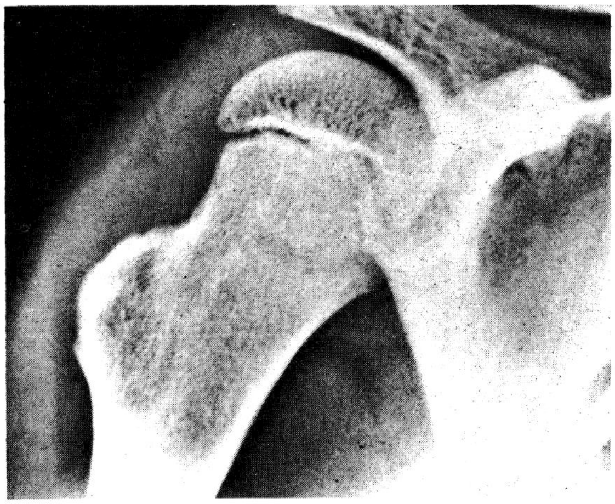

Fig. 14-4. Osteochondroma involving the upper end of the humerus.

The radiographic appearance is entirely characteristic and diagnostically reliable. A solitary osteochondroma within a long bone may appear in two ways:

Osteochondroma with a narrow stalk (Fig. 14-3). The bony stalk shows the presence of two cortical areas in continuity with the cortex of the adjacent bone. The origin of these lesions is always from the metaphysis and the direction always towards the diaphysis. They are shaped like a club. At its origin the metaphysis often lacks normal local modeling. The tip of the stalk is covered by a bony mass like a "cauliflower," and also by cartilaginous material, which blends in with the adjacent soft tissues. Sometimes this can be recognized in between layers of fat under the facia. Such a finding can most frequently be noted at the metaphyses of the distal femur and of the proximal tibia.

Osteochondroma with large sessile origin will present as a swelling of the bone at the metaphyseal or metaphyseodiaphyseal region. This bony prominence is covered by cortex, which continues from the normal bone but thins out as it reaches towards the tip of the lesion where cartilage persists. If seen in the AP view, this type of exostosis can present as a lacunar image surrounded by a narrow sclerotic zone (Fig. 14-4). Associated with this finding is often a modeling defect in the area of exostosis implantation, most frequently located at the proximal end of the humerus.

Occasionally, the cartilaginous portion which caps the exostosis may contain calcific deposits forming within the cartilage a matrix. They usually are punctate or finely granular and if, larger, may have the appearance of "popcorn."

Such a lesion has an entirely benign prognosis. The great majority of these osteochondromas are tolerated well, but occasionally one may require surgical removal. It is unusual that a tumor recurs locally after resection requiring reoperation. Should this, however, be the case a second intervention may be a definitive one. If there is local recurrence one should think of the possibility that this is no longer a real osteochondroma, but that there is already local degeneration, and possibly a primitive chondrosarcoma is present. One of the risks in such a patient is sarcomatous degeneration. This should always be suspected if there are numerous calcific densities located within the cartilaginous portion, and they are located at a considerable distance from the bony portion of the exostosis. A very strong diagnostic argument would be a rapid local expansion and a marked increase in numbers from one examination to the next. Such malignant degeneration is very rarely seen and it hardly ever occurs before 14 years of age. This development is most unusual in a solitary osteochondroma, and is more likely to occur in the syndrome of multiple cartilaginous exostoses.

There are some patients, where such a lesion does not occur alone, and the patient is affected by many exostoses of the skeleton. These patients may be suffering from multiple cartilaginous exostoses, a familial disorder which is inherited as a dominant trait (see p. 90). The incidence of solitary versus familial types is about nine to one in favor of the solitary osteochondroma. The lesions are entirely identical in appearance. The prognosis, however, is somewhat different, since the incidence of chondrosarcomatous degeneration is higher than 10 per cent, according to Dahlin.

The differential diagnosis should not offer any difficulties. In an occasional situation, where a slightly calcified cartilaginous mass develops in the immediate neighborhood of a joint, there may be some hesitation between an osteosarcoma or synovial osteochondromatosis, both rare lesions occurring during childhood. Subungual exostoses should not be included among this form of osteochondromas because this lesion is often a local bony reaction to repeated trauma or infection (Dahlin).

CHONDROMAS

This benign tumor considered by Levy and others to be a hamartoma is composed of mature hyaline cartilage. The most frequent site of origin is within the

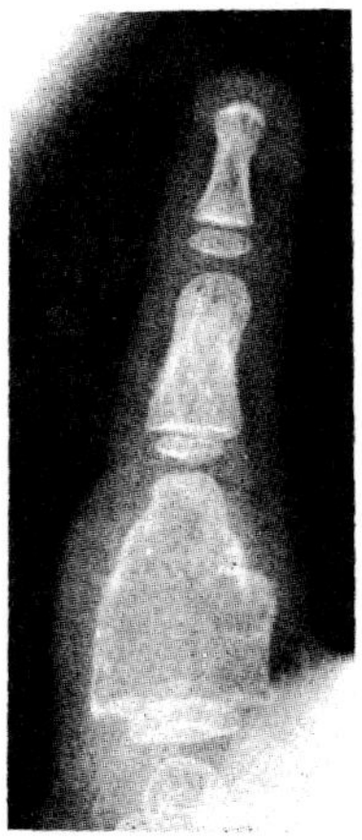

Fig. 14-5. Chondroma involving the 1st phalanx of the small finger.

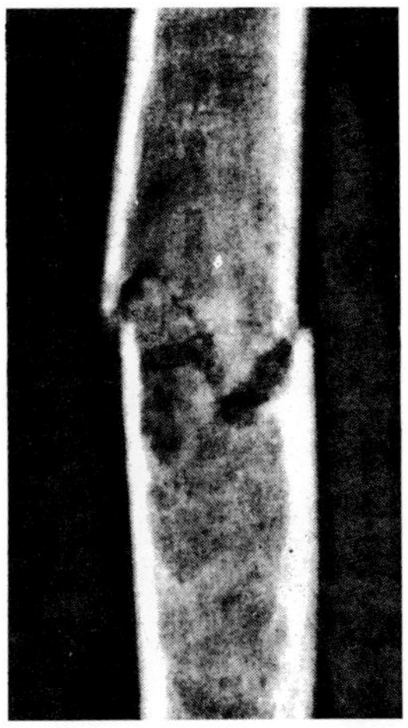

Fig. 14-6. Chondroma in the diaphysis of the humerus after a spontaneous fracture in an 11-year-old girl.

medullary cavity of bone, thus the term enchondroma is applicable. On rare occasions, however, it can be eccentric and develop under the periosteum. We would then call this a periosteal chondroma, preferable to the term ecchondroma, which is sometimes used. This benign tumor can occur in only one location, however, patients have been known to develop several chondromatous lesions. If chondromas are widely disseminated throughout the skeleton, with the tendency for unilateral distribution, this condition is called Ollier's enchondromatosis (see p. 93). Where multiple chondromatosis is associated with soft tissue angiomatosis, we have the Kast-Maffuci's syndrome (see p. 96).

The incidence of chondromas is relatively high, according to Dahlin, making up 10 per cent of benign tumors, and 3 per cent of all bone tumors. This incidence may actually be even higher, because many chondromas not subjected to surgery and anatomic verification are not included in these statistics.

There is no sex predilection. The lesion may be recognized at any age with the maximum found during the second and third decade, especially in multiple locations. Clinical symptomatology is limited to spontaneous, local swelling, possible local pain, with additional swelling following trauma, especially if we are dealing with a peripheral lesion involving the parts of the hands or feet. Local pain or a pathological fracture may lead to the recognition of a more centrally located chondroma within a long bone. Recognition is sometimes accidental when an examination is done for unrelated reasons.

The location is somewhat peculiar since more than 50 per cent of these tumors are found within the hands and feet, mostly in the phalanges. Ninety per cent of chondromas located on the phalanges are found in the hands (Fig. 14-5). This is, by far, the most frequently encountered tumor of the hand. Much less frequent locations are the humerus (Fig. 14-6) and the femur.

The radiographic appearance of an enchondroma, as it is typically manifested, is unusual. It assumes a transparent appearance with a geographic, polycyclic outline located in the middle of bone, most frequently towards its distal end. A small tubular bone such as a phalanx or metacarpal bone may be totally involved with a degree of expansion. The cortex although it may be thin, is maintained and not destroyed. There is often no peripheral sclerosis around the defect, and even if it is present, it is minimally so and forms a very fine border. The periosteum and the adjacent soft tissues are entirely normal with the exception of a local callus formation after a fracture. The tumoral center sometimes contains flaky, punctate, or lumpy calcifications (Fig. 14-7).

In the long bones close to the diaphyseometaphyseal region an accumulation of flaky calcifications may be present in a "smoky curls" or "popcorn" arrangement. They may be isolated, without associated osteolytic lesions, giving rise to an image very similar to that of bone infarcts. Calcifications within chondromas, however, are central within a tumor, whereas infarcts are located peripherally separating healthy and necrotic bone. This type of chondroma is quite unusual during childhood and occurs primarily in the older and aged patient.

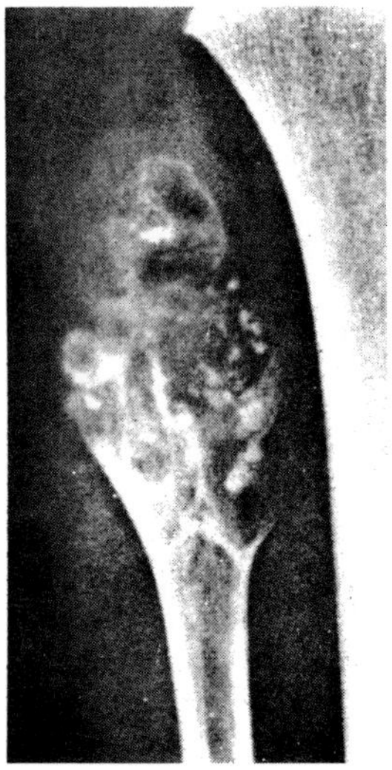

Fig. 14-7. Chondroma of the proximal end of the fibula in the localization of Ollier's Disease. Note the punctate calcifications which are characteristically present within the cartilaginous stroma.

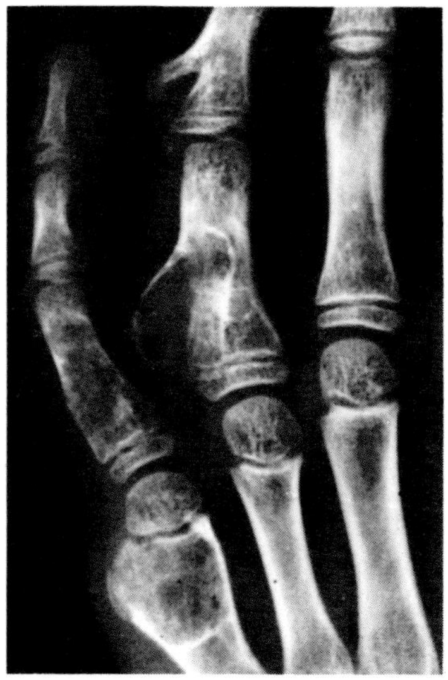

Fig. 14-8. Subperiosteal chondromas of a finger.

Subperiosteal chondromas (Fig. 14-8) present as a lacunar defect within the diaphyseal cortex or metaphysis. These lesions are well defined, and are encircled by a dense border on their bony side which elevates the cortex towards the soft tissues, more so here than in a nonossifying fibroma. There is no direct invasion of the adjacent soft tissues. At the level of the phalanges and metacarpals the subperiosteal localization is usually in the neighborhood of the growth cartilage, frequently leading to a modeling defect.

Anatomopathologic study of a surgical biopsy reveals an often lobulated and partially mineralized tumor. The chondrocytes are small and usually possess a single nucleus. The clinical and radiographic signs of local degeneration associated with abnormal nuclei might result in the fear of a local chondrosarcoma.

The differential diagnosis is usually easily made. Regarding the hands one can discuss a chondromyxoid fibroma, an epidermoid inclusion cyst, localized fibrous dysplasia. However, in this case, one is generally faced with polyostotic involvement. It is sometimes difficult to define it clearly if such a cartilaginous tumor does have a malignant tendency, or if it has already undergone degeneration into chondrosarcoma. This rare possibility must be suspected, especially if there is rapid local expansion, a marked cortical sclerosis, and the local lesion is noticeably painful. Malignant degeneration is hardly ever present in chondromas of the hands or feet. Though it still occurs rarely, there is a higher incidence in chondromas of the long bones of the extremities, the trunk, and the pelvis. Such degeneration is seen somewhat more frequently in multiple chondromatosis, which occurs in older patients, and only exceptionally during childhood.

Overall chondromas are generally benign tumors and usually do well without special attention or therapy. It is only an exceptional patient that will require surgery because of local pain, mechanical interference, or a fracture. Intervention is either by total excision through the ribs or subperiosteal locations in the long bones, or by local curettage and grafting. Local recurrence may follow these interventions. Where the acetabular region is the site of local chondromas, Stewart, Dahlin and Pugh emphasize the danger of chondrosarcoma development and recommend local treatment.

BENIGN CHONDROBLASTOMAS

Defined as a pathologic entity by Jaffe and Lichtenstein in 1942 benign chondroblastoma is a rare lesion with an incidence, according to Dahlin, below 1 per cent among all bone tumors. The incidence was higher of boys in the proportion of approximately two to one (Dahlin). Three out of four cases were recognized during the second decade and some at the end of the first. The rest of the patients were between 20 and 60 years old.

Leg pains of long standing are the main symptom of a benign chondroblastoma. Frequently an adjacent joint is incriminated. The localization of this tumor is unusual. The long bones are most frequently involved, and in particular the proximal epiphysis of the humerus, the distal portion of the femur, and the uppermost region of the tibia. In some cases the lesion is located at an extra center of ossification, such as the trochanter or the greater tuberosity of the humerus. The flat bones, the pelvis, and the scapula can also be involved.

The radiographic appearance (Fig. 14-9) is that of a geographic rounded or oval defect, usually less than 6 cm in diameter and sometimes surrounded by dense borders. If large, a chondroblastoma can expand throughout the bone, but it will not destroy the cortex although it may be thin. Occasionally, there is mild benign cortical and periosteal thickening. In extensive lesions parietal trabeculation may occur. In 50 per cent of the patients there are punctate or irregularly cloudy flocular calcifications representing calcific deposits within the cartilaginous matrix. This finding, if present, is very helpful in arriving at the diagnosis.

The diagnosis is somewhat more difficult to make in flat bones, since the epiphyseal origin of the tumor, so characteristically recognizable in other localizations is not evident.

Thus the radiographic diagnosis is usually suggested by radiologists if long bones are involved. During childhood, the other only possible considerations might be geodes of an infectious origin which, however, have a tendency, to localize on both sides of the growth cartilage and enchondromas or chondromyxoid fibromas. However, even if the radiographic diagnosis is possible, it is still necessary to confirm this by biopsy (Monat and Meary). Treatment is by curettage of the lesion followed by local grafting. Histology will show a mass of grossly chondroid tissue with partial calcification, or zones with giant cells within groups of very dense chondroblasts, and in some places irregular calcific foci.

The prognosis for this lesion is good with only a rare patient requiring further intervention, because of local recurrence after surgical removal. Chondrosarcomatous degeneration is highly unusual (Levy et al.) and occasionally seems to be the result of a patient who underwent radiotherapy. Levy and collaborators mention a single patient with spontaneous chondrosarcomatous degeneration and they feel that chondroblastoma has not been defined and followed long enough to be certain that it is an entirely benign lesion. They propose the theory that chondroblastomas possibly are malignant tumors with an extremely slow growth potential.

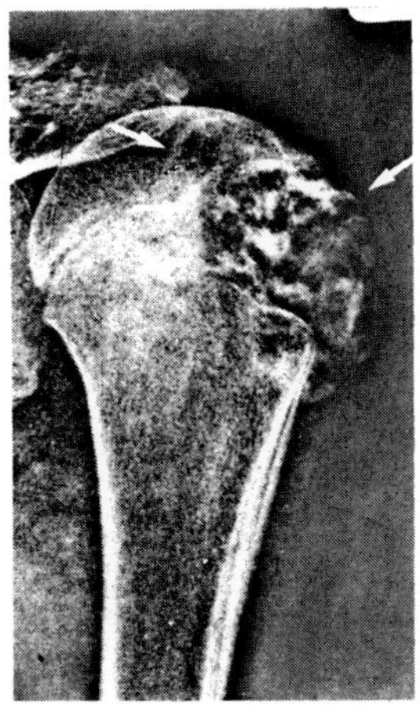

Fig. 14-9. Benign chondroblastoma.

CHONDROMYXOID FIBROMA

This well defined entity was first recognized by Jaffe and Lichtenstein in 1948. It is a benign tumor which originates from connective tissue and eventually forms cartilage. According to Dahlin, this is a rare tumor, with an incidence of 1 per cent in his entire material. If one considers the data of the literature it would appear that it might even have a lower incidence, probably lower than that of chondroblastomas. There is no sex predilection.

This tumor is discovered primarily during the second and third decade, since about two-thirds of all the cases occur in these age groups (Stewart et al.). The youngest patient in Dahlin's series was six years old. Still, it is most unusual to encounter this lesion during the first decade. This leads to the conclusion that a priori one would doubt the diagnosis in an infant (Nézelof).

Sometimes local swelling which is noted by the patient or his physician will lead to the recognition of such a tumor located in a bone which is accessible to direct palpation. Frequently there is pain. Quite often this tumor is recognized accidentally in an asymptomatic individual.

Eighty per cent of these tumors are found in the long bones (Stewart et al.). The most frequently involved bone is the tibia. Within long bones it is the metaphyseal region around the growth cartilage that is most frequently the site of involvement. Sometimes, as in chondroblastoma, the lesion can extend beyond the growth cartilage leading to the suspicion that it had its origin within this structure. Other localizations can be found in the small bones of the hands and feet, the iliac wing, and, more rarely, in the vertebrae, the ribs, the scapula, and even the mastoid.

The radiographic appearance is suggestive only because of the localization. There is a geographic lacunar rounded or ovoid appearance with the great axis parallel to the bone. Its size is usually less than 6 cm. The periphery is polycyclic showing a dense, sometimes thick border on the medullary, as well as on the cortical side of the lesion. Within the sclerotic surroundings one can recognize septal cristae expressing the multilobulated character of the lesion. This finding can be verified microscopically.

This lesion develops eccentrically towards the cortex and pushes it outwards. This cortical expansion connects with the normally preserved cortex. The cortex will become somewhat thin, although without local destruction, sometimes being difficult to recognize at the peak of the tumor. At the point where the healthy cortex joins the tumor its local thickening reaches over to a flying buttress. In the center of the tumor the matrix may show calcific degeneration of a cartilaginous type with punctate, lobular, or granular calcifications. In other locations within the flat or short bones there is a less characteristic appearance. Whatever the location, a definitive diagnosis without biopsy is not possible. The pathologist can only confirm the lesion's benign character. The differential diagnosis during childhood must consider an aneurysmal bone cyst, a benign chondroblastoma, an enchondroma, a simple bone cyst, a nonossifying fibroma, and monostotic fibrous dysplasia.

Therapy involves complete curettage which removes the dense bony cavity filled with spongiosa. Cortical grafting is also performed if there is heavy diaphyseal involvement (Monat and Meary).

Pathologic study is required to firmly establish the diagnosis. Microscopically this tumor is lobulated and largely cartilaginous, and may be well separated from the adjacent bone. Histologic study reveals a characteristic mixture of chondroid, myxoid, and fibrous elements. Nuclear anomalies may, in some areas, simulate a chondrosarcoma. For this reason it is important that the radiologist informs the pathologist that the radiographic appearance may be that of a chondromyxoid fibroma, thus avoiding any aggressive intervention.

Prognosis is good as this tumor is usually benign. However, local recurrences have been observed after surgical intervention and sarcomatous degeneration is possible as has been documented by individual observations reported within the last few years. Levy and his collaborators propose that we might be forced in the future to modify our understanding of this tumor, and change our concept of it from a benign tumor to a cartilaginous tumor. This would be like the chondroblastoma with a malignant potential of very slow evolution.

BENIGN OSTEOGENIC TUMORS

OSTEOMAS

Osteomas are benign, mesenchymal osteoblastic tumors, essentially composed of mature bony tissue which is dense and compact in nature. We are excluding from this discussion bony reactions to a number of stimuli, especially bone formation subsequent to the organization of a traumatic, subperiosteal hematoma, condensing bone islands and lesions during healing of bone cysts and other varieties of osteolytic benign lesions. This tumor is very rare during childhood and warrants only short description here.

Osteomas are usually asymptomatic, however, if they develop within a very superficial bone, such as the vault of the skull or the mandible, they present as a hard swelling. They have a predilection for the facial sinuses, especially the frontal sinus, the cranial vault and mandible, and only rarely involve long bones.

Radiographically they appear to be dense, homogeneous, uniform bony islands, sometimes with a lobulated contour. They are well delineated. If they are located in the vault of the skull, tangential films will show that they develop within the external table.

In spite of their rare occurrence during childhood and adolescence, an occasional patient suffering from Gardner's syndrome may present with an osteoma of the cranial vault and the mandible along with intestinal polyps and disseminated fibromas within the organism. The presence of an osteoma in a child should lead to radiographic study of the colon.

The prognosis of this lesion is good. Its development is very slow and is marked only by local progressive growth. There has never been degeneration, but these osteomas may block off sinus drainage. They generally do not require surgical intervention. If one is noted during childhood and involves the skull, the possibility of a meningioma, although very rare, must be considered. In our experience the nature of condensing lesions of the vault of the skull, and the sinus region, as well as the mandible during infancy and adolescence, most frequently are an expression of fibrous dysplasia, generally polyostotic, although it may occasionally be monostotic.

OSTEOID OSTEOMA

In 1935 Jaffe proposed the term osteoid osteoma to designate a lesion of osteoblastic mesenchymal origin, characterized by a more or less extensive osteoid nidus, and often surrounded by secondary, reactive, bony sclerosis of varied importance. The specific nature of this disorder has been repeatedly discussed as

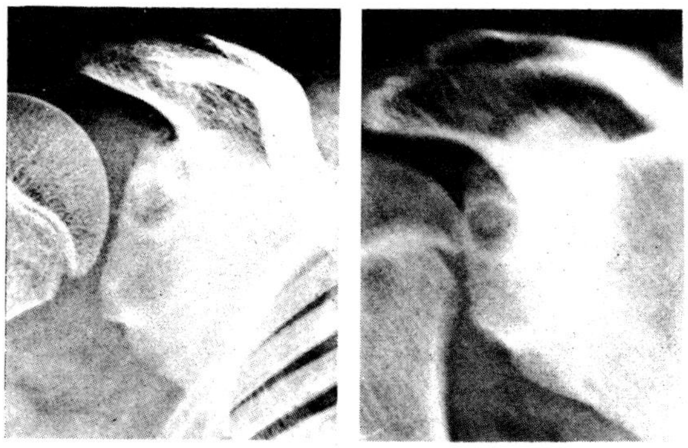

Fig. 14-10. Osteoid osteoma involving the glenoid of the scapula. *(Left)* A geode in the middle of an extensive condensation. *(Right)* This tomogram presents a better picture of the geode. One can actually see the small opacity within it.

to whether it is truly a tumor. A number of authors consider this to be simply a slowly growing, sclerosing nonsuppurative form of osteomyelitis, such as Garré's osteomyelitis, or as a reaction to a foreign body.

The incidence of osteoid osteoma is high, and in Dahlin's material which is supported by others, it represents 10 per cent of all benign tumors. Incidence in relation to age is interesting. In Dahlin's material 87 per cent of all patients were between 5 and 25 years of age with a clear peak in the second decade. It is our experience that this is one of the most frequently seen tumors in childhood, with our youngest patient being 18 months old.

Males are clearly more prone with a preponderance ranging from two through four to one depending on the statistics.

The clinical symptomatology is in itself of special interest. Osteoid osteomas often present with severe pain of nocturnal predominance and with increasing intensity. Such local pain is often localized to the nearest, adjacent joint. Neither exercise, nor rest will influence the pain. Aspirin, however, has a remarkable effect, and may aid in the diagnosis. Local pain may precede by several weeks or months the first radiographic manifestation. If a very superficial bone is involved, it may be possible to recognize local swelling and palpate a very painful lesion. Muscular atrophy with hypotonia may be noted along with an absence of tendon reflexes (Rushton et al.). Increased local sweating has occasionally been noted.

If there is spinal involvement, the local pain will also cause rigidity and scoliosis with concavity towards the lesion. Involvement of the cervical spine may result in painful torticollis with contracture of the sternocleidomastoid muscle of one side.

All laboratory investigations, in particular, blood studies and sedimentation rate are normal. An analysis of the skeletal location reveals that there is a favored location for the proximal end of the femur, the neck, and the upper diaphyseal region. Involvement of the femur and tibia together represent about 60 per cent of all patients. Any other skeletal location is a possible site. Aside from the long bones this may include the pelvis, the scapula, and the mandible. Vertebral involvement, according to the statistics may be as high as 10 per cent, especially in the posterior arches. However, as Dahlin emphasizes, although these lesions may be called osteoid osteomas they are probably often benign osteoblastomas. When long bones are in-

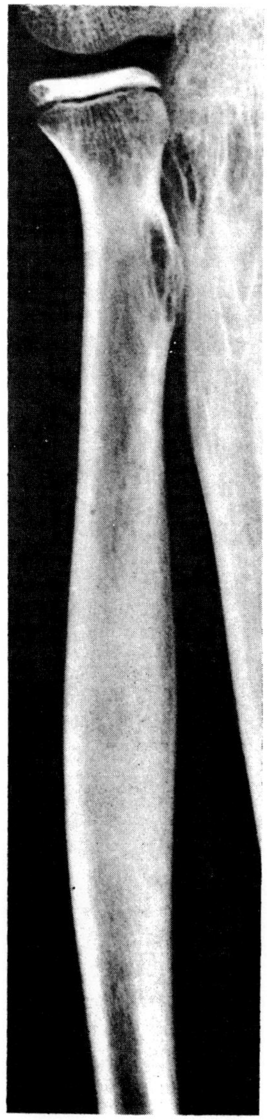

Fig. 14-11. Osteoid osteoma of the radius.

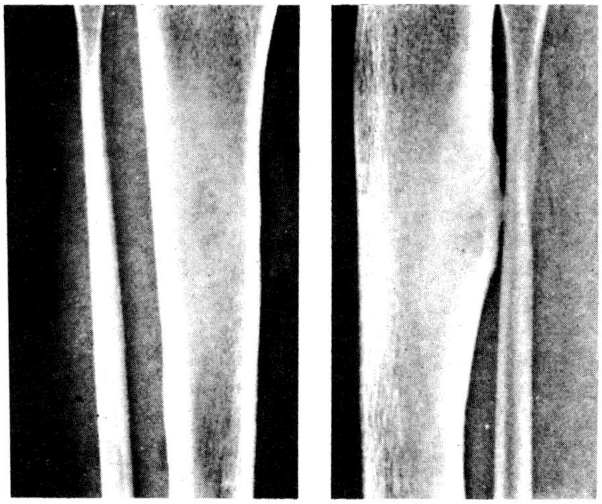

Fig. 14-12. Osteoid osteoma of the tibia.

volved the location is usually at either end of the diaphysis.

The characteristic radiographic appearance (Figs. 14-10, 14-11 and 14-12) is a radiolucent defect surrounded by a dense, sclerotic, extensive zone. The nidus, centrally located within this sclerosis, is round or oval, and is relatively small. Their size ranges from between several millimeters up to one but usually less than 2 cm. The large size of this lesion suggests that it is a benign osteoblastoma. In all of the lesions one or several areas of calcification can at times be noted within the center of the nidus. This finding might be better appreciated on tomograms.

The sclerosis surrounding the lesion may appear as a narrow ring or it may extend at some distance under the form of a large dense band with homogenous and elliptic characteristics. If tangentially shown, it may appear as an often marked fusiform protruberance which is fused, without a clearcut border, with the adjacent unaffected cortex. Active hyperostosis is especially marked in children. Diaphyseal involvement is sometimes so dense that it may almost completely mask the nidus on plain films. In such a situation tomograms are required to properly bring out this finding. Peripheral reactive condensation may be somewhat more discrete if the lesion is located within spongy bone. This is especially true within the spine. As in other similar involvements where the bone is relatively thick, one may run the risk of overlooking the actual lesion on plain films and will only be able to fully appreciate their presence on tomograms. This is particularly true in spinal involvement.

Besides these types where radiographic diagnosis is simple, there are atypical ones where the nidus is either totally dense or eccentric in its location with respect to the dense bony area. This finding may be present in involvement of the femoral neck. Here the nidus may present as a small subperiosteal notch within the cortex, with or without peripheral sclerotic reaction, and types with lamellar corticoperiosteal osteosclerosis.

These variants have led some authors (Edeiken et al., Schajowicz et al.) to differentiate osteoid osteomas into three types. These are cortical osteoid osteoma, the most frequently seen classical type, osteoid osteoma of spongy tissue, and subperiosteal osteoid osteoma. In chronic cases there may also be local osteoporosis. In locations close to joints, local decalcification along with changes in the joint space, may appear similar to local arthritis. Lindbom and collaborators were able to show by angiography that there is often hypervascularity of the nidus within the osteoid osteoma. This may be a helpful aid in differentiating an osteoid osteoma from a local infection or chronic abscess.

In its usual presentation the radiographic diagnosis of an osteoid osteoma does not offer any difficulty. It may be difficult to differentiate Brodie's central abscess of the bone from Garré's sclerosing osteomyelitis. However, we have seen that this apparently rare condition can be properly differentiated. In patients with the relatively unusual local finding of lamellar periosteal cortical location, there may be a slight problem in differentiating this from Ewing's tumor, histiocytosis X, or a chronic march or fatigue fracture.

If left to itself, an osteoid osteoma will develop over many months and even years. A spontaneous cure, although rare, may occur. When located within the long bones, bone length may be increased (Giustra and Freiberger).

In spite of the aspirin's effectiveness, which may decrease progressively, local surgical excision is the rule due to the persistence and progression of local pain. In order to be fully effective the nidus must be completely removed. If there is local pain persistence, the excision was probably incomplete. In order to avoid this, the surgeon often requests that the radiologist performs a careful radiographic study of the operative specimen. Recurrence outside of the original location is unusual, but has been reported (Karlsberg and Kittleson). The pathologist will have to confirm the identity of this nidus and its complete excision. The diagnosis does not offer any problem to the pathologist if he is given the nidus and the surrounding dense bone. The radiograph of the specimen may help him in his appraisal. Microscopically the nidus is composed of a network of osteoid tissue covered by benign osteoblasts which contain, in its meshwork, a fibrovascular tissue with in some rare places giant cells.

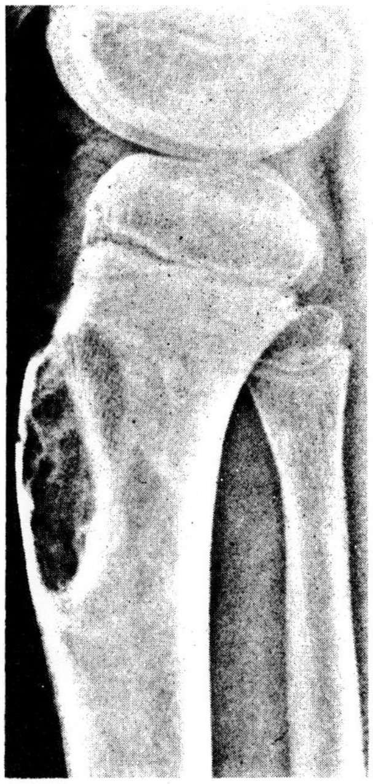

Fig. 14-13. Benign osteoblastoma involving the proximal end of the tibia.

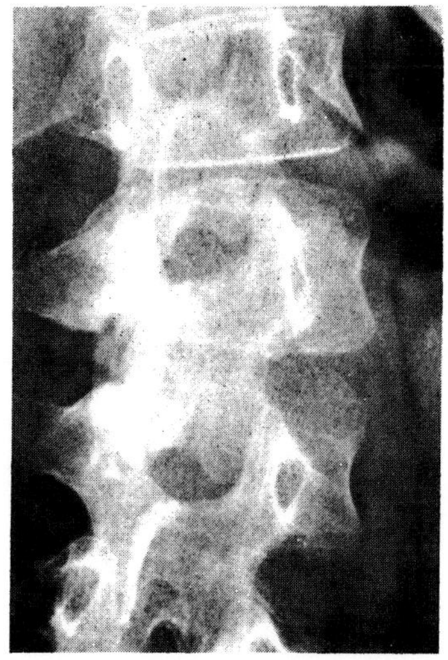

Fig. 14-14. Benign osteoblastoma of the right lamina and the spinous process L2. (Courtesy of Meary and Queneau)

The histologic diagnosis, as well as the radiographic evaluation, may occasionally encounter difficulties in differentiating the osteoid osteoma from a benign osteoblastoma which is a very similar tumor. As a result, some authors call these lesions giant osteoid osteomas.

BENIGN OSTEOBLASTOMA

This term was independently proposed by Lichtenstein and by Jaffe in 1956 to designate a benign lesion. It is composed of numerous osteoblasts and other cells which produce osteoid and bone in the center of a highly vascularized connective tissue stroma. The terms of giant osteoid osteoma and osteogenic fibroma were previously used for this lesion.

This is a relatively rare tumor and represents less than 1 per cent of tumors in the material of Dahlin. However, this author maintains that its incidence may be somewhat higher. It is very likely that in the future, when better known to pathologists, this tumor will be more often differentiated from osteoid osteoma and other histologically similar benign tumors.

A male predilection is noted in most statistics. Benign osteoblastoma is almost exclusively encountered within the second and third decade.

Clinically the patients complain of local pain, especially during the night. Aspirin is less beneficial than it is in osteoid osteoma. Vertebral localization usually results in a painful scoliosis, and sometimes exhibits symptoms resulting from radicular or even medullary compression.

Spinal localization, especially at the posterior vertebral arch, is most frequent. In the statistics of Dahlin which focus on the spine and the pelvis, 11 cases among 28 have this localization. Further involvement, in order of decreasing incidence are the long bones, the short bones, and eventually the flat bones which include the patella, ribs, cranial vault, and the orbits.

The radiographic appearance (Figs. 14-13 and 14-14) is not uniform. In some patients the diagnosis can be suspected because of a geographic lacunar defect. This is frequently of considerable size with the largest diameter being at least 2 cm, however, it may sometimes reach 5 or 6 cm. The contours are often polycyclic. The bone may be widened and the cortex thin (Fig. 14-13). Sclerosis around this lesion is more or less pronounced, but is usually less extensive than in an osteoid osteoma. There may be irregular calcifications at the center of the defect.

It is relatively easy to delineate the normal cortex in such patients. This and the cortical expansion are indications of a benign lesion. There are local forms with a radiographic aspect of a more complex nature leading to difficulties in clarifying the benign character of the lesion. There are other cases, where a very marked similarity with an osteoid osteoma exists, but with an unusually large and irregularly formed nidus, which may lead to the proper recognition of a benign osteoblastoma. In spongy bone for instance, a vertebra orametaphysis of the long bone, may have very little local sclerosis if any at all (Fig. 14-14). Because of local corticoperiosteal expansion, the tumor may actually resemble an aneurysmal bone cyst.

The possibility of subperiosteal localization with osteoblastic development under the periosteum towards the exterior of the bone offers special problems. Locally, the tumor will be separate from the cortex. Lichtenstein and Sawyer have reported two observations in children, one affecting the humerus and the other the femur. Radiographically both resembled an osteochondral exostosis, however, this exostosis remains separate from the bone by the bony cortex. In a true osteochondroma the bony cortex is interrupted at the base of the exostosis with continuation of the cortex on to the latter.

A radiographic differential diagnosis is difficult, due to the different appearances of a benign osteoblastoma and because of our limited experience with this unusual lesion. Still, we agree with Stewart et al. that this diagnosis must be considered in a patient with an unusual bizarre bony spinal lesion. This localized lesion appears to have benign characteristics and has at least some radiographic characteristics mentioned here. The presence of a benign osteoblastoma can be suspected on this basis. The diagnosis will not be a radiographic one and histologic verification is required. Surgical intervention is the rule either by total removal depending on the location and access – such as part of a rib – or by local curettage followed by bone grafting. Radiotherapy alone is not successful, but has been proposed by some authors as additional therapy when resection has been incomplete (Meary et al.). The effectiveness of this additional form of therapy is not proven (Dahlin). There are some observations in the literature of spontaneous healing which has occurred after a number of years where there has been no local surgical excision but only a biopsy (Aegerter et al., Dahlin).

Surgical approach is indicated in order to obtain a biopsy for microscopic study which will show the good limitation of the lesion. The tumor has a reddish-grey appearance and is hypervascularized. Although the surrounding cortex may be eroded and thin it always remains intact. The tumor itself is composed of a network of osteoid tissue which is somewhat larger and longer than that found in osteoid osteoma. Its vascularity is richer and, in some instances, there may be a large number of mitotic figures. This may present problems in differentiating it from osteosarcoma. These problems also result from the numerous multinucleated cells which are similar to a giant cell tumor. Differentiation from an osteoid osteoma can also be difficult. Many authors see a very close relationship between these two lesions.

The prognosis is good and there is only a rare recurrence after surgery. Malignant sarcomatous degeneration is very unusual although it has been reported (Dahlin, Mayer, Schajowicz and Lemos).

BENIGN TUMORS AND PSEUDOTUMORAL PROCESSES OF VARYING AND UNKNOWN ORIGINS

BENIGN TUMORS AND PSEUDOTUMORAL PROCESSES OF UNKNOWN ORIGIN

Giant Cell Tumors

True giant cell tumors are rarely seen before the age of 20 and never before 15 years-of-age. The presence of a growth zone is practically incompatible with the diagnosis (Merle D'Aubigné and Thomine). This diagnosis, made in a child prior to puberty or at puberty, can only be accepted after a number of specialists in bone tumor pathology have reviewed the biopsy material and after the exclusion of those tumors, frequently confused histologically with this lesion, because of the presence of multinucleated cells (Edeiken and Hodes). This refers, in particular, to aneurysmal bone cysts, benign metaphyseal fibrous lacunae, nonossifying fibromas, and chondromyxoid fibromas. As has been emphasized by Merle D'Aubigné and Thomine the presence of giant cells is required, but is not in itself sufficient for the diagnosis of giant cell tumor. Among the 155 cases reported by Dahlin there were only five patients between the ages of 12 and 14. The reader is referred to the articles mentioned in the bibliography (Merle D'Aubigné and Thomine, Edeiken and Hodes).

Aneurysmal Bone Cyst

Considered for a long time to be a variant of giant cell tumor, aneurysmal bone cysts were recognized as a well defined entity in 1942 by Jaffe and Lichtenstein. Aneurysmal bone cysts are lesions which occur mainly in childhood and adolescence with a peak incidence in the second decade. Females are more frequently affected with a ratio of six to eight for one boy depending on the statistical data. Dahlin, however, denies such a sex predilection.

These patients do not present with any striking clinical characteristics. There may be a vague night-

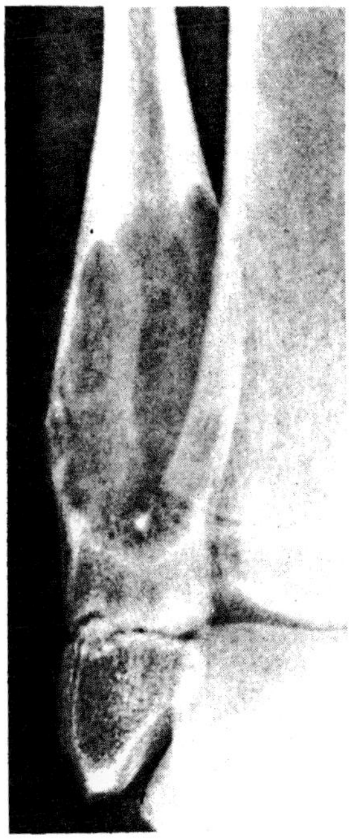

Fig. 14-15. Aneurysmal bone cyst at the distal end of the fibula.

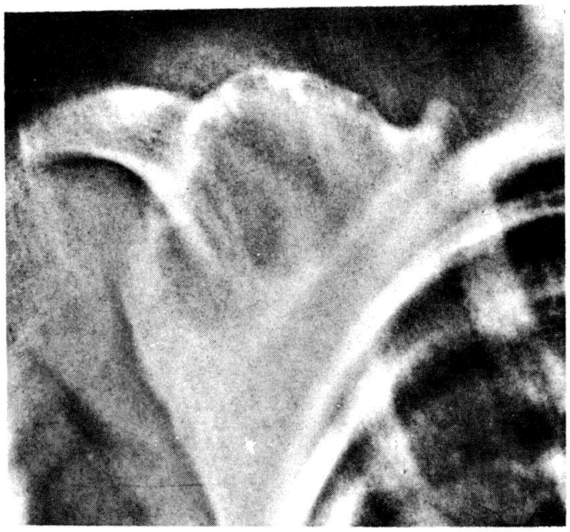

Fig. 14-16. Tomographic view of an aneurysmal bone cyst which was verified as being located within the scapula.

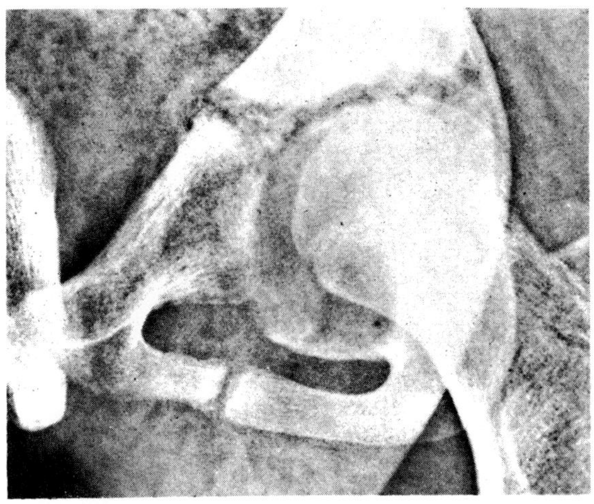

Fig. 14-17. Aneurysmal bone cyst of the ischium and the supraacetabular region. (Courtesy Institut Gustave-Roussy)

time pain without predilection, sometimes pulsating, and increasing after effort. Some patients have a local palpable mass, in particular when an extremity is involved. Pathological fractures are rarely noted. Vertebral lesions can result in thoracolumbar pain, spinal stiffness, even neurologic findings, occasionally as a radicular syndrome or paraplegia.

The most frequently involved area of the skeleton is the metaphyseal region of the long bones along with a high incidence of spinal involvement. The radiographic signs vary depending on the size and location of the lesion (Figs. 4-15, 4-16 and 4-17).

If small, an aneurysmal bone cyst will appear as a homogeneously osteolytic defect with clearcut and regular borders. In the somewhat larger forms, there will still be a geographic defect which is occasionally larger than 6 cm in its long axis with a tendency towards expansion. This will also manifest itself by an eccentrically widened bone. The cortex is eroded, and thin and is at times hardly recognizable below the periosteum. If the eccentric portion is documented in a tangential view, the area within the soft tissues which surround and border the lesion in its most peripheral parts may look like a spider's web. The periosteum can be noted to possess a mild degree of thickening, usually of regular, benign characteristics. Towards the spongy bone, the borders of this lesion are usually clearcut without any adjacent condensation. In small, short bones it is usually not possible to recognize an eccentric growth tendency, as there is a relatively quick expansion within the bone which leads to complete filling and expansion in all directions.

There are several superficial locations which leads to the theory (Edeiken and Hodes, Slowick et al., Tillman et al.) that there are two different types of aneurysmal bone cysts. The first type would be of intraosseus origin that expanded the bone and a second more superficial type would erode the cortex towards the medullary cavity, thus elevating the periosteum. In this second group the tangential view will reveal the described fine, reticular network simulating a periosteal spiculated reaction. This finding can best be seen at the point where the tumor joins the normally preserved bone, forming a spur and an angle of Codman. Some believe that the superficial types result from trauma (Edeiken and Hodes).

In its spinal location or within flat bone (Fig. 14-16 and 14-17) aneurysmal cysts have the greatest tendency to demonstrate their characteristic expansion, since the defects often extend throughout the involved bone elevating and "ballooning out" the cortex. Some more aggressive types do not respect the natural limits of an involved vertebra and will extend by erosion to neighboring bones, thereby destroying several vertebrae.

The pathological appearance of this lesion is characteristic. Under the microscope there is a cystic lesion with loss of local substance in closely arranged spaces, surrounded in a clear fashion by a thin periosteal layer, and subperiosteal new bone. This cavity usually contains uncoagulated blood, which immediately surges forward once the cyst is opened. In some older patients this liquid will be either a clear color or yellowish. In some regions a fleshy, fibrous, tissue will be in this location. Histologic studies reveal cavernous spaces which lack the normal color of blood vessels. The solid portions consist of fibrous tissue, sometimes containing osteoid trabeculations. A large number of multinucleated cells are normally present, which explains the earlier confusion with giant cell tumors.

According to Edling there is a close relationship between giant cell tumors, aneurysmal bone cysts, and simple cysts.

Therapy is surgical by curettage and is followed by bone grafting. Radiotherapy with weak doses (1500 rads) may be useful in approaching an inoperable site, or where surgery is particularly difficult, as in a vertebra or the femoral neck.

Solitary Bone Cyst

There is recent agreement that solitary bone cysts are not bony neoplasias, but are the result of cystic distrophy. Pathogenesis is still under discussion, thus, there are a number of differing therapeutic approaches. Incidence is relatively high and these lesions are the most frequently encountered benign bone lesions of the peripheral skeleton during childhood.

Age distribution is of special interest because this lesion occurs almost exclusively during the growth period. According to different statistics 80 to 90% of all cases occur between the ages of 3 and 19. It is quite unusual to encounter this lesion after the age of 20 and it is only an exceptional patient seen after the age of 30. Jaffe and Lichtenstein report of a case in a 42-year-old and Lefranc and Nézelof in a 59-year-old patient. At the other end of the spectrum it is most unusual to see a solitary bone cyst in a patient under the age of two. Several exceptions are on record. Males are involved two to three times more frequently than females. Clinical signs vary and a bone cyst may remain asymptomatic for a very long time. Occasionally, vague pains or the sensation of a local mass may lead to radiographic examination. If local pain leads to examination it is commonly the result of a pathological fracture which has resulted from progressive cortical erosion by a cyst. Often the detection of a cyst occurs inadvertently on an examination performed for unrelated reasons.

The distribution of the lesions is quite typical, since the solitary bone cyst usually occurs within long bones, and in particular, the femur and humerus. The humerus appears to be involved more than any other bone, especially at its proximal end. Almost 50 per cent of all cases are located here. Aside from the humerus and femur there are other relatively frequent locations, with the tibia being the site of 13 per cent of all cases. Both ends are equally involved. Not only located within long bones there are some in short bones, especially the calcaneus—3 per cent—or the flat bones.

Within long bones the lesions are primarily located at the metaphyseal end—52 per cent—and develop close to the growth zone which they never cross. While the cyst is active, it will increase in size and remains immediately adjacent to the growth zone. Once it stops to be active, its size will no longer increase and there is a migration towards the diaphysis with a zone of newly formed normal bone tissue separating it from the physis. Using these criteria it is possible to differentiate between two types, an active evolving type, which remains directly adjacent to the growth cartilage, and inactive cysts with no further activity or growth.

The radiographic appearance varies depending on the activity of the cyst (Figs. 14-18 and 14-19). The geographic defect is always oval or spherical, is centrally located, and has clear and well delineated contours. Frequently, the defect will occupy the complete metaphyseal diameter, eroding the cortex without local destruction. Occasionally, the bone expands in a symmetrical fashion. At both poles the ends of the

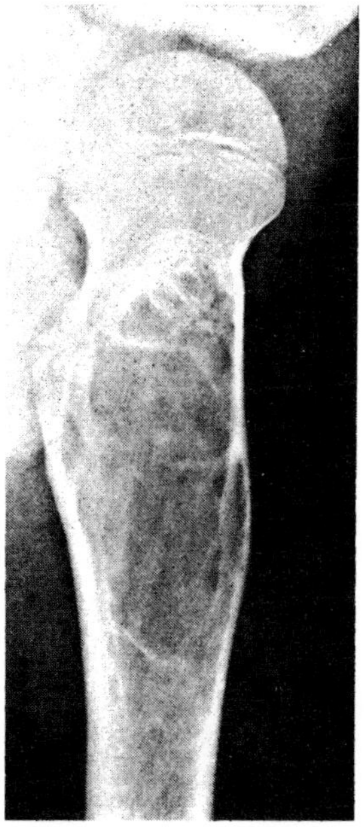

Fig. 14-18. Benign bone cyst of the femur.

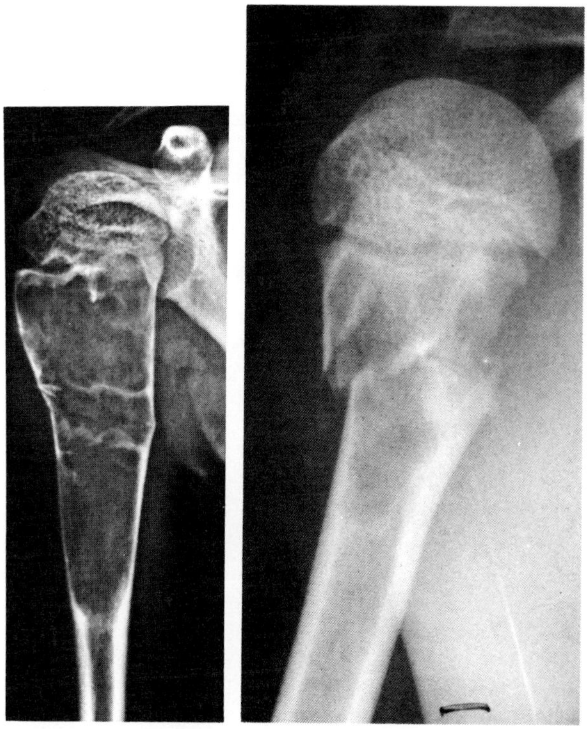

Fig. 14-19. Bone cysts at the upper end of the humerus. Its first clinical symptoms were precipitated by a fracture.

defect are somewhat condensed with slightly less involvement towards the growth zone which is never crossed. Towards the diaphyseal side, however, the described condensation which is often dense results in a very clear border between the cyst and the uninvolved diaphysis. This defect is usually homogeneous and consists of a unilocular cavity. It is unusual to have dense trabecular bands subdividing the cyst. These lines may only represent small crista-like structures which protrude into the lumen of a single cyst from the walls. The cortex is always present although sometimes it is extremely thin. There is never a periosteal reaction, but if there has been a fracture, there may be minimal callus formation in that location.

The radiographic appearance is characteristic and usually leads to the correct diagnosis without arteriography, which will only show normal vasculature. The appearance is so striking that if, in particular, the proximal humerus is involved, the diagnosis is so reliable that it is not necessary to perform biopsy or histologic study.

The anatomic diagnosis is without a problem and the cyst is usually formed by a single large cavity with very thin bluish walls covered by normal periosteum. The inner wall is outlined by fine irregular ridges and is covered by a fine greyish or whitish membrane. The cyst usually contains a clear, sometimes serous-hemorrhagic fluid. On rare occasions, a mass of fibrous tissues fills part of the cyst.

Histologically the wall of the cyst is formed by new bony lamellae, bordering on distended vessels. The conjunctival inner wall-cover is only a pseudomembrane formed by connective tissue, which in places is thick and highly vascularized. Either within this membrane or within phagocytes we find free hemoglobin. These cells may also contain cholesterol or fatty acids. In the parietal ridges, we find osteoblasts and osteoclasts in a varying proportion.

According to Lefranc and Nézelof the walls of cysts often contain an aseptic necrosis with an irregular center. This necrosis is said to be a characteristic finding for a solitary bone cyst. According to these authors, reliable pathologic significance may be attached to this lesion. It is felt that this cyst is the result of circulatory problems which cause local ischemia. However, we still do not have a good pathogenetic understanding of solitary bone cysts. Unanimity on this point is far from a reality, as there are many other theories on inflammatory or traumatic processes, as well as on preexisting chondromatous or fibrous lesions.

Prognosis is good. There is, however, no agreement as to therapy. Surgery is advisable on cysts of the leg, due to the local problems of weight bearing, but a con-

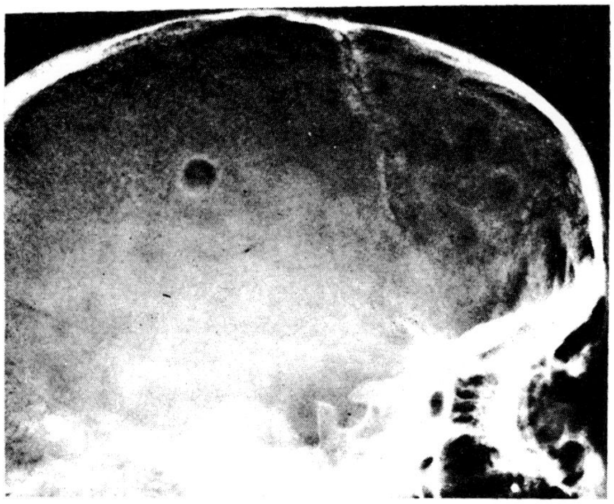

Fig. 14-20. Epidermoid cyst of the cranial vault.

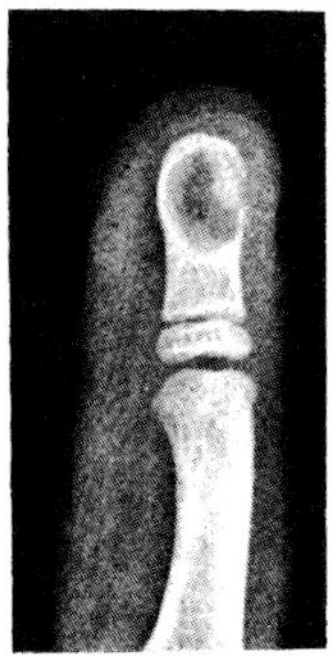

Fig. 14-21. Epidermoid cyst after a posttraumatic inclusion.

servative approach may be better when the arms are involved. This approach is also desirable, when a cyst appears active and is close to the growth cartilage. In many cases of this type local recurrences have developed after surgery.

The direct approach consists of curettage or a partial resection of the lesion which preserves the cortical wall. The cavity is then filled with bone grafts or muscle fibers (Estève). Recurrence may occur, especially active cysts close to the growth zone, but there is no absolute rule about this. In the absence of therapy, a cyst may continue to enlarge, but it also may stabilize and slowly migrate towards the diaphysis. Some cysts actually heal by filling the cavity. This healing mechanism appears to occur most frequently after local fracture. However, this is not always so.

Radiotherapy should be firmly rejected as it has no beneficial results and entails the risk of local growth arrest. This is due to the fact that the growth cartilage is contained in the primary field of radiation.

OTHER BENIGN PSEUDOTUMORAL LESIONS

Epidermoid Cysts

Intraosseus epidermoid cysts are characterized by the presence of squamous epiphelial cells within bone. They tend to expand through local evolution of low intensity and slow growth. This is a benign lesion seen during childhood with its two preferred locations being within the cranial vault and the most distal phalanges of fingers.

Epidermoid cysts of the cranial vault are by far the most common. Often the patient or their parents will note a small, smooth, rounded, and firm lesion which is palpable. It is attached to the bone over which the scalp can be moved. There is no local pain, and it is only in a very unusual case that the cyst will develop into the deep region of the vault. This could then compress the underlying brain and provoke epilepsy. However we are generally dealing here with an entirely benign asymptomatic lesion. Frequently such an epidermoid cyst is unrecognized and is discovered by chance at the time of radiographic examination for unrelated, possibly traumatic reasons.

The common location is close to the pterion and lateral region of the coronal sutures. Many other locations, however, are possible. Its radiographic appearance is practically uniform (Fig. 14-20). The appearance is that of a round or ovoid radiolucent homogeneous defect, surrounded by a clearcut, peripherally dense border. In some patients there is a gutter-like depression at one point on this circle. Tangential views may reveal that a cyst is sometimes located within the external table. In other cases it is located within the diploe pushing aside both tables. In rare situations there is development along the internal table with local thinning. Most of the time its appearance is stable and does not show any evolution. An exceptional case displays a slow increase in size. This is a benign tumor with reliable radiographic symptomatology allowing for correct diagnosis. The pathologist will find that this is a well delineated and limited tumor formed by a whitish keratinizing pearly tissue.

These benign tumors do not require surgery except for esthetic reasons and in the unusual situation of cerebral compression.

The pathogenesis of this tumor is unknown. We have observed a patient who developed such a lesion immediately below a scar of the scalp in the supramas-

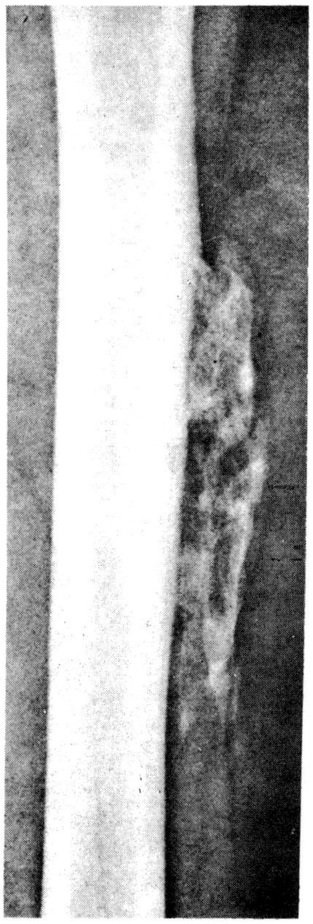

Fig. 14-22. Ossified musculoperiosteal hemtoma. This post-traumatic myositis ossificans follows direct muscular and periosteal trauma.

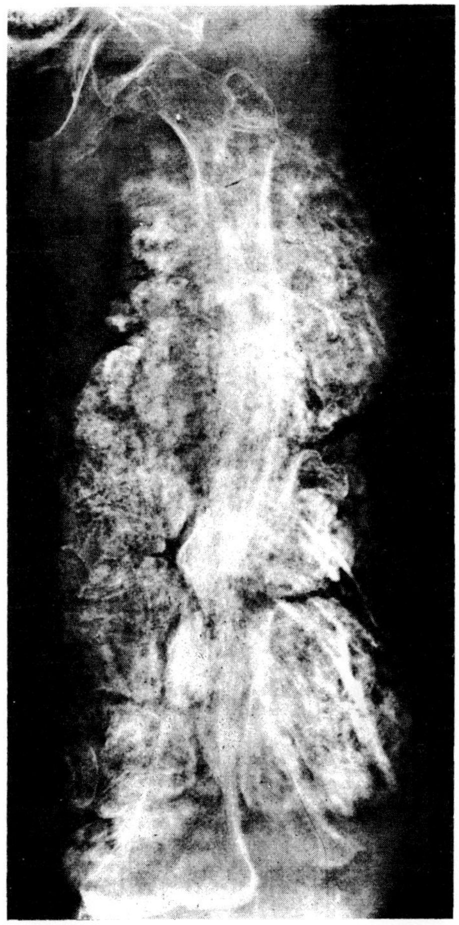

Fig. 14-23. Exuberant hypertrophic callus formation with a pseudo-tumor appearance in a patient suffering from osteogenesis imperfecta.

toid region. This was the result of an episiotomy performed at birth. This may represent an analogous pathogenetic mechanism as that postulated for the phalangeal localization.

We are always dealing with intraosseus inclusions of dermal cells in this second predilection. These are the result of local perforating trauma, especially by puncture injury. The intraosseus lesions can be mildly painful. Its radiographic appearance (Fig. 14-21) is that of a rounded defect of the most distal phalanx which is uniform in density and limited by a dense sclerotic bony border. This lesion is seen much less frequently than the cranial vault involvement. The local lesion is benign and has a good chance of healing after curettage.

Pigmented Villonodular Synovitis

This is an osteoarticular inflammatory lesion of unknown etiology seen in young adults. Occasionally, however, it occurs during adolescence and in children over 12 years of age.

The villonodular synovial formations, if present in sufficient numbers, will eventually erode the bone by progressive local impression. This may actually lead to the disappearance of the cortex and can penetrate into spongy bone leading to the formation of true local defects. The knee, as well as the hip, are the favored localizations of this disorder. The radiographic appearance reveals geodes right next to the articular surface. The articular soft tissue is swollen and is similar to osteoarthritis or rheumatoid arthritis. Still, the presence of relatively large and isolated geodes within an epiphysis should lead to the diagnosis of a local tumor. This must then be verified under the microscope.

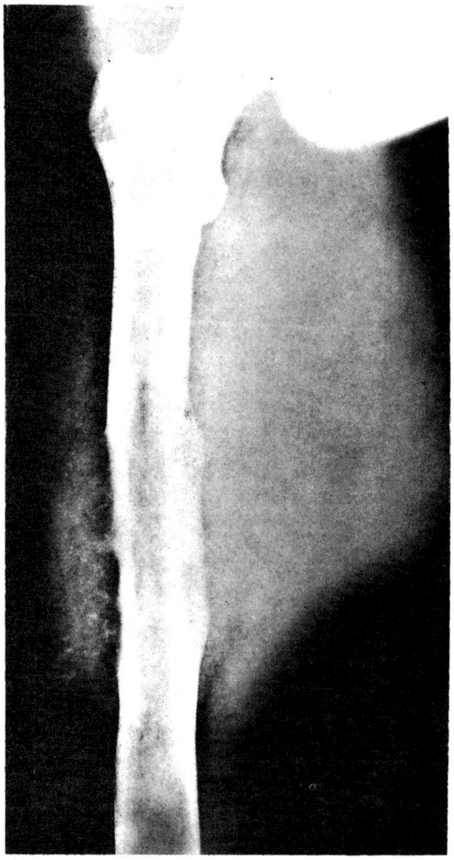

Fig. 14-24. Periosteal spiculation resulting from a pseudotumoral, periosteal hematoma in a hemophiliac patient. (Courtesy of P. Caen)

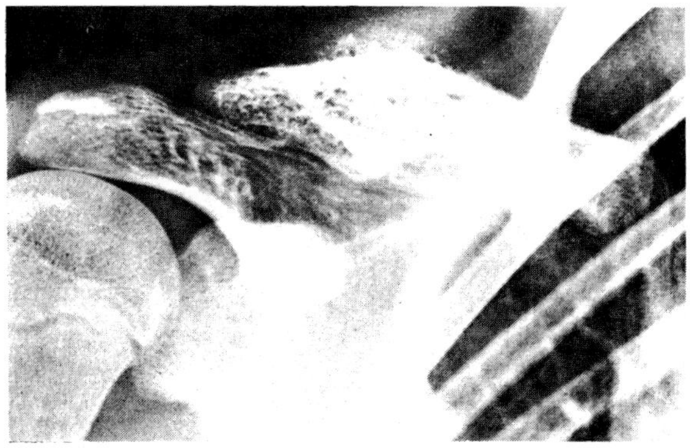

Fig. 14-25. Angioma of the clavicle. (Courtesy Institut Gustave-Roussy)

Hypertrophic Callus Formation and Periosteal Hematomas

Observed as (Fig. 14-22) the result of a fatigue fracture or after unrecognized fractures in osteogenesis imperfecta (Fig. 14-23; Banta et al.) or in the course of hemophilia (Fig. 14-24; Caen et al., Kubicz, Serve et al.) these lesions may clinically and radiographically simulate the presence of a bone tumor, especially an osteosarcoma. We are not dealing here with a problem of differential diagnosis, but with pseudotumoral local reactions. Similar problems can arise during the course of progressive myositis ossificans (Kaplan et al.), which early along may present clinically as a hot and painful tumor in a paraosseus intramuscular location. Secondly, in this region dense calcific and, in part, cloudy opacities will appear close to the periosteum in a fashion similar to a local tumor. Even histologically this muscular lesion while in its early active developing phase may be strongly similar to a malignant lesion (see p. 319).

BENIGN VASCULAR TUMORS AND CLOSELY RELATED DISORDERS (MASSIVE OSTEOLYSIS)

This chapter deals with hemangiomas, lymphangiomas, and extensive osteolysis. Hemangiomas and lymphangiomas are only seen rarely and more often in adults than in children. It involves twice as many females than males. Hemangiomas are localized either within the cranial vault or in the vertebrae. The radiographic characteristics in the skull are lacunae. If seen in the AP view they present as many small defects with clear surrounding borders. In the tangential view they look like radiating rays which are originating from the external table. If a vertebra is involved, hemangiomas will look like a "bee's nest," often with longitudinal striations and a slight degree of increased vertebral size. This same appearance can be recognized if other bones are affected (Fig. 14-25).

These benign angiomatous lesions are usually isolated. There are, however, children on record (Modeley et al., Wallis et al.), with multiple angiomatosis of the long bones (Fig. 14-26), the skull, the spine, which all reveal well delineated lacunar defects.

Lymphangiomatosis of the skeleton (Cohen et al., Reilly et al., Rosenquist et al., Sauvegrain et al., Schopfner et al., Wittenberger) is a rare lesion leading to a similar appearance. This condition is sometimes associated with lymphedema. These cystic skeletal lesions are often hard to differentiate from other diffuse osteolytic, skeletal involvement. It may be impos-

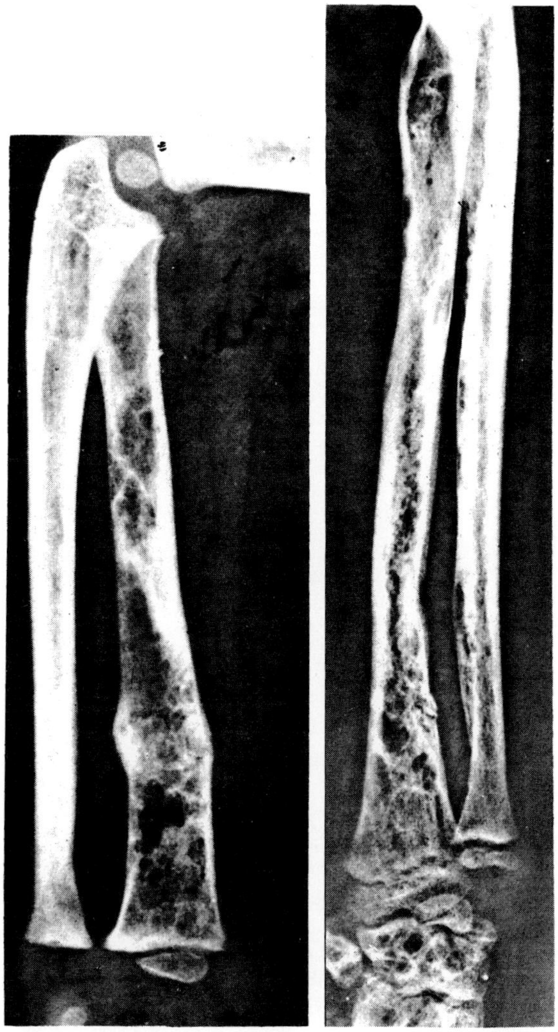

Fig. 14-26. Angiomatosis of the bone with multiple involvement of the radius and ulna. *(Left)* at 4 years. *(Right)* at 13 years.

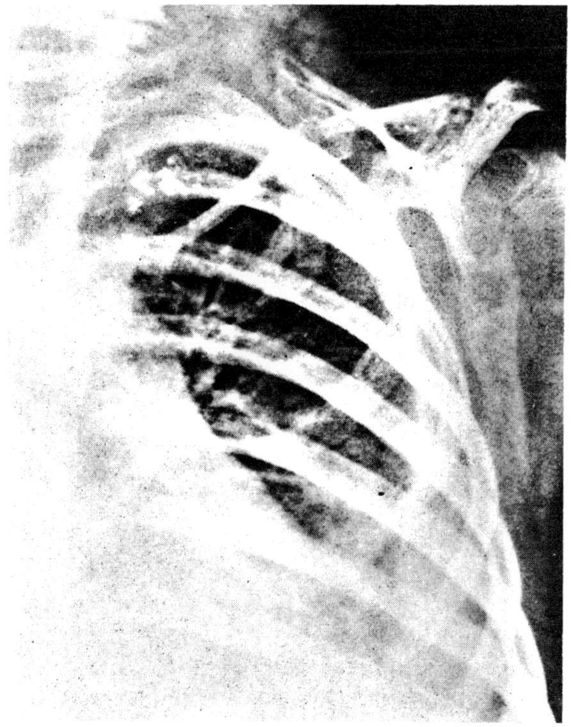

Fig. 14-27. Osteolysis due to unexplained "vanishing bone disease" involving the 1st and 2nd ribs and the acromion in a 5-year-old child who is suffering from a chylothorax. Note that some lipiodol remains after a lymphography which was done at the level of the supraclavicular region.

sible to differentiate between angiomatosis or lymphangiomatosis, thus, in order to describe such lesions of a hamartoma type some authors do not attempt to define its exact nature and prefer the terms cystic angiomatosis of bone.

Massive osteolysis (Gorham's disease, "vanishing bone disease") (Gorham et al., Halliday et al., Touraine et al.) is a rare disorder, noted especially during infancy, childhood and adolescence. Sometimes young adults are affected. The thorax and pelvis are most frequently involved, but other bones can be affected. This disease usually begins after trauma and has a severe progressive character which totally destroys the involved bone. It may sometimes also destroy neighboring bones, spearing joints and eventually leading to death. Radiographically (Fig. 14-27) we note progressive destruction of either a part or all of a bone until it simply disappears. There is no local reaction in the vicinity or of the periosteum. The bony portion, which is not yet destroyed, will simply become thin and ill-defined and will not exhibit expansion. This osteolytic process does not stop at the joints and invades neighboring bones.

The course can extend over several months or years. Osteolysis has been attributed to a hemangioma or an extensive lymphangioma which destroys the bone and then replaces it with fibrous tissue. There is no effective therapy available.

BONE LIPOMAS

Intraosseus lipomas are very unusual tumors and primarily affect adults. Still, there have been some unusual observations during childhood (Cohen-Solal and Herrault).

If we eliminate from this discussion osteoperiosteal lipomas which originate from the periosteum and have the tendency to eventually erode the neighboring cortex, there are two types originating within bone. Medullary lipomas are characterized by a benign appearing centroosseus lesion without cortical or periosteal involvement. The other type is a lipoma or fibrolipoma of corticomedullary origin which develops a cortical defect which consists of a number of juxtaposed abnormalities separated by dense streaks and often a mild expansion of the involved bone.

These benign lesions have only a very slow tendency to develop and do not require active treatment. There are several cases on record where local intervention and curettage was performed on the basis of a questionable diagnosis and where surgery had the primary diagnostic aim of obtaining a biopsy.

SKELETAL NEURILEMMOMAS AND NEUROFIBROMAS

Neurilemmoma is an exceedingly rare nervous tissue tumor. In Dahlin's data of 4000 tumors, there were only seven such patients. This has been observed in the adult as an osteolytic well delineated pseudocystic defect.

Neurofibromatosis involving parts of the skeleton occurs with a low incidence. It is well known that the corticoperiosteal erosions and bony destruction taking place in this disorder by external pressure can be observed in the areas of contacts between skeletal parts and neurofibromas or a plexiform neuroma (see p. 323). Intraosseus neurofibromas or malignant schwannomas are almost never seen (Dahlin).

REFERENCES

General References

LICHTENSTEIN (L.). Bone tumors. *3e édit., Saint-Louis, 1965, C. V. Mosby Co., éd.*

STEWART (J. R.), DAHLIN (D. C.) et PUGH (D. G.). The pathology and radiology of solitary benign tumors. *Seminars Roentgenol., 1966,* **1**, *268-292.*

Benign Fibrogenic Tumors

CAFFEY (J.). Pediatric X-ray diagnosis. *5e édit., Chicago, 1967, Year Book, éd.*

CÉDARD (C.), RAINAUT (J. J.) et AUBRIOT (J.). Fibrome non ostéogénique (maladie de Jaffé-Lichtenstein). *Ann. Chir., 1965,* **19**, *1416-1425.*

DAHLIN (D. C.). Bone tumors. *2e édit., Springfield, Ill., 1967, Ch. C. Thomas, éd.*

DAHLIN (D. C.) et HOOVER (N. W.). Desmoplastic fibroma of bone. Report of two cases. *J. amer. med. Ass., 1964,* **188**, *685-687.*

DUHAMEL (A.), COHEN-SOLAL (J.) et HERRAULT (A.). Lacunes corticales métaphysaires des os longs. *Méd. infant. (Paris), 1965,* **72**, *415-420.*

FERGUSON (A. B.). Benign tumors of bone in childhood. *Pediat. Clin. N. Amer., 1967,* **14**, *683-704.*

FIRAT (D.) et STUTZMAN (L.). Fibrous dysplasia of the bone. Review of 24 cases. *Amer. J. Med., 1968,* **44**, *421-429.*

GORDON (L. R. S.). Fibrous lesions of bone in childhood. *Brit. J. Radiol., 1964,* **37**, *253-259.*

HARDY (R.) et LEHRER (H.). Desmoplastic fibroma v.s. desmoid tumor of bone. *Radiology, 1967,* **88**, *899-901.*

JAFFÉ (H. L.) et LICHTENSTEIN (L.). Non-osteogenic fibroma of bone. *Amer. J. Pathol., 1942,* **18**, *205-215.*

LEFEBVRE (J.), NÉZELOF (C.), FAURÉ (C.), HUC (M.) et ERRERA (A.). Les lacunes corticales métaphysaires des os longs chez l'enfant et l'adolescent. Rapports avec le fibrome non ostéogénique. A propos de 32 observations. *J. Radiol. Electrol., Paris, 1956,* **37**, *300-307.*

LEFEBVRE (J.) et HASSAN (M.). Fibromes non ossifiants. *Rev. Prat., Paris, 1969,* **19**, *2133-2141.*

LÍCHTENSTEIN (L.). Polyostotic fibrous dysplasia. *Arch. Surg., 1938,* **36**, *874-898.*

LICHTENSTEIN (L.) et JAFFÉ (H. L.). Fibrous dysplasia of bone. A condition affecting one, several or many bones, the graver of which may present abnormal pigmentation of skin, premature sexual development, hyperthyroidism or still other extraskeletal abnormalities. *Arch. Path., 1942,* **33**, *777-816.*

LOUYOT (P.), GAUCHER (A.), JEANBLANC (J.) et FRESSE (B.). Neuf cas de dysplasie fibreuse des os de Jaffé-Lichtenstein. *Rev. Rhum., Paris, 1965,* **32**, *745-751.*

NILSONNE (U.) et GOTHLIN (G.). Desmyeloplastic fibroma in bone. *Acta orthop. scand., 1969,* **40**, *205-215.*

PADOVANI (P.), RAINAUT (J. J.), CÉDARD (C.) et AUBRIOT (J.). Les fibromes non ostéogéniques. *Rev. Chir. orthop., Paris, 1965,* **51**, *595-603.*

PRITCHARD (J. E.). Fibrous dysplasia of the bones. *Amer. J. med. Sci., 1951,* **222**, *313-332.*

RABHAN (W. N.) et JUAN ROSAI. Desmoplastic fibroma (report of 10 cases and review of the literature). *J. Bone Jt Surg., 1968,* **50-A**, *3, 487-502.*

RIGAULT (P.) et KLISOWSKI (H.). Les fibromes non ossifiants de l'extrémité inférieure du tibia chez l'enfant et l'adolescent. Rapport de 5 cas et revue de la littérature. *Rev. Chir. orthop., 1969,* **55**, *533-541.*

SKREDE (O.). Non osteogenic fibroma of bone. *Acta orthop. scand., 1970,* **41**, *369-380.*

SONTAG (L. W.) et PYLE (S. I.). The appearance and nature of cyst-like areas in the distal femoral metaphyses in children. *Amer. J. Roentgenol., 1941,* **46**, *185-188.*

Benign Chondrogenic Tumors

DAHLIN (D. C.). Bone tumors. *2e édit., Springfield, Ill., 1967, Ch. C. Thomas, éd.*

FELDMAN (F.), HECHT (H. L.) et JOHNSTON (A. D.). Chondromyxoid fibroma of bone. *Radiology, 1970,* **94**, *249-260.*

HAMLIN (J. A.), ADLER (L.) et GRENNHAUM (E. I.). Central enchondroma. A precursor to chondrosarcoma. *J. canad. Ass. Radiol., 1971,* **22**, *206-209.*

JAFFÉ (H. L.) et LICHTENSTEIN (L.). Benign chondroblastoma of bone : a reinterpretation of the so-called calcifying or chondromatous giant-cell tumor. *Amer. J. Path., 1942,* **18**, *969-983.*

JAFFÉ (H. L.) et LICHTENSTEIN (L.). Chondromyxoid fibroma of bone : a distinctive benign tumor likely to be mistaken especially for chondrosarcoma. *Arch. Path., 1948,* **45**, *541-551.*

LEVY (W. M.), AEGERTER (E. E.) et KIRKPATRICK (J. A.). The nature of cartilaginous tumors. *Radiol. Clin. N. Amer., 1964,* **2**, *327-336.*

MAROTEAUX (P.). Aspects tumoraux des maladies constitutionnelles du squelette. *Rev. Prat., Paris, 1969,* **19**, *2093-2104.*

MIDDLEMISS (J. H.). Cartilage tumours. *Brit. J. Radiol., 1964,* **37**, *277-286.*

MONAT (Y.) et MEARY (R.). Chondromes, chondroblastomes, fibromes chondromyxoïdes. *Rev. Prat., Paris, 1969,* **19**, *2177-2184.*

NÉZELOF (C.). Communication personnelle.

NÉZELOF (C.), MAZABRAUD (A.) et JOBARD (L.). Le chondroblastome bénin; à propos de 4 observations. *Arch. Anat. path., 1962,* **10**, *111-117.*

PLUM (G. E.) et PUGH (D. G.). Roentgenologic aspect of benign chondroblastoma of bone. *Amer. J. Roentgenol., 1958,* **79**, *584-591.*

RAVAULT (P. P.) et coll. Le chondroblastome bénin des os (à propos de six observations anatomo-cliniques). *Rev. Rhum., Paris, 1969,* **36**, *215-224.*

SCHAJOWICZ (F.) et GALLARDO (H.). Epiphyseal chondroblastoma of bone. A clinico-pathological study of sixty nine cases. *J. Bone Jt Surg., 1970,* **52-B**, *205-226.*

SCHAJOWICZ (F.) et GALLARDO (H.). Chondromyxoid fibroma (fibromyxoid chondroma) of bone. A clinico-pathological study of thirty two cases. *J. Bone Jt Surg., 1971,* **53-B**, *198-216.*

SIRSAT (M. V.) et DOCTOR (V. M.). Benign chondroblastoma of bone. Report of a case of malignant transformation. *J. Bone Jt Surg., 1970,* **52-B**, *741-745.*

STEWART (J. R.), DAHLIN (D. C.) et PUGH (D. G.). The pathology and radiology of solitary benign tumors. *Seminars Roentgenol., 1966,* **1**, *268-292.*

TURCOTTE (B.), PUGH (D. G.) et DAHLIN (D. C.). The roentgenologic aspects of chondromyxoid fibroma of bone. *Amer. J. Roentgenol., 1962,* **87**, *1085-1095.*

Benign Osteogenic Tumors

AEGERTER (E.) et KIRKPATRICK (J. A.). Orthopedic diseases. Physiology, pathology, radiology. *Toronto, 1968, Saunders, éd.*

BYERS (P. D.). Solitary benign osteoblastic lesions of bone. Osteoid osteoma and benign osteoblastoma. *Cancer, 1968,* **22**, *43-57.*

DAHLIN (D. C.). Bone tumors. *2e édit., Springfield, Ill., 1967, Ch. C. Thomas, éd.*

DAHLIN (D. C.) et JOHNSON (E. W., Jr.). Giant osteoid osteoma. *J. Bone Jt. Surg., 1954,* **36-A**, *559-572.*

EDEIKEN (J.) et HODES (Ph. J.). Roentgen diagnosis of diseases of bone. *Baltimore, 1967, Williams and Wilkins, éd.*

FOWLES (S. J.). Osteoid osteoma. *Brit. J. Radiol., 1964,* **37**, *245-252.*

FREIBERGER (R. H.), LORTMAN (B. S.), HELPERN (M.) et THOMPSON (T. C.). Osteoid osteoma : a report on 80 cases. *Amer. J. Roentgenol., 1959,* **82**, *194-205.*

GIUSTRA (P. E.) et FREIBERGER (R. H.). Severe growth disturbance with osteoid osteoma (a report of two cases involving the femoral neck). *Radiology, 1970,* **96**, *285-288.*

GOLDING (J. S. R.). The natural history of osteoid osteoma; with a report of 20 cases. *J. Bone Jt Surg., 1954,* **36-B**, *218-229.*

GOLDING (J. S. R.) et SISSONS (H. A.). Osteogenic fibroma of bone. A report of two cases. *J. Bone Jt Surg., 1954,* **36-B**, *428-435.*

GOUTTIÈRES (Fr.) et coll. Ostéome ostéoïde. *Ann. Pédiat. (Sem. Hôp. Paris), 1967,* **61**, *793-797.*

JAFFÉ (H. L.). Osteoid osteoma : a benign osteoblastic tumor composed of osteoid and atypical bone. *Arch. Surg., 1935,* **31**, *709-728.*

JAFFÉ (H. L.). Benign osteoblastoma. *Bull. Hosp. Jt Dis. (N. Y.), 1956,* **17**, *141-151.*

KARLSBERG (R. C.) et KITTLESON (A. C.). Osteoid osteoma. *Radiol. Clin. N. Amer., 1964,* **2**, *337-345.*

LANCE (P.). Les ostéomes. *Rev. Prat., Paris, 1969,* **14**, *2143-2151.*

LAWRIE (T. R.) et coll. Painless osteoid osteoma. A report of two cases. *J. Bone Jt Surg. (Amer.), 1970,* **52-A**, *1357-1363.*

LICHTENSTEIN (L.). Benign osteoblastoma : A category of osteoid- and bone-forming tumors other than classical osteoid osteoma, which may be mistaken for giant-cell tumor or osteogenic sarcoma. *Cancer, 1956,* **9**, *1044-1052.*

LICHTENSTEIN (L.) et SAWYER (W. R.). Benign osteoblastoma. Further observations and report of twenty additional cases. *J. Bone Jt Surg., 1964,* **46-A**, *755-765.*

LIÈVRE (J. A.) et LIÈVRE (Mme J. A.). Ostéoblastome bénin. *Rev. Rhum., 1961,* **28**, *95-100.*

LINDBOM (Å.), LINDVALL (N.), SÖDERBERG (G.) et SPJÜT (J.). Angiography in osteoid osteoma. *Acta radiol., 1960,* **54**, *327-333.*

MAYER (L.). Malignant degeneration of so-called benign osteoblastoma. *Bull. Hosp. Jt Dis. (N. Y.), 1967,* **28**, *4-13.*

MEARY (R.), MERLE-D'AUBIGNÉ (R.) et MAZABRAUD (A.). Ostéoblastome bénin. *Mém. Acad. Chir., Paris, 1965,* **91**, *911-925.*

POULSEN (J. O.). Osteoid osteoma. *Acta orthop. scand., 1969,* **40**, *198-204.*

RUSHTON (J. G.), MULDER (D. W.) et LIPSCOMB (P. R.). Neurologic symptoms in osteoid osteoma. *Neurology, 1955,* **5**, *794-797.*

SALMON (M.) et coll. Ostéoblastome du rachis cervical chez un enfant. Problèmes diagnostiques et thérapeutiques. *Mém. Acad. Chir., 1970,* **96**, *723-730.*

SCHAJOWICZ (F.) et LEMOS (C.). Osteoid osteoma and osteoblastoma. Closely related entities of osteoblastic derivation. *Acta orthop. scand., 1970,* **41**, *272-291.*

STEWART (J. R.), DAHLIN (D. C.) et PUGH (D. G.). The pathology and radiology of solitary benign tumors. *Seminars Roentgenol., 1966,* **1**, *268-292.*

TRIFAUD (A.), PAYAN (H.), BUREAU (H.) et ARGENSON (C.). Les ostéoblastomes bénins. A propos de 5 observations. *Mém. Acad. Chir. Paris, 1965,* **91**, *890-895.*

TULLOH (M. P.) et HARRY (D.). Osteoblastoma in a rib in childhood. *Clin. Radiol., 1969,* **20**, *337-338.*

VICKERS (C.), PUGH (D. C.) et IVINS (J. C.). Osteoid osteoma; a fifteen-year follow-up of an untreated patient. *J. Bone Jt Surg., 1959,* **41-A**, *357-358.*

Various Other Benign Tumors

BANTA (J.), SCHREIBER (R. R.) et KULIK (W. J.). Hyperplastic callus formation in osteogenesis imperfecta simulating osteosarcoma. *J. Bone Jt Surg., 1971,* **53-A**, *1, 115-122.*

BENSAHEL (H.). Kyste solitaire des os. Etude diagnostique et thérapeutique. *Rev. Prat., Paris, 1969,* **19**, *2121-2130.*

BRODER (H. M.). Possible precision of unicameral bone cyst. *J. Bone Jt Surg., 1968,* **50-A**, *503-507.*

CAEN (J.) et coll. Pseudo-tumeurs hémophiliques (à propos de 3 cas). *Nouv. Rev. fr. Hémat., Paris, 1964,* **4**, *695-699.*

CÉDARD (C.) et RAINAUT (J. J.). Le kyste anévrysmal de l'os. *Ann. Chir., 1965,* **19**, *1104-1113.*

COHEN (J.) et CRAIG (J. M.). Multiple lymphangiectases of bone. *J. Bone Jt Surg., 1955,* **37-A**, *585-596.*

COHEN-SOLAL (J.) et HERRAULT (A.). Un cas de fibrolipome osseux. *In* Journées parisiennes de Pédiatrie. *Paris, 1967, Flammarion, éd.*

DAHLIN (D. C.). Bone tumors. *2e édit., Springfield, Ill., 1967, Ch. C. Thomas, éd.*

DAUDET (M.), MARION (J.), FRAYSSE (R.), VAUZELLE (J. L.), BAULIEU (J.), REBOUILLAT (J.) et LAPRAS (C.). Le kyste anévrysmal osseux chez l'enfant (à propos de 8 observations). *Ann. Chir. infant., 1971,* **12**, *7-34.*

EDEIKEN (J.) et HODES (P. J.). Giant-cell tumors vs with giant-cells. *Radiol. Clin. N. Amer., 1963,* **1**, *75-100.*

EDEIKEN (J.) et HODES (Ph. J.). Roentgen diagnosis of diseases of bone. *Baltimore, 1967, Williams and Wilkins, éd.*

EDLING (N. P. G.). Is the anevrysmal bone cyst a true pathologic entity ? *Cancer, 1965,* **18**, *1127-1130.*

ESTÈVE (P.). Plombage des kystes solitaires des os par un lambeau musculaire. *Mém. Acad. Chir., 1962,* **88**, *585-590.*

GARCEAU (G. J.) et GREGORY (C. F.). Solitary unicameral bone cyst. *J. Bone Jt Surg., 1954,* **36-A**, *267-280.*

GORHAM (L. W.) et STOUT (A. P.). Massive osteolysis (acute spontaneous absorption of bone, Phantom bone, Disappearing bone) : its relation to hemangiomatosis. *J. Bone Jt Surg., 1955,* **37-A**, *985-1004.*

HALLIDAY (D. R.), DAHLIN (D. C.), PUGH (D. G.) et YOUNG (H. H.). Massive osteolysis and angiomatosis. *Radiology, 1964,* **82**, *637-644.*

HARRIS (R.) et PRANDOWI (A. G.). Primary generalized lymphangiomas of bone : report of a case associated with congenital lymphedema of the forearm. *Ann. intern. Med., 1950,* **33**, *1302-1313.*

JAFFE (H. L.). Aneurysmal bone cyst. *Bull. Hosp. Jt Dis., 1950,* **11**, *3-13.*

JAFFE (H. L.) et LICHTENSTEIN (L.). Solitary unicameral bone cyst with emphasis of the roentgen picture, pathologic appearance and pathogenesis. *Arch. Surg., 1942,* **44**, *1004-1025.*

KAPLAN (M.) et coll. A propos d'un cas de myosite ossifiante progressive. *Ann. Pédiat. (Sem. Hôp. Paris), 1963,* **39**, *356-365.*

KUBICZ (S.). Aspect radiologique du kyste osseux anévrysmal chez l'enfant. *Ann. Radiol., 1970,* **13**, *211-218.*

LAPEYRIE (M.), PICARD (J. J.) et POUS (J. G.). Le kyste anévrysmal des os. Problèmes diagnostiques et thérapeutiques. *Rev. Chir. orthop., 1965,* **51**, *545-556.*

LAZAROVITS (P.) et GRIEM (M. L.). Radiotherapy of hemophilia pseudotumors. *Radiology, 1968,* **91**, *1026-1027.*

LEFRANC (J.) et NÉZELOF (C.). Les kystes essentiels des os longs. Etude anatomo-pathologique et traitement chirurgical. *Rev. Chir. orthop., 1957,* **43**, *385-406.*

LICHTENSTEIN (L.). Aneurysmal bone cyst, a pathological entity commonly mistaken for giant-cell tumor, and occasionally for hemangioma and osteogenic sarcoma. *Cancer, 1950,* **3**, *279-289.*

LICHTENSTEIN (L.). Aneurysmal bone cyst; observations on 50 cases. *J. Bone Jt Surg., 1957,* **39-A**, *873-882.*

LODWICK (G. S.). Juvenile unicameral bone cyst; a roentgen reappraisal. *Amer. J. Roentgenol., 1958,* **80**, *495-504.*

MERLE D'AUBIGNÉ (R.) et THOMINE (J. M.). Les tumeurs osseuses à cellules géantes. *Rev. Prat., Paris, 1969,* **19**, *2163-2174.*

MORCHOISNE (Ph.) et MASSE (P.). Evolution radiologique des kystes essentiels des os. *Ann. Radiol., 1970,* **13**, *811-826.*

MOSELEY (J. E.) et STAROBIN (S. G.), Cystic angiomatosis of bone : manifestation of a hamartomatous disease entity. *Amer. J. Roentgenol., 1964,* **91**, *1114-1120.*

NÉZELOF (C.), MICHEL (J.) et D'AMATO (J.). Le kyste anévrysmal de l'os. Ses principaux caractères anatomo-radiologiques. A propos de six observations personnelles. *Rev. Chir. orthop., 1960,* **46**, *369-383.*

OTTOLENGHI (C. E.), SCHAJOWICZ (F.) et RAFFA (J.). Le kyste osseux essentiel uniloculaire. Etude clinique et anatomo-pathologique de 123 cas. *Rev. Chir. orthop., 1969,* **55**, *287-303.*

POUS (J. G.). Hémangiome et kyste anévrysmal des os. *Rev. Prat., Paris, 1969,* **19**, *2153-2160.*

REILLY (B. J.), DAVIDSON (J. W.) et BAIN (H.). Lymphangiectasis of the skeleton. A case report. *Radiology, 1972,* **103**, *385-386.*

RIGAULT (P.), BENEUX (J.) et DESVIGNES (P.). Le kyste anévrysmal des os chez l'enfant. A propos de 16 cas. *Ann. Pédiat., 1972,* **19**, *223-234.*

ROSENQUIST (C. J.) et WOLFE (D. C.). Lymphangioma of bone. *J. Bone Jt Surg., 1968,* **50-A**, *158-162.*

ROTH (S. I.). Squamous cysts involving the skull and distal phalanges. *J. Bone Jt Surg., 1964,* **46-A**, *1442-1450.*

SAUVEGRAIN (J.), PARSA (G.), AICARDI (J.) et MANLOT (G.). Lymphangiectasies intra-osseuses et lymphœdème congénital. *Ann. Radiol., 1973,* **16**, *1-10.*

SCHOPFNER (C. E.) et ALLEN (R. P.). Lymphangioma of bone. *Radiology, 1961,* **76**, *449-453.*

SERRE (H.), IZARN (P.) et SIMON (L.). Forme pseudotumorale de l'hémophilie. *Rev. Rhum., 1966,* **33**, *555-561.*

SHERMAN (R. S.) et WILNER (D.). Roentgen diagnosis of hemangioma of bone. *Amer. J. Roentgenol., 1961,* **86**, *1146-1159.*

SLOWICK (F. A.), CAMPBELL (C. J.) et KETTELKAMP (D. B.). Aneurysmal bone cyst. An analysis of thirteen cases. *J. Bone Jt Surg., 1968,* **50-A**, *1142-1151.*

TILLMAN (B. P.) et coll. Aneurysmal bone cyst : An analysis of ninety five cases. *Mayo Clin. Proc., 1968,* **43**, *478-495.*

TOURAINE (R.), BERNARD (J. P.), TROULLIER (J. P.) et BALANDREAU (Mlle A. M.). Chylothorax et maladie de Gorham. *J. franç. Méd. Chir. thor., 1971,* **25**, *315-326.*

TRIFAUD (A.) et ROUX (H.). Aspects tumoraux des dystrophies osseuses. *Rev. Prat., Paris, 1969,* **19**, *2107-2118.*

VENOUIL (J.), FISCHER (L.) et BOCHU (M.). Le kyste anévrysmal des os (à propos de 7 cas). *J. Radiol. Electrol., Paris, 1970,* **51**, *186-187.*

WALLIS (L. A.), ASCH (T.) et MAISEL (B. W.). Diffuse skeletal hemangiomatosis. Report of two cases and review of literature. *Amer. J. Med., 1964,* **37**, *545-563.*

WITTENBERGER (A. R.). Radiographic diagnosis of lymphangiomatosis of bone. *Radiology, 1972,* **102**, *321-324.*

15 Malignant Tumors

PRIMARY MALIGNANT BONE TUMORS

Due to their very serious prognosis this group of tumors is given special attention in this chapter, in spite of the fact that they are rare in comparison to benign tumors and secondary malignant tumor-lesions. A special place will be given to osteosarcoma on the one hand and Ewing's reticuloendothelial sarcoma and reticulosarcoma on the other. Mention will be given to fibrosarcoma. Only a relatively short discussion will follow on the skeletal involvement by chondrosarcoma, juxtacortical sarcoma, and a few other tumors as they are seen infrequently during childhood.

In every patient the serious prognosis demands that an absolutely reliable diagnosis has been established. This can only be reached through a joint radiographic and anatomic investigation. Even with this approach there will occasionally be a patient in whom it will be almost impossible to properly classify a lesion. This does not even enable one to define it as malignant or benign. Only further development will eventually allow for the proper classification of the tumor.

OSTEOGENIC SARCOMA

Osteogenic sarcomas or osteosarcomas originate from bone-forming connective tissue. During its evolution osteoid tissue or bone is produced as well as some chondroid or fibroid cellular groups. This has led some observers to subdivide osteogenic sarcomas into the following three groups—osteoblastic, chondroblastic, and fibroblastic.

Osteosarcomas must be differentiated from fibrosarcomas and chondrosarcomas, on the basis of age of onset, and their entirely different behavior and anatomic appearances as they do not produce osteoblastic tissue.

There is no need to maintain the old subdivision for osteosarcomas as sclerosing, osteolytic, subperiosteal, medullary, or teleangiectatic. Only a few variants, for example, multiple sclerosing osteosarcoma, should be retained as this is a tumor seen primarily during childhood. Juxtacortical osteogenic sarcoma should also be retained. Osteosarcomas diagnosed on the basis of preexisting lesions, as Paget's disease, irradiated bone, fibrous dysplasia, and others will be mentioned briefly because they usually involve adults.

Incidence

Osteosarcoma without question, is the most frequently encountered primary malignant tumor of bone, with a 21.9 per cent incidence in the material of Dahlin and 30 per cent among the primary malignant tumors according to Calle and Chavanne. Only myeloma has a higher incidence but this is not a childhood tumor. We thus conclude that in the pediatric practice osteosarcoma is by far the most frequently seen primary malignant skeletal tumor.

Sex

There is a higher incidence among males, about 60 to 70 per cent depending on the statistics.

Age

This tumor occurs in young individuals. In spite of the fact that only relatively few cases are noted during the first decade, its maximum incidence is between the ages of 10 and 20 with subsequent rapid decline of the curve. The statistical data of the Fondation Curie indicate that among 54 patients, 51 were between 6 and 33 years of age and 43 between the ages of 10 and 20. In Dahlin's material the youngest patient was 4 years old.

Clinical Findings

Pain and local swelling are the two main findings in osteosarcomas. Pain is virtually constant, initially intermittent and very intensive. The interval from the appearance of the first local pain until the first medical examination and the first radiographic examination varies from days to several weeks, if not months. It is,

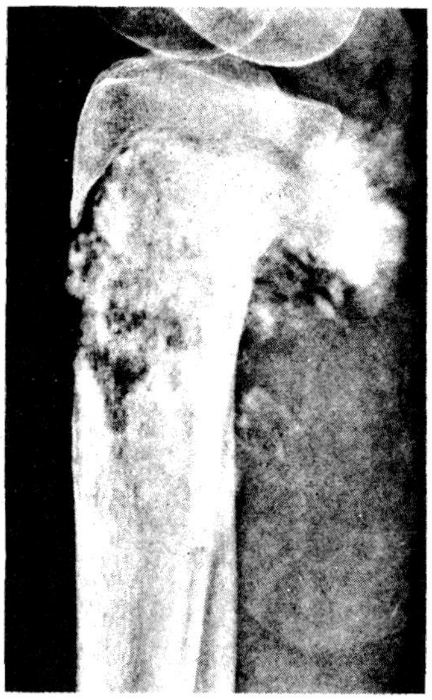

Fig. 15-1. Osteosarcoma. Note the diffuse appearance of calcification within the bony tumeral matrix.

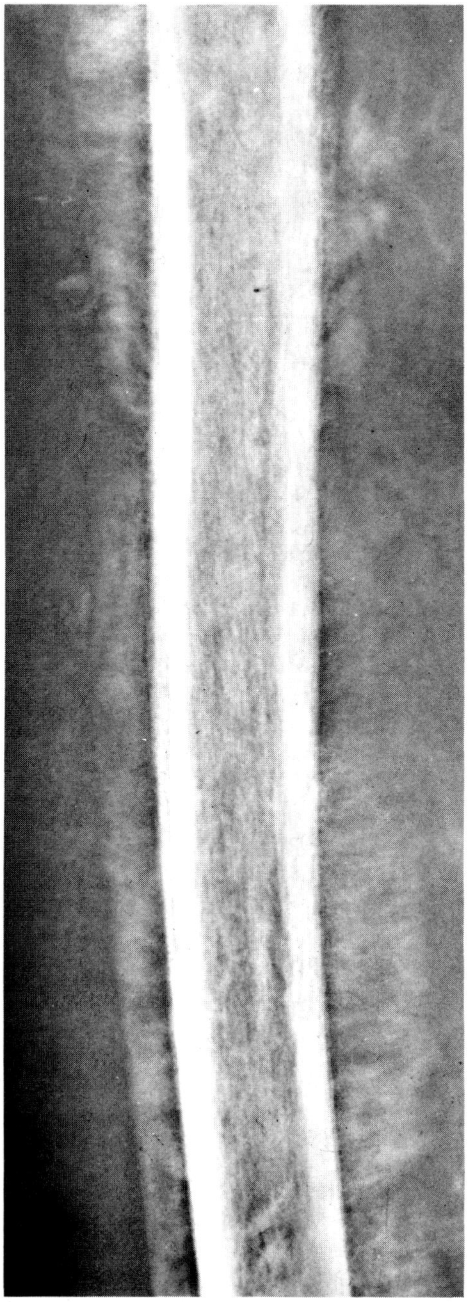

Fig. 15-2. Osteosarcoma. The degree and type of periosteal spiculation, with "hair on end" appearance, is unusual and is seen most frequently in Ewing's sarcoma. (Courtesy Institut Gustave-Roussy)

however, unusual to have local pain for more than one year. If located sufficiently close to the skin, even a deep seated tumor can be palpated. In slow growing types the tumor can become recognizable by a deformity of the involved limb, presenting a variable consistency and sometimes appearing pulsatile. The overlying skin is reddish, tense, and warm with a marked collateral circulation.

Pathologic factors are unusual except during the late stages. The general condition of affected patients is completely normal for a very long time. Laboratory tests are of little interest, since they are usually not significantly affected, with the possible exception of the elevated alkaline phosphatase in an occasional patient above 20 units. Such an elevation in alkaline phosphatase is an expression of the osteoblastic activity of the tumor. Thus, the values may be normal or only mildly elevated during early phases of tumor development. After radical treatment the values return to normal, but there may be a new increase, if metastases with osteoblastic activity develop within the lung.

Localization

Long bones are usually the site in 80 to 90 per cent of cases. In the order of decreasing incidence this refers to the distal end of the femur, the proximal portion of the tibia and the proximal end of the humerus. Almost three-quarters of all cases are affected in the knee area. Localization beyond the thigh or the wrist is an exception. Within the long bones the point of origin of the tumor is usually the metaphysis, and only rarely the diaphysis. The epiphysis as this site is very unusual.

Among the flat bones the iliac bone and the mandible are most frequently involved.

Radiographic Findings

Depending on the degree of ossification and mineralization of the sarcomatous lesion there is a high degree of variability in radiographic appearance. Some tumors are completely osteolytic, whereas others contrary to this are sclerosing. The majority of tumors combine these two features. All transitional appearances and combinations are possible between early condensing and purely osteolytic types. In the usual presentation there are two main appearances, the mixed types with a varying degree of condensation and the purely osteolytic types.

The mixed or condensing type (Figs. 15-1, 15-2 and 15-3). This tumor is characterized by a loss of density in the metaphyseal spongiosa where the tumor originates. This region is replaced by local condensation, often of increased density, somewhat eccentric and more or less expansile. The diameter will rapidly go beyond 6 cm in the long axis of the lesion. The condensation is rarely uniform. This will only happen in a pure condensing type, which is rare. Most frequently we note individual areas of osteolysis next to the condensation, more or less numerous and with a varying tendency to confluence. Condensation usually predominates within the center of such a lesion. In those persistently dense zones the tumoral stroma appears homogeneous and uniformly opaque.

The borders of the lesion are fuzzy and ill-defined. Extension towards the diaphysis is without a clear border. It develops much slower in the direction of the epiphysis, whether the growth cartilage is still intact or already beginning to fuse. The epiphysis, usually at its periphery, may be involved. Destruction of articular cartilage is not uncommon.

From its point of eccentric origin in the metaphysis the tumor has a tendency to extend transversely until it occupies a deeper area of the metaphyseal spongiosa. It will then develop towards the exterior and soon involve the cortex. In spite of the fact that it has already been infiltrated, the cortex in the early stages may still appear radiographically intact, while the periosteum and adjacent soft tissues are already visibly involved. The cortex will rapidly become demineralized revealing punctate osteolysis with a tendency to progressively enlarge. This leads to cortical destruction of varying degrees. This invasion and destruction is well visualized, especially in the mixed or predominantly osteolytic types. In the condensing type, this process will engulf the cortex, although this

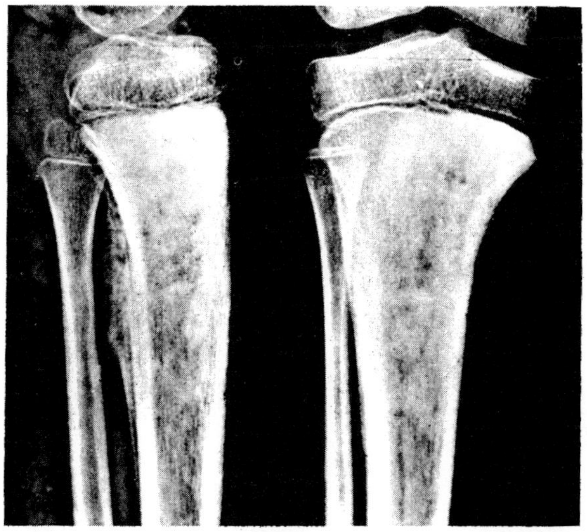

Fig. 15-3. Osteosarcoma. Typical aspect of the calcification of the bony tumoral matrix and clearly defined borders of the tumor's extent at the level of the growth zone. (Courtesy Institut Gustave-Roussy)

may not be evident on the radiograph. Once the tumor has penetrated the cortex the periosteum is stimulated in an attempt to build up a barrier of bone against the progression of the tumor. The invasion by the tumor, however, is so rapid that there is progressive infiltration into the newly formed periosteal bone which will also be destroyed. The periosteal reaction initially laid down in lamellar layers, soon shows signs of destruction at its center. However, the lamellar appearance of the periphery can still be seen along with its connection with the normal cortex. This peripheral layered periosteal reaction will be pushed out and eroded towards the center of the tumor. This represents the periosteal spur or Codman's triangle. It is well known that as an isolated finding no pathognomonic significance can be attached to this lesion.

Once the tumoral development has extended all the way across the cortex, periosteal involvement will become organized in a different manner. A number of fine bony calcified trabeculae will appear as fine lines perpendicular to the cortical direction and will eventually result in the "sunburst" phenomenon or a "hair on end" appearance. Occasionally, tumoral invasion of the soft tissues may be excessive, pushing aside the intermuscular fascial fat planes. This portion of the tumor developing within the soft tissues may occasionally undergo mineralization of its stroma and, as in the case presented here, this mineralization can proceed in large amorphous, almost homogeneous masses (Fig. 15-2).

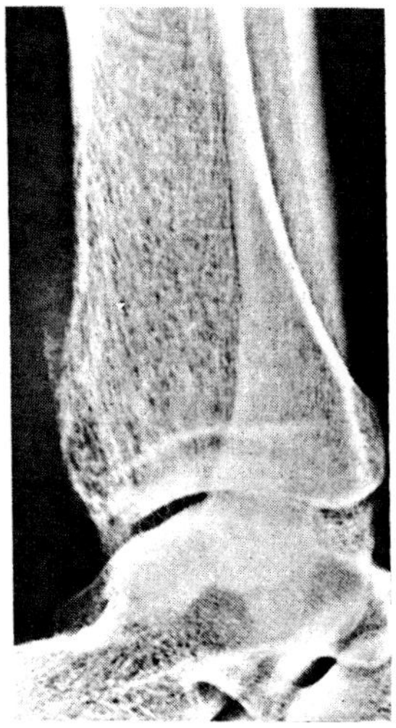

Fig. 15-4. Osteosarcoma with lytic characteristics in a purely cortical location at the distal end of the tibia. (Courtesy Institut Gustave-Roussy)

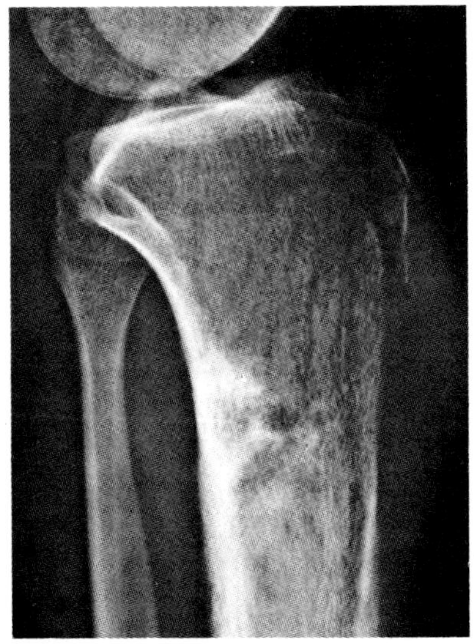

Fig. 15-5. Osteosarcoma of the upper end of the tibia with osteolytic characteristics and rupture of the anterior cortex and extension into the soft tissues. Biopsy of the tumor resulted in severe local bleeding due to the high degree of local vascularity. This could not be controlled and immediate amputation was unavoidable. (Courtesy Institut Gustave-Roussy)

This is the radiographic appearance of the mixed type of osteosarcoma. There is no need to await further development and rapid expansion of the mass lesion in order to radiographically confirm the suspicion of a malignancy. This presentation is that of a malignant bone tumor, most likely an osteosarcoma. A biopsy should be obtained as soon as possible.

The osteolytic type (Figs. 15-4 and 15-5), is characterized by a considerable radiolucent defect with a diameter above 6 cm due to its very rapid development. The borders are undefined towards the diaphysis and are mottled or punctate. The growth cartilage forms for a long time an insurmountable barrier to this tumor. Epiphyseal invasion occurs less frequently than in the condensing types.

The cortex is rapidly destroyed without bony expansion. The soft tissues are easily invaded with marked periosteal involvement along with periosteal and peripheral spurs. The tumor may develop within the soft tissues pushing peripherally on some bony cortical fragments which have not been lysed yet. Spiculation in the form of the "sunburst phenomenon" is frequently present within the soft tissues.

Pathologic fractures occur frequently and in such patients there is a lack of mineralization of the tumoral stroma. The diagnosis of a malignant tumor is obvious in these types. There may be some degree of difficulty in eliminating the possibility of a chondrosarcoma, a fibrosarcoma, Ewing's sarcoma, or even metastatic tumor.

These are the two principal types of radiographic manifestation of osteosarcoma. Other appearances are possible and von Ronnen differentiates from the radiographic appearance among 245 verified osteosarcomas, a normal type seen in 135 patients which corresponds to the mixed type, an osteosclerotic type seen 28 times, and a subperiosteal type seen nine times with an appearance characterized by superficial cortical erosion and periosteal proliferation. The cystic type was noted in 11 patients with an osteolytic appearance analogous to what we have described here. Finally, he reports on 62 unclassifiable cases, based on the analysis of the radiographic manifestations. This approach to differentiation appears to be somewhat arbitrary. Its author suggests that there might be some possible prognostic merit here and that, in particular, the subperiosteal types would have a better prognosis. But couldn't there have been some histologic errors here? The author refers to the observation that certain types of so-called periosteal manifestation also have radiographic evidence of fatigue fractures. If one considers the histologic appearance of callus formation with an appearance that can simulate an osteosarcoma (Nézelof) it becomes very difficult to accept this classification even with reservations. Other authors have attempted to differentiate central and superficial osteosarcomas.

We have more interest in questions of agreement of the radiologic images in a tentative differentiation between osteoblastic condensing types and the differentiation in chondroblastic hypoplastic or anaplastic forms of the last one appearing mostly osteolytic. Most authors agree that there is too often a lack of concordance between the anatomic and radiographic appearances.

Scintigraphy with ^{47}Ca or ^{67}Ga can help as a biopsy guide by pointing to the most active tumor zone, thus avoiding the confusion caused by the removal of an uninterpretable piece (Marsh and Choi).

What is the place of angiography in investigations of an osteosarcoma? Since the publication of Lagergren et al. it is known that most of the osteogenic sarcomas have marked hypervascularity demonstrated by arteriography (Fig. 15-6) with pathologic vessels present. The hypervascularity can be more or less pronounced and would seem to be more important in osteolytic types. It will certainly be very prominent if the soft tissues are involved and resulting in a much better appreciation of tumor involvement. The arteriographic appearance, however, is not constant and, therefore, not entirely pathognomonic. Other malignant tumors may have similar arteriographic appearances (Johnson et al., Geschickter). Benign tumors, for example, an osteoid osteoma (Lindbom et al.) can have marked local hypervascularization of a similar type.

If the diagnosis of a malignant primary tumor is unquestionable and if one is even sure of the presence of an osteogenic sarcoma, considering the severe prognosis, it is still impossible to rely solely on radiographic findings. Therefore, biopsy with subsequent histologic study, is needed.

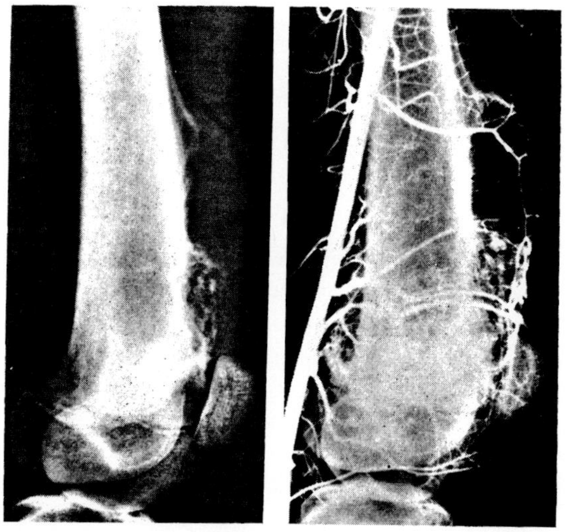

Fig. 15-6. Osteogenic sarcoma of the femur in a 15-year-old boy (*Left*) regular lateral view. (*Right*) femoral arteriography. (Courtesy of Chérigie, Bigot and Monnier)

Anatomic Findings

When the pathologist receives the operative specimen, the tumor is already highly developed. The cortex and periosteum are perforated and the soft tissues have been invaded. Thus, it is somewhat difficult to decide on the exact point where the malignant process originates. Intensity of central involvement in early stages leads to a reliable assumption of the actual point of origin. Only rarely will a highly malignant tumor be detected at the external cortical surface where it invades and develops subsequently within the bone suggesting a periosteal origin. In all cases extension occurs rapidly in different directions towards the diaphysis, this is while this is fundamentally different in the direction of the epiphysis where the growth cartilage offers a strong resistance to extension. When this barrier is finally broken, invasion is often only partial. Transversely the central forms extend quite rapidly allowing the tumor to attain the cortex and erode its structure. The periosteum will offer resistance to local tumoral invasion by actively forming new bone in subsequent layers. However, these will soon also be destroyed. Once this final barrier is broken down invasion into the soft tissues follows and the tumor may be surrounded for a limited time by a fibrous layer.

Microscopically, the tumor offers varying appearances. At times it is extremely soft with fibrous granular elements and then sometimes very firm with islands of irregular ossification and chondroid tissue. Thus, there are markedly varying local findings with partly dense and sclerotic zones. In the mixed types hard and sclerotic areas are located essentially in the central portions, and the necrotic, cystic, and teleangiectatic lesions, for example, hemorrhagic zones, can be adjacent especially in the osteolytic forms.

Microscopically the appearance of osteosarcomas varies from one case to the next and even from a lesion in one area to a lesion in another. According to Lichtenstein there are two essential criteria for the positive diagnosis of osteosarcoma. The first is the presence of a frankly sarcomatous stroma and second is the direct formation of osteoid and bony tumor tissue from this malignant connective tissue stroma. Actually, besides osteoid and bony tumoral tissue there are often more or less extensive areas of cartilaginous tissue or neoplastic fibrous tissue. Along with Dahlin, and depending on the predominant tissue present, one can differentiate the following tumor types—osteoblastic, chondroblastic, fibroblastic, and even in some cases a more highly undifferentiated and anaplastic pattern.

Aegerter and Kirkpatrick have attempted to divide osteosarcomas in four groups on the basis of histologic criteria. *Group I* corresponds to an osteoblastic tumor with direct tumor formation from abnormal osteoblasts without a cartilage or collagen formation. This type occurs most frequently. *Group II* is formed by tumors with a more or less abundant cartilage formation. Chondroid tissue is, in all likelihood, an intermediary step in the formation of the bone tumor. These types can sometimes be difficult to delineate from a chondrosarcoma. *Group III* is composed of tumors forming neither osteoid nor cartilage, but rather a collagenous substance which could be misinterpreted as the stroma of a fibrosarcoma. Metastatic lesions of such a tumor often contain osteoid and can actually form bone. *Group IV,* the rarest one, is characterized by osteosarcomas containing cells incapable of forming intercellular substances. For this reason there is no formation of cartilage or bone and only very little collagen. Cells vary and the diagnosis may be so difficult that it is often made in retrospect after metastatic lesions have occurred. According to Aegerter and Kirkpatrick two variants of osteosarcomas should especially be mentioned because of their histology. The first is the sclerosing form, which leads to an area of radiographic condensation and which is characterized histologically by the presence of osteoid tissue containing only occasional, thick tumor cells with relatively few nuclear anomalies. The second is the type described by Hutter et al. combining histologic findings typical for osteosarcoma and Ewing's sarcoma.

Generally speaking histologic examinations may offer real difficulties, however, they remain an essential diagnostic technique without which, as will be shown it is impossible, if not dangerous to begin any form of therapy.

Evolution and Prognosis

Left to itself the tumor will continue to grow, invading the soft tissues and the skin with local ulcer formation. Pain will become intolerable. There will be fever and after several months death will ensue, often precipitated by pulmonary metastases.

Prognosis for the survival of the patient has not significantly changed with modern therapy. Still, the survival has been considerably prolonged for many months and often years. Death is rarely due to local recurrence but usually results from pulmonary metastases, most frequently occurring within six or eight months after the onset of treatment. Usually several lesions will appear simultaneously along with pleural effusion, occasionally manifested by a pneumothorax. Once present, death will occur after several weeks or months. Some pulmonary metastases may calcify.

Skeletal metastases occur in about 15 per cent of the patients, mainly in flat bones such as ribs, skull, and vertebrae.

Only rarely will a patient survive longer than five years. The risk to develop metastases will diminish but does not disappear during the ensuing five, seven or more years.

Pathogenesis

Pathogenesis is unknown. It is possible that osteosarcomas are due to an oncogenic virus, but contrary to animal experimentation, it has so far been impossible to prove such a mechanism in man (Jasmin and Mathé).

The possible role of trauma has been discussed for a long time. Frequently incriminated, it does not play a more significant role than that it frequently leads to the recognition of the tumor's presence. There are, however, some very unusual cases where the possibility of a role of trauma as the causative factor has been postulated utilizing careful criteria (Padovani). If we consider some of the available information about osteosarcomas in animals, especially in the dog (Parodi), the role of trauma and repeated microtrauma cannot entirely be overlooked. Local defects favoring the influence of an oncogenic virus should at least be considered.

Clinical Types

We do not encounter osteosarcomas during childhood within a bone affected by Paget's disease. Osteosarcoma of the maxilla, frequently seen in adults, occurs only rarely during childhood. Osteosarcomas within portions of the skeleton after local irradiation occur rarely. An occasional extraskeletal osteosarcoma has been described, most frequently within myositis ossificans. Such a diagnosis, however, must be made with great caution, since this disorder can manifest clinically and histologically as a "pseudotumor" (Kaplan et al.).

Periosteal sarcoma is a special type and will be discussed in a separate chapter (see p. 404).

Multicentric sclerosing osteosarcoma, although rare, does have a tendency to occur in young patients under 15 years of age (Mosely and Bass, Singleton et al.). Several bony lesions are present simultaneously, involving both long and flat bones. Pain is the major presenting symptom, initially in one area of the bone and later becoming multifocal. Alkaline phosphatase is soon markedly elevated. In the long bones uniformly dense metaphyseal lesions are present radiographically, mostly bilaterally and symmetrically. These local lesions may be either few or many in number and they may involve any bone. In the early stages, there is a tendency to consider such findings simply benign condensing islands. They will, however, expand rapidly with cortical breakdown and invasion of the soft tissues in the immediate neighborhood which is proof of the malignant nature of this process. This special type is different from simple osteosarcoma with bone metastases because of the fact that aside from long bones, flat and short bones are similarly affected and the local lesions are of the same size throughout.

This type has a very rapid downhill course with early pulmonary metastases leading to death.

Treatment

Therapy attempts to combine two aims which are not compatible with one another to save the patient's life or at least to make the survivor comfortable. In order to achieve the first aim, mutilating and dangerous forms of therapy are required which is in direct contrast to the second aim. In order to meet this second aim one should limit a surgically aggressive course and preserve as much as possible the physical and psychological integrity of the patient. Our therapy directed against the tumor itself combines the following methods of surgical intervention, radiation therapy, and chemotherapy.

Surgery will attempt the removal in a block of the involved extremity at some distance from the tumor.

Amputation is performed after carefully ligating the vessels. Removal of the limb at the joint above the tumor is recommended. However, at times it is decided to simply remove the segment of the limb where the tumor has its seat if it is possible to resect at least 6 to 10 cm above the upper limit of the macroscopically recognizable tumor.

Exarticulation of the hip or shoulder, if the femur or humerus are involved, are the preferred procedures. Radiotherapy can be applied alone or prior to surgery. Today cobalt therapy or megavolt therapy, by betatron or cyclotron deliver a tumor dose of 7,000 to 10,000 rads over a period of eight to ten weeks.

Chemotherapy by intraarterial infusion is presently under intensive study. It is not yet part of the routine therapy for osteogenic sarcoma.

The approach to a single pulmonary metastasis or several closely clustered lesions within the same lobe is frequently surgical. At the time of surgery other smaller radiographically invisible metastases are often noted (Merlier). This can be missed even by tomography.

Radiotherapy has been proposed as curative therapy for pulmonary metastases since it sometimes prolongs life considerably. Some authors propose preventive irradiation of both lung fields at the time of therapy for the primary lesion in order to sterilize neoplastic emboli at an infraclinical microscopic stage (Trifaud et al., Roy-Camille et al.). This approach must be undertaken with extreme precaution and the dosage is limited to 1,750 rads given over a period of 16 to 20 days. This therapy is not without adverse effects.

Patients with multiple pulmonary or bony metastases can only be treated with chemotherapy which may slow down the eventual outcome. Indications and details of the approach depend to an extent on the school of thought and differ from case to case.

We repeat our earlier statement that any form of therapy must be based on reliable histological diagnosis after local biopsy, and in patients where the surgeon plans immediate removal, diagnosis from a frozen section. The danger of dissemination at the time of the biopsy is negligible, especially when compared to the conservative expectations brought about by a lesion considered erroneously to be benign, or, if a mutilating surgical approach is executed for a lesion that proves to be benign by subsequent careful histologic study.

Finally, the choice of the therapeutic approach must also be guided by whether there are pulmonary metastases or not. This is accomplished after a careful search on chest films and tomographies in addition to bony metastases detected on a skeletal survey possibly by tomography and isotope uptake study.

The overall results unfortunately are most disappointing. Aggressive initial surgery by amputation or disarticulation results in the best statistics in a 20- per cent survival of five years (Dahlin: 20.3% at 5 years, 17.3% at 10 years). Radiotherapy given alone results in a similar survival of about five years, but this statistical evaluation may be slightly misleading since one is often forced to amputate at a later time because of postirradiation damage by trophic local disturbance. Radiotherapy as an isolated measure will be the only possible form of therapy which can be offered a patient with an osteosarcoma of the iliac bone. Many oncologists today prefer a combined approach by initial radiotherapy to the tumor bed followed by resection or amputation of the primary lesion after four to eight months. Some advocate preventive irradiation of the lungs. The survival figures after two years are the same as in the group which offers surgery alone (26%, Institut Gustave-Roussy, Denoix et al.), and only slightly inferior at five years (Institut Gustave-Roussy; surgery alone 25% after radiotherapy 23%).

The approach combining local chemotherapy, surgery by resection or amputation, irradiation of the lungs, and systemic chemotherapy is interesting and will have to be adequately tested and statistically evaluated. The hoped for immunologic form of therapy promises a better survival rate. Actually, the healing rates of 10 to 25 per cent should result in a categorical rejection of the entirely pessimistic attitude expressed by some who refuse to offer or accept aggressive therapy. This argument should help the specialist and the family physician create a comforting and constructive approach to the family and the patient.

PAROSTEAL SARCOMA

This special type of osteosarcoma is typically an adult lesion. Thus, we will not spend much time on its discussion and direct attention to a number of respective references in our bibliography. This diagnosis should be made with only the greatest caution during childhood or adolescence, since it is a common error to attach this diagnosis to a patient suffering from ossifying traumatic myositis.

EWING'S SARCOMA

Originally described by Ewing in 1921 as diffuse endothelioma of the bone this tumor merits, according to the original author, a separate identification because of its diaphyseal localization, its uniform histologic appearance, and its high sensitivity to radiation. In fact, this lesion has resulted in many discussions with respect to its individual characteristics, and especially, its relationship with reticulosarcoma. Ewing was of the opinion that the underlying cells this tumor originates from are endothelial cells bordering on the vascular or lymphatic intraosseus canals. Osling was the first in 1928 to oppose this theory by considering that the tumor cells result from the primary cellular element of the bone marrow, the reticular cells. This opinion was later also voiced by Stout, by Lichtenstein, by Jaffe, and by McCormack et al. Oberling even proposed that in bone sacromas originating from the reticuloendothelial system one can recognize some lesions with an undifferentiated appearance, some however, are highly differentiated in the direction of a reticular, endothelial, or hematopoetic appearance. In 1939 Parker and Jackson isolated from this confusing group of tumors called Ewing's sarcoma a differentiated reticular variety. This disorder now bears their names. Histologic identification of Ewing's sarcoma is actually difficult and can lead to serious disagreements in interpretation resulting from necrosis, hemorrhage, sometimes inflammatory local reaction, and occasionally by simple chronic irritation. The tumor cells have only a mildly specific appearance and confusion with other malignant tumors can easily result, especially with metastases from a neuroblastoma. Willis, for instance, has for a long time questioned the actual existence of Ewing's sarcoma as he assumes that, especially during childhood, this was the metastatic form of a neuroblastoma.

This has resulted in a progressive reduction of the parameters of Ewing's sarcoma and the identification of a group of different metastatic lesions and the reticulosarcomas.

Does Ewing's sarcoma actually originate from an endothelial cell? Doesn't this tumor rather develop from a reticular cell which would lead to its being mixed in with the entire group of reticular bony sarcomas? Don't they both originate from the same cell, but at a differing degree of differentiation? This theory appears most acceptable, because of the evidence offered by patients where the histological appearance is transitional between the two, making a definitive classification difficult.

Even though some authors and institutions continue to classify all the reticulosarcomas including Ewing's sarcoma into the same statistical group, it is our opinion that this type of tumor should be studied separately, since the great majority of publications and institutions specializing in oncology accept this entity. If one plans to compare statistical data it is important to adhere to the same classification.

Incidence

If one carefully excludes from consideration with Ewing's sarcoma reticulosarcomas and other varieties of metastases, the incidence will be about 10 per cent among all tumors according to Ridings and 7 per cent according to Dahlin.

Age

The majority of patients are between 5 and 14 years old. In a literature review, Riding states that the youngest patient was seven months old, and in several statistics there is reference to an occasional case in the fifth decade. It is advisable to be cautious in accepting these cases at both ends of the age distribution since one should first consider the presence of metastatic lesions, especially from a neuroblastoma in an infant.

Sex

There is a male predilection (Bhansali and Desai, Dahlin et al., Sherman and Soong) whereas some other authors favor an equal distribution among the sexes (Aegerter and Kirkpatrick).

Clinical Findings

Pain is always present, but initially more or less impressive. By history this pain may have been noted for several weeks or months and initially there is improvement at rest. Almost invariably one can find a palpable mass, often of considerable size, painful to local pressure and of firm consistency. There is often some degree of local redness and warmth, sometimes combined with markedly dilated vessels in the neighborhood of the mass. Spontaneous fracture is rarely noted. General symptoms are fever, up to 38-38.5° C, leukocytosis, increased sedimentation rate, which together with the local symptoms may sometimes lead to the impression of a local inflammatory bone disease.

Localization

Any bone may be involved. The skull, the bones of the hands and those of the foot are only rarely involved. The calcaneus does however make an exception. Long bones are most frequently affected, most especially the femur and then the tibia, humerus, and fibula, which is relatively more frequently affected in comparison with other varieties of bone sarcomas. Several flat bones, the ribs, the pelvis, the scapulae, and the clavicles are also frequently involved. According to Dahlin 61.4 per cent of all Ewing's tumors in his statistics show leg or pelvic localization. Aegerter and Kirkpatrick claim that localization within long bones of the extremities is more frequently encountered during childhood and up to 20 years of age – 54 in long bones, 21 in flat bones and beyond 20 years this proportion is reversed – 19 in flat versus 6 in long bones. These authors conclude that this distribution is an expression of the tumor's point of origin to the disadvantage of the bone marrow cells within bone.

If a long bone is involved, the point of origin is either the metaphysis or the diaphysis. More frequently it is the latter and never the epiphysis. This structure may be secondarily involved after the growth cartilage has disappeared and fusion with the metaphysis has taken place.

Radiographic Findings

The radiographic findings of Ewing's tumor are not uniform. Not a single radiographic finding is pathognomonic, but a combination of certain symptoms makes this diagnosis highly suggestive. The most helpful findings are the following – extensive local osteolysis with a diameter above 6 cm, and a moth-eaten, riddled or punctate appearance along with a geographic border of undefined punctate character (Fig. 15-7). This destruction is located on the medullary side of the diaphysis of long bone, close to one end of the diaphysis. Secondarily, it invades the metaphysis itself at some length. The cortex is being destroyed

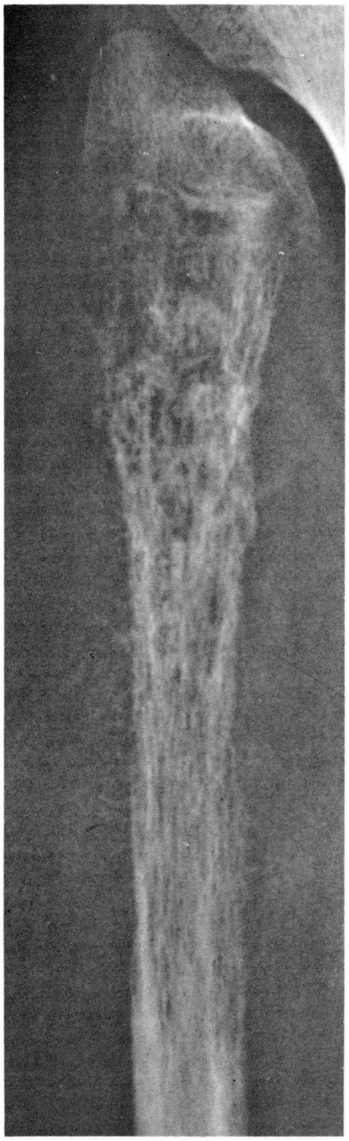

Fig. 15-7. Ewing's sarcoma of the proximal fibula. Note the spotty osteolysis and spiculation. The tumor does not spread across the growth plate.

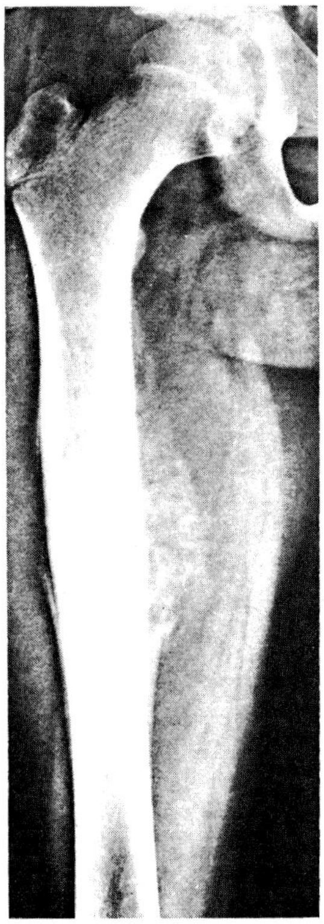

Fig. 15-8. Ewing's sarcoma. Note the radiating spiculation and periosteal spindle. The radiating type of spiculation is most frequently noted in osteosarcomas. (Courtesy Institut Gustave-Roussy)

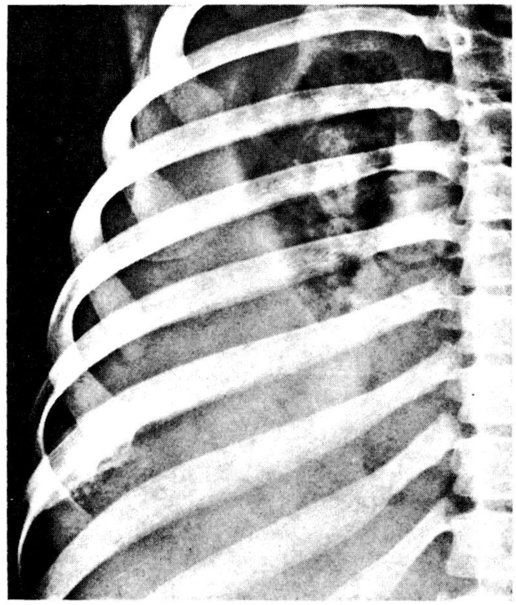

Fig. 15-9. Ewing's sarcoma of the 7th rib. There is a remarkable discrepancy between the involvement of the subpleural soft tissues and the relatively mild and localized involvement of the bone itself. (Courtesy Institut Gustave-Roussy)

and at times is blown up in places. Corticoperiosteal proliferation in either a lamellar or parallel striated fashion is usually present. If the cortex is partially destroyed there are fine poorly calcified spicules (Fig. 15-8) in an arrangement perpendicular to the axis of the bone. At the end of the spicula formation, in the location where the lesion is joined to the still normal cortex, a Codman's triangle can be found. There can be considerable invasion of the adjacent soft tissues with signs at some distance from the bone. This is the case especially of rib tumors often with endothoracic development (Fig. 15-9). Occasionally, there may be indirect signs by displacement of neighboring organs, in particular, of the ureters or the bladder during urography resulting from the pelvic localization of the tumor (Fig. 15-10). In the case of osteoblastic involvement this will only be found in a bone close to the lesion which has not yet undergone destruction.

Several radiographical appearances can be found.

Within long bones:

A purely central diaphyseal form (Fig. 15-11): The point of origin is within the medullary canal and the tumor itself is symmetrically expansile, purely lytic with a lamellar periosteal reaction, occasionally showing spiculation, a "sunburst phenomenon" adjacent to the central region of the tumor (Fig. 15-12). This appearance can be suggestive of an osteomyelitis or even an eosinophilic granuloma.

Diaphyseal cortical type: Characterized by a partial subperiosteal cortical erosion, this is an asymmetrical development with marked invasion of soft tissues. The periosteal proliferation can be of two different types. Towards the periphery by lamellar apposition and the formation of Codman's triangle or in the center spiculation with a "sunburst phenomenon" often of a fine, irregular, and poorly visible character.

Metaphyseal type: The lesion with a metaphyseal or metaphyseodiaphyseal point of origin is extensive reaching towards the diaphysis with ill-defined borders. On the other hand it is close to the growth cartilage and hardly ever invades the epiphysis. Its appearance may be purely lytic or may combine lytic and sclerotic findings. Reactive sclerosis involves the bony tissues, that have not yet been destroyed. Occasionally, periosteal reaction can be noted in lamellar or spiculated forms in bones together, depending on the individual

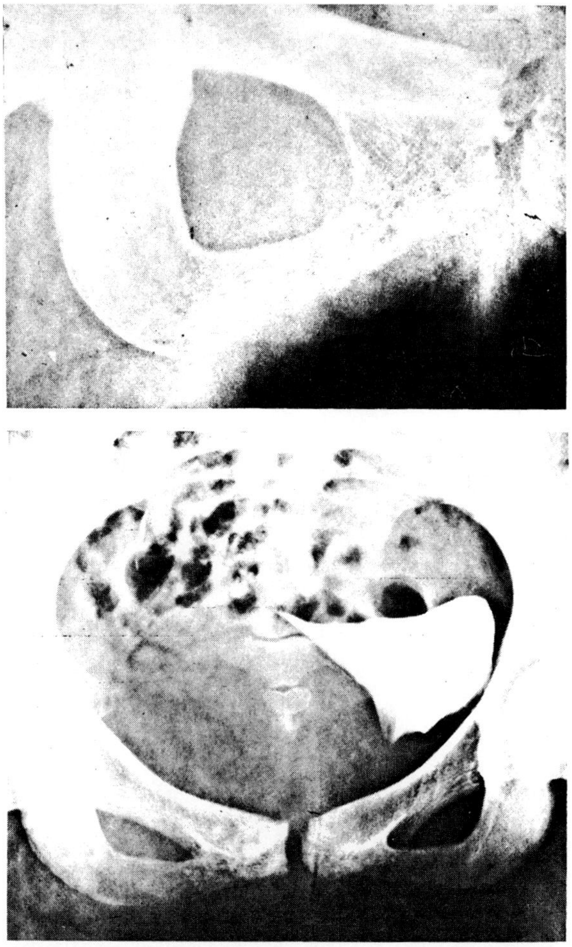

Fig. 15-10. Ewing's sarcoma of the pubis. *(Top)* punctate osteolysis. *(Bottom)* Note the considerable involvement of the neighbouring soft tissues around the inner surface of the pubis, displacing the bladder filled by intravenous urography.

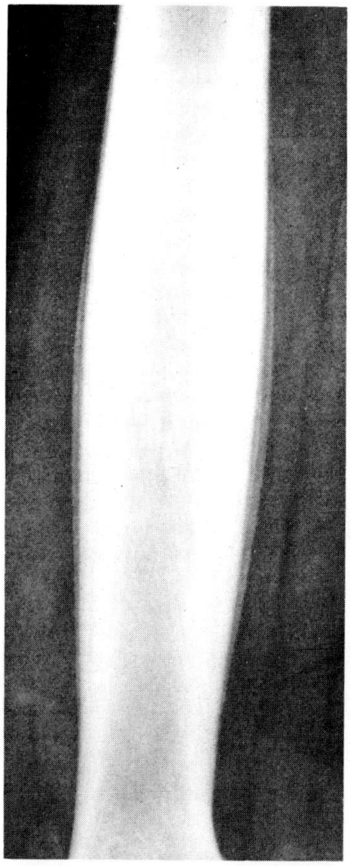

Fig. 15-11. Ewing's sarcoma. (Courtesy Institut Gustave-Roussy)

case. The radiographic appearance may simulate osteosarcoma or osteomyelitis (Fig. 15-13).

In flat or short bones (Figs. 15-9 and 15-10): Osteolysis is more important than condensation. This may, however, be very mild and hardly noticeable over a period of time with an appearance of a somewhat reduced bony density, slightly ill-defined in its detail and contours. This is particularly the case where the ribs and the pubis are involved. After some time osteolysis becomes more defined, often punctate with ill-defined borders. Periosteal reaction may also be difficult to recognize. Contrary to this, however, a marked extension of the tumor into the adjacent soft tissues may be noted. This finding is particularly prominent when the ribs are involved because the endothoracic extension will produce local opacification and push the pulmonary parenchyma aside. In patients with involvement of the lower ribs, the spine, the sacrum, or pelvis, this soft tissue component of the tumor can often be recognized by indirect signs resulting from displacement of the kidneys, ureters, or the bladder during intravenous urography.

Irrespective of the actual localization angiography is an important diagnostic technique revealing different findings of malignant hypervascularity (Kittredge). These changes are not specific. Such studies have their value in determining the exact location for a biopsy, and in a case of nonsurgical treatment, the exact territory for radiotherapy can be determined.

The malignant characteristics of the lesion can usually be recognized without much problem. However, one should be cautious with this diagnosis on purely radiographic evidence. Histologic study after biopsy is a "sine qua non."

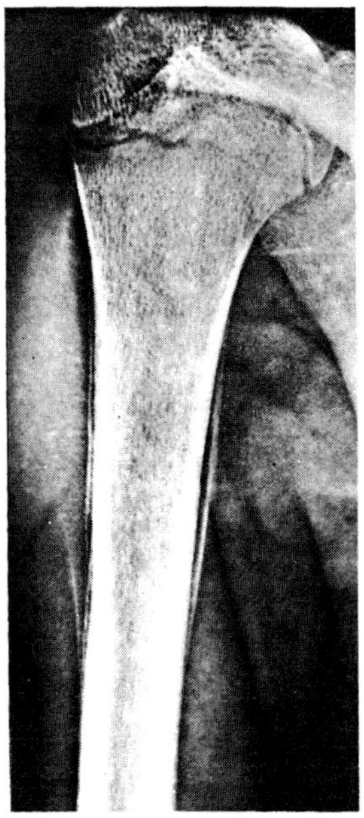

Fig. 15-12. Ewing's sarcoma involving the proximal end of the humerus. There is layered periosteal reaction at the medial and lateral surface of the humeral diaphysis. Note the spiculation—"sunburst phenomenon"—and Codman triangle at the lateral surface as well as the punctate osteolysis of the cortex adjacent to the striated periosteal reaction. (Courtesy Institut Gustave-Roussy)

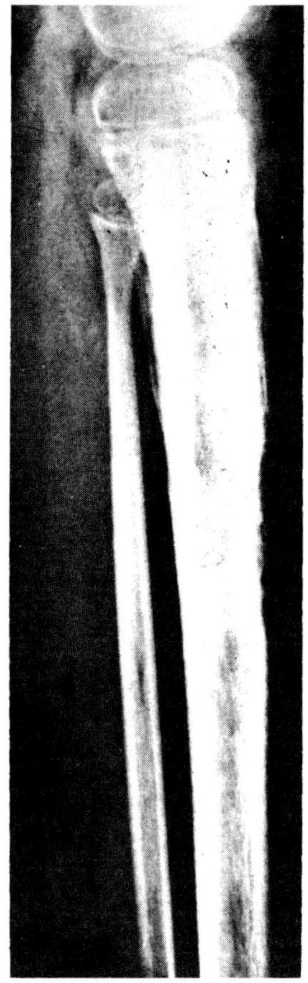

Fig. 15-13. Ewing's sarcoma of the upper tibial region developing an appearance which mimicks an operated osteomyelitis. Earlier this lesion was curetted, but not histologically verified. The diagnosis was not properly made until 8 months later, and this was due to antibiotic failure and the appearance of pulmonary metastases.

Pathologic Findings

Macroscopically the tumor is solid, but in some places it may appear somewhat soft because of local necrosis or hemorrhage. Occasionally it even contains fluid-filled cysts. The cut surface is greyish white or greyish red, usually glistening. Its extent within the diaphysis is always much more extensive than one would expect from simple palpation or radiographic study. Usually there is a rich vascularization. The tumor seems to be composed of uniformly arranged closely packed small round cells with only minimal cytoplasma and ill-defined borders. Mitotic figures can be found but they are not abundant. Using different stains one can show that the tumor appears to have a lobular structure with some rare reticular fibers outlining the globules and some of these penetrating into the tumor cells. In some patients there is a somewhat different appearance with larger cells of varying sizes sometimes resembling the cell of a reticulosarcoma. The cells may be round and arranged like a crown, but such pseudo-rosettes actually are cellular relics around vessels within necrotic zones. Sometimes it may be difficult, if not impossible, to eliminate on a biopsy specimen the possibility of a metastatic neuroblastoma or leukemic infiltration (Dahlin).

Evolution and Prognosis

Left alone this tumor will rapidly expand locally and will result in distant metastases. Metastases occur early and may be recognized as early as the first presentation. Frequently they are the result of hematogenous spread. There is still some controversy, if lymphatic spread also exists. Lichtenstein and Jaffe claim that this occurs only rarely and they would classify this tumor with the reticulosarcomas. Metastases are pulmonary in 60 per cent of the patients or skeletal in location.

Early treatment, in particular radiotherapy, will often result in an arrest of further local tumoral development. Unfortunately, recurrence is frequent and this form of therapy can rarely prevent distant metastases which will eventually lead to the death of the patient after several months or years.

Treatment

The excellent response to radiation therapy has been generally accepted. Cobalt or megavolt therapy by cyclotron or betatron is recommended using a relatively large field including besides the tumor also a good portion of the involved diaphysis from either side with a local dose of 5 to 6000 rads.

Several weeks after radiation we can note progressive recalcification of the osteolytic areas. The reactive ossification becomes more and more incorporated within normal bony architecture. The spiculated or lamellar corticoperiosteal involvement will widen and slowly fuse with the neighboring bone. After termination of this local repair process there may be very little local radiographic sequelae, at the most, slight cortical thickening. If radiotherapy is given to a growing bone there may be swelling or growth may be completely arrested. Surgical intervention by amputation or disarticulation is still advocated by some, especially in distal extremity location (Dahlin). Surgical removal subsequent to tumor eradicating radiotherapy is rarely recommended. It is only contemplated to alleviate the discomfort that the patient who has a limited survival period, is experiencing.

Radiotherapy of some metastatic lesions and tumor chemotherapy are further measures offered to these patients. Their exact effectiveness is presently under study. Systemic chemotherapy is certainly more effective here than for osteogenic sarcoma.

The association of local tumor eradicating radiotherapy in combination with total body irradiation and chemotherapy forms another new approach which has definite potential.

Ewing's sarcoma, unfortunately, still has a very serious prognosis with a 15 per cent 5-year survival rate under whatever therapy. The disturbing fact remains that late metastases may appear as late as 12 years thereafter (Dahlin). Ten-year survival rates are close to 10 per cent.

RETICULAR OSTEOSARCOMA

This type of bone tumor has been defined by Parker and Jackson under the name of "reticulum cell sarcoma." Its skeletal localization occurs, according to Dahlin, only in 3.4 per cent of all malignant tumors. There is a clear male preponderance.

This tumor can be seen at all ages, but only rarely in young individuals. It is mainly noted in patients older than 20 years of age and has its maximum incidence during the sixth decade. For this reason we will not discuss it here.

CHONDROSARCOMA

This malignant tumor had its origin in cartilaginous cells and it differs from other sarcomas, not only in its histology, but also by its clinical appearance and evolution. The tumor is seen almost exclusively in adults, even where it complicates a benign preexisting cartilaginous lesion, such as an enchondroma or osteochondroma.

FIBROSARCOMA

This malignant fibroblastic tumor has a matrix which produces neither bone nor cartilage. From this relatively simple definition fibroblastic osteosarcoma of all malignant bone tumors is the one most frequently questioned or debated, because of the difficulties in properly delineating its individual character. Some (Geschickter, Stout) are of the opinion that its central form is none other than an undifferentiated purely osteolytic osteosarcoma or invasion of the medullary canal after cortical destruction by a fibroblastic sarcoma from the adjacent soft tissues. Others (Dahlin) offer the same explanation in order to refute a periosteal peripheral type. However, the majority of authors (Aegerter and Kirkpatrick, Dahlin, Jaffe, Lichtenstein) still accept this entity by not only confirming the individual character of this lesion, but also because of its histologic characteristics, its clinical appearance, and special evolution. Fibrosarcomas can develop within preexisting lesions, such as Paget's disease, benign irradiated disorders, and osteomyelitis (Dahlin and Ivins).

Incidence

This is a rare tumor with a 3.4 per cent incidence among all primary malignant bone tumors in Dahlin's statistics and it is seen six times less frequently than osteosarcoma.

Sex Distribution

There seems to be an equal distribution among both sexes.

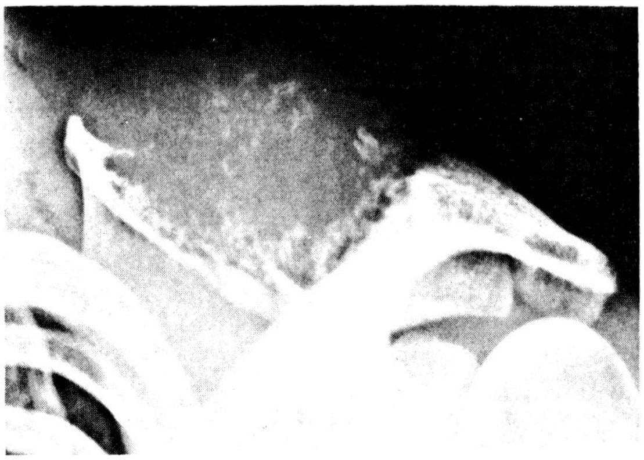

Fig. 15-14. Fibrosarcoma. Mixed osteolysis with a geographic appearance in its center and a spotty periphery. (Courtesy Institut Gustave-Roussy)

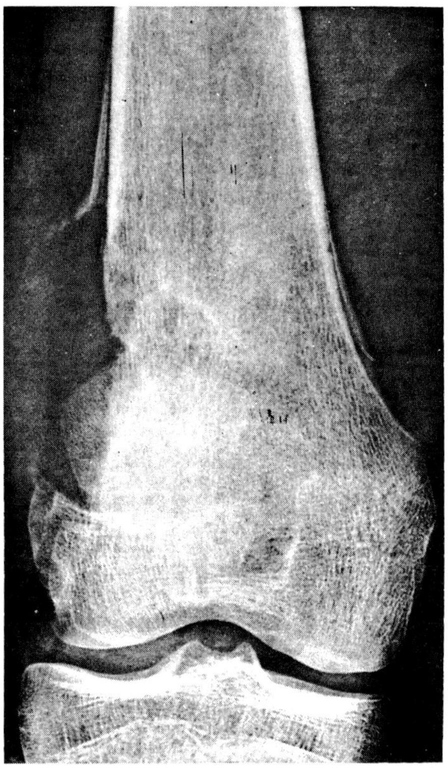

Fig. 15-15. Fibrosarcoma of the femur. (Courtesy Institut Gustave-Roussy)

Age

Fibrosarcomas are only rarely seen during the first decade. There is an even distribution of the incidence from the second to the sixth decade with a peak around 30 years (Aegerter and Kirkpatrick, Dahlin).

Clinical Signs

Pain is usually the presenting symptom and is sometimes present for many months and up to two years before the first consultation. This pain is often localized to a joint. The tumor is locally palpated in some patients. Pathological fractures occur somewhat more frequently than in osteosarcoma, and their evolution varies. Some types have a very slow development while others undergo rapid change.

Localization

As has been stated for osteosarcoma, about 50 per cent of all these tumors are located in long bones and in Dahlin's material 40 per cent of all patients had metaphyseal involvement—either of their distal femur or proximal tibia. Long bone involvement seems to be more frequent in younger patients, while the flat and short bones are more frequently involved in the older individual (Jaffe, cited by Edeiken). Maxillary and mandibular localization is said to occur frequently (Aegerter and Kirkpatrick), whereas Dahlin excludes such patients since he is of the opinion that in such cases the point of tumoral origin is not primarily within bone.

Radiographic Findings

Central type: According to Dahlin there is no radiographic difference between a central fibrous sarcoma and a purely osteolytic sarcoma. This is true, especially in the presence of a rapidly developing anaplastic fibrosarcoma. In well differentiated types there may be a degree of cortical sclerosis, the bone may be widened and the appearance may have similarities with an aneurysmal bone cyst. The widening of the bone however is seen all around and symmetrical in fibrosarcoma whereas an aneurysmal bone cyst would lead to an excentric lesion.

Peripheral fibrosarcomas (Figs. 15-14 and 15-15) are characterized by the presence of a mass lesion within soft tissues adjacent to bone, totally lacking ossification. The adjacent cortex may be thickened or eroded. Occasionally, it is even destroyed and the tumor invades the medullary canal. There are some cases, where the destruction of the cortex in the neighborhood of the tumor is not complete with some local remaining sequestra of cortical fragments. According to Edeiken "few other malignant tumors than a fibrosarcoma can bring about such a sequestration."

Pathology

Histologically these tumors are composed of fusiform cells, sometimes arranged in trabeculae or whirls.

As in other connective tissue lesions histology may encounter great difficulties in attempts at classification. There are all the different extremes and shades between a clearly benign and a clearly malignant tumor. If one is faced with great difficulties, or if there is hesitation in deciding whether one is dealing with a benign tumor or a differentiated fibrosarcoma with a slow evolution, then the radiographic appearance and the clinical course may offer important additional information for the pathologist.

Treatment and Prognosis

Fibrosarcomas are resistant to radiotherapy. The only reliable form of therapy is surgery. Aggressive surgical removal by amputation is recommended. If amputation at some distance from the lesion is possible, the results are far better than in patients with only partial removal. The 5-year survival rate varies from 25 to 30 per cent, but a quarter of the surviving patients will later succumb to their tumor. The slowly evolving well differentiated types have a far better prognosis (Dahlin).

UNUSUAL PRIMARY MALIGNANT BONE TUMORS DURING CHILDHOOD

Chordomas

Chordomas are rare tumors, hardly ever seen during childhood, and usually occur in adults over 30 years of age. This is a malignant tumor, developing from notochordal remnants located at both ends of the spine, the sacrum, and the coccyx as well as the base of the skull close to the sphenooccipital synchondrosis and the cervical spine. Radiographically chordomas are characterized by frequent asymmetrical osteolysis with a soft tissue tumor of equal density as the surrounding soft tissue sometimes containing small areas of ossification.

Adamantinomas of Long Bones

This is one of the rarest malignant tumors, almost exclusively involving the tibia. This can be noted during childhood as well as in the adult. Radiographically there is a slightly expansile osteolytic and sometimes multilocular lesion. The cortex is thin but rarely destroyed. Periosteal reaction is usually minimal.

This tumor is essentially a localized malignancy in spite of the fact that in an occasional patient there may be regional and even pulmonary metastases. Surgical treatment should be recommended including amputation, since more conservative management leads to recurrence.

Angiosarcomas and Liposarcomas

Angiosarcomas—angioblastoma, hemangio-endothelioma, hemangiosarcoma and malignant hemangioma and liposarcoma—lipofibrosarcoma, lipomyxosarcoma and lipoblastic sarcoma have their point of origin within bone and are only rarely encountered. These lesions are only diagnosed by histology and usually have a bad prognosis.

Among the nervous system tumors which occasionally have malignant characteristics, malignant schwannomas originate frequently from a juxtaperiosteal location with secondary bony involvement.

METASTATIC MALIGNANT TUMORS OF THE SKELETON

Secondary skeletal involvement by a malignant tumor during childhood or in the adult may be the result of local propagation or of distant dissemination by hematogenous or lymphatic spread.

Direct invasion as seen at the base of the skull or the facial bones in certain lymphosarcomas, reticulosarcomas, or rhabdomyosarcomas will not be discussed here. We will devote our attention to tumor metastases by distant spread. During infancy and childhood we are mainly dealing with neuroblastomas. Other primitive tumors can spread to the skeleton, but their incidence is significantly lower—nephroblastoma, rhabdomyosarcoma or embryonal sarcoma, retinoblastoma, medulloblastoma, osteosarcoma, and Ewing's sarcoma.

As in the adult a certain number of characteristics are common to all metastatic localizations, whatever the underlying primary tumor. Most frequently we find osteolytic lesions—either one or several. If we are in the presence of a neuroblastoma these may be indicative of the underlying pathology even when the primary lesion cannot be recognized. Cytologic study of bone marrow frequently reveals invasion by tumor cells. Hypercalcemia and elevated alkaline phosphatases are sometimes encountered in multiple metastases in the adult but rarely during childhood. Skeletal metastases always aggravate the prognosis and frequently are the hallmark of the terminal phase of the disorder. However, there are patients on record with at least 5-year survival rates after skeletal metastases in neuroblastoma.

Depending on the underlying tumor several peculiarities can be noted.

SKELETAL METASTASES OF NEUROBLASTOMA

By far the most frequently encountered metastatic tumors involving the skeleton in childhood result from neuroblastomas, aside from local dissemination of leukemia. Among patients with neuroblastoma there is a very high incidence varying from 38 to 74 per cent depending on the statistical data. Among 187 patients this finding was noted in 109 of them (58%) in the material of the Institut Gustav-Roussy (Rambert). Skeletal metastases are seen less frequently under one year of age. Later the incidence is much higher, even in the somewhat older child (Rambert). The metastatic tendency seems to be less marked if the primary tumor has an intrathoracic location rather than an intraabdominal one (Rambert). However there is no direct relationship between the early age of a patient, that is, less than one year, and the point of origin within the thorax of the primary tumor. The incidence of metastatic lesions is the same in a sympathogonioma or a sympathoblastoma. It is less, if the primary tumor shows a tendency to differentiation towards a ganglioneuroma (ganglioneuroblastoma; Bodian, Dargeon, Koop and Hernandez, Rambert, Rice, Salle et al., Stowens).

The timing of the manifestations of metastases varies. They are frequently present at the time of the first examination as in 59 patients among 187 in the material of the Institut Gustave-Roussy (Rambert). Nineteen times among 59 patients, it was the presence of skeletal metastases, which first brought the patient to medical attention while the primary tumor was unknown. Fourteen of these patients suffered from a cranial tumor of the vault, the orbit, or of the mandible and five patients presented with pain and tumors of long bones. This high incidence of metastatic presentation has been emphasized by a number of authors (Bodian, Koop and Hernandez, Reiquam et al., Richard et al.). Busfield emphasizes the high incidence of neuroblastomas with initial presentation clinically combining with skeletal metastases and actually presenting problems of differential diagnosis with orthopaedic lesions. The subsequent appearance of skeletal metastases may be noted in half of the cases before six months – 28 patients out of 50 in the data of the Institut Gustave-Roussy. Still, the risk of sudden skeletal involvement persists during the entire first year following the recognition of the basic disorder. In the following year metastatic complications are much less frequently encountered. Later development of metastases after 18 months is unusual but has been observed. In the material of the Institut Gustave-Roussy three patients presented such late lesions two, four, and six years after the onset of their disease (Rambert).

The clinical presentation is that of pain in a febrile infant, which sometimes leads to the suspicion of acute rheumatoid arthritis, osteomyelits, or arthritis. Such a suspicion should be based also on an elevated sedimentation rate. Local soft tissue tumors, and occasionally spontaneous fractures may be present. This, however, is usually at a somewhat later stage of the disease. Often a myelogram is performed in such pale and anemic infants, because of evidence for local invasion. The cytologic differentiation from acute leukemia may sometimes be difficult.

Intraspinal metastases may result in neurologic signs due to spinal compression. Such spinal symptomatology is most frequently the result of local compression by the primary tumor after local expansion into the spinal canal as an "hourglass tumor."

If there is cranial or orbital localization, patients frequently have all the findings of Hutchinson's syndrome with palpebral ecchymoses, which can rapidly disappear or recur and unilateral or bilateral exophthalmus, tumors of the cranial vault, or facial bones. These would be somewhat hard in consistency combined with a collateral venous circulation. In some patients intracranial hypertension may be combined with vomiting, headaches, and hypertensive eyegrounds. Optic nerve compression may lead to blindness.

Skeletal localization varies. The skull is most frequently involved with 91 per cent of all patients; followed by the proximal long bones, femur 83 per cent, humerus 79 per cent and the pelvis 71 per cent. Involvement of other skeletal elements, such as distal long bones, the ribs, the spine, the mandible, is not uncommon. The distal long bones are practically always involved at the same time as the proximal ones. If present, most frequently there are multiple metastases, either at the first workup or during subsequent evolution. This was the case in 91 out of 109 patients studied at the Institut Gustave-Roussy (Rambert). Among the other patients isolated involvement was noted, sometimes involving the skull, the pelvis twice and only once the femur. The predilection for the skull, femur, humerus, and the pelvis, along with the very high incidence of multiple involvement are emphasized in the majority of statistical presentations (Barrett and Toye, Hansman and Girdany, Kindcaid et al., Mardsen and Stewart, Scherman and Leaming).

Radiographic findings vary (Figs. 15-16 and 15-17).

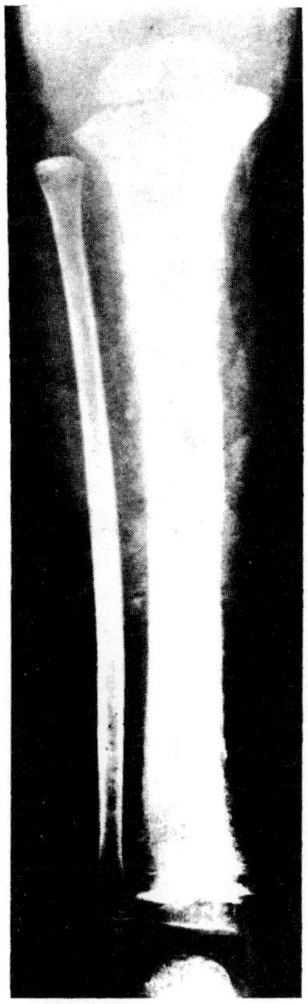

Fig. 15-16. Metastases of a sympathoblastoma involving the entire tibial diaphysis.

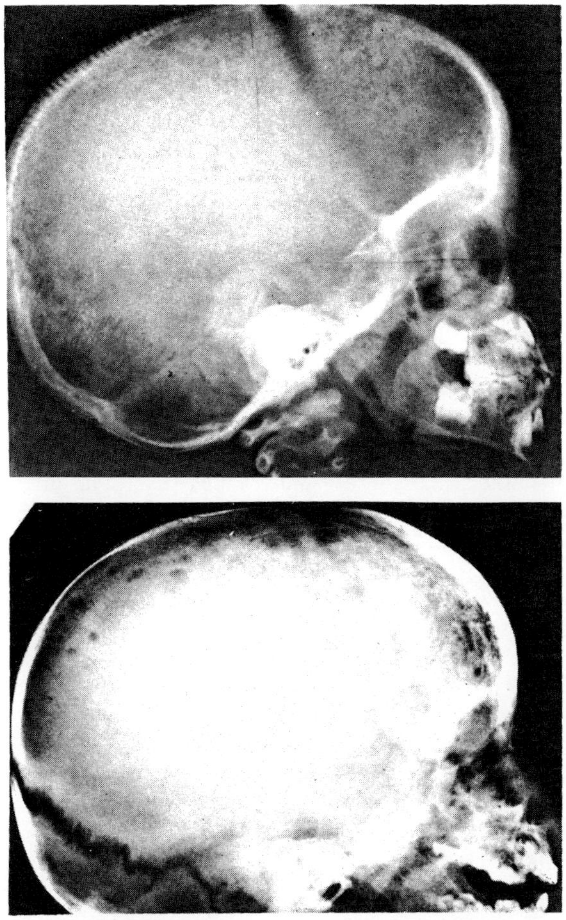

Fig. 15-17. Metastatic lesions from a sympathoblastoma to the skull. (*Top*) Minimal punctate lytic lesions of the frontal bones and widening of the coronal sutures. (*Bottom*) Somewhat larger lytic areas within the vault, with a motheaten appearance and more or less confluent progressive widening of sutures. (Courtesy Institut Gustave-Roussy)

Their appearance may be somewhat delayed with respect to the onset of local pain.

Osteolysis is the usual manifestation with metastatic foci. There may be a local motheaten or punctate appearance early, which will become more extensive and defined, eventually assuming a more lacunar character with ill-defined borders. These defects extend by effacing the bony structure and destroying the cortex. Condensation of bone can sometimes be noted, but never in an isolated fashion, since it is always associated with osteolysis and its proportion is usually relatively discrete. This mixed appearance is occasionally seen in involvement of flat bones, such as the pelvis, the skull or ribs, but relatively infrequently in the extremities. A periosteal reaction above a metastatic lesion is frequently present, most often of the lamellar type or like "onion peels." Sometimes this is the most striking radiographic expression and is more prominent than the osteolytic local involvement. At a late stage there may be perforation of this periosteal layer with the subsequent appearance of spiculated local reaction, the "hair on end" appearance with invasion of the adjacent soft tissues, resulting in an appearance similar to that of Ewing's sarcoma (Fig. 15-16).

Pathologic fractures may appear, especially involving the neck of the femur or the humerus, but also at the level of the diaphyses of the radius or ulna and even of the femur. Depending on the location within the skeleton some radiographic findings may have peculiar characteristics.

The proximal metaphyses of the proximal bones of the limbs are usually the first and the most frequently involved long bones. If the femur is more extensively involved, metastases can also be situated near the diaphysis and the distal metaphysis, but in the humerus the distal metaphysis is rarely involved. If the distal portion of a limb is involved, then the metastases are located within the proximal metaphyses. The epiphyses are usually spared and the growth cartilage is always free of pathology. Hands and feet are rarely affected. If metastases are generalized, there is frequently a tendency towards bilateral and symmetrical involvement (Rambert).

Skull lesions (Fig. 15-17) are on the whole characterized by small discrete osteolytic defects, located in the parietal and frontal bone. During their early stages it may be difficult to properly differentiate them from physiologic lacunae due to Pacchioni's granulations. Sometimes the lacunae are somewhat coarse and numerous and present a porous aspect like "a honey cake" or simply have a mottled form. There may also be involvement of the temporal bone and of the occipital squama, but these usually appear late. The orbits may be affected by small defects or more frequently by a clearcut local osteolysis completely replacing a portion of the orbital rim, either the roof or the external or medial wall, the floor or the lesser or major wing of the sphenoid.

The base of the skull is often affected as a late manifestation and the local lesions are, on the whole, osteolytic. Local lesions in the area of the sella are never accompanied by hypophyseo-hypothalamic pathology.

Splitting of cranial sutures is a frequent manifestation of metastasizing neuroblastoma. The sutures are wide and are bordered by marked serration. This widening is most prominent in the area of the sagittal and coronal sutures and results from intracranial hypertension. This is caused by extradural and intracranial tumors developing from the bone and the internal table, but which are stopped by the dura. There is no direct cerebral involvement and no invasion into the basal cisternae. Finally, in the area of the cranial vault, fine radiating spiculae, which create the "hair on end" appearance may be seen as one sign of diffuse osteolytic skeletal involvement, which is so characteristic for neuroblastoma.

All facial bones may be affected, usually by osteolytic lesions. Metastases to the mandible are not rare and they are practically always combined with cranial involvement as evidenced by 19 among 21 patients in the statistics of the Institut Gustave-Roussy (Rambert). There may be marked swelling of the gingiva and radiographic findings may be absent. If present, there are usually local osteolytic or finally punctate defects with destruction of aleolar walls giving the appearance of "floating teeth." A marked local periosteal reaction can be noted with invasion of adjacent soft tissues.

The shoulder girdle is usually combined in its involvement with lesions of the humerus.

In the early stages pelvic involvement may be difficult to differentiate from a false image of overlying intestinal gas. The lesions are usually composed of discrete osteolytic motheaten or punctate lesions predominating in the vicinity of the acetabulum. Often there is also a reactive bony condensation resulting in a cottony appearance of the lesion.

Costal involvement is often difficult to prove, because of a summation effect of the pulmonary images with those of the ribs. For this reason it is easier to recognize involvement of the midportion of the ribs on an AP film.

Spinal metastases are usually osteolytic and may involve several vertebral bodies and the posterior arches without much change in form. Collapse, especially of the anterior portion of a body, can occur resulting in a wedged vertebra or in a biconcave appearance between two normal intervertebral discs. It is not always easy to differentiate a local metastasis from a postcorticosteroid therapy platyspondyly.

Metastases to the ribs and spine must be carefully differentiated from skeletal manifestations which result from direct invasion of the primary tumor. In such patients the ribs are pushed out and thinned but are not destroyed. There is widening of the intercostal spaces. In the spine the spinal canal and the foramina may be enlarged.

Depending on whether the primary tumor is known or not, the diagnostic approach is different. If a primary neuroblastoma has been recognized, the clinical signs, and especially the radiographic findings, result in certainty that we are dealing with bony metastatic lesions. Confirmation can also be obtained by proving the presence of an elevated value for VMA or HVA in the urine and by the finding of tumor cells in bone marrow smears.

If on the other hand the diagnosis of neuroblastoma is still open, the differential diagnosis of bony involvement must clinically consider acute rheumatoid arthritis, osteomyelitis or leukemia. If one recognizes one or several osteolytic lesions of the skeleton, the radiographic findings lead one to consider in the presence of a single local finding, an osteomyelitis or Ewing's sarcoma and if there are several lesions present an acute leukemia with bony involvement or other tumors of the pediatric age group resulting in metastases (see p. 415). The primary tumor is usually found by urography and by the presence of elevated values for VMA and HVA which offer strong diagnostic support. Radiographically the most difficult problem is the differentiation of acute leukemia with multiple skeletal involvement from neuroblastoma with generalized metastases. If there are radiolucent metaphyseal bands we would rather tend towards the diagnosis of leukemia or neuroblastoma if there is spiculation or a "hair on end" appearance of the skull.

The prognosis of patients with skeletal metastases of neuroblastoma is especially poor. The 5-year survival rate in all statistics is close to 50 per cent in all forms without metastases, while there is a dramatic drop to 1 to 5 per cent in patients complicated by metastases. Everyone agrees that neuroblastomas have the best prognosis when diagnosed prior to one year of age. This is not only the result of the lower incidence of metastases in the first year of life. The number of survivors having had skeletal metastases is actually greater in infants affected during their first year than in the other age groups (Rambert).

The spontaneous evolution of the bony metastases is towards aggravation and extension. Spontaneous remissions are unusual. Under therapy associating chemotherapy using cyclophosphamide and vincristine, cortico-steroids and radiotherapy, the latter especially directed against the local pain, three possible courses can be expected.

1. Temporary disappearance of pain, possibly for a prolonged period of time, but with a complete lack of objective improvement, especially by radiographic study.
2. Complete clinical remission with persisting abnormal biochemical and radiographic findings for a number of weeks or months, followed by a progressive unrelenting course towards death.
3. Complete clinical, biological, and subsequently radiographic remission with definitive healing and the possible risk of one or more late recurrences.

There is no way to predict which evolution a given patient will have.

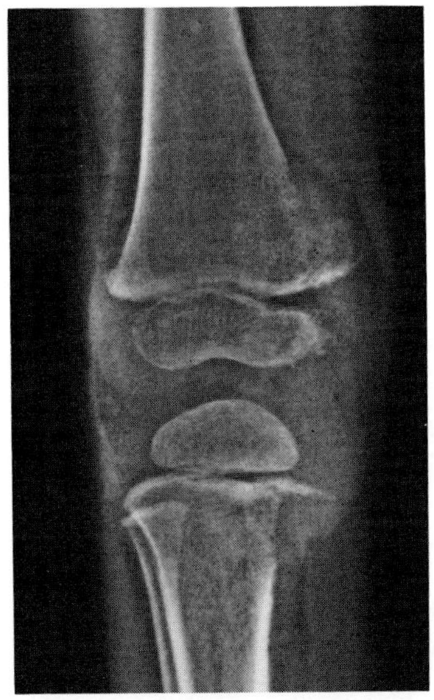

Fig. 15-18. Osteolytic metastases from a nephroblastoma involving the upper tibial metaphyses—mainly here on the right—and the right distal femoral metaphysis. (Courtesy Institut Gustave-Roussy)

SKELETAL METASTASES FROM NEPHROBLASTOMAS-WILMS TUMOR

Nephroblastoma is one of the most frequently encountered malignant tumors during infancy having almost the same incidence as neuroblastoma. Skeletal metastases are seen with a much lower frequency. The long term prognosis is dominated by the intraabdominal local situation and developments and by the occurrence of pulmonary metastases. In the statistical material of the Institut Gustave-Roussy (Masselot et al.) this incidence has been established as 4.5 per cent among all patients with nephroblastoma and with a slight predilection for boys. The incidence for skeletal metastases is the same, whatever the age of discovery of the nephroblastoma. The interval until such metastases appear is usually less than one year, but can be between two and three years. Such skeletal metastases rarely occur alone, since in the great majority—16 out of 19 patients in the statistics of the Institut Gustave-Roussy (Masselot et al.) there were also other metastatic manifestations, most frequently within the lungs. Bony involvement is usually recognized because of local pain and sometimes local swelling. Spinal localization may present as a paraplegia. Most frequently, however, the diagnosis of skeletal involvement results from a systematic and routine skeletal survey.

The highest incidence of metastases will be found in the femur, ribs, the pelvis, the skull, and the face. Within the long bones, lesions usually are in the diaphyseal or diaphyseometaphyseal region and only exceptionally within epiphyses. Single bone metastases can be encountered, but more often several are present. There are often three to six and even generalized dissemination throughout the skeleton can be encountered (Masselot et al.).

The radiographic appearance (Figs. 15-18 and 15-19) is essentially that of osteolytic lesions, some with relatively defined defects of a geographic type or more often microlacunar, with disseminated punctate characteristics and lacking confluence. A defect of the cortex in the osteolytic area is often noted.

Local bony condensation occurs only rarely as an isolated finding. Most frequently it is associated with osteolysis and leads to a mixed appearance.

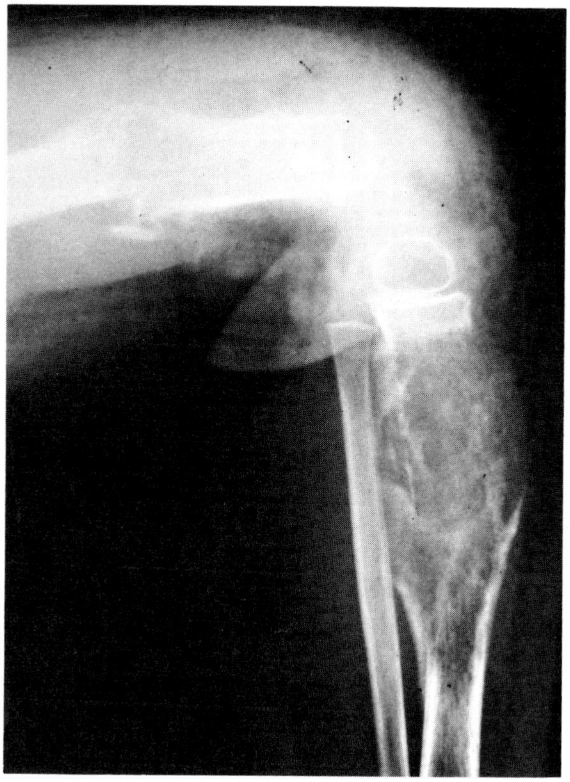

Fig. 15-19. Metastases of a nephroblastoma to the tibia and femur. This patient suffered a pathologic fracture. (Courtesy Institut Gustave-Roussy)

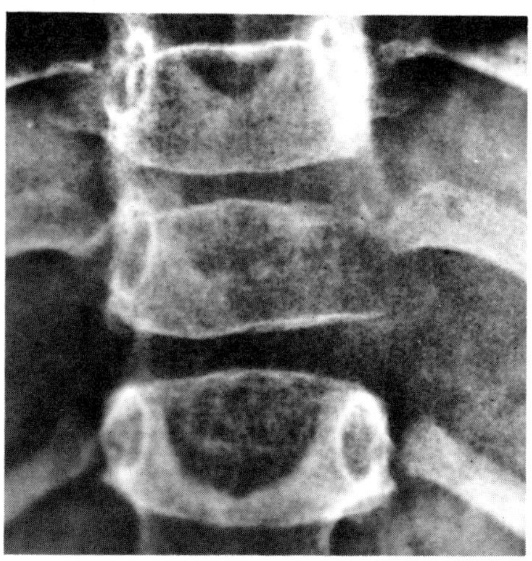

Fig. 15-20. Metastasis of a rhabdomyosarcoma of Th 11. Note the disappearance of the left pedicle and the neighbouring region of the vertebral body along with the left half of the posterior arch. (Courtesy Institut Gustave-Roussy)

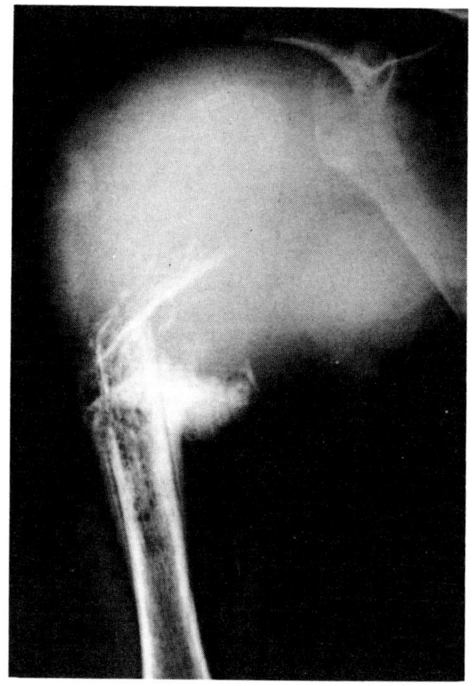

Fig. 15-21. Metastases of a rhabdomyosarcoma to the humerus. This is the same patient who is in Fig. 15-20.

Periosteal reaction can be present, usually of the lamellar type, with periosteal spurs and spicula formation in some rare instances. Adjacent soft tissue structures can also be invaded by the tumor. Metastatic bone involvement can lead to pathologic fractures.

In patients with rib involvement there may be an accompanying deep seated intrathoracic opacity which results from tumor invasion of extrapleural soft tissues. Vertebral localization is usually characterized by a mild degree of flattening and occasionally, by an unusually dense vertebra or "eburnization."

The radiographic appearances of nephroblastoma metastases are not specific. They are all part of an underlying primary tumor which has a tendency to form generalized metastases. The differential diagnosis should not offer any difficulties because in every case recorded, once metastases have occurred in nephroblastoma, the patient had already been subjected to a nephrectomy.

The evolution and prognosis for these patients is grave. Chemotherapy combined with radiotherapy in palliative dose range often only has a temporary effect which may aid in suppressing pain. Survival subsequent to the recognition of skeletal metastases is generally less than seven months, occasionally it may be eight to 14 months. Longer survival is unusual. This poor prognosis is considerably different from that of patients with pulmonary metastases of a nephroblastoma which can be curable.

SKELETAL METASTASES FROM RHABDOMYOSARCOMA

In the past these metastases were considered to be extremely rare, and the disease led to the demise of the patient in a few months after extensive and rapid local evolution. Progress in therapeutic approaches utilizing local aggressive surgery, radiotherapy, and chemotherapy has resulted in prolonged survival, but also of skeletal metastases which are generally of the osteolytic type (Figs. 15-20 and 15-21).

SKELETAL METASTASES FROM RETINOBLASTOMAS

This type of skeletal generalization is seen relatively frequently during childhood. The lesions are of the osteolytic type.

SKELETAL METASTASES FROM CEREBELLAR MEDULLOBLASTOMAS

These metastases are unusual, but there are a number of such observations recorded in the literature. They usually involve the axial skeleton, such as the skull, spine, ribs, pelvis, scapulae, and the proximal portions of the femora and humeri. These frequently multiple localizations usually combine osteolytic and osteoblastic foci. Periosteal reaction may be present and, on occasion, some degree of speculation is found. In a number of patients the osteoblastic type of metastases predominates. This results in diffuse skeletal condensation (Fig. 15-22; Black and Keats).

SKELETAL METASTASES OF OSTEOGENIC SARCOMAS AND EWING'S SARCOMA

These are generally of the osteolytic type. The discovery of osteosarcomas with multiple sclerosing foci should lead one to consider multiple localization rather than the presence of metastases. The diagnosis should be oriented towards osteogenic sclerosing osteosarcomatosis.

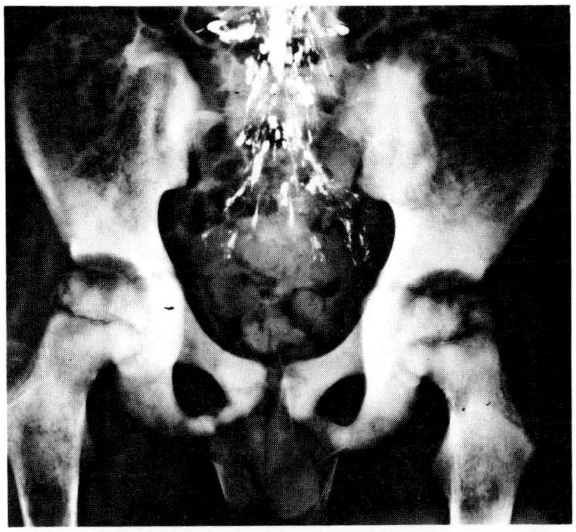

Fig. 15-22. Sclerosing metastases from a medulloblastoma involving the pelvis and the neighbouring bones. In this patient almost the entire skeleton was involved by this unusual condensation. The condensations tend to localize in the metaphyses of the limbs, but not exclusively. (Courtesy Institut Gustave-Roussy)

REFERENCES

Osteogenic Sarcomas and Related Malignant Tumors

AEGERTER (E.) et KIRKPATRICK (J. A.). Orthopedic diseases. Physiology, pathology, radiology. *Toronto, 1968, Saunders, éd.*

AMSTUTZ (H. C.). Multiple osteogenic sarcomata. Metastatic or multicentric ? Report of two cases and review of literature. *Cancer, 1969,* **24**, *923-931.*

CALLE (R.) et CHAVANNE (G.). Tumeurs osseuses. *In* R. Trial, Traité de radiodiagnostic, vol. 10; Os, Pathologie générale. *Paris, 1969, Masson et Cie, éd.*

CHIGOT (P. L.) et THUILLEUX (G.). Sarcomes ostéogéniques, ostéolytiques, ostéo-plastiques. Ostéofibrosarcomes. *Rev. Prat., Paris, 1969,* **19**, *2397-2412.*

DAHLIN (D. C.). Bone tumors. *2e édit., Springfield, Ill., 1967, Ch. C. Thomas, éd.*

DARGENT (M.), PAPILLON (J.), DUTOUL (L.) et MAYER (M.). Notre position actuelle dans le problème thérapeutique de l'ostéo-chondro-sarcome (d'après l'expérience du Centre Léon-Bérard). *Chirurgie, 1970,* **96**, *68-72.*

DENOIX (P.), GENIN (J.), KISSOUS (J.), SARRAZIN (D.), SCHWEISGUTH (O.) et WEILER (J.). Considérations sur le traitement des sarcomes ostéogéniques (à propos de 80 observations). *Chirurgie, 1970,* **96**, *63-67.*

GESCHICKTER (C. F.). So-called fibrosarcoma of bone. Bone involvement by sarcoma of the neighbouring soft parts. *Arch. Surg., 1932,* **24**, *231-291.*

GUÉRIN (R. A.). La scintigraphie dans l'ostéosarcome. *Chirurgie, 1970,* **96**, *50-52.*

HASTRUP (J.) et SKOV JENSEN (T.). Osteogenic sarcoma arising in a non-osteogenic fibroma of bone. *Acta path. microbiol. scand., 1965* **63**, *493-499*.
HUTTER (R. V. P.), FOOTE (F. W.), FRANCIS (K. C.) et SHERMAN (R. S.). Primitive multipotential primary sarcoma of bone. *Cancer, 1966,* **19**, *1-25*.
JASMIN (C.) et MATHÉ (G.). Perspectives virologiques et immunologiques des ostéosarcomes humains. *In* A. Trifaud et R. Meary, Pronostic et traitement des sarcomes ostéogéniques. *Paris, 1972, Masson et Cie, éd., p. 105*.
JOHNSON (R. E.), SENYSZYN (J. J.), RABSON (A. S.) et PETERSON (K. A.). Treatment of Ewing's sarcoma with local irradiation and systemic chemiotherapy. A progress report. *Radiology, 1970,* **95**, *195-197*.
LAGERGREN (C.), LINDBOM (Å.) et SÖDERBERG (G.). Blood vessels of osteogenic sarcomas : histologic, angiographic and microradiographic studies. *Acta Radiol., 1961,* **55**, *161-176*.
LICHTENSTEIN (L.). Bone tumors. *3e édit., Saint-Louis, 1965, C. V. Mosby Co., éd.*
LINDBOM (Å.), LINDVALL (N.), SÖDERBERG (G.) et SPJÜT (J.). Angiography in osteoid osteoma. *Acta radiol., 1960,* **54**, *327-333*.
LINDBOM (Å.), SÖDERBERG (G.) et SPJUT (H. J.). Osteosarcoma. A review of 96 cases. *Acta radiol., 1961,* **56**, *1-19*.
MARSH (H. O.) et CHOI (C. B.). Primary osteogenic sarcoma of the cervical spine orinally mistaken for benign osteoblastoma. A case report. *J. Bone Jt. Surg., (Amer.), 1970,* **52-A**, *1467-1471*.
MERLIER (M.). *In* A. Trifaud, P. Groulier et G. Roux. Le pronostic pulmonaire des ostéosarcomes. *Chirurgie, 1970,* **96**, *73*.
MOOKHERJEE (P. K.). A case of osteogenic sarcoma invading a paired bone. *Brit. J. Radiol., 1971,* **44**, *393-395*.
MORASCA (L.), ROY-CAMILLE (R.) et POULIQUEN (J. C.). Ostéosarcomes ostéogéniques de chimiothérapie. Etude *in vitro* de la sensibilité des ostéosarcomes vis-à-vis des agents chimiothérapiques. Applications thérapeutiques. *Chirurgie, 1970,* **96**, *53-62*.
MOSELEY (J. E.) et BASS (M. H.). Sclerosing osteogenic sarcomatosis. *Radiology, 1956,* **66**, *41*.
NÉZELOF (Ch.). Communication personnelle.
PADOVANI (P.). Problèmes médico-légaux posés par les ostéosarcomes. *Chirurgie, 1970,* **96**, *41-44*.
PARODI (A. L.). L'ostéosarcome (sarcome ostéogénique) chez le chien. *Chirurgie, 1970,* **96**, *75-80*.
ROSS (F. G. M.). Osteogenic sarcoma. *Brit. J. Radiol., 1964,* **37**, *259-276*.
ROY-CAMILLE (R.), ROY-CAMILLE (M.), SAILLANT (G.), DEMEULENAERE (C.) et LA CAFFINIÈRE (J. Y. de). Notre expérience actuelle du traitement des ostéosarcomes ostéogéniques. *Presse méd., 1971,* **79**, *1455-1458*.
SINGLETON (E. B.), ROSENBERG (H. S.), DODD (G. O.) et DOLAN (P. A.). Sclerosing osteogenic sarcomatosis. *Amer. J. Roentgenol., 1962,* **88**, *483-490*.
TRIFAUD (A.). Symposium sur l'ostéosarcome. Introduction. *Chirurgie, 1970,* **96**, *37-40*.
TRIFAUD (A.), GROULIER (P.) et ROUX (G.). Le pronostic pulmonaire des ostéosarcomes. *Chirurgie, 1970,* **96**, *73-74*.
VAN RONNEN (J. R.). Diagnostic radiologique de l'ostéosarcome. Classification des types radiologiques. Fidélité du diagnostic radiologique. L'examen radiologique peut-il remplacer la biopsie ? *Ann. Radiol., 1970,* **13**, *465-482*.

Parosteal Sarcoma

AEGERTER (E.) et KIRKPATRICK (J. A.). Orthopedic diseases. Physiology, pathology, radiology. *Toronto, 1968, Saunders, éd.*
DAHLIN (D. C.). Bone tumors. *2e édit., Springfield, Ill., 1967, Ch. C. Thomas, éd.*
DWINNEL (L. A.), DAHLIN (D. C.) et GHORMLEY (R. K.). Parosteal (juxtacortical) osteogenic sarcoma. *J. Bone Jt. Surg., 1954,* **36-A**, *732-744*.
EDEIKEN (J.), FARRELL (C.), ACKERMAN (L. V.) et SPJUT (H. J.). Parosteal sarcoma. *Amer. J. Roentgenol., 1971,* **111**, *579-583*.
GESCHICKTER (C. F.) et COPELAND (M. M.). Parosteal osteoma of bone; a new entity. *Ann. Surg., 1951,* **133**, *790-807*.
LAURENCE (G.). Sarcomes juxta-corticaux. *Rev. Prat., Paris, 1969,* **19**, *2461-2465*.
MERLE D'AUBIGNÉ (R.), MEARY (R.) et MAZABRAUD (A.). Sarcome ostéogénique juxta-cortical. *Rev. Chir. orthop., 1959,* **45**, *873-884*.
MERLE D'AUBIGNÉ (R.) et THOMINE (J. M.). A propos de 9 cas de sarcomes juxta-corticaux. *Chirurgie, 1970,* **96**, *45-49*.
STEVENS (G. M.), PUGH (D. G.) et DAHLIN (D. C.). Roentgenographic recognition and differentiation of parosteal osteogenic sarcoma. *Amer. J. Roentgenol., 1957,* **78**, *1-12*.

Ewing's Sarcoma and Reticulo-sarcoma

AEGERTER (E.) et KIRKPATRICK (J. A.). Orthopedic diseases. Physiology, pathology, radiology. *Toronto, 1968, Saunders, éd.*
BHANSALI (S. K.) et DESAI (P. P.). Ewing's sarcoma. Observations on 107 cases. *J. Bone Jt. Surg., 1963,* **45-A**, *541-553*.
COLVILLE (H. C.) et WILLIS (R. A.). Neuroblastoma metastases in bones with a criticism of Ewing's endothelioma. *Amer. J. Path., 1933,* **9**, *421-429*.
DAHLIN (D. C.). Bone tumors. *2e édit., Springfield, Ill., 1967, Ch. C. Thomas, éd.*
DAHLIN (D. C.), COVENTRY (M. B.) et SCANLON (P. W.). Ewing's sarcoma. A critical analysis of 165 cases. *J. Bone Jt. Surg., 1961,* **43-A**, *185-192*.
EWING (J.). Diffuse endothelioma of bone. *Proc. N. Y. path. Soc., 1921,* **21**, *17-24*.
GOUIN (J. L.). Endothélioréticulosarcomes d'Ewing et réticulosarcomes. *Rev. Prat., Paris, 1969,* **19**, *2431-2439*.
HOURTOULLE (F. G.). Réticulosarcomes osseux. *Encyclopédie méd.-chir. : Appareil loco-moteur, 14030 E1*.
JENKIN (R. D. T.), RIDER (W. D.) et SONLEY (M. J.). Ewing's sarcoma. A trial of adjuvant total-body irradiation. *Radiology, 1970,* **96**, *151-155*.
JOHNSON (R. E.), SENYSZYN (J. J.), RABSON (A. S.) et PETERSON (K. A.). Treatment of Ewing's sarcoma with local irradiation and systemic chemiotherapy. A progress report. *Radiology, 1970,* **95**, *195-197*.
KITTREDGE (R. D.). Arteriography in Ewing's tumor. *Radiology, 1970,* **97**, *609-610*.
LICHTENSTEIN (L.) et JAFFÉ (H. L.). Ewing's sarcoma of bone. *Amer. J. Path., 1947,* **23**, *43-77*.
MAC CORMACK (J. L.), DOCKERTY (M. B.) et GHORMLEY (R. K.). Ewing's sarcoma. *Cancer, 1952,* **5**, *85-99*.
MORGAN (S. K.) et THURDMAN (W. G.). Ewing's sarcoma in children. Lessons from four cases. *Clin. Pediat., 1970,* **9**, *37-41*.
NACCACHE (G.). Aspects radiologiques des sarcomes

osseux réticulaires (tumeurs d'Ewing et réticulosarcomes). Etude analytique de 114 observations. *Thèse Méd., Paris, 1967.*

Oberling (C.). Les réticulosarcomes et les réticulo-endothélio-sarcomes de la moelle osseuse. *Bull. Ass. franç. Cancer, 1928,* **17**, *259-296.*

Parker (F.) et Jackson (H.). Primary reticulum-cell sarcoma of bone. *Surg. Gynec. Obstet., 1939,* **68**, *45-53.*

Phelan (J. T.) et Cabrera (A.). Ewing's sarcoma. *Surg. Gynec. Obstet., 1964,* **118**, *795-800.*

Philips (R. F.) et Higinbotham (N. L.). The curability of Ewing's endothelioma of bone in children. *J. Ped., 1967,* **70**, *391-397.*

Ridings (G. R.). Ewing's tumor. *Radiol. Clin. N. Amer., 1964,* **2**, *315-325.*

Schajowicz (F.). Ewing's sarcoma and reticulum-cell sarcoma of bone. With special reference to the histochemical demonstration of glycogen as an aid to defferential diagnosis. *J. Bone Jt Surg., 1959,* **21-A**, *349-356.*

Sherman (R. S.) et Soong (K. Y.). Ewing's sarcoma. Its roentgen classification and diagnosis. *Radiology, 1956,* **66**, *529-539.*

Stout (A. P.). A discussion of the pathology and histogenesis of Ewing's tumor of bone marrow. *Amer. J. Roentgenol., 1943,* **50**, *334-342.*

Willis (R. A.). Metastasis neuroblastoma in bone presenting the Ewing's syndroma. With a discussion of « Ewing's sarcoma ». *Amer. J. Path., 1940,* **16**, *317-331.*

Chondrosarcoma

Aegerter (E.) et Kirkpatrick (J. A.). Orthopedic diseases. Physiology, pathology, radiology. *Toronto, 1968, Saunders, éd.*

Dahlin (D. C.). Bone tumors. *2e édit., Springfield, Ill., 1967, Ch. C. Thomas, éd.*

Chavanne (G.), Calle (R.) et Schlienger (P.). A propos des chondrosarcomes osseux (étude radioclinique de 44 observations). *J. Radiol. Electrol., Paris, 1971,* **52**, *425-438.*

Henderson (D.) et Dahlin (D. C.). Chondrosarcoma of bone. A study of two hundred and eighty eight cases. *J. Bone Jt Surg., 1963,* **45-A**, *1450-1458.*

Lagersen (C.), Lindbom (Å) et Söderberg (G.). The blood vessels of chondrosarcoma. *Acta radiol., 1961,* **55**, *321-328.*

Lindbom (Å), Söderberg (G.) et Spjüt (H. J.). Primary chondrosarcoma of bone. *Acta radiol., 1961,* **55**, *81-96.*

Merle d'Aubigné (R.), Meary (R.), Gauthier-Villars (P.) et Nézelof (C.). A propos du diagnostic de malignité dans les tumeurs cartilagineuses. *Mém. Acad. Chir., 1958,* **84**, *83-92.*

Phelan (J. T.) et Cabrera (A.). Chondrosarcoma of bone. *Surg. Gynec. Obstet., 1964,* **119**, *42-46.*

Roger (A.) et Meary (R.). Les chondrosarcomes. *Rev. Prat., Paris, 1969,* **19**, *2415-2422.*

Fibrosarcoma

Aegerter (E.) et Kirkpatrick (J. A.). Orthopedic diseases. Physiology, pathology, radiology. *Toronto, 1968, Saunders, éd.*

Dahlin (D. C.). Bone tumors. *2e édit., Springfield, Ill., 1967. Ch. C. Thomas, éd.*

Dahlin (D. C.) et Ivins (J. C.). Fibrosarcoma of bone. A study of 114 cases. *Cancer, 1969,* **23**, *35-41.*

Edeiken (J.) et Hodes (Ph. J.). Roentgen diagnosis of diseases of bone. *Baltimore, 1967, Williams and Wilkins, éd.*

Geschickter (C. F.). So-called fibrosarcoma of bone. Bone involvement by sarcoma of the neighbouring soft parts. *Arch. Surg., 1932,* **24**, *231-291.*

Jaffé (H. L.). Tumors and tumorous conditions of bones and joints. *Philadelphie, 1958. Lea and Febiger, éd.*

Lagergren (C.), Lindbom (Å) et Söderberg (G.). Vascularization of fibromatous and fibrosarcomatous tumors : histopathologic, microradiographic and angiographic studies. *Acta radiol., 1960,* **53**, *1-15.*

Laurence (G.). Fibrosarcomes. *Rev. Prat., Paris, 1969,* **19**, *2425-2429.*

Lichtenstein (L.). Bone tumors. *3e édit., Saint Louis, 1965, C. V. Mosby Co., éd.*

Stout (A. P.). Fibrosarcoma. The malignant tumor of fibroblasts. *Cancer, 1948,* **1**, *30-63.*

Other Malignant Tumors

Bundens (B. W., Jr.) et Brighton (C. T.). Malignant hemangioendothelioma of bone. Report of two cases and review of literature. *J. Bone Jt Surg., 1965,* **47-A**, *762-772.*

Christensen (E.), Hojgaard (K.) et Winkel-Smith (C. C.). Congenital malignant mesenchymal tumors in a two months old child. *Acta path. microbiol. scand., 1961,* **53**, *237-242.*

Delarue (J.), Chomette (G.) et Brocheriou (C.). Adamantinome du tibia et dysplasie fibreuse. *Ann. Anat. path., 1964,* **9**, *373-378.*

Evans (R. W.), Thomas (C. E.) et Walker (N. M.). A congenital malignant synovial tumour of bone. *J. Bone Jt Surg., 1960,* **43-B**, *742-748.*

Hartmann (W. H.) et Stewart (F. W.). Hemangioendothelioma of bone. Unusual tumor characterized by indolent course. *Cancer, 1962,* **15**, *846-854.*

Merle d'Aubigné (R.). Adamantinome du tibia. *Rev. Chir. orthop., 1960,* **46**, *92-96.*

Otis (J.). Hemangioendothelioma of bone. *Surg. Gynec. Obstet., 1968,* **127**, *295-305.*

Retz (L. D., Jr.). Primary liposarcoma of bone. Report of a case and review of the literature. *J. Bone Jt Surg., 1961,* **43-A**, *123-129.*

Ross (C. F.) et Hadfield (G.). Primary osteoliposarcoma of bone (malignant mesenchymoma). Report of a case. *J. Bone Jt Surg., 1968,* **50-B**, *639-643.*

Rosenquist (H.) et Saltzman (G. F.). Sacro-coccygeal and vertebral chordomas and their treatment. *Acta radiol., 1959,* **52**, *177-193.*

Slavens (J. J.). Congenital fibromyxosarcoma of os calcis. *Pediatrics, 1953,* **11**, *617-621.*

Wells (H. G.). Occurrence and significance of congenital malignant neoplasms. *Arch. Path., 1940,* **30**, *535-601.*

Metastatic Tumors

Banna (M.), Lassman (L. P.) et Pearce (G. W.). Radiological study of skeletal metastases from cerebellar medulloblastoma. *Brit. J. Radiol., 1970,* **43**, *173-179.*

Barrett (A. F.) et Toye (D. K. M.). Sympathoblastoma : radiological findings in forty-three cases. *Clin. Radiol., 1963,* **14**, *33-42.*

BLACK (P. W.) et KEATS (T. E.). Generalised osteosclerosis secondary to metastatic medulloblastoma of the cerebellum. *Radiology, 1964,* **82**, *395-400.*

BODIAN (M.). Neuroblastoma. *Pediat. Clin. N. Amer., 1959,* **6**, *449-472.*

BUSFIELD (P. I.). Neuroblastoma in orthopaedic practice. *J. Bone Jt Surg., 1958,* **40-B**, *47-57.*

CHAPTAL (J.) et coll. Sympathoblastome de l'enfant à forme osseuse; à propos de cinq observations. *Arch. franç. Pédiat., 1961,* **18**, *969-980.*

DARGENT (M.), BRUNAT (M.), COLON (J.), DUTOU (L.), LAHNÈCHE (B.), MAYER (M.), NOËL (P.) et POMMATAU (E.). Les métastases osseuses. *Rev. Prat., Paris, 1969,* **19**, *2467-2502.*

DARGEON (H. W.). Neuroblastoma. *J. Pediat., 1962,* **61**, *456-471.*

FORTNER (J.), NICASTRI (A.) et MURPAY (L.). Neuroblastoma : natural history and results of treating 133 cases. *Ann. Surg., 1968,* **167**, *132-142.*

GROSS (R. E.), FARBER (S.) et MARTIN (L. W.). Neuroblastoma sympathicum : a study and report of 217 cases. *Pediatrics, 1959,* **23**, *1179-1191.*

HANSMAN (C. F.) et GIRDANY (B. B.). The roentgenographic findings associated with neuroblastoma. *J. Pediat., 1957,* **51**, *621-633.*

HELSON (L.), WATSON (R. C.), BENUA (R. S.) et MURPHY (M. L.). 18 F Radioisotope scanning of metastatic bone lesions in children with neuroblastoma. *Amer. J. Roentgenol., 1972,* **115**, *191-199.*

HUTCHINSON (R.). On suprarenal sarcoma in children with metastases in the skull. *Quart. J. Med., 1907,* **I**, *621-633.*

KINDCAID (O. W.), HODGSON (J. R.) et DOCKERTY (M. B.). Neuroblastoma : A roentgenologic and pathologic study. *Amer. J. Roentgenol., 1957,* **78**, *420-436.*

KOOP (C. E.) et HERNANDEZ (J. R.). Experience with 100 cases in children neuroblastoma. *Surgery, 1964,* **56**, *726-733.*

MARDSEN (H. B.) et STEWART (J. K.). Ewing's tumours and neuroblastomas. *J. clin. Path., 1964,* **17**, *411-417.*

MASSELOT (J.), BERGIRON (C.), TCHERNIA (G.), TOURNADE (M. F.) et MARKOVITS (P.). Etude radioclinique des métastases du néphroblastome. *Ann. Radiol., 1972,* **15**, *1-12.*

RAMBERT (Ch.). Etude radiologique des métastases osseuses dans 193 cas de neuroblastomes. *Thèse Méd. Paris, 1968.*

REIQUAM (C. W.), BEATTY (E. S., Jr.) et ALLEN (R.). Neuroblastomas in infancy and childhood; a review of 10 years' experience. *Amer. J. Dis. Child., 1956,* **91**, *588-592.*

RICE (M. J.). Neuroblastoma in childhood. A review of 69 cases. *Aust. paediat. J., 1966,* **2**, *1-15.*

RICHARD et coll. Neuroblastoma : a review of 28 cases and presentation of two cases with metastases and long survival. *Amer. J. Roentgenol., 1961,* **85**, *733-747.*

RUDHE (U.). Skeletal metastases in Wilms' tumour. A roentgenographic study. *Ann. Radiol., 1969,* **12**, *337-342.*

SALLE (B.), FEROLDI (J.) et BRUNAT (M.). Pronostic des sympathomes chez l'enfant. *Rev. lyon. Méd., 1965,* **14**, *661-671.*

SCHERMAN (R. S.) et LEAMING (E.). The roentgen findings in neuroblastoma. *Radiology, 1953,* **60**, *837-849.*

SCHWEISGUTH (O.) et BAMBERGER (J.). Les métastases dans le néphroblastome de l'enfant. *Arch. franç. Pédiat., 1965,* **22**, *939-948.*

STOWENS (D.). Neuroblastoma and related tumors. *Arch. Path., 1957,* **63**, *451-459.*

SUTOW (W.). Prognosis in neuroblastoma of childhood. *Amer. J. Dis. Child., 1958,* **96**, *299-305.*

Index

Numbers in *italics* indicate a figure; "t" following a page number indicates a table.